W9-AFD-454

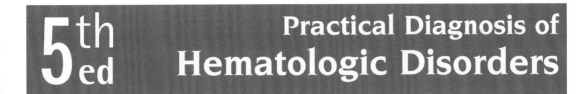

5th ed Practical Diagnosis of Hematologic Disorders

Vol 1
Benign Disorders

Authors

Carl R Kjeldsberg, MD
Professor of Pathology, University of Utah Health Sciences Center
Chairman of the Board, ARUP Laboratories, Inc

Sherrie L Perkins, MD, PhD
Professor of Pathology, University of Utah Health Sciences Center
Chief Medical Officer, Director of Laboratories, Medical Director of Hematopathology, ARUP Laboratories, In

John Anastasi, MD
Associate Professor, Associate Director Hematopathology
Department of Pathology
University of Chicago Medical Center

Daniel A Arber, MD
Professor and Associate Chair of Pathology for Clinical Services
Stanford University

David W Bahler, MD, PhD
Associate Professor of Pathology, University of Utah
Director, Hematologic Flow Cytometry Laboratory, ARUP Laboratories, Inc

Robert C Blaylock, MD
Professor of Pathology, Medical Director of University Hospital Transfusion Services and ARUP Blood Services
Medical Director of the Immunohematology Reference Laboratory, ARUP Laboratories, Inc
Co-Director of University Hospital Clinical Laboratories

Kojo S J Elenitoba-Johnson, MD
Professor of Pathology, Director of Division of Translational Research
Director of Molecular Diagnostics Laboratory
Director, Molecular Genetic Pathology Program
University of Michigan

Kathryn Foucar, MD
Professor of Pathology, Vice Chair for Clinical Affairs
University of New Mexico Health Sciences Center and TriCore Reference Laboratories

Amy Heerema-McKenney, MD
Clinical Assistant Professor, Department of Pathology
Stanford University

Megan S Lim, MD, PhD
Associate Professor of Pathology, Director of Hematopathology
Director, Hematopathology Fellowship Training Program
University of Michigan

Robert W McKenna, MD
Professor and Vice Chair for Academic Affairs
Senior Consultant in Hematopathology, Department of Laboratory Medicine and Pathology
Richard D Brunning Professor of Laboratory Medicine and Pathology
University of Minnesota

LoAnn C Peterson, MD
Paul E Steiner Research Professor of Pathology, Feinberg Medical School
Northwestern University, Northwestern Memorial Hospital

George M Rodgers, MD, PhD
Professor of Medicine and Pathology, University of Utah Health Sciences Center
Medical Director, Coagulation Laboratory, ARUP Laboratories, Inc

Mohamed E Salama, MD
Assistant Professor of Pathology, University of Utah Health Sciences Center
Assistant Medical Director, Hematopathology, ARUP Laboratories, Inc

James W Vardiman, MD
Professor of Pathology
University of Chicago Medical Center

Practical Diagnosis of Hematologic Disorders

5th Edition

Vol 1
Benign Disorders

Carl R Kjeldsberg, MD
Sherrie L Perkins, MD, PhD
Editors
et xiii alia

ASCP Press
American Society for Clinical Pathology
Chicago, IL

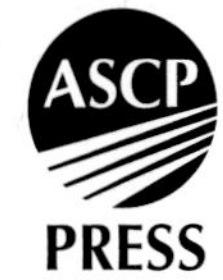

Publishing Team

Erik Tanck (production manager/designer)
Tae Moon (production)
Joshua Weikersheimer (publishing direction)

Notice

Trade names and equipment and supplies described herein are included as suggestions only. In no way does their inclusion constitute an endorsement or preferences by the American Society for Clinical Pathology. The ASCP did not test the equipment, supplies, or procedures and, therefore, urges all readers to read and follow all manufacturers' instructions and package insert warnings concerning the proper and safe use of products.

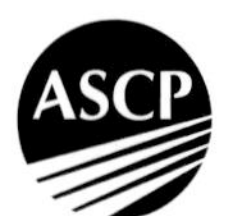

Printed in Singapore

14 13 12 11 10

Contents

Vol 1 Benign Disorders

Part III Reactive Disorders of Granulocytes and Monocytes

Part IV Reactive Disorders of Lymphocytes

Part V Reactive Disorders of Lymph Nodes

Part VI Bleeding Disorders

Part VII Thrombotic Disorders

Part VIII Anticoagulant Therapy

List of Tables

Preface

The goal of this book, beginning with the first edition in 1989, has been to provide an up-to-date, concise source of guidelines to the selection, use and interpretation of laboratory tests, while at the same time providing an overview of the pathogenesis and clinical features of the most common hematologic disorders.

Though the size and scope of this book have increased considerably, keeping pace with the expansion of the knowledge and diagnostic complexity in hematopathology, the focus on providing practical information has not changed. Each chapter follows a practical format to make finding specific information easy. This fifth edition contains substantial new information, particularly with regard to molecular modalities and utilization of ancillary testing in the diagnosis of hematologic disorders. The new edition uses the framework of the 2008 WHO classification for malignancies, and provides up-to-date diagnostic approaches, correct usage of laboratory testing, and algorithms for diagnosis of both benign and malignant disorders.

We hope that this newest edition will be an even more valuable tool and resource for a broad audience, including pathologists, residents and fellows in pathology and medicine, hematologists/oncologists, internists, pediatricians, medical students and medical technologists, as well as for those preparing for board examinations in pathology and internal medicine.

We welcome your comments or suggestions for future editions and trust that this book will provide the quality information and education you've come to expect.

Acknowledgements

We wish to express our appreciation to Joshua Weikersheimer of the ASCP Press, for his assistance in all aspects of publication, and to Susan Flinders for administrative assistance.

We want to also thank our colleagues in the Department of Pathology at the University of Utah, and the staff at ARUP Laboratories for their support. Present and former hematopathology fellows have provided much inspiration

Most of all, we are grateful for the support and love from our families, Gillean, Tanya, Kristina, Don, Rachel and Jessica.

Dedication

We dedicate this book to our co-authors
John Anastasi, MD
Daniel A Arber, MD
David W Bahler, MD, PhD
Robert C Blaylock, MD
Kojo S J Elenitoba-Johnson, MD
Kathryn Foucar, MD
Amy Heerema-McKenney, MD
Megan S Lim, MD, PhD
Robert W McKenna, MD
LoAnn C Peterson, MD
George M Rodgers, III, MD, PhD
Mohamed Salama, MD
James Vardiman, MD
With much respect and admiration.

Part I

Anemias

Chapter 1
Diagnosis of Anemia

Sherrie Perkins, MD, PhD

The bone marrow contains pluripotential stem cells that have the capacity for self-renewal as well as differentiation into mature cells, including red blood cells. Erythropoietin stimulates primitive stem cells to undergo four rounds of cellular division—over 6 to 7 days—and differentiation to form pronormoblasts and normoblasts. During the final step of differentiation the nucleus is extruded from the red blood cell precursor to form a reticulocyte, that still retains cytoplasmic RNA. Reticulocytes enter the peripheral circulation, appearing as faintly blue-gray polychromatophilic cells in Wright stained blood smears that persist for about 24 hours. Upon the loss of cytoplasmic RNA, a mature red blood cell is formed. A red blood cell remains in the peripheral circulation for 120 days before being removed via hemolysis by the spleen and reticuloendothelial system.

Usually red blood cell numbers remain relatively constant with removal from the peripheral circulation balanced by proliferation and differentiation within the marrow. However, many disease states will disrupt red blood cell homeostasis, leading to possible alterations in red blood cell number, appearance, or hemoglobin concentration. The most common pathologic process associated with red blood cells is the decrease in overall red blood cell numbers. Morphologic characteristics and the complete blood count (CBC) performed by an automated hematology analyzer will provide important information that will direct further laboratory testing to allow diagnosis and characterization of a red blood cell disorder.

1.1 Normal and Pathologic Red Blood Cells

The normal red blood cell is a biconcave disk, 6 to 9 µm in diameter and 1.5 to 2.5 µm thick. In the peripheral smear, red blood cells are anucleate and contain predominantly hemoglobin that is distributed to form a dense outer rim with a paler center that occupies approximately one third of the diameter of the cell. The hemoglobin imparts a uniform pink to orange-red color to the cytoplasm that is typically without inclusions. Normally all red blood cells are relatively uniform in size and shape. Numerous disease states affect the size, shape, and hemoglobin content of red cells. Variation in size is referred to as "anisocytosis," and variation in shape is termed "poikilocytosis." Pathologic red cells may be larger or smaller than normal, may be abnormally shaped, or may contain inclusions. Knowledge of the disease states associated with specific appearances of red blood cells will provide important diagnostic clues that aid in the diagnosis of hematologic disorders. **t1.1** presents a summary of morphologic red blood cell abnormalities that may be seen in blood smears, including those associated with specific disease states.

t1.1 Pathologic Red Blood Cells in Blood Smears

RBC Type	Description	Underlying Change	Disease States
Acanthocyte (spur cell)	Irregularly speculated cells with projections of varying length and dense center	Altered cell membrane lipids	Abetalipoproteinemia, parenchymal
Basophilic stippling	Punctate basophilic inclusions	Precipitated ribosomes (RNA)	Coarse stippling; lead intoxication, thalassemia; fine stippling; many anemias
Bite cell (degmacyte)	Smooth semicircle taken from one edge	Heinz body "pitting" by spleen	G6PD deficiency, drug-induced oxidant hemolysis
Burr cell (echinocyte), or crenated cell	Cells with short, evenly spaced spicules and preserved central pallor	May be associated with altered membrane lipids	Usually artifactual; seen in uremia, bleeding ulcers, gastric carcinoma, artifact
Howell-Jolly bodies	Small, discrete basophilic dense inclusions; usually single	Nuclear remnant	Postsplenectomy, hemolytic anemia, megaloblastic anemia
Hypochromic cell	Prominent central pallor	Diminished hemoglobin synthesis	Iron deficiency anemia, thalassemia, sideroblastic anemia
Macrocyte	Cells larger than normal (>8.5 μm), well-filled hemoglobin	Reticulocytes, abnormal cell DNA maturation	Increased erythropoiesis, oval macrocytes in megaloblastic anemia, round macrocytes in liver disease
Microcyte	Cells smaller than normal (<7 μm)	Abnormal hemoglobin production	Iron deficiency anemia, thalassemia, sideroblastic anemia
Ovalocyte (elliptocyte)	Elliptical cell	Abnormal cytoskeletal proteins	Hereditary elliptocytosis
Pappenheimer bodies	Small, dense basophilic granules	Iron-containing mitochondrial remnant or siderosome	Sideroblastic anemia, postsplenectomy
Polychromatophilia	Gray or blue hue frequently seen in reticulocytes	Ribosomal material	Reticulocytosis, premature marrow release of red blood cells
Rouleaux	Cell aggregates resembling stack of coins	Cell clumping by red cell interactions with paraprotein	Paraproteinemia, artifact
Schistocyte	Distorted, fragmented cell, two or three pointed ends	Mechanical destruction in microvasculature by fibrin strands, mechanical damage or prosthetic heart valve	Microangiopathic hemolytic anemia (DIC, TTP), prosthetic heart valves, severe burns
Sickle cell (drepanocyte)	Bipolar, speculated forms, sickle-shaped, pointed at both ends	Molecular aggregation of hemoglobin S	Sickle cell disorders excluding S trait
Spherocyte	Spherical cell with dense hemoglobin and absent central pallor; usually decreased in diameter	Decreased membrane redundancy	Hereditary spherocytosis, immunohemolytic anemia, transfusion, artifact
Stomatocyte	Mouth- or cup-like deformity	Membrane defect with abnormal cation permeability	Hereditary stomatocytosis, immunohemolytic anemia
Target cell (codocyte)	Target-like appearances hypochromic with central hemoglobin	Increased redundancy of cell membrane	Liver disease, postsplenectomy, thalassemia, hemoglobin C disease, iron deficiency
Teardrop cell (dacrocyte)	Distorted, drop-shaped cell	Mechanical distortion of red cell	Myelofibrosis, myelophthisic anemia

1.2 Automated Hematology

In both office and hospital settings, most patients' blood is evaluated with an automated electronic blood cell counter. Most instruments analyze individually and combine data to characterize the entire cell population. Analysis of cell characteristics is achieved by various methods including voltage pulse-impedance analysis and low- or high-angle light scatter from a coherent or laser light source. In an impedance counter, the passage of a particle through an orifice of standard size and volume displaces conductive electrolyte solution within the orifice. If an electric current is applied across the orifice, a change in resistance and conductivity of the electrolyte solution occurs as the particle passes through it. A detector notes a pulse when the particle passes through the orifice; this pulse is proportional to the volume of the electrolyte solution displaced by the particle. Thus, the counter counts and sizes particles simultaneously. In a light scatter counter, interruption of the light beam by a particle produces an electronic pulse. The angle of light scatter and the intensity of the light scattered at a particular angle delineates several physical properties of the cell, including cell size, volume, shape, and internal complexity. Many modern hematology analyzers utilize a combination of these two approaches to provide accurate data about red blood cells.

With the physical data collected, a hematology analyzer can generate a histogram of size distribution on the x-axis and relative number of particles on the y-axis. From these data, the red cell number (RBC) and mean corpuscular volume (MCV) can be determined, and other indices, such as mean corpuscular hemoglobin concentration (MCHC), can be calculated. Newer instruments also generate an index that provides the degree of dispersion of red blood cell sizes (anisocytosis) compared with a "normal" size distribution histogram, referred to as a "red cell distribution width" (RDW).

1.3 Evaluation of the Blood Smear

Examination of the blood smear by a physician who is aware of the patient's clinical condition is extremely useful in evaluating the patient with anemia, as some red cell disorders may have subtle changes that are easily overlooked, such as minimal hypersegmentation of neutrophils in patients with combined folate and iron deficiency (masked macrocytosis) or basophilic stippling in a patient with thalassemia and other complicating causes of anemia. Electronically derived red blood cell indices, although useful, are simply representations of the mean and overall degree of dispersion of the cellular population and provide little information about specific red blood cell shapes and the presence or absence of minor populations of abnormal red cells. Examination of the blood smear for specific shape variations, such as those listed in **t1.1**, can provide valuable information to aid in the diagnosis of a patient's underlying disease.

1.4 Anemia

The primary function of the red blood cell is to deliver oxygen to the tissues. Anemia is defined as a reduction in the total number of red blood cells, amount of hemoglobin in the circulation, or circulating red blood cell mass. This results in impaired oxygen delivery to tissues, giving rise to physiologic consequences of tissue hypoxia as well as compensatory mechanisms initiated by the organism to correct anoxia. Signs and symptoms of anemia include fatigue, syncope, dyspnea, or impairment of organ function due to decreased oxygen; pallor or postural hypotension due to decreased blood volume; and palpitations, onset of heart murmurs, or congestive heart failure due to increased cardiac output. Anemia is not a diagnosis, but a sign of underlying disease. Hence, the evaluation of a patient with anemia is directed at elucidating the causes for the patient's decreased red blood cell mass. A thorough history and physical examination are crucial for an intelligent, directed approach to the differential diagnosis of anemia. **t1.2** and **t1.3** show important features in a patient's history and physical examination that can yield diagnostic clues as to the cause of anemia, and efficiently direct further laboratory testing.

t1.2 Patient History in the Diagnosis of Anemia

Historical Information	Possible Causes of Anemia
Age of onset	Inherited or acquired disorder, continuous or recent onset
Duration of illness	Results of previous examinations and blood counts
Prior therapy for anemia	Vitamin B_{12}, iron supplementation, and how long ago
Suddenness or severity of anemia	Symptoms of dyspnea, palpitations, dizziness, fatigue, postural hypotension
Chronic blood loss	Menstrual and pregnancy history, gastrointestinal symptoms, black or bloody stools
Hemolytic episodes	Episode of weakness with icterus and dark urine
Toxic exposures	Drugs, hobbies, and occupational exposures
Dietary history	Alcohol use, unusual diet, prolonged milk ingestion in infants
Family history and racial background	Possible inherited disorder: family members with anemia, gallbladder disease, splenomegaly, splenectomy
Underlying diseases	Uremia, chronic liver disease, hypothyroidism

t1.3 Physical Signs in the Diagnosis of Anemia

Physical Sign	Associated Disease
Skin and mucous membranes	
Pallor	Any anemia
Scleral icterus	Hemolytic anemia
Smooth tongue	Pernicious anemia, severe iron deficiency
Petechiae	Thrombocytopenia and bone marrow replacement or aplastic anemia
Ulcers	Sickle cell disease
Lymph nodes	
Lymphadenopathy	Infectious mononucleosis, lymphoma, leukemia
Heart	
Cardiac dilatation, tachycardia, loud murmur	Severe anemia
Soft murmurs	Anemia, usually mild
Abdomen	
Splenomegaly	Infectious mononucleosis, leukemia, lymphoma, hypersplenism
Massive splenomegaly	Chronic myelogenous leukemia, myelofibrosis
Hepatosplenomegaly with ascites	Liver disease
Central nervous system	
Subacute combined degeneration of spinal cord	Pernicious anemia (vitamin B_{12} deficiency)
Delayed Achilles tendon reflex	Hypothyroidism

1.4.1 Examination of the Blood

Anemia has been classified by several different approaches, none of which is completely satisfactory. For practical purposes, an initial morphologic classification of anemia with integration of red blood cell indices and morphologic characteristics is probably most useful. With use of the MCV and the RDW or red cell morphologic index (RCMI), anemia may be classified into six categories **t1.4**. The anemia may be characterized by cell size as microcytic, normocytic, or macrocytic. The absence or presence of anisocytosis (as measured by RDW) further subdivides these three size categories. In general, anemia caused by nutritional deficiencies (such as iron, folate, or vitamin B_{12}) tend to have a greater degree of anisocytosis than anemia caused by genetic defects or primary bone marrow disorders. However, difficulties arise in classification using this scheme, particularly with regard to anemia of chronic disease.

t1.4 Classification of Anemia Based on Red Blood Cell Size and Distribution Width

Cell Size	Normal RDW	High RDW
Microcytosis (MCV <70 μm^3 [70 fL])	Thalassemia minor, anemia of chronic disease, some hemoglobinopathy traits	Iron deficiency, hemoglobin H disease, some anemia of chronic disease, some thalassemia minor, fragmentation hemolysis
Normocytosis	Anemia of chronic disease, hereditary spherocytosis, some hemoglobinopathy traits, acute bleeding	Early or partially treated iron or vitamin deficiency, sickle cell disease
Macrocytosis (MCV >100 μm^3 [100 fL])	Aplastic anemia, some myelodysplasias	Vitamin B_{12} or folate deficiency, autoimmune hemolytic anemia, cold agglutinin disease, some myelodysplasias, liver disease, thyroid disease, alcohol

RDW = red cell distribution width; MCV = mean corpuscular volume

In addition to pure morphologic criteria, anemia also may be classified by the degree of bone marrow response or peripheral blood reticulocytosis as hyperproliferative, normoproliferative, or hypoproliferative. This often provides insights into the pathogenesis of the process. Thus, patients with defects in red blood cell proliferation or maturation tend to have little or no increase in reticulocytes, reflecting the inability of the bone marrow to increase red blood cell production in response to the anemia (hypoproliferative anemia). In contrast, patients with anemia caused by decreased survival of red blood cells with a normal bone marrow proliferative response often exhibit increased peripheral blood reticulocytes (normoproliferative or hyperproliferative anemia) (see **f1.1**). If the degree of reticulocytosis is adequate to replace the loss of red blood cells, the anemia is termed "compensated." If the bone marrow response is inadequate, the anemia will progressively worsen.

Finally, anemia caused by decreased red blood cell survival are often subdivided by pathogenetic mechanism into those caused by intrinsic or inherited defects and those that are acquired or caused by extrinsic factors. This classification is often useful in understanding the underlying disease processes and may facilitate the evaluation and diagnosis of anemia that arises secondary to extrinsic processes.

1.4.2 Differential Diagnosis of Anemia

Anemia may be either relative (due to increased plasma volume with a normal red blood cell mass) or absolute (due to a decreased red blood cell mass). It is important to rule out causes of relative anemia, such as pregnancy, excessive hydration, or macroglobulinemia, as they represent disturbances in plasma volume rather than a true decrease in red blood cell mass. Similarly,

f1.1 Classification of macrocytic anemia by reticulocyte count

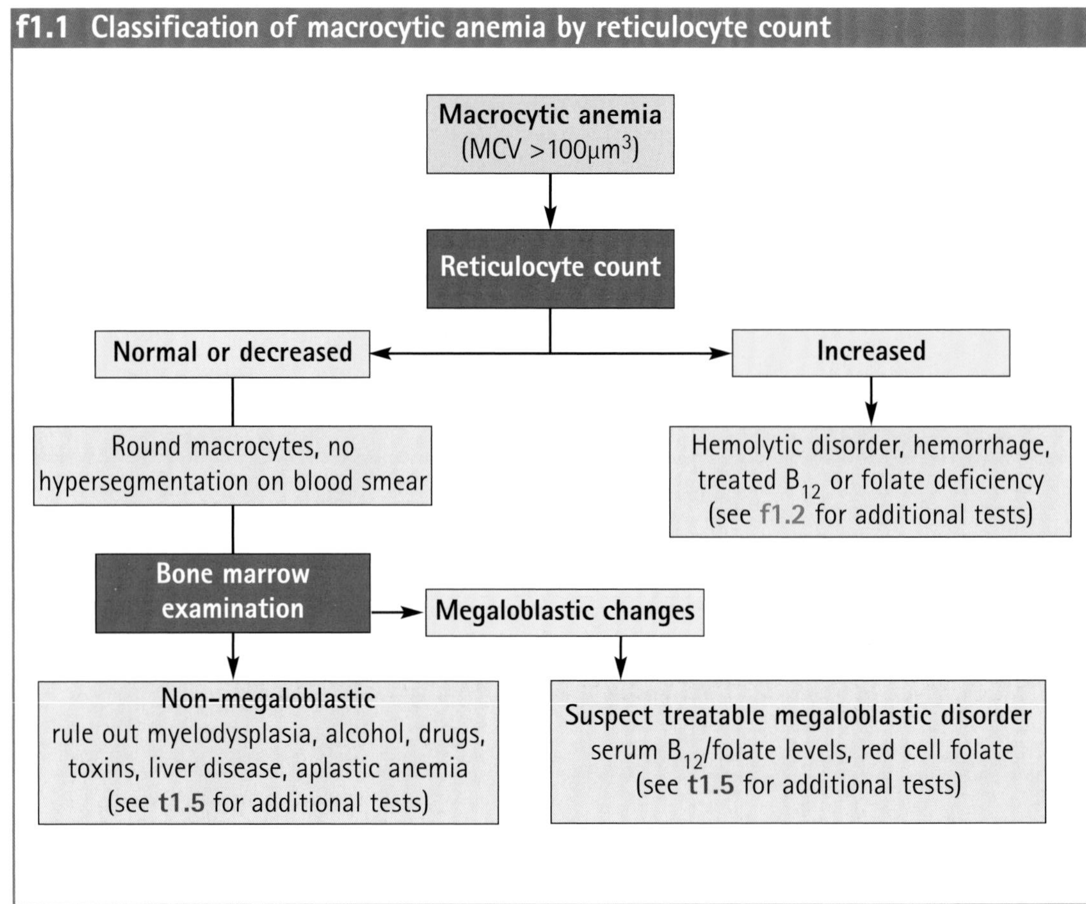

decreased plasma volume, caused by dehydration, may mask a real decrease in circulating red blood cell mass.

Use of a morphologic classification scheme in combination with red blood cell indices and the reticulocyte count allows for practical classification of anemia into broad groups. This will facilitate selection of additional laboratory tests to determine the underlying cause of the anemia.

1.4.3 Macrocytic Anemia

Macrocytic anemia (MCV >100 μm^3 [>100 fL]) is less common than normocytic or microcytic anemia. Macrocytic anemia may be subdivided into those with a normal RDW (principally those caused by bone marrow failure, such as aplastic anemia and myelodysplasia) and those with a high RDW (caused by deficiencies of either vitamin B_{12} or folic acid, autoimmune hemolysis, or cold agglutinins). However, many exceptions to this general classification scheme exist. For example, a mild degree of macrocytosis with a normal RDW is relatively common as a direct toxic effect of alcohol. Similarly, some cases of myelodysplasia may have a high RDW.

Further classification of a macrocytic anemia based on the presence or absence of a reticulocyte response is also helpful (see f1.1). Hemolytic anemia, blood loss, and partially treated vitamin B_{12} or folic acid deficiencies will demonstrate an increased reticulocyte count. Normal to increased reticulocyte counts are more likely to be associated with autoimmune hemolysis, disorders of membrane structural proteins (eg, elliptocytosis or spherocytosis), paroxysmal nocturnal hemoglobinuria, and fragmentation hemolysis f1.2. For those patients with a normal or decreased corrected reticulocyte count, disorders associated with decreased bone marrow function—including untreated vitamin deficiency, drugs, toxins, liver and thyroid disease, or primary bone marrow

f1.2 Classification of normocytic or megaloblastic anemias with elevated reticulocyte counts

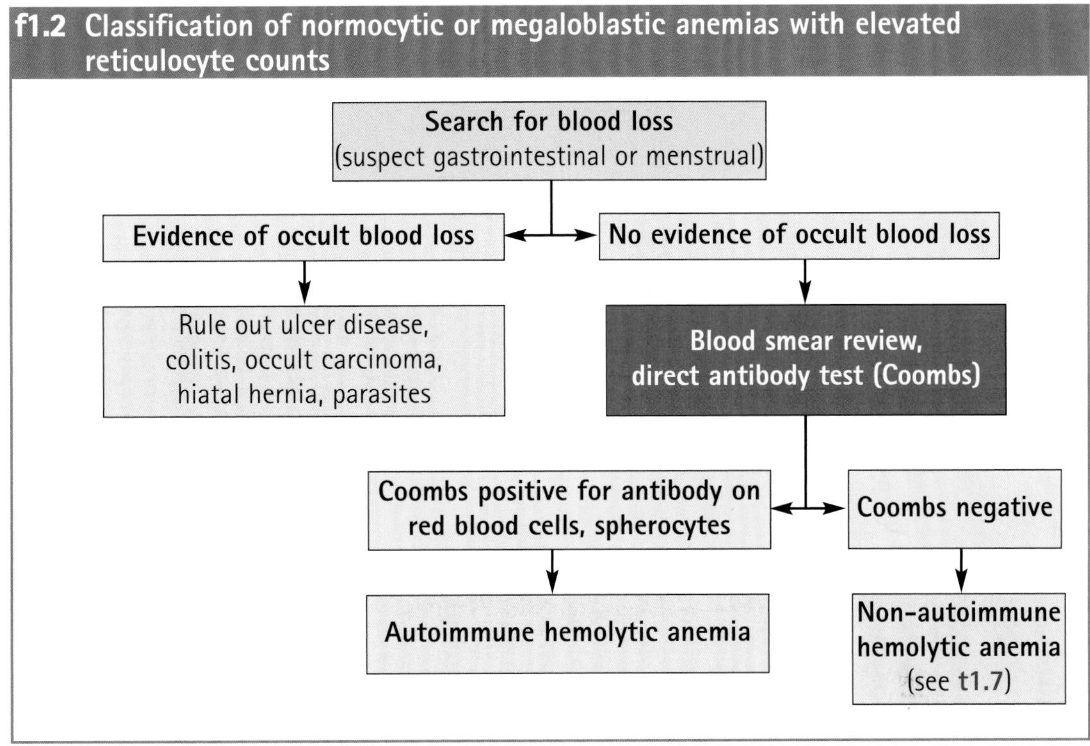

failure—should be suspected. Blood smears that show morphologic features compatible with megaloblastic anemia (oval macrocytes and hypersegmented neutrophils) may warrant further evaluation with vitamin assays but not bone marrow examination. When megaloblastic changes are present without signs of vitamin B_{12} or folate deficiency, bone marrow examination and additional testing **t1.5** may be needed. A more extensive discussion of the diagnosis and evaluation of macrocytic anemia is found in Chapter 5.

t1.5 Ancillary Tests for Macrocytic Anemia Without Increased Reticulocyte Response

Megaloblastic bone marrow changes present only in erythroid line:
Thyroid function tests
Cytogenetic analysis—evaluate for myelodysplasia

Megaloblastic bone marrow changes present in more than one cell line:
Dietary and drug history
Malabsorption studies
Schilling test if vitamin B_{12} deficiency

1.4.4 Microcytic Anemia

The three most common causes of microcytic anemia (MCV <70 µm^3 [<70 fL]) are iron deficiency, thalassemia minor, and anemia of chronic disease **f1.3**. The RDW is useful in distinguishing thalassemia, which generally (but not invariably) produces elevated red blood cell counts and a lower RDW than would be expected for the degree of anemia. Iron deficiency is almost always associated with a high RDW. The values seen in anemia of chronic disease are extremely variable, with some being normocytic, while others are microcytic (particularly in patients with renal disease). By using additional laboratory testing to determine body iron stores, such as serum iron and

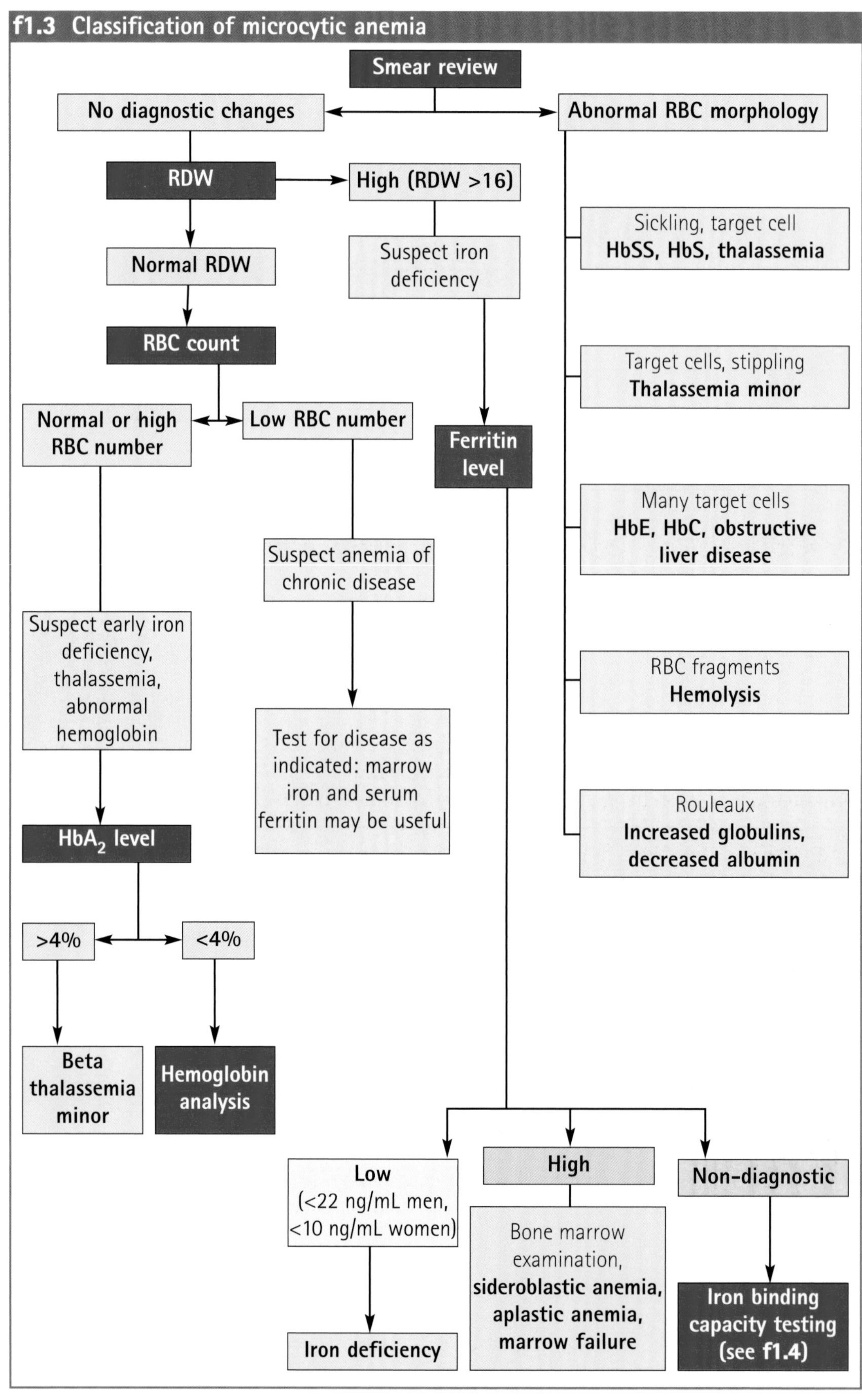
f1.3 Classification of microcytic anemia
Smear review
No diagnostic changes
Abnormal RBC morphology
RDW
High (RDW >16)
Normal RDW
Suspect iron deficiency
Sickling, target cell
HbSS, HbS, thalassemia
RBC count
Target cells, stippling
Thalassemia minor
Normal or high RBC number
Low RBC number
Ferritin level
Many target cells
HbE, HbC, obstructive liver disease
Suspect anemia of chronic disease
Suspect early iron deficiency, thalassemia, abnormal hemoglobin
RBC fragments
Hemolysis
Test for disease as indicated: marrow iron and serum ferritin may be useful
Rouleaux
Increased globulins, decreased albumin
HbA2 level
>4%
<4%
Beta thalassemia minor
Hemoglobin analysis
Low (<22 ng/mL men, <10 ng/mL women)
High
Non-diagnostic
Bone marrow examination, sideroblastic anemia, aplastic anemia, marrow failure
Iron deficiency
Iron binding capacity testing (see f1.4)

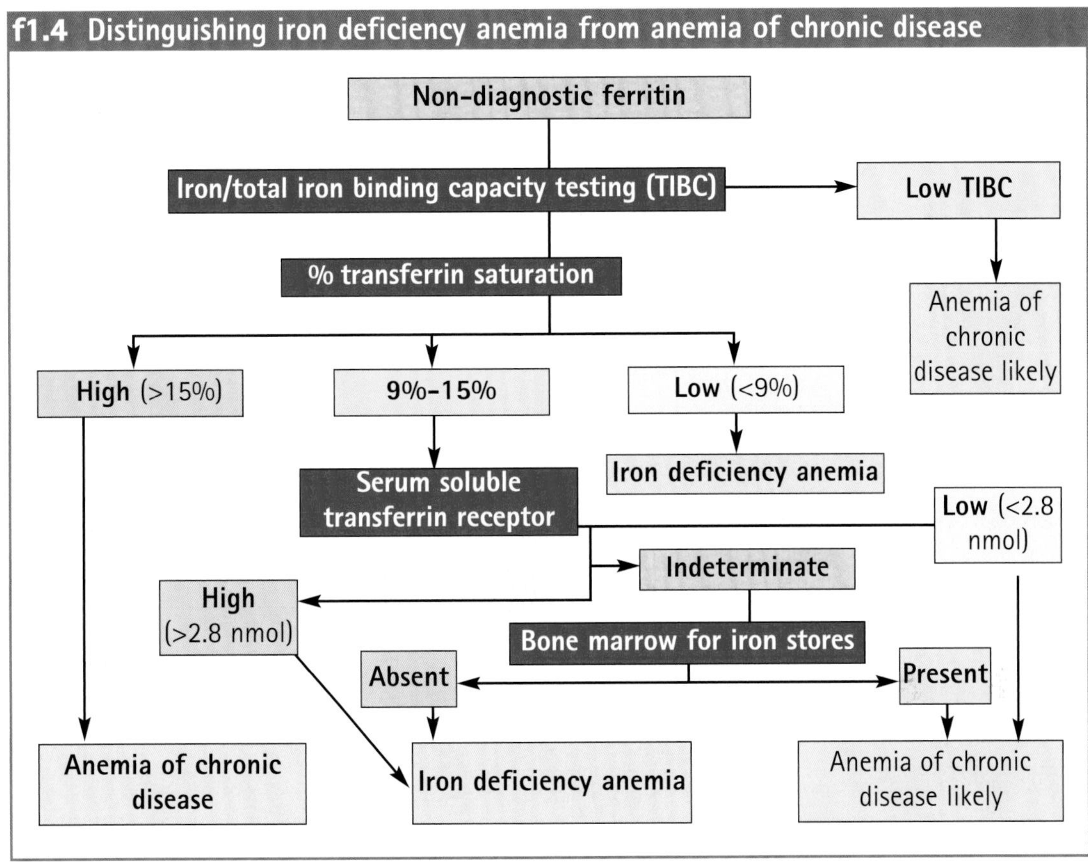

total iron binding studies, iron deficiency anemia and anemia of chronic disease may usually be distinguished without a bone marrow examination f1.4. A more detailed consideration of the evaluation and diagnosis of microcytic anemia is found in Chapter 2.

1.4.5 Normocytic, Normochromic Anemia

Patients with normal or hypoproliferative reticulocyte counts and normocytic, normochromic anemia generally require bone marrow evaluation. A peripheral blood smear may provide valuable clues for the differential diagnosis **t1.6**. Patients with normocytic anemia and an elevated reticulocyte count should undergo the same general evaluation as patients with macrocytosis and an elevated reticulocyte count (see f1.2). Normocytic, normochromic anemia with an elevated reticulocyte count can be divided into those with positive direct antiglobulin test results (DAT or Coombs test) and those lacking evidence of red blood cell-bound

t1.6 Normochromic, Normocytic Anemia Without High Reticulocyte Response

Findings on Peripheral Blood Smear	Further Workup
Leukoerythroblastosis	**Suspect myelophthisic process**—bone marrow examination for space-occupying lesion (metastatic tumor, lymphoma, myelofibrosis) in children suspect infection
Abnormal white blood cells	**Suspect leukemia, lymphoma**—bone marrow examination
Rouleaux	**Suspect myeloma**—serum and urine electrophoresis, radiographs to look for lytic lesions, bone marrow examination
No abnormal cells	**Suspect anemia of chronic disease or sideroblastic anemia**—bone marrow examination; rule out chronic disease processes, ferritin, total iron-binding capacity, and percent transferrin saturation as indicated

antibodies. Coombs-negative hemolytic anemia is a heterogeneous group of disorders. The blood smear and patient history often suggest possible causes for the anemia **t1.7**. A more detailed discussion of non-hemolytic normocytic anemia may be found in Chapter 3, and discussion of different causes of hemolytic anemia are presented in Chapters 6 through 15.

t1.7 Workup of Coombs-Negative Anemia

Feature of Anemia	Possible Process	Tests
Episodic anemia	Enzyme deficiency Paroxysmal nocturnal hemoglobinuria	G6PD, other RBC enzymes Sucrose hemolysis, Ham's test, flow cytometry
RBC fragmentation	DIC, TTP, HUS	Coagulation tests, serum haptoglobin levels
Abnormal RBC stippling	Lead poisoning Thalassemia	Lead levels Hemoglobin electrophoresis
Abnormal shapes or increased target cells	Hemoglobinopathy, thalassemia	Hemoglobin analysis
Spherocytes	Hereditary spherocytosis	Osmotic fragility test

G6PD = glucose-6-phosphate dehydrogenase; DIC = disseminated intravascular coagulation; TTP = thrombotic thrombocytopenic purpura; HUS = hemolytic-uremic syndrome

The differential diagnosis of anemia is often tempered or modified by knowledge of other patient data. All algorithmic classification schemes should be qualified by the pragmatic knowledge of the physician in considering the probable causes of anemia in an individual patient or patient population. For example, as 98% or more of anemia in children under the age of 4 years is caused by iron deficiency, many pediatricians simply treat all children with this type of anemia with iron supplementation and perform workups only for those who fail to respond to this therapy. In many situations, clinical knowledge can suggest several possible causes of anemia. Thus, the provided algorithms are suggested pathways for physicians to use for determining test utilization and should not be considered required clinical work-ups.

1.5 Laboratory Tests

Test 1.5.1 Manual Reticulocyte Count

Purpose. This test enumerates the number of reticulocytes, indicating bone marrow production of new red blood cells.

Principle. Residual RNA in immature red blood cells is precipitated and stained with a supravital dye.

Specimen. Venous or capillary blood may be used for this test.

Procedure. A blood smear is made, and the red blood cells are stained with brilliant cresyl blue or methylene blue. Cells containing stained reticular material are enumerated per 1000 red blood cells and expressed as percent reticulocytes (absolute number per 100 red cells). Many automated hematology analyzers now analyze reticulocyte counts based on staining and light-scatter properties as an optional function of the complete blood count.

Interpretation. Reticulocytes are immature red blood cells that contain at least two dots of stainable reticulin material in their cytoplasm. More immature forms have multiple dots and small networks or skeins of bluish-staining material. Intra-observer variation and uneven distribution of reticulocytes introduce a high analytic variation in manual reticulocyte counting, with interlaboratory coefficients of variation often in the range of 20%. Duplicate reticulocyte counts or 3-day average values may help to reduce the imprecision of the raw reticulocyte count. Automated reticulocyte counts (see **Test 1.5.2**), owing to larger sample analysis and mechanically defined criteria, tend to be more reproducible.

Effective red blood cell production is a dynamic process, and the number of reticulocytes should be compared with the expected number to be released in a patient without anemia. This is calculated as 1% of $5 \times 10^6/mm^3$ ($5 \times 10^{12}/L$) red cells daily for an absolute reticulocyte production of $50 \times 10^3/mm^3$ ($50 \times 10^9/L$). The corrected reticulocyte count takes into account normal red blood cell proliferation for a specific hematocrit and may be calculated with the following formula:

$$\text{Corrected Reticulocyte Count} = (\%\ \text{Observed Reticulocytes} \times \text{Hematocrit}) \div 45$$

Another complicating factor in reticulocyte count correction is that patients with anemia may release reticulocytes prematurely into the circulation. Reticulocytes are usually present in the blood for 24 hours before they extrude the residual RNA and become erythrocytes. If they are released early from the bone marrow, immature reticulocytes may persist in peripheral blood for 2 or 3 days. This is most likely to occur when severe anemia causes a marked acceleration in erythropoiesis and release. Some authors have advocated correction of the reticulocyte count for immature reticulocytes (thought to be the best reflection of bone marrow response to anemia), called the "reticulocyte production index" (RPI):

$$\text{RPI} = [(\%\ \text{Reticulocyte} \times \text{Hematocrit Value}) \div 45] \times [1 \div \text{Correction Factor}]$$

The correction factor calculation is shown in **t1.8**.

t1.8 Correction Factor Calculation

Patient's Hematocrit Value, %	Correction Factor
40-45	1.0
35-39	1.5
25-34	2.0
15-24	2.5
<15	3.0

In cases of low erythropoietin (often seen in patients with renal or hepatic disease), application of an RPI correction may mask a failure of bone marrow response, because the shift does not take place fully or at all. In general, RPI values less than 2 indicate failure of bone marrow red blood cell production or a hypoproliferative anemia. Reticulocyte production indexes of 3 or greater indicate marrow hyperproliferation or appropriate response to anemia.

Test 1.5.2 Automated Reticulocyte Count

Purpose. Determination of reticulocyte numbers provides insight into the underlying pathophysiology of an anemia. Use of automated staining and determination of reticulocytes in a hematology analyzer provides accurate reticulocyte enumeration by allowing evaluation of many more red blood cells than can be studied with manual supravital staining and also can provide information as to time since release from the bone marrow (reticulocyte maturity stage) by the staining patterns.

Principle. Reticulocytes are immature red blood cells in the final stage of differentaition that have been recently released from the bone marrow and still retain intracellular protein and RNA. They may be stained with RNA avid dyes that can be detected by fluorescence, light scatter properties or absorbance characteristics. Specific, proprietary dyes vary between types of hematology analyzers, but show similar reticulocyte staining patterns. The maturity level of the reticulocytes can be determined by the amount and intensity of staining, with the most immature reticulocyte fraction having the highest staining (highest RNA levels). Usually reticulocytes are fractionated into two to three different populations (immature, intermediate and mature), with the immature reticulocyte fraction being the most accurate reflection of erythropoietic activity that provides insight into the bone marrow proliferative response to an anemia.

Specimen. Anti-coagulated whole blood, usually in EDTA.

Procedure. Whole blood is stained with the RNA avid dye and analyzed in the hematology analyzer using the reticulocyte enumeration program. Data are provided as a percentage of red blood cell reticulocytes. The instrument will also fractionate the reticulocytes into an immature and mature fraction, with some instruments providing an intermediate reticulocyte fraction based on levels of staining.

Problems and Pitfalls. Automated reticulocyte counts may vary widely dependent on the methodology and instrumentation used, and monitoring should be done using the same methodology over time. Methods using fluorescence and argon laser detection may be more sensitive at detecting low numbers of reticulocytes. There is significant imprecision at very low reticulocyte numbers, reflecting limitations of analytic sensitivity in the method. Samples with significant numbers of reticulocytes are usually reproducible on the same instrument over time, both in determination of total numbers of reticulocytes and the immature fraction.

Test 1.5.3 Bone Marrow Examination

Purpose. Bone marrow examination allows assessment of the cellularity, maturation, and composition of the hematopoietic elements in the bone marrow, as well as evaluation of iron stores. Some infections also may be cultured from the bone marrow.

Principle. The cortical bone is penetrated and a sample of the bone marrow is aspirated. In most cases, a small biopsy specimen of the medullary bone and marrow is obtained. The most common sites for the procedure are the posterior or anterior iliac crest and the sternum.

Specimen. Bone marrow aspiration and biopsy samples.

Procedure. Bone marrow aspiration and biopsy are innocuous procedures when performed by experts. Several sites in the skeleton have been used for bone marrow sampling. Because active hematopoiesis occurs in the long bones of the arms and legs in infants under the age of 8 months, aspiration from the anterior aspect of the tibial tuberosity is useful. For adults, the posterior iliac crest is the recommended site. Patients who are unable to lie on their stomachs may be approached through the anterior iliac crest or sternum. The sternum is aspirated relatively easily, but its structure does not allow biopsy. In elderly patients, sternal bone marrow may be most representative of the patient's hematopoietic status and superior to that of the relatively acellular iliac crest. Sternal aspiration also may be most appropriate for patients who have lesions in the sternum or ribs.

Notes and Precautions. Processing and interpretation have significant technical variables and require experienced personnel. Bone marrow examination should be limited to situations in which noninvasive procedures do not yield clear answers. **t1.9** gives the most common indications for bone marrow examination.

t1.9 Indications for Bone Marrow Examination in Anemia

Abnormalities in blood counts and/or peripheral blood smear
Unexplained cytopenias
Unexplained leukocytosis or abnormal white blood cells
Teardrop cells or leukoerythroblastosis
Rouleaux
No or low reticulocyte response to anemia
Evaluation of systemic disease
Unexplained splenomegaly, hepatomegaly, lymphadenopathy
Tumor staging: solid tumors, lymphomas
Monitoring of chemotherapy effect
Fever of unknown origin (with bone marrow cultures)
Evaluation of trabecular bone in metabolic disease (use undecalcified bone)

Interpretation. When both a Wright-stained aspirate preparation and a histologic core needle biopsy are available, optimal evaluation may be performed. The false-negative rate for metastatic carcinoma using aspiration alone is about 25%; for lymphomas it seems to be somewhat higher—30% to 40%—depending on the cell type. Because of the small nature of the biopsy specimen, sampling errors still may be a problem, causing false-negative results. Additional testing, such as iron stains to evaluate iron stores, immunohistochemical staining, flow cytometric analysis, and cytogenetic analysis, may be performed on aspirated bone marrow specimens to provide additional information about the disease process.

1.6 Treatment

Treatment of anemia is usually aimed at correcting the underlying abnormality. This may involve identification of a source of blood loss, iron or vitamin supplementation, or discontinuation of a drug that predisposes a patient to hemolysis. Acquired anemia associated with hematopoietic abnormalities (such as myelodysplasia or aplastic anemia) or inherited anemia (such as red blood cell membrane defects, enzymopathies or hemoglobinopathies) may require transfusions when symptoms arise due to decreased oxygen delivery to the tissues. The benefit of transfusion therapy must be balanced carefully against the risks of disease transmission and iron overload. Usually transfusions are not required unless the hemoglobin concentration falls below 7 g/dL (70 g/L), unless significant cardiac or pulmonary disease is present and hypoxia would be exacerbated by even modest decreases in oxygen delivery. Long-term transfusion therapy may cause iron overload, leading to subsequent organ iron deposition and failure of function as patients are unable to appropriately decrease gut mucosal iron absorption when iron loading occurs via transfusion.

1.7 References

Asare K. Anemia of critical illness. *Pharmacotherapy.* 2008 Oct;28(10):1267-82.

Aslan D, Gumruk F, Gurgey A, et al. Importance of RDW value in differential diagnosis of hypochromic anemias. *Am J Hematol.* 2002;69:31-33.

Bain BJ. Bone marrow aspiration. *J Clin Pathol.* 2001;54:657-663.

Borgna-Pignatti C, Marsella M. Iron deficiency in infancy and childhood. *Pediatr Ann.* 2008 May;37(5):329-37.

Brugnara C. Iron deficiency and erythropoiesis: new diagnostic approaches. *Clin Chem.* 2003, 49:1573-1578.

Brugnara C. Use of reticulocyte cellular indices in the diagnosis and treatment of hematological disorders. *Int J Clin Lab Res.* 1998;28:1-11.

Carmel R. Nutritional anemias and the elderly. *Semin Hematol.* 2008 Oct;45(4):225-34.

Carmel R. Cassileth PA. A focused approach to anemia. *Hosp Pract.* 1999;34:71-91.

Clark SF. Iron deficiency anemia. *Nutr Clin Pract.* 2008 Apr-May;23(2):128-41.

Cotelingham JD. Bone marrow biopsy: interpretive guidelines for the surgical pathologist. *Adv Anat Pathol.* 2003;10:8-26.

Galloway M, Hamilton M. Macrocytosis: pitfalls in testing and summary of guidance. *BMJ.* 2007 Oct 27;335(7625):884-6.

Gehrs BC, Friedberg RC. Autoimmune hemolytic anemia. *Am J Hematol.* 2002;69:258-271.

Gulati G. *Blood Cells: An Atlas of Morphology.* Chicago, IL: ASCP Press;2007:20-101.

Kaferle J, Strzoda CE. Evaluation of macrocytosis. *Am Fam Physician.* 2009;79(3):203-8.

Means RT, Glader B. Anemia: general considerations in: Greer JP, Foerster J, Rodger GM, et al eds. *Wintrobe's Clinical Hematology. 12th ed.* Baltimore, MD: Lippincott Williams & Wilkins; 2009:779-809.

Pierre RV. Reticulocytes. Their usefulness and measurement in peripheral blood. *Clin Lab Med.* 2002; 22:63-79.

Tefferri A. Anemia in adults: a contemporary approach to diagnosis. *Mayo Clin Proc.* 2003;78:1274-1280.

Wians FH Jr., Urban JE, Keffer JH, Kroft SH. Discriminating between iron deficiency anemia and anemia of chronic disease using traditional indices of iron status vs transferring receptor concentration. *Am J Clin Pathol.* 2001;115:112-118.

Chapter 2

Hypochromic, Microcytic Anemias

Sherrie Perkins, MD, PhD

Due to deficiencies in either heme or globin chain synthesis, decreased hemoglobin synthesis gives rise to a hypochromic, microcytic anemia. The quantitative defect in hemoglobin production may arise due to abnormal heme production due to insufficient amounts of iron or abnormal iron utilization, abnormalities in heme synthesis, or hereditary abnormalities in globin protein synthesis (thalassemias). The most common cause of hypochromic, microcytic anemia is iron deficiency.

2.1 Pathophysiology

Hypochromic, microcytic anemias are characterized by normal cellular proliferation and DNA synthesis but decreased red blood cell hemoglobin production. The erythroid precursors divide normally, but lack of sufficient hemoglobin production leads to formation of paler, small hypochromatic red blood cells **i2.1**. Hemoglobin makes up approximately 98% of the cytoplasmic protein in a red blood cell and functions to bind and transport oxygen. Hemoglobin is composed of four globin protein chains: two α-globins and 2 non-α-globin chains (usually β-globin in adults) that are conjugated to four heme molecules that each contain an iron atom. Each hemoglobin molecule is capable of reversibly binding and transporting four oxygen molecules. The principal causes of decreased hemoglobin production include defective synthesis of heme secondary to decreased iron availability, abnormal iron utilization or disordered heme synthesis (sideroblastic anemias), and disorders of globin synthesis that give rise to the thalassemic disorders. The common causes of hypochromic, microcytic anemia are listed in **t2.1**.

Iron deficiency, the most common cause of anemia, is one of the most common human diseases. The etiology of iron deficiency varies with the age of the patient **t2.2** but usually arises from inadequate intake for metabolic demands, poor absorption, or increased losses through bleeding. In infants and children, a negative iron balance usually occurs because the dietary intake of iron is inadequate to meet the requirements for growth. In adults, iron deficiency is usually the result of insufficient intake for metabolic demands of pregnancy and lactation or blood loss. Because normal daily losses of iron are very small, insufficient dietary intake usually plays only a contributory role in the development of anemia in most adults. Blood loss is by far the most common cause of iron deficiency in an adult. The first sign of a malignant lesion of the gastrointestinal or genitourinary tract is often occult blood loss and resultant hypochromic, microcytic anemia. To effectively treat the anemia, the source of blood loss must be identified and corrected. Less likely causes of iron deficiency are linked to poor absorption of iron due to gastric surgery and intestinal malabsorption syndromes.

i2.1 Iron deficiency anemia

The red blood cells are hypochromic and microcytic with notable anisocytosis. *(Wright stain)*

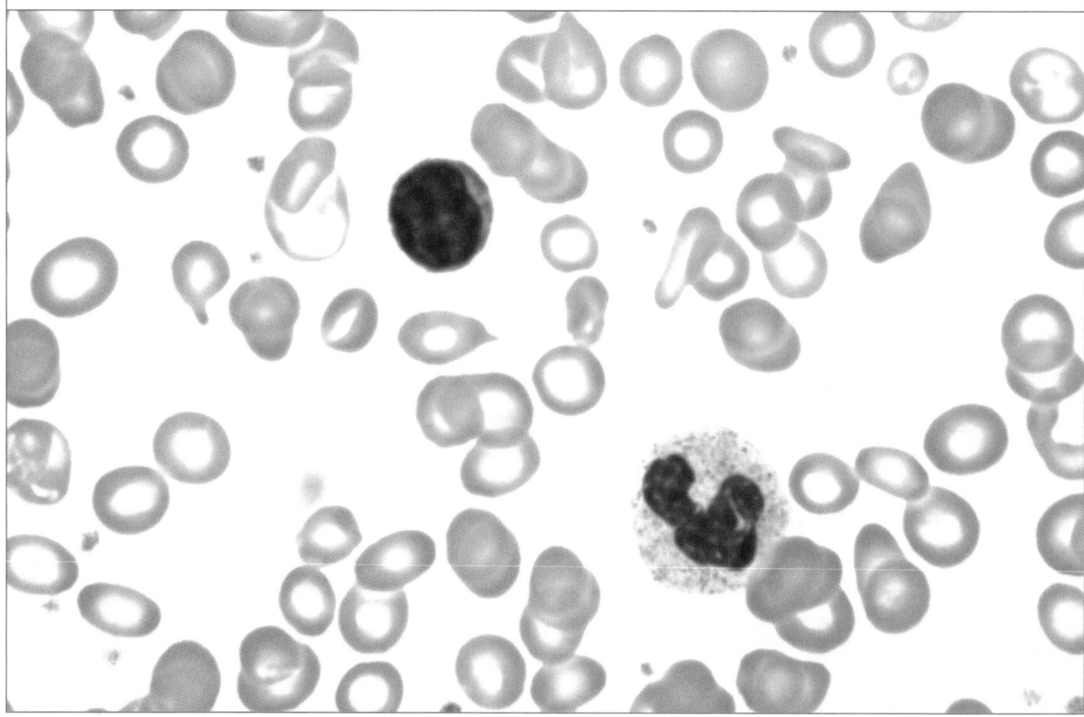

t2.1 Causes of Hypochromic Anemia

Disorders of iron metabolism
Iron deficiency
Blood loss
Poor intake with increased growth or pregnancy requirements
Malabsorption
Chronic infections or inflammatory states
Neoplasia

Disorders of heme synthesis
Sideroblastic anemias
  Hereditary (X-linked or autosomal)
  Acquired idiopathic (myelodysplasia)
  Acquired toxic (lead, drugs, alcohol)

Disorders of globin synthesis
Thalassemic syndromes
  α-Thalassemia
  β-Thalassemia
  γδ-Thalassemia

Iron metabolism may be deranged in many people with chronic inflammatory diseases or malignancies that do not cause overt blood loss. These patients exhibit defective iron cycling between macrophages and erythroid precursors, so iron becomes trapped within macrophages and is unavailable for heme synthesis. This gives rise to "anemia of chronic disease" that is

t2.2 Common Causes of Iron Deficiency Anemia by Age

Infants and children	Inadequate intake Growth spurts with increased iron requirements
Premenopausal women	Menstrual blood loss Pregnancy with inadequate intake
Adult men and postmenopausal women	Blood loss due to tumor, peptic ulcer, gastrointestinal or genitourinary bleeding Malabsorption

most often normochromic and normocytic, but may also be a hypochromic, microcytic anemia. Diagnosis of this entity is discussed further in Chapter 3.

Another group of disorders, sideroblastic anemias, is characterized by abnormal iron metabolism and heme synthesis within the red blood cell. In these disorders, iron is sequestered in erythroid cell mitochondria, making it unavailable for heme synthesis. The iron deposition swells and distorts the mitochondria. Because the mitochondria in a developing bone marrow erythrocyte are found in a perinuclear distribution, iron stains in these disorders show a characteristic pattern of iron staining with siderotic granules distributed around the red blood cell precursor nucleus, forming ringed sideroblasts i2.2. Sideroblastic anemias may be hereditary (either X-linked or autosomal) or acquired later in life. Acquired sideroblastic anemias arise from idiopathic causes (usually as part of a myelodysplastic disorder) and toxic insults (drugs, lead, or alcohol). Hereditary sideroblastic anemias are very rare in comparison with acquired forms.

i2.2 Ringed sideroblasts

Bone marrow aspirate iron stain demonstrating ringed sideroblasts. The siderotic granules extend around the normoblast nucleus. *(Prussian blue stain)*

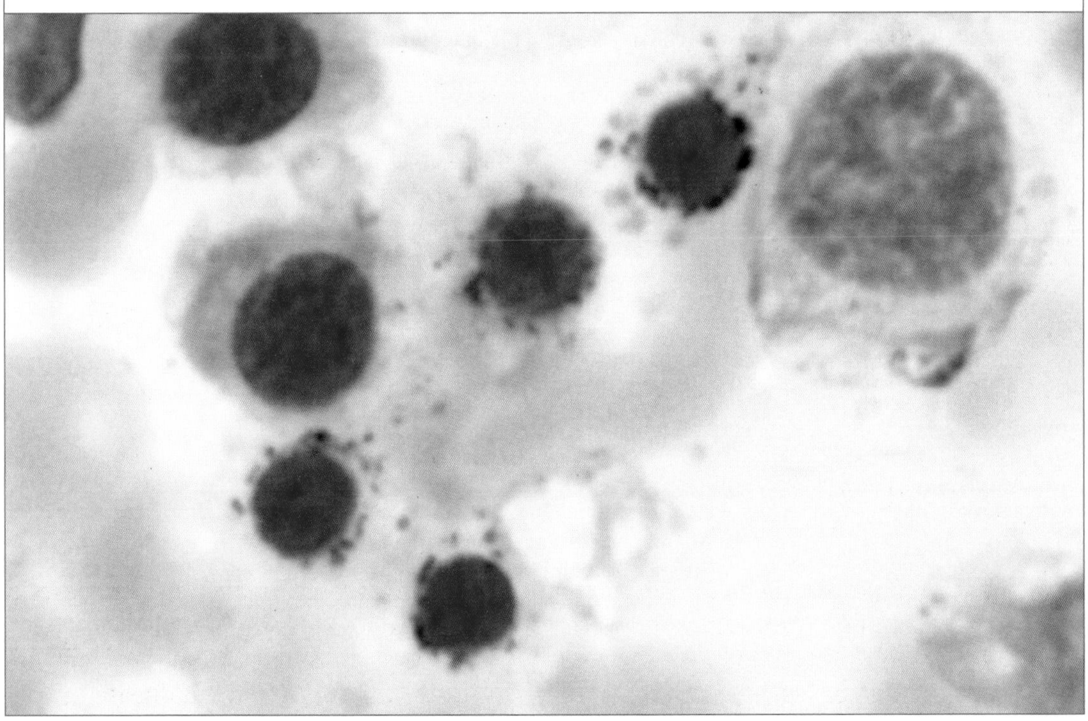

Hereditary disorders of globin synthesis, or thalassemic syndromes, are common hemoglobinopathies seen primarily in Asian, Mediterranean, and black populations. They rival iron deficiency as the cause of hypochromic, microcytic anemia in these ethnic groups. Evaluation and diagnosis of thalassemias are discussed in further detail in Chapter 10.

2.2 Clinical Aspects

The clinical findings of hypochromic anemias depend on the severity of the anemia and its underlying cause. Severe anemia is associated with pallor, weakness, dizziness, palpitations, and even dyspnea. Mild to moderate chronic anemia is well tolerated by most, particularly younger, patients. Moderate to severe anemia may be life threatening in patients when superimposed on other clinical conditions that affect blood circulation or oxygenation, such as heart or pulmonary disorders. Some patients with iron deficiency may have cheilitis or spooning of the nails (koilonychia). Food cravings for ice, clay (pica), dirt, starch, or pickles are common.

For a patient with a hypochromic, microcytic anemia, evaluation of clinical features in conjunction with laboratory testing is required to determine the etiology of the anemia and allow for proper treatment. Laboratory test selection is determined by the clinical situation. Thus, new onset of anemia in an elderly person triggers a workup for iron deficiency secondary to blood loss, anemia of chronic disease, or acquired sideroblastic anemia and is unlikely to be associated with a thalassemic syndrome. Similarly, an infant with hypochromic, microcytic anemia would require consideration of iron deficiency due to insufficient intake to support increased demands secondary to growth or thalassemia as the most probable causes for the anemia while myelodysplasia would be unlikely. Various tests may be used to evaluate hypochromic anemias (see **t2.3**). Judicious selection of laboratory testing allows for definitive diagnosis in a cost-effective manner.

t2.3 Commonly Used Tests to Evaluate Hypochromic, Microcytic Anemias

Test	Uses
Complete blood count (CBC)	
RBC count, hematocrit, hemoglobin concentration	Document anemia. Normal or increased RBC count in face of microcytosis may suggest thalassemia.
MCV	Used to classify anemia as microcytic.
RDW	Measures red blood cell anisocytosis Useful to differentiate between thalassemia (normal RDW) and iron deficiency (increased RDW). Sideroblastic anemia may also have increased RDW.
Iron studies	
Serum iron, TIBC, ferritin saturation	Measures body iron stores. Useful in documenting iron deficiency.
Serum ferritin	Correlates with iron stores but may be increased with infection, tissue damage, or malignancy.
Serum soluble transferrin receptor	Measurement of iron stores that is not altered in inflammatory states.
Free erythrocyte protoporphyrin	Increased in iron deficiency and lead poisoning, but normal in thalassemia.
Blood and bone marrow morphology	
Anisocytosis	Variability in red blood cell size. More prominent in iron deficiency than in thalassemic traits.
Target cells	Seen in hemoglobinopathies and liver disease.
Basophilic stippling	Associated with thalassemia and lead poisoning.
Bone marrow iron stains	Used to distinguish iron deficiency (absent iron), thalassemia (increased iron), and sideroblastic anemia (ringed sideroblasts).

RBC=red blood cell; MCV=mean corpuscular volume; RDW=red cell distribution width; TIBC=total iron-binding capacity

2.3 Diagnostic Approach

Following a clinical history and physical examination, the evaluation of hypochromic anemia may be undertaken as follows, with test selection mediated by the clinical findings for each patient:

1. Examination of red blood cell morphology and evaluation of red blood cell indices and size distribution **t2.4**.

t2.4 Pertinent Findings in Hypochromic, Microcytic Anemia

Cause of Anemia	Red Blood Cell Number	Red Blood Cell Distribution Width	Aniso-poikilo-cytosis	Basophilic Stippling	Bone Marrow Iron Staining
Iron deficiency	Decreased	Increased	Yes	No	Decreased
Thalassemia minor	Normal or increased	Normal	No	Yes	Increased
Sideroblastic anemias					
Hereditary	Decreased	Variable	Variable	Yes	Increased RSB
Acquired	Decreased	Dimorphic population	Yes	Yes	Increased RSB
Chronic disease	Decreased	Variable	Variable	No	Decreased in siderocytes; increased in RE cells

RE = reticuloendothelial; RSB = ringed sideroblasts

2. Estimation of serum iron levels and total iron-binding capacity (TIBC), ferritin, or serum transferrin receptor levels. These measurements reflect body iron stores and help to distinguish iron deficiency from other causes of hypochromic, microcytic anemia **t2.5**.

t2.5 Iron Studies in Hypochromic Anemias

Cause of Hypochromic Anemia	Serum Iron	TIBC	Percent Saturation	Soluble Serum Transferrin Receptor	Bone Marrow Storage Iron
Iron deficiency	Decreased*	Increased*	Decreased*	High	Decreased
Thalassemia	Increased or normal	Decreased or normal	Increased or normal	Variable, may be high	Increased
Sideroblastic anemia	Increased	Decreased or normal	Increased	Variable, may be high	Increased
Chronic disease	Decreased	Decreased	Decreased	Normal	Increased

**Serum iron and TIBC (total iron-binding capacity) are occasionally normal in early iron deficiency.*

3. Measurement of free erythrocyte protoporphyrin. This is valuable as a screening test in distinguishing iron deficiency from thalassemia minor.
4. Examination of aspirated bone marrow for stainable iron is the most direct assessment of iron stores. Associated dysplasia or demonstration of ringed sideroblasts may reflect a sideroblastic anemia. Bone marrow examination is usually not required for diagnosis of iron deficiency or thalassemia.
5. Hemoglobin analysis by electrophoresis or HPLC (high-performance liquid chromatography) when thalassemia is suspected. This will allow measurement of hemoglobin A_2 levels (increased in most patients with β-thalassemia) and determination of globin-chain synthetic ratios (often the only means of making a positive diagnosis of mild forms of α-thalassemia).
6. Cytogenetic analysis to support a diagnosis of an acquired sideroblastic anemia secondary to a myelodysplastic syndrome. Cytogenetic abnormalities may be seen in 20-80% of patients with myelodysplasia and include complex chromosomal defects, abnormalities of chromosomes 5 and 7, and trisomy 8.
7. Documentation of a hematologic response to iron supplementation therapy, thereby confirming a diagnosis of iron deficiency.

2.4 Hematologic Findings

Initial workup of a hypochromic, microcytic anemia usually is aimed at distinguishing iron deficiency anemia from thalassemia. Sideroblastic anemia and anemia of chronic disease may also be considered. Pertinent red blood cell findings may help to narrow this differential **t2.4**. Significant hypochromia, microcytosis, and anisocytosis are usually present in well-developed iron deficiency anemia. However, in early or mild iron deficiency, morphologic abnormalities of the red blood cells may be absent. Hypochromia and microcytosis are found uniformly in the thalassemia syndromes, and the reductions in mean corpuscular volume (MCV) and mean corpuscular hemoglobin concentration (MCHC) are generally greater than those observed in the same degree of anemia in iron deficiency. Microcytosis with significant elevations of the red blood cell count to greater than $6 \times 10^6/\text{mm}^3$ ($6 \times 10^{12}/\text{L}$) are common in thalassemia minor. Basophilic stippling of red blood cells is commonly seen in thalassemia but is unusual in iron deficiency anemia. Hypochromia is often present in patients with sideroblastic anemia, but it also occurs in patients with chronic inflammatory or neoplastic disorders and the associated anemia of chronic disease. Characteristically, the variability of red blood cell size (anisocytosis) is increased in iron deficiency, but variability is much less than in thalassemia. The size distribution in sideroblastic anemias varies, but a characteristic dimorphic population of normocytic or microcytic cells and macrocytes is often seen, particularly in acquired sideroblastic anemia.

2.4.1 Blood Cell Measurements

The MCV is decreased in severe iron deficiency anemia and thalassemias, but may be normal in patients with hemoglobin levels greater than 10 g/dL (100 g/L). The MCV may be normal to increased in sideroblastic anemia due to the dimorphic population, although microcytosis is more common in the hereditary types. The reticulocyte count may be modestly decreased, normal, or modestly increased. Red blood cell number is often a useful distinguishing feature as it is usually not decreased and may be significantly increased in patients with thalassemia with normal red blood cell distribution width (RDW) values reflecting less anisocytosis. In contrast, iron deficiency anemia usually shows concordant decreases in red blood cell number, hemoglobin levels, and MCV, with a characteristic increase in RDW.

2.4.2 Peripheral Blood Smear Morphology

Hypochromia and microcytosis are present in severe iron deficiency anemia (see i2.1) but may be lacking or comprise a minor component of the red blood cells in patients with less severe iron depletion. Sideroblastic anemias usually have notable anisocytosis and poikilocytosis, giving rise to the characteristic dimorphic population of hypochromic, microcytic cells and normocytic, normochromic red blood cells (see i2.3). Occasionally, dysplastic features may be noted in neutrophils or other cytopenias may be noted in idiopathic cases of sideroblastic anemia associated with myelodysplasia. Target cells and basophilic stippling may be prominent in the thalassemias (see i2.4).

2.4.3 Bone Marrow Examination

Bone marrow examination, usually not required for the diagnosis of iron deficiency anemia or thalassemia, is important in diagnosis of a sideroblastic anemia. Erythroid hyperplasia will usually be present in association with all of the hypochromic, microcytic anemias, but is usually not as prominent as in hemolytic anemia. The only specific bone marrow finding in hypochromic, microcytic anemias that may be useful diagnostically is the pattern of marrow iron staining. Stainable iron, both sideroblastic and reticuloendothelial storage forms, is decreased or absent in iron deficiency. In contrast, anemia of chronic disease will demonstrate increased reticuloendothelial iron with decreased sideroblastic iron (see i2.5). The presence of ring sideroblasts and increased reticuloendothelial iron is required for diagnosis of a sideroblastic anemia (see i2.2). Marrow reticuloendothelial iron stores are often increased in thalassemia due to ineffective erythropoiesis.

i2.3 Sideroblastic anemia

Dimorphic red blood cell population of hypochromic, microcytic red blood cells and normochromic, normocytic cells in a patient with sideroblastic anemia. *(Wright stain)*

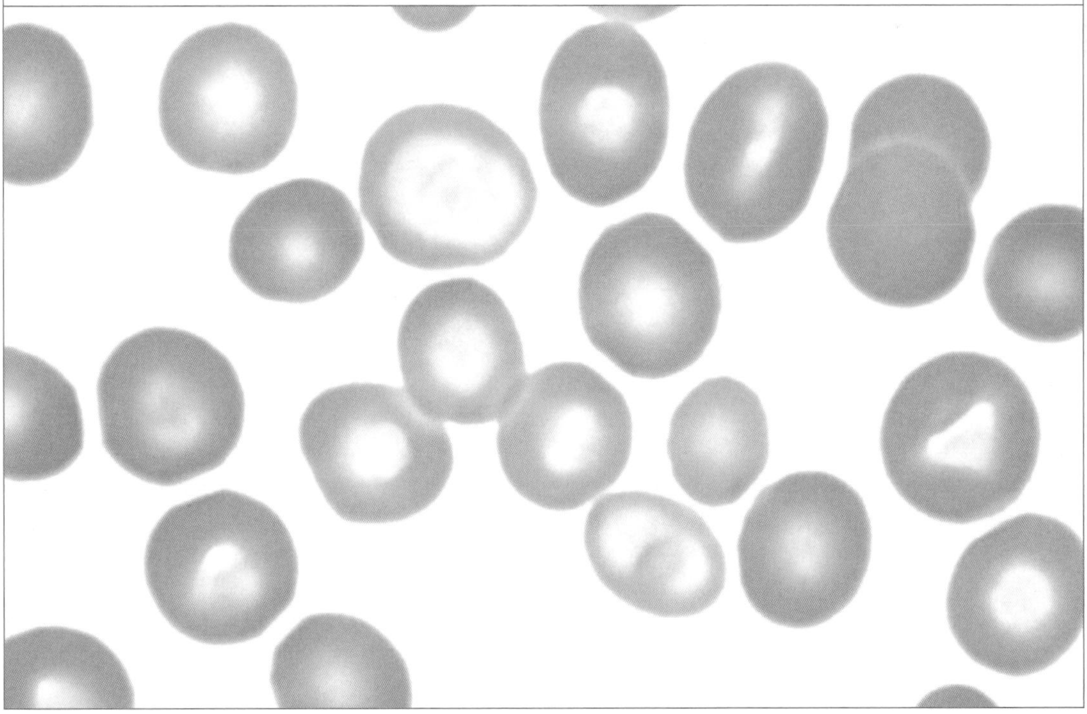

i2.4 Beta-thalassemia

Hypochromic, microcytic anemia with associated target cells and basophilic stippling in a patient with β-thalassemia. *(Wright stain)*

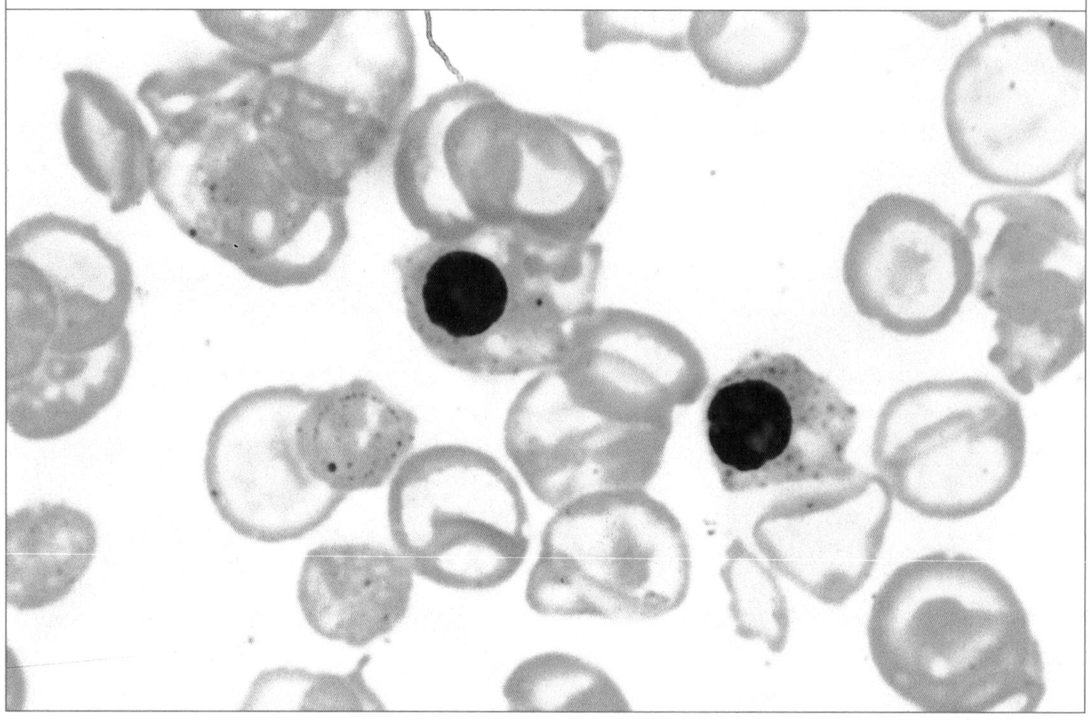

i2.5 Anemia of chronic disease

Iron staining of bone marrow in a patient with anemia of chronic disease demonstrating increased reticuloendothelial iron stores. *(Prussian blue stain)*

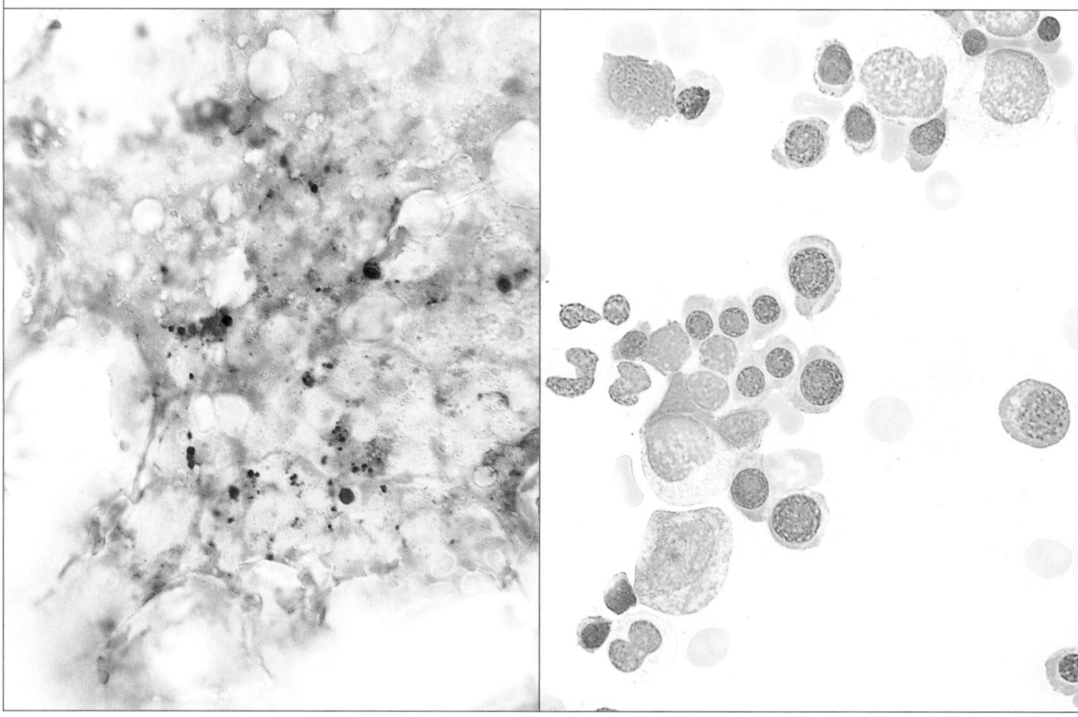

2.5 Other Laboratory Tests

Laboratory testing plays an important part of the evaluation of hypochromic, microcytic anemia as it provides important insights into the patient's iron stores and may help to identify the cause of the anemia. Testing may also identify early iron depletion or deficiency as depletion of body iron stores can be recognized before development of frank anemia (see **t2.5**). Furthermore, the pattern of results observed in the CBC (see **t2.4**) and iron studies usually will help to indicate the underlying disease process (see **t2.5**) and help to direct further testing.

Test 2.5.1 Serum Iron Quantitation and Total Iron-Binding Capacity

Purpose. Serum iron and total iron-binding capacity (TIBC) determinations help differentiate iron deficiency anemia from other types of hypochromic, microcytic anemia. In mild iron deficiency anemia, decreased serum iron levels and increased TIBC usually precede changes in red blood cell morphology or CBC indices.

Principle. All iron transported in the plasma is bound in the ferric form to the specific iron-binding protein transferrin. Serum iron measures the transferrin-bound iron. Total iron-binding capacity—the iron concentration necessary to saturate the iron-binding sites of transferrin—is a measure of transferrin concentration. Saturation of transferrin is calculated by the following formula:

$$\% \text{ Transferrin Saturation} = [\text{Serum Iron (mol/L)} \div \text{TIBC } (\mu\text{mol/L}) \times 100$$

Normal mean transferrin saturation is approximately 30%. Unsaturated iron-binding capacity (UIBC) is the difference between TIBC and serum iron.

Specimen. A specimen of blood should be drawn in the morning owing to diurnal variations in serum iron levels. Serum is used for the determination.

Procedure. Serum iron is freed from transferrin by acidification of the serum and is reduced to the ferrous form. After the protein has been precipitated out, the iron in the filtrate is detected spectrophotometrically after reaction with a chromogen such as bathophenanthroline sulfonate. The TIBC is measured by adding iron to the serum and then removing excess unbound iron by magnesium carbonate absorption. The bound iron is then released from transferrin and reduced, and its concentration is measured as in the serum iron test. The TIBC also can be determined by measuring transferrin with immunodiffusion.

Interpretation. The representative normal range of values for serum iron is 60-180 μg/dL (12.7-35.9 μmol/L); for TIBC, the range is 250-410 μg/dL (45.2-77.7 μmol/L). The range for percent saturation is 20%-50%. The serum iron level and percent saturation is low in both iron deficiency anemia and anemia of chronic disease. Although the value for percent saturation is often reduced to levels below 16% in iron deficiency anemia and is frequently more than 16% in anemia of chronic disease, values for the two conditions overlap. The TIBC is uniformly increased in severe uncomplicated iron deficiency anemia and is decreased or normal in microcytic anemia of chronic disease. In mild iron deficiency anemia, both the serum iron and TIBC may be normal. Serum iron concentration is increased in the sideroblastic anemias and in some cases of thalassemia (see **t2.5**).

Notes and Precautions. Serum iron concentrations show wide diurnal variations, with highest levels in the morning. Thus, specimens should be collected in the morning and oral iron therapy should be withdrawn 24 hours before the blood sample is drawn. Iron dextran administration causes plasma iron levels to be elevated for several weeks. A normal plasma iron level and iron-binding capacity do not rule out the diagnosis of iron deficiency when the hemoglobin level of the blood is above 9 g/dL (90 g/L) in women and 11 g/dL (110 g/L) in men.

Test 2.5.2 Stainable Bone Marrow Iron

Purpose. The most direct means for assessing body iron stores is by histochemical examination of aspirated bone marrow for storage iron.

Principle. Iron is stored in reticuloendothelial cells, and iron granules are formed in developing normoblasts. Normoblasts that contain one or more particles of stainable iron are known as "sideroblasts." Iron is stored as ferritin (iron complexed to the apoferritin protein) and hemosiderin (iron-protein complexes with a high iron content and denatured ferritin aggregates). Hemosiderin is the stainable form of storage iron that appears blue when treated with an acid potassium ferricyanide solution used in the Prussian blue reaction.

Specimen. Either sectioned bone marrow aspirate fragments (clot section) or particle smears are used for the assessment of reticuloendothelial iron, but bone marrow aspirate films must be used to detect sideroblasts. Iron staining may be decreased in decalcified sections due to leaching out of iron during the decalcification process.

Procedure. The bone marrow aspirate is stained with the Prussian blue reaction. Heating the staining mixture to 56°C increases its sensitivity. The search for sideroblasts is aided by a counterstain such as basic fuchsin.

Interpretation. Normally, hemosiderin granules are seen in reticuloendothelial cells in every third or fourth oil immersion field. With reduced iron stores, either no or only a few hemosiderin granules are seen in the entire preparation. With increased iron stores, hemosiderin granules are seen in every oil immersion field, often deposited in clumps.

The appraisal of reticuloendothelial iron is extremely helpful in the differential diagnosis of anemia (see **t2.4**, **t2.5**). Because iron from the breakdown of red blood cell heme cannot be excreted, it is diverted to the storage compartment. Thus, increased iron is generally present in the marrow of patients with anemia who are not iron deficient due to ineffective erythropoiesis. An exception may exist in myeloproliferative disorders in which bone marrow iron stores may be absent without other evidence of iron deficiency, perhaps resulting from impaired storage function. When storage iron is present in the bone marrow, anemia cannot be a result of iron deficiency, unless the patient has recently received parenterally administered iron treatment.

Normally, 20%-40% of red blood cell precursors are iron-containing sideroblasts. Although a sideroblast count is not ordinarily necessary for the diagnosis of iron deficiency anemia, it may be useful when an inadequate number of bone marrow particles have been obtained and in patients who have received parenterally administered iron. Decreased bone marrow sideroblasts are seen in iron deficiency anemia, after acute blood loss when reticuloendothelial stores have not yet been depleted, and in anemia of chronic disease. Sideroblastic anemia is characterized by the presence of ring sideroblasts, normoblasts that contain iron granules that surround at least two thirds of the nuclear circumference (see i2.2).

Notes and Precautions. Some practice is required to distinguish stainable reticuloendothelial iron from artifacts. When a patient has received iron parenterally, either as iron dextran or in the form of blood transfusions, histochemically stainable iron particles may be seen in the bone marrow in the presence of iron deficiency anemia. A well-prepared bone marrow aspirate film is essential for the detection of iron granules in normoblasts, and appropriate positive control slides should be performed simultaneously to ensure adequate staining.

Test 2.5.3 Serum Ferritin Quantitation

Purpose. Small amounts of ferritin or the antigenically equivalent apoferritin normally circulate in the plasma. Estimating serum ferritin levels provides a semiquantitative, less invasive test for iron store determination than the histochemical examination of aspirated bone marrow.

Principle. Ferritin is a storage complex of the protein apoferritin and iron. The largest quantities of ferritin are found in the liver and reticuloendothelial cells. Ordinarily, serum ferritin concentration reflects the amount of stored iron.

Specimen. Serum is used for testing.

Procedure. Reliable estimation of serum ferritin levels has been achieved with a sensitive radioimmune method using a sandwich technique. Ferritin is removed from the serum by solid phase antiferritin antibodies, and radioactively labeled antiferritin antibodies are then permitted to bind to the removed ferritin.

Interpretation. The normal concentration of serum ferritin varies from 10 to 500 ng/mL (10 to 500 μg/L). In iron deficiency anemia, serum ferritin level is diminished, making it a relatively sensitive and reliable indicator. Serum ferritin levels may be low in iron deficiency that is not associated with overt anemia. Elevated ferritin levels are common in iron overload states, including sideroblastic anemia and hemochromatosis. Serum ferritin levels are also elevated in patients with inflammatory diseases and, for poorly understood reasons, in patients with Gaucher's disease.

Notes and Precautions. When iron deficiency and inflammatory disease coexist, serum ferritin levels may be in the normal range.

Test 2.5.4 Serum Soluble Transferrin Receptor

Purpose. Measurement of serum soluble transferrin receptor levels provides an additional means to quantitate iron deficiency, which is proportional to red blood cell-associated transferrin receptor levels. These levels do not appear to be altered by inflammatory states and may provide a sensitive means to quantify iron stores when borderline values for iron deficiency are obtained by other tests. Serum soluble transferrin levels are increased in iron deficiency.

Principle. The transferrin receptor is a transmembrane protein that transfers iron from plasma transferrin into the red blood cell. Most transferrin receptors are found in the cell membrane, but a truncated form of the tissue receptor that is bound to transferrin is found in soluble form in the serum. Transferrin receptor levels reflect iron status, with receptor synthesis being rapidly induced by decreased iron levels. Thus, measurement of the soluble transferrin receptor (which mirrors cellular transferrin receptor levels) provides an additional measurable parameter of iron balance.

Specimen. Serum is used.

Procedure. Serum transferrin receptors are assayed with a sandwich enzyme immunoassay that uses a polyclonal antibody against the serum transferrin receptor protein. Commercially available kits can detect the protein in ranges from 0.85-20 mg/L.

Interpretation. Levels of serum soluble transferrin receptors >3.1 mg/L can indicate iron deficiency in most studies. This test is best used in combination with other tests of iron status (ferritin, total iron-binding capacity, and serum iron).

Notes and Precautions. Elevated serum soluble transferrin receptor levels have been noted, irrespective of patient iron status, in patients with hematologic malignancies or conditions with increased effective or ineffective hematopoiesis (ie, hemolytic anemia, hemoglobinopathies, or deficiencies of vitamin B_{12} or folate). Normal ranges for pregnant women and pediatric patients are not well established. Blacks and those living at high altitudes may have normal serum soluble transferrin levels 6% higher than upper normal limits. This may be additive (blacks living at high altitudes may have levels up to 12% above upper limits). The observation that serum soluble transferrin receptor levels are not increased in patients with inflammatory disease may help distinguish iron deficiency from anemia of chronic disease in these patients.

Test 2.5.5 Free Erythrocyte Protoporphyrin

Purpose. Free erythrocyte protoporphyrin (FEP) levels are elevated in patients with anemias associated with failure of iron incorporation into heme.

Principle. When insufficient iron is available for developing erythroblasts, excess protoporphyrin that was destined to be converted to heme accumulates as FEP. This substance is elevated both in iron deficiency and in conditions associated with an internal block in iron utilization, such as anemia of chronic disease, lead poisoning, and sideroblastic anemias.

Specimen. Whole anticoagulated blood is collected. There is also a spot test for blood specimens collected on filter paper.

Procedure. Free erythrocyte protoporphyrin is extracted from red blood cells with ethyl acetate/acetic acid and is quantitated fluorometrically.

Interpretation. Free erythrocyte protoporphyrin is normally less than 100 µg/dL (1.7 µmol/L) in packed red blood cells. Elevated levels are seen in patients with iron deficiency, chronic disease states associated with decreased transferrin saturation, and acquired idiopathic sideroblastic anemia. Marked elevation of FEP is seen in patients with sideroblastic anemia secondary to lead intoxication with FEP values of about 1000 µg/dL (17 µmol/L) packed red blood cells. In patients with microcytic anemias associated with abnormal globin synthesis rather than abnormal heme synthesis (such as thalassemia minor), FEP levels are normal. Because iron deficiency anemia and thalassemia minor are the first and second most common causes of hypochromic, microcytic anemia, measurement of FEP may be particularly useful as a screening test to distinguish between these two disorders.

2.6 Test Selection

Examination of the peripheral blood smear and red blood cell indices is essential for determining the etiology of a microcytic anemia. The red blood cell number, hemoglobin content, MCV, and RDW provide important diagnostic clues as to the etiology of the anemia (see **t2.4**). If iron deficiency is suspected on the basis of a high RDW and low red blood cell numbers, iron studies such as serum iron, total iron binding capacity (TIBC), serum ferritin, and/or soluble serum transferrin receptor may be ordered. If a thalassemia is suspected on the basis of a high red blood cell count for the degree of microcytosis and a normal RDW or the presence of target cells, testing can be aimed at determining FEP levels, quantifying hemoglobin A_2 levels, and possible hemoglobin analysis. If a dimorphic population of red blood cells or dysplastic changes are seen in the other blood cells, a bone marrow examination with iron staining for demonstration of ringed sideroblasts is indicated.

2.7 Course and Treatment

Ultimately, the diagnosis of iron deficiency depends on demonstration of an adequate response to iron therapy. Treatment usually consists of the oral administration of a ferrous iron salt, such as ferrous sulfate, in a dosage providing 0.06 to 0.12 g of iron three times a day. In some circumstances, the parenteral administration of iron dextran may be preferred. Reticulocytosis and a significant rise in blood hemoglobin concentration may occur as early as the third or fourth day after treatment, particularly in children, but is usually seen after 7 or 8 days. The hemoglobin concentration in the blood may not rise significantly until 10 days after treatment begins. Thereafter, complete restoration of the hemoglobin level to normal should be rapid (essentially complete by the sixth week after institution of therapy), regardless of the initial severity of the anemia.

Infection, inflammatory disease, or neoplastic disease may prevent an adequate response, and continued bleeding may blunt the therapeutic effect of iron administration. The most common cause of failure of iron therapy in patients with a hypochromic, microcytic anemia is an incorrect diagnosis. It is important to identify the cause of the iron deficiency (almost always blood loss or pregnancy in adults) and to correct it, if possible. Iron deficiency is often an indication of an underlying gastrointestinal or genitourinary tract cancer.

Sideroblastic anemias, other than the acquired idiopathic forms, may respond to treatment with pyridoxine. Many of the drugs that cause toxic sideroblastic anemias are pyridoxine antagonists. If a toxic etiology is suspected, removal of the drug or alcohol often leads to rapid improvement in the anemia. Some hereditary sideroblastic anemias are pyridoxine resistant, indicating heterogeneous metabolic abnormalities in affected patients. In both the acquired idiopathic form of the disease and hereditary forms, repeated transfusions may be required to treat severe anemia. The acquired idiopathic form of the disease is a myelodysplastic syndrome, and small numbers of the patients develop progressive bone marrow failure, cytopenias, or overt acute myelogenous leukemia. However, most patients have stable anemia and disease-associated symptoms over many years.

The thalassemic syndromes also have a wide range of symptoms and clinical severity. The traits often have mild anemia. In β-thalassemia major, transfusions are required to maintain life. Splenectomy may help to ameliorate the anemia in these patients. In both sideroblastic anemias and thalassemias, long-term transfusion therapy may lead to iron overload, requiring chelation therapy.

2.8 References

Bain BJ. Diagnosis from the blood smear. *New Engl J Med.* 2005;353:498-507.

Brugnara C. Iron deficiency and erythropoiesis: new diagnostic approaches. *Clin Chem.* 2003;49:1573-1578.

Brugnara C. Reticulocyte cellular indices: a new approach in the diagnosis of anemias and monitoring of erythropoietic function. *Crit Rev Clin Lab Sci.* 2000, 37:93-130.

Eldinbany MM, Totonchi KF, Joseph NJ, et al. Usefulness of certain red blood cell indices in diagnosing and differentiating thalassemia trait from iron-deficiency anemia. *Am J Pathol.* 1999;111:676–682.

Furuyama K, Sassa S. Multiple mechanisms for hereditary sideroblastic anemia. *Cell Mol Biol* (Noisy-le-grand). 2002;48:5-10.

Hermiston ML, Mentzer WC. A practical approach to the evaluation of the anemic child. *Pediatr Clin North Am.* 2002;49:877-891.

Irwin JJ, Kirchner JT. Anemia in children. *Am Fam Physician.* 2001;64(8):1379-86.

Koc S, Harris JW. Sideroblastic anemias: variations on imprecision in diagnostic criteria, proposal for an extended classification of sideroblastic anemias. *Am J Hematol.* 1998;57:1–6.

Mast AE, Blinder MA, Gronowski AM, et al. Clinical utility of the soluble transferrin receptor and comparison with serum ferritin in several populations. *Clin Chem.* 1998;44:45–51.

Pierre RV. Reticulocytes. Their usefulness and measurement in peripheral blood. *Clin Lab Med.* 2002;22:63-79.

Riley RS, Ben-Ezra JM, Goel R, Tidwell A. Reticulocytes and reticulocyte enumeration. *J Clin Lab Anal.* 2001;15:267-294.

Tefferi A. Anemia in adults: a contemporary approach to diagnosis. *Mayo Clin Proc.* 2003;78:1274-1280.

Waters HM, Seal LH. A systematic approach to the assessment of erythropoiesis. *Clin Lab Haematol.* 2001, 23:271-283.

Worwood M. The laboratory assessment of iron status—an update. *Clin Chim Acta.* 1997;259:3–23.

Worwood M. Serum transferrin receptor assays and their application. *Ann Clin Biochem.* 2002;39:221-230.

CHAPTER 3

Anemia of Chronic Disease and Normochromic, Normocytic, Non-Hemolytic Anemias

Kathryn Foucar, MD

Anemia is the most common hematologic abnormality in patients with chronic diseases. These chronic diseases are highly diverse and include neoplasms, infections, other inflammatory processes, and end organ failure. Despite this heterogeneity of primary disorders, the anemias that occur in these patient populations exhibit many common features; most of these anemias can be attributed to chronic disease, nutritional deficiency, blood loss, or a combination thereof.

3.1 Anemia of Chronic Disease

Anemia of chronic disease (ACD) is defined by a constellation of clinical, morphologic, and laboratory features **t3.1** and is second only to iron deficiency anemia in incidence. In a tertiary care setting, ACD may be the most frequently encountered type of anemia. Affected patients usually develop normocytic, normochromic anemia that is mild and non-progressive 1 to 2 months after the onset of chronic disease. This anemia is associated with multiple iron-related abnormalities, including decreased serum iron level, decreased transferrin level, decreased transferrin saturation, and increased storage iron (ferritin). The bone marrow examination reveals that erythroid precursors are generally present in normal numbers; erythroid iron is decreased, whereas storage iron is increased i3.1.

Various inflammatory, infectious, and neoplastic disorders are associated with ACD **t3.2**. Because the etiologies of anemias are considerably more complex in patients with renal failure, endocrine disorders, hepatic failure, and AIDS, these conditions are discussed separately at the end of this chapter. However, even in this patient group, ACD may be a dominant type of anemia in these patients.

3.1.1 Pathophysiology

Although incompletely understood, the overall picture of ACD appears to result from an immunologic response to protect the host from invading organisms and developing neoplasms. In this scenario, an immune-driven cytokine response induces hepcidin release by hepatocytes which ultimately results in iron deprivation to proliferating cells such as organisms and/or tumor cells. However, when this physiologic response is sustained, ACD is the consequence **t3.1**. Through the multifactorial actions of various inhibitory cytokines as tumor necrosis factor-β (TNF-β), interleukins (IL) 1 and 6, interferon γ (IFNγ), and the hepatic hormone, hepcidin, a cascade of events occur, adversely impacting erythropoiesis. These events include disturbances in iron homeostasis (decreased intestinal absorption plus increased shunting of iron

t3.1 Characteristics of Anemia of Chronic Disease

Clinical
Development of anemia 1-2 months after onset of chronic disease

Blood
Usually normocytic, normochromic anemia with normal mean corpuscular volume, mean corpuscular hemoglobin concentration, and red cell distribution width
Inappropriately low reticulocyte count

Iron studies
Decreased serum/plasma iron
Decreased transferrin (total iron-binding capacity)
Decreased transferrin saturation
Increased ferritin
Normal to slightly increased serum transferrin receptor levels
Increased hepcidin levels

Bone marrow
Variable numbers of erythroid precursors, usually normal, but sometimes reduced
Decreased sideroblasts (iron-containing erythroid precursor cells)
Increased storage iron within macrophages/ histiocytes

Pathophysiologic mechanisms
Chronic inflammation triggers pro-inflammatory cytokines (eg, IL-1, IL-6, TNF-a, which induce hepcidin release by hepatocytes and inhibit erythropoietin production
Increased hepcidin results in iron retention by macrophages, hepatocytes, and small bowel mucosa, reducing availability for erythropoiesis
Hepcidin also directly inhibits erythropoiesis by reducing proliferation and survival of erythroid progenitor cells
Decreased erythrocyte survival time due to sustained IL-1 production, fever, and other factors

TNF-α = tumor necrosis factor-α; IL = interleukin

into macrophages compounded by decreased macrophage release of iron), inhibition of erythroid progenitor cell proliferation and differentiation (blunted erythropoietin response in conjunction with increased apoptosis of erythroid precursor cells), and probable decreased erythrocyte survival time.

3.1.2 Clinical Findings

Because ACD is generally mild, the patient's symptoms are primarily related to the underlying disease. There are no physical examination findings unique to ACD.

3.1.3 Approach to Diagnosis

In a patient with anemia and a chronic illness, the contribution of ACD to this condition can vary from major to insignificant. Because multifactorial anemia in such a patient population is the rule rather than the exception, the patient's evaluation should identify other concomitant anemia-inducing factors. For example, a patient with a neoplasm may suffer from iron deficiency anemia secondary to chronic blood loss, myelophthistic anemia secondary to bone marrow replacement by tumor, hypoplastic anemia secondary to bone marrow suppression by chemotherapeutic agents, or even microangiopathic hemolytic anemia secondary to drug treatment or mucin production by tumor. **t3.3** lists these and other possible factors that may contribute to anemias that occur in patients with neoplasms. During the course of the clinical and hematologic evaluation of the patient, it is often readily apparent that one or more of these additional causes of anemia is present. In clinical practice, the distinction between ACD and iron deficiency anemia is the most frequent diagnostic dilemma **t3.4**.

Another increasing medical challenge is chronic anemia in elderly patients. The incidence of anemia increases with age and exceeds 20% in patients 85 years or older; this incidence doubles in elderly nursing home patients. In over one third of these patients the cause of the anemia cannot be determined; about one third have anemia of chronic disease, while the remaining third have nutritional deficiencies. Alcohol ingestion may be a factor in indeterminant cases. Significant

i3.1 Increased macrophage storage iron

Markedly increased macrophage storage iron is evident in this bone marrow aspirate smear, while adjacent erythroid elements do not contain iron. *(Prussian blue stain)*

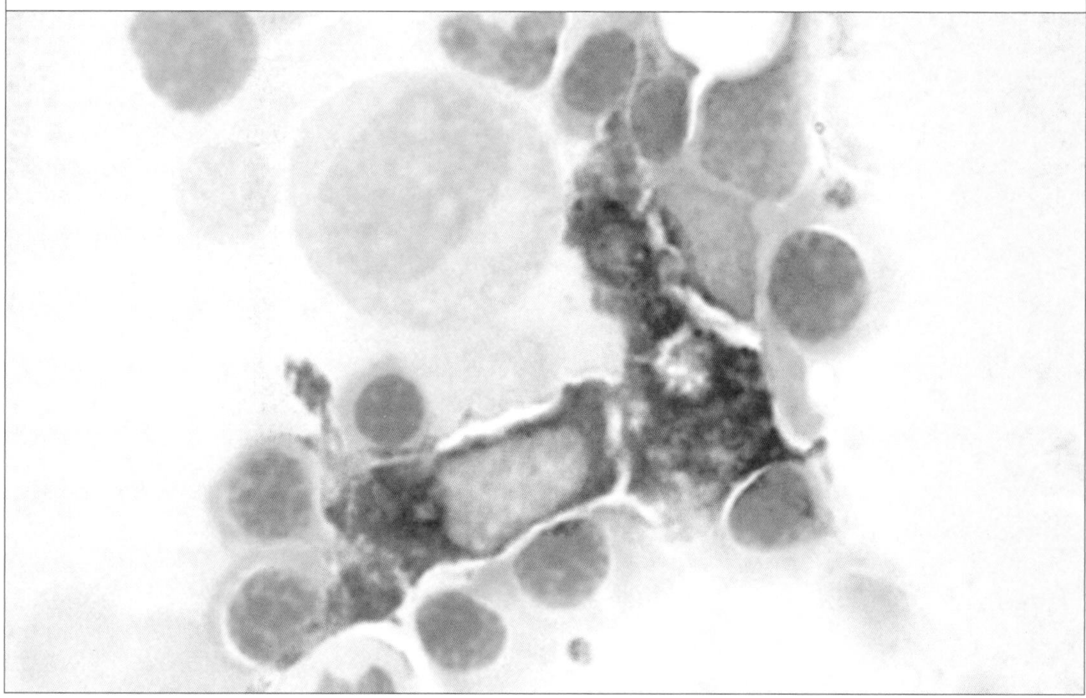

t3.2 Diseases Commonly Associated With Anemia of Chronic Disease*

Chronic inflammatory disorders
Rheumatoid arthritis
Systemic lupus erythematosus
Inflammatory bowel disease
Other connective tissue disorders
Sarcoidosis
Trauma
Vasculitis
Chronic rejection (solid organ transplantation)

Chronic infections
HIV-1 infections
Other viral infections†
Tuberculosis
Pyelonephritis
Osteomyelitis
Chronic fungal infections
Subacute bacterial endocarditis

Neoplasms
Malignant lymphoma
Carcinomas
Chronic leukemias

End organ failure
Chronic liver disease
Endocrinopathies
Chronic inflammatory kidney disease

**Patients often have multiple concurrent types of anemia*
†Usually in patients with underlying immunodeficiency
HIV-1 = human immunodeficiency virus-1

t3.3 Causes of Anemia in Patients With Malignancies*

Anemia of chronic disease
Myelotoxic effects of chemotherapy
Blood loss
Nutritional deficiencies, especially iron, less often folate/vitamin B_{12}
Bone marrow replacement by tumor/fibrosis
Chemotherapy-related myelodysplasia
Hypersplenism
Microangiopathic hemolytic anemia secondary to drug treatment, disseminated intravascular coagulation, tumor products (eg, mucin)
Secondary infection, inflammation
Immune-mediated hemolysis (warm or cold antibodies)
Red cell aplasia
Florid hemophagocytic syndrome

**Treatment with recombinant human erythropoietin successful in some patients, especially those in whom anemia of chronic disease is the dominant cause of anemia.*

t3.4 Comparison of Parameters Useful in Distinguishing Iron Deficiency Anemia From Anemia of Chronic Disease*

	Iron Deficiency	Chronic Disease
Serum iron	↓	↓ to Nl
TIBC (transferrin)	↑	↓
% Transferrin saturation	↓ (< 10%)	↓ (> 10%)
Serum ferritin	↓	↑
Serum transferrin receptor	↑	Nl to sl ↑
Bone marrow storage iron	↓	↑
MCV	↓	Nl
MCHC	↓	Nl
RDW	↑	Nl to sl ↑

**Modified from Wians 2001, Weiss 2002, Baillie 2003, Das Gupta 2003.*
Sl = slight; Nl = normal range; MCV = mean corpuscular volume; MCHC = mean corpuscular hemoglobin concentration; RDW = red cell distribution width; ↑ = increased; ↓ = decreased

reductions in erythropoietin production noted in some studies on elderly patients may be linked to decreased renal function and/or chronic inflammation.

The laboratory evaluation of patients for ACD usually includes the following steps:

1. Measurement of standard hematologic parameters with reticulocyte count.
2. Evaluation of peripheral blood smear for "clues" suggesting other specific types of anemia.
3. Iron studies, including assays of serum iron, transferrin level, percentage of transferrin saturation, and serum ferritin **t3.4**.
4. Appropriate laboratory testing to establish or exclude diagnoses of other types of anemia.
5. Bone marrow aspiration, with iron stains, and biopsy in selected cases that are not clear-cut after routine blood and laboratory evaluation or in patients in whom bone marrow examination is indicated for other reasons.

The laboratory approach to the evaluation of these patients must always be correlated with the clinical findings. The approach should be tailored to each case, using clues from the patient's history, disease course, and physical examination to direct the sequence of tests used.

3.1.4 Hematologic Findings

There are no pathognomonic findings in the peripheral blood in patients with ACD. These patients generally have a mild to moderate anemia that is not associated with an appropriate compensatory increase in the reticulocyte count.

Blood Cell Measurements

In ACD, the hemoglobin level ranges from 7.0-11.0 g/dL (70-110 g/L). The RBCs vary little in size, as indicated by their normal or near-normal red cell distribution width (RDW). The mean corpuscular volume (MCV), mean corpuscular hemoglobin (MCH), and mean corpuscular hemoglobin concentration (MCHC) are generally normal, although the MCV and MCHC may be mildly decreased. Reticulocyte quantitation is below the predicted level for the degree of anemia. WBC and platelet counts are usually normal; decreases in these parameters may be attributable to therapy or other factors.

Peripheral Blood Smear Morphology

Erythrocytes are generally normocytic and normochromic without significant anisopoikilocytosis or polychromasia, although they are occasionally mildly hypochromic. There are usually no morphologic abnormalities of WBCs or platelets.

Bone Marrow Examination

Erythroid elements in the bone marrow are generally morphologically normal and present in normal numbers. Sideroblasts are decreased, while storage iron is increased substantially. Myeloid and megakaryocytic elements usually are unremarkable. Depending on the underlying chronic disease, additional bone marrow abnormalities, ranging from granulomas in patients with chronic infections to foci of metastatic tumor in cancer patients, may be detected.

3.2 Laboratory Tests

Although no single laboratory test is specific for ACD, a well-established laboratory profile includes serum iron, iron transport protein (transferrin or "iron-binding capacity"), transferrin saturation, and storage iron measurements (serum ferritin) **t3.4**.

Test 3.2.1 Serum Iron Quantitation

Purpose. The determination of serum iron, in conjunction with other iron studies described later, is important in distinguishing ACD from other types of anemia that may develop in patients.

Principle. Specimen, Procedure, Notes, and Precautions. See Test 2.5.1.

Interpretation. A prompt decline in serum iron level is associated with infection and other types of tissue injury. This decrease precedes the development of anemia, which occurs only if the infection or injury is sustained. A low serum iron level also is seen in patients with iron deficiency anemia.

Test 3.2.2 Serum Transferrin Measurement (Total Iron-Binding Capacity)

Purpose, Principle, Specimen, Procedure, Notes, and Precautions. See Test 2.5.4.

Interpretation. Transferrin is characteristically decreased in patients with ACD, in contrast to the substantial elevation of this protein level in patients with iron deficiency anemia. This test, however, is neither specific nor sensitive enough to consistently distinguish between the two types of anemia.

Test 3.2.3 Transferrin Saturation

Purpose. The percent saturation of transferrin reflects the availability of iron for erythropoiesis and can be calculated by dividing the serum iron level by the transferrin level.

Interpretation. The percent saturation of transferrin is generally decreased in patients with ACD, in whom a range of 10% to 25% saturation is usually found. Although in iron deficiency anemia the percent saturation of transferrin is usually less than 15%, there is some overlap between the percent saturation ranges found in these two disorders.

Test 3.2.4 Serum Ferritin Quantitation

Purpose. The serum ferritin level is a measure of the patient's total body iron stores.

Principle, Specimen, Procedure, Notes, and Precautions. See Test 2.5.1.

Interpretation. The serum ferritin level usually is increased in patients with ACD, reflecting their abundant storage iron. The serum ferritin level in patients with iron deficiency anemia generally is markedly decreased.

Notes and Precautions. Ferritin is an acute phase reactant that may be elevated spuriously in patients with acute inflammatory processes. Despite this problem, serum ferritin levels are still of value in patients with possible ACD because they can help distinguish such patients from those with iron deficiency anemia. If results of serum ferritin assays are correlated with erythrocyte sedimentation rate, the distinction between ACD and iron deficiency anemia is enhanced.

3.3 Ancillary Tests

The free erythrocyte protoporphyrin level is elevated in patients with ACD because the iron available for hemoglobin synthesis is decreased. Measuring free erythrocyte protoporphyrin, however, is not generally done in the initial evaluation for this disorder (See Test 2.5.5). Likewise, more recently developed tests such as assays of soluble serum transferrin receptor concentration may provide additional information in distinguishing ACD (normal to mildly increased) from overt iron deficiency anemia (increased). Recent studies document excellent correlation between the bone marrow storage/erythroid precursor iron picture and serum transferrin receptor levels. Patients with concomitant iron deficiency and ACD exhibited a hybrid picture when serum transferrin receptor, MCV, and MCHC were correlated. If further studies confirm the use of serial serum transferrin receptor level assessment in distinguishing iron deficiency anemia from ACD, this test may obviate the need for bone marrow examination in some patients. In addition, measurement of serum/urine hepcidin levels may prove useful in the identification of patients with ACD, although studies are currently preliminary.

3.4 Course and Treatment

Treatment of the underlying disease is of paramount importance in the care of patients with ACD, because eradication or control of the underlying disorder results in improvement of the anemia. Anemia of chronic disease is often mild and usually does not require specific treatment. Transfusion results in temporary improvement but is not recommended unless the patient is symptomatic. Recent evidence suggests that some patients with ACD respond at least partially to recombinant human erythropoietin, while anti-TNFa therapy resulted in improved hemoglobin/hematocrit levels in some rheumatoid arthritis patients.

3.4.1 Anemia With Chronic Renal Failure

The anemia that often occurs in patients with chronic renal disease shares some characteristics with ACD. As individuals age, the incidence of both renal insufficiency and anemia increases. This anemia generally is normocytic and normochromic, and its severity roughly parallels the severity of the underlying renal disease. As in ACD, multiple factors contribute to the development of anemia in patients with renal disease; however, some important pathophysiologic differences exist between the two disorders. The primary pathophysiologic mechanism for anemia in renal failure patients is decreased erythropoiesis secondary to either decreased or non-functional eythropoietin **t3.5**. The bone marrow usually shows erythroid hypoplasia. Azotemia exacerbates the anemia by both direct suppression of bone marrow and decreased RBC survival. Other manifestations of the anemia associated with chronic renal disease include burr cells in the blood and decreased serum iron and transferrin levels. Sustained secretion of inhibitory cytokines may be responsible for these iron and transferrin abnormalities.

t3.5 Causes of Anemia in Patients With Chronic Renal Failure
Hypoproliferation secondary to decreased erythropoietin production (dominant factor)
Decreased bone marrow sensitivity to erythropoietin
Hemolysis (decreased erythrocyte survival)
Iron or folate deficiency
Hemorrhage
Red blood cell toxins introduced by dialysis
Chronic infections, other inflammatory processes (concomitant anemia of chronic disease)
Bone marrow suppression from azotemia*
Bone marrow fibrosis from advanced osteitis fibrosa cystica*†
Red cell aplasia secondary to antierythropoietin antibodies (patients receiving recombinant erythropoietin)
Dilutional anemia from fluid imbalance*

**Rarely significant contributing factors in anemia of chronic renal failure*
†From secondary hyperparathyroidism

Several additional factors can exacerbate anemia in these patients. For example, patients may have long-term blood loss because of both platelet and vessel defects secondary to the underlying renal disease. Patients undergoing long-term hemodialysis can readily become folate deficient; red blood cell toxins (eg, aluminum, copper, formaldehyde, chlorine) can be introduced by dialysis. Finally, patients with renal disease are prone to fluid overload, which can further decrease the hematocrit value.

The treatment of the underlying renal disease is of primary importance in these patients. Treatment with recombinant human erythropoietin, often in conjunction with intravenous iron therapy, has resulted in amelioration of the anemia in many patients with chronic renal failure. However, the development of pure red cell aplasia secondary to antierythropoietin antibodies has been described in chronic renal failure patients receiving recombinant erythropoietin.

3.4.2 Anemia With Chronic Endocrine Disease

Anemia is common in patients with chronic endocrine diseases such as diabetes mellitus and hypothyroidism. The anemia in patients with diabetes is characteristically multifactorial. In addition to ACD, such patients may develop enteropathy, which leads to poor absorption of iron, vitamin B_{12}, and folate. They also may suffer from chronic blood loss and chronic renal insufficiency. In addition, secondary effects on hematocrit are produced by abnormalities in plasma volume. The relative contribution of all of these abnormalities to an anemia varies from patient to patient and varies over time in the same patient.

Patients with chronic hypothyroidism also are frequently anemic. The possible factors contributing to an anemia in these patients include decreased oxygen requirements, concurrent pernicious anemia, iron deficiency secondary to menorrhagia, and impaired iron absorption. Treatment of the underlying endocrine disorder is of primary importance, but the anemia generally does not require treatment.

3.4.3 Anemia Associated With Liver Diseases

The prototypic liver disease linked to anemia is alcoholism, and anemia is a very common finding in patients with chronic alcoholism. Although this anemia is generally mild to moderate, it can periodically become more severe, corresponding to the patient's alcohol ingestion and the severity of the patient's liver disease. Although anemia in alcoholic patients is at least partially attributable to ACD, many other mechanisms are operative concurrently, including direct toxic effects of alcohol, various nutritional deficiencies, RBC survival defects, abnormal iron metabolism, and hemodilution. The predominant mechanism causing anemia may vary with time, and production, maturation, and survival defects may all play a role in the development of anemia in these patients. The pathogenesis and morphologic features of the various causes of anemia in patients with alcoholism are highlighted in **t3.6**.

Alcohol, especially when ingested in large amounts, has a direct toxic effect on hematopoietic elements, resulting in decreased bone marrow cellularity and vacuolization of

t3.6 Pathogenesis and Morphologic Features of Anemia in Patients With Alcoholism

Mechanism	Morphologic Features	Etiology/Cause
Chronic disease	Normocytic/normochromic anemia	See earlier discussion in this chapter
Folate deficiency* (rarely vitamin B_{12} deficiency)	Megaloblastic anemia with oval macrocytes and hypersegmented neutrophils Macrocytosis may be masked by concurrent iron deficiency	Decreased ingestion, impaired absorption, and antagonistic action of alcohol on folate function Alcohol-induced chronic pancreatitis can lead to vitamin B malabsorption
Iron deficiency†	Hypochromia present but microcytosis often masked by concurrent macrocytosis from hepatic disease	Decreased ingestion of iron and chronic blood loss via gastrointestinal tract
Decreased red blood cell survival (including hemolysis and acute blood loss)	Target cells, spherocytes, sometimes spur cells and microspherocytes	Extracorpuscular erythrocyte defects due to: Congestive splenomegaly and portal hypertension Lipoprotein abnormalities causing target and spur shapes Severe hypophosphatemia
Toxic suppression	Hypocellular bone marrow with vacuolated erythroid precursors	Alcohol toxic to hematopoietic elements
Abnormal iron metabolism	Ring sideroblasts in bone marrow	Complex etiology, not completely known Caused in part by decreased functional pyridoxine and inhibition of enzymes involved in hemoglobin synthesis
Hemodilution	None	Portal hypertension associated with fluid overload leading to dilutional anemia

**See Chapter 5 for more details.*
†See Chapter 2 for more details.

erythroid precursors. Nutritional deficiencies often found in patients with chronic alcoholism include folate and iron deficiency; vitamin B_{12} deficiency can also occur in alcoholic patients who develop chronic pancreatitis. Folate deficiency is particularly common in such patients because of decreased ingestion, impaired folate absorption by alcohol, and antagonism of folate function by alcohol. Although typical morphologic features of megaloblastic anemia may be identified in the blood and bone marrow of patients with alcoholism, these changes are often masked by concurrent RBC abnormalities from iron deficiency, hemolysis, or both. Iron stores may be decreased in patients with chronic alcoholism because of both decreased ingestion and chronic gastrointestinal blood loss. Hypochromasia is generally present, but the microcytosis of iron deficiency may be masked by counteracting macrocytosis caused by liver disease, folate deficiency, acute alcohol ingestion, or a combination of these. Decreased RBC survival is seen frequently in alcoholic patients with significant hepatic disease. The target cells, spherocytes, spur cells, and microspherocytes that may be identified in the peripheral blood of patients with chronic alcoholism are secondary to extracorpuscular RBC defects caused by congestive splenomegaly, lipoprotein abnormalities in the blood, and severe hypophosphatemia. In addition to iron deficiency, patients with chronic alcoholism may have abnormal iron metabolism manifested by ring sideroblasts in the bone marrow. Although the etiology of this phenomenon is not completely understood, the ring sideroblasts are caused in part by decreased functional pyridoxine and decreased activity of the enzymes involved in hemoglobin synthesis. Finally, portal hypertension is often associated with an increase in plasma volume that leads to dilutional anemia.

It is beyond the scope of this chapter to detail the clinical findings and laboratory features of patients with chronic alcoholism. Details of the laboratory evaluation of patients for possible iron deficiency and folate deficiency can be found in Chapters 2 and 5, respectively. Except for patients with pronounced spur cell formation, marked nutritional deficiency, or gastrointestinal tract bleeding, the anemia associated with chronic alcoholism is generally mild to moderate and does not require treatment. Management of the portal hypertension and congestive splenomegaly is important in ameliorating the RBC survival defects.

3.4.4 Anemia With AIDS

Cytopenias are common peripheral blood abnormalities in patients with AIDS, and the severity of these cytopenias is roughly correlated with disease status. Consequently, patients with the most severe cytopenias tend to be those with advanced disease. As with the other disorders presented in this chapter, the anemia in patients with AIDS is multifactorial, although ACD often predominates **t3.7**.

In addition, evidence suggests that HIV-1 may invade bone marrow progenitor cells, resulting in multilineage suppression of hematopoiesis. Likewise, immune aberrations characteristic of this disease may result in defective regulation of hematopoiesis. The anemia in patients with AIDS is frequently exacerbated by zidovudine therapy, which is also linked to marked macrocytosis. Bone marrow infiltration by secondary tumors may result in impaired hematopoiesis, and bone marrow suppression also may be the consequence of either various secondary infections or drug treatments required for secondary infections and/or neoplasms.

Various nutritional deficiencies can develop in patients with AIDS secondary to gastrointestinal blood loss, poor intake, or drugs that act as folate antagonists. One of the secondary infections that patients with AIDS can acquire is parvovirus, which invades erythroid progenitor cells and causes profound red cell aplasia (see Chapter 4). Because patients with AIDS are often unable to mount an immune response to parvovirus, the red cell aplasia is often sustained. Gamma globulin therapy is generally required to ameliorate this secondary viral infection.

t3.7 Causes of Anemia in Patients With AIDS

Anemia of chronic disease
Bone marrow suppression by virus (HIV-1)
Ineffective regulation of hematopoiesis (T-cell/monocyte defects)
Secondary infections and neoplasms
Myelotoxic effects of various drug treatments
Immune mechanisms (autoantibody production)
Sustained parvovirus infection resulting in prolonged red cell aplasia
Iron deficiency, other nutritional deficiencies
Thrombotic thrombocytopenic purpura-like picture
Chronic alcoholism, hepatitis, or other associated disorders
Advanced serous fat atrophy from inanition

3.5 References

Adamson JW. Renal disease and anemia in the elderly. *Semin Hematol.* 2008;45:235-241.

Andrews NC. Forging a field: the golden age of iron biology. *Blood.* 2008;112:219-230.

Baillie FJ, Morrison AE, Fergus I. Soluble transferrin receptor: a discriminating assay for iron deficiency. *Clin Lab Haematol.* 2003;25:353-357.

Casadevall N, Nataf J, Viron B, et al. Pure red-cell aplasia and antierythropoietin antibodies in patients treated with recombinant erythropoietin. N *Engl J Med.* 2002;346:469-475.

Dallalio G, Fleury T, Means RT. Serum hepcidin in clinical specimens. *Br J Haematol.* 2003;122:996-1000.

Dallalio G, Law E, Means RT, Jr. Hepcidin inhibits in vitro erythroid colony formation at reduced erythropoietin concentrations. *Blood.* 2006;107:2702-2704.

Das Gupta A, Abbi A. High serum transferrin receptor level in anemia of chronic disorders indicates coexistent iron deficiency. *Am J Hematol.* 2003;72:158-161.

Ferrucci L, Balducci L. Anemia of aging: the role of chronic inflammation and cancer. *Semin Hematol.* 2008;45:242-249.

Fitzsimons EJ, Sturrock RD. The chronic anaemia of rheumatoid arthritis: iron banking or blocking? *Lancet.* 2002;360:1713-1714.

Foucar K. Non-neoplastic erythroid lineage disorders. In: King D, Gardner W, Sobin L, et al., eds. *Non-Neoplastic Disorders of Bone Marrow* (AFIP fascicle). Washington, DC: American Registry of Pathology; 2008:75-124.

Foucar K. Noninfectious systemic diseases and miscellaneous bone marrow conditions. In: King D, Gardner W, Sobin L, et al., eds. *Non-Neoplastic Disorders of Bone Marrow* (AFIP fascicle). Washington, DC: American Registry of Pathology; 2008:371-396.

Hockenberry MJ, Hinds PS, Barrera P, et al. Incidence of anemia in children with solid tumors or Hodgkin disease. *J Pediatr Hematol Oncol.* 2002;24:35-37.

Keeling DM, Isenberg DA. Haematological manifestations of systemic lupus erythematosus. *Blood Rev.* 1993;7:199-207.

Lewis G, Wise MP, Poynton C, Godkin A. A case of persistent anemia and alcohol abuse. *Nat Clin Pract Gastroenterol Hepatol.* 2007;4:521-526.

Makoni SN, Laber DA. Clinical spectrum of myelophthisis in cancer patients. *Am J Hematol.* 2004;76:92-93.

Means RT, Jr. Hepcidin and anaemia. *Blood Rev.* 2004;18:219-225.

Moore RD. Anemia and human immunodeficiency virus disease in the era of highly active antiretroviral therapy. *Semin Hematol.* 2000;37:18-23.

Papadaki HA, Kritikos HD, Valatas V, et al. Anemia of chronic disease in rheumatoid arthritis is associated with increased apoptosis of bone marrow erythroid cells: improvement following anti-tumor necrosis factor-alpha antibody therapy. *Blood.* 2002;100:474-482.

Paradkar PN, De Domenico I, Durchfort N, et al. Iron depletion limits intracellular bacterial growth in macrophages. *Blood.* 2008;112:866-874.

Patel KV. Epidemiology of anemia in older adults. *Semin Hematol.* 2008;45:210-217.

Remacha AF, Cadafalch J. Cobalamin deficiency in patients infected with the human immunodeficiency virus. *Semin Hematol.* 1999;36:75-87.

Samol J, Littlewood TJ. The efficacy of rHuEPO in cancer-related anaemia. *Br J Haematol.* 2003;121:3-11.

Siebert S, Williams BD, Henley R, et al. Single value of serum transferrin receptor is not diagnostic for the absence of iron stores in anaemic patients with rheumatoid arthritis. *Clin Lab Haematol.* 2003;25:155-160.

Spivak JL. The blood in systemic disorders. *Lancet.* 2000;355:1707-1712.

Theurl I, Theurl M, Seifert M, et al. Autocrine formation of hepcidin induces iron retention in human monocytes. *Blood.* 2008;111:2392-2399.

Weiss G, Goodnough LT. Anemia of chronic disease. *New Engl J Med.* 2005;352:101.

Wians FH, Jr., Urban JE, Keffer JH, et al. Discriminating between iron deficiency anemia and anemia of chronic disease using traditional indices of iron status vs transferrin receptor concentration. *Am J Clin Pathol.* 2001;115:112-118.

CHAPTER 4

Aplastic and Hypoplastic Anemias and Miscellaneous Types of Anemia

Kathryn Foucar, MD

This chapter reviews aplastic and hypoplastic anemias, bone marrow replacement disorders, and congenital dyserythropoietic anemias.

4.1 Aplastic, Hypoplastic Anemias and Miscellaneous Types of Anemia

Both constitutional and acquired disorders of RBC production have been well delineated **t4.1**. These production defects can involve the erythroid lineage (ie, pure red cell aplasia), two cell lines (ie, bicytopenia), or production of all hematopoietic cells (ie, aplastic anemia). The constitutional (hereditary) types of aplastic anemia primarily include Fanconi anemia, dyskeratosis congenita, and occasional cases of Shwachman-Diamond syndrome. Diamond-Blackfan anemia is the only well-established constitutional pure red cell aplasia; recent reports suggest that evolution to aplastic anemia is a feature of long-standing disease **t4.2**. In general, these constitutional disorders are associated with abnormalities in other organ systems, including skeletal and mucocutaneous defects, or mental retardation. In addition to the obvious loss of one or more bone marrow lineages, biochemical abnormalities in erythrocytes are characteristic of both Diamond-Blackfan and Fanconi anemia. These RBC defects include increased fetal hemoglobin, increased expression of i antigen on the surface membrane, and abnormalities of cytoplasmic enzyme levels. Although Diamond-Blackfan anemia (constitutional red cell aplasia) is generally evident at birth or shortly thereafter, the constitutional aplastic anemias tend to manifest more gradually with the progressive development of trilineage hypoplasia.

Both pure red cell aplasia and aplastic anemia can be acquired, and these acquired hypoplastic disorders are substantially more common than their constitutional counterparts (see **t4.1** and **t4.2**). Acquired pure red cell aplasia can be classified as three general types: transient erythroblastopenia of childhood, parvovirus-induced red cell aplasia (usually transient), and acquired (sustained) pure red cell aplasia. Transient erythroblastopenia of childhood is a self-limited disorder that is likely linked to an antecedent viral infection, although a specific cause has not been well documented. Spontaneous recovery occurs; affected children are otherwise entirely normal. When erythroblastopenia occurs in a young child, the chief differential diagnostic considerations are Diamond-Blackfan anemia and parvovirus-induced red cell aplasia. The distinction among these disorders can be achieved by the integration of clinical findings, family history, documentation of anemia since birth, and viral serologic/PCR studies. The subsequent spontaneous resolution of transient erythroblastopenia of childhood confirms this diagnosis if parvoviral studies are negative.

Clinically significant parvovirus infection affects two general categories of patients—those with constitutional anemias associated with decreased erythrocyte survival time and immunocompromised patients who are unable to mount an antibody response to clear the infection.

t4.1 Types of Constitutional and Acquired Aplastic Anemia and Red Cell Aplasia

Constitutional aplastic anemia	Constitutional red cell aplasia
Fanconi anemia Dyskeratosis congenita Shwachman-Diamond syndrome	Diamond-Blackfan anemia
Acquired aplastic anemia	**Acquired red cell aplasia (RCA)**
Idiopathic Secondary to drugs, toxins, infections, and miscellaneous disorders/conditions Paroxysmal nocturnal hemoglobinuria (clonal)	Transient erythroblastopenia of childhood Parvovirus infection* (usually transient) Idiopathic pure red cell aplasia Sustained pure red cell aplasia secondary to neoplasms, immune disorders, infections, and drug treatment Antierythropoietin antibody-induced RCA in patients receiving recombinant erythropoietin

**Parvovirus infection may be sustained in immunocompromised host*

Children and adults who have underlying constitutional RBC survival disorders, such as hereditary spherocytosis or sickle cell anemia, can develop dramatic exacerbation of the underlying anemia secondary to acute parvovirus infection. Because of shortened RBC survival times, baseline production of erythrocytes greatly exceeds normal levels in patients with these constitutional hemolytic anemias. Consequently, the hemoglobin and hematocrit levels plummet when RBC production is halted, even temporarily, by parvovirus invasion and destruction of erythroid progenitor cells. Even though thalassemia is both an RBC maturation and an RBC survival disorder, the identical clinical "aplastic crisis" occurs as a consequence of acute parvovirus infection. Viral inclusions within the residual erythroblasts generally can be identified, but the diagnosis should be confirmed by serologic or molecular studies i4.1. Once the patient mounts an immune response to the parvovirus, the infection is eliminated and erythropoiesis returns to baseline levels. In immunocompromised patients, unless treated, parvovirus infections are typically sustained with prolonged red cell aplasia; rare reports describe multilineage hypoplasia in this patient population.

In addition to the acquired transient red cell aplasias, both primary and secondary types of acquired (sustained) pure red cell aplasia have been described t4.3. Disorders linked to acquired pure red cell aplasia include T-cell large granular lymphocytic leukemia, other hematopoietic and non-hematopoietic neoplasms, drug treatments (notably diphenylhydantoin), immune disorders, and chronic viral infections.

Although most cases of acquired aplastic anemia are idiopathic, the causes of acquired aplastic anemia include drug and toxin exposures, various viral infections, immune aberrations, and radiation t4.4. In addition, some patients with paroxysmal nocturnal hemoglobinuria (PNH) develop an aplastic picture. All hematopoietic lineages are either absent or severely attenuated in affected patients.

4.1.1 Pathophysiology

For erythropoiesis to occur, the necessary components include adequate stem cells (which are capable of renewal and differentiation), erythropoietin and other growth factors, appropriate immunoregulation of hematopoiesis, and an adequate microenvironment. Deficiencies or defects in all of these components have been suggested in the pathophysiology of the diverse spectrum of congenital and acquired erythropoietic production disorders. Mutations in genes encoding DNA repair proteins are responsible for the generalized DNA repair defects that characterize Fanconi anemia. Defects in telomere maintenance occur in dyskeratosis congenita,

t4.2 Features of Constitutional and Acquired Aplastic Anemias and Red Cell Aplasia

Type	Clinical Features/Mechanisms	Blood	Bone Marrow
Constitutional aplastic anemia**			
Fanconi	Autosomal recessive disease with associated bone, skin, and renal abnormalities Mental retardation Underlying DNA repair defect	Thrombocytopenia is typically initial abnormality Pancytopenia deve-lops by mid-childhood Decreased reticulocytes	Initially normo/hypercellular with variable megaloblastic changes Eventual aplasia Substantial late development of myelodysplasia or acute myeloid leukemia
Dyskeratosis congenita	X-linked recessive disorder with skin, nail, and mucosal abnormalities (other genetic types noted) Mental retardation Defect in telomere maintenance/ ribosome biogenesis	Gradual development of pancytopenia Decreased reticulocytes	Initially normo/hypercellular Eventual aplasia in one half of patients Reports of late development of acute myeloid leukemia
Shwachman-Diamond syndrome	Autosomal recessive; exocrine pancreas deficiency, some patients have associated bone abnormalities Defect in ribosome biogenesis	Neutropenia predominates 1/4 of cases progress to pancytopenia Decreased reticulocytes	Initial abnormalities are granulocytic Eventual aplasia in one fourth of patients Some patients develop acute myeloid leukemia
Constitutional red cell aplasia			
Diamond-Blackfan anemia	Onset of anemia at birth or early infancy Autosomal dominant Defect in ribosome biogenesis Short stature, hypertelorism, retardation Likely intrinsic progenitor cell defect	Macrocytic anemia with decreased reticulocytes	Only rare erythroblasts evident Other lineages unremarkable Increased hematogones Increased incidence of AML in long-term survivors
Acquired aplastic anemia			
Aplastic anemia	Onset at any age Most cases idiopathic Other cases linked to infections, toxins, drugs, radiation, immune disorders Activated T cells induce apoptosis of precursor cells, suppress hematopoiesis Some PNH cases evolve into aplastic anemia	Pancytopenia Normal morphology Decreased reticulocytes	Panhypoplasia Variable lymphoid infiltrates
Acquired red cell aplasia			
Transient erythroblastopenia of childhood	Patient usually over 1 year old Presumed transient viral suppression of erythroid lineage	Normocytic, normochromic anemia Decreased reticulocytes	Only rare erythroblasts evident Other lineages unremarkable Variable lymphocytosis, hematogones
Parvovirus-induced red cell aplasia*	Any age Patient typically has either underlying constitutional anemia or immunodeficiency Virus selectively infects and kills erythroblasts	Variable RBC morphology depending on underlying chronic anemia Decreased reticulocytes	Only erythroblasts evident; these cells may contain intranuclear inclusions† Other lineages usually unremarkable Infection transient in immunocompetent, sustained in immunocompromised patients
Acquired sustained pure red cell aplasia	Adolescence through adulthood Both idiopathic and secondary types Likely immune-mediated mechanism Strongest neoplastic association is T-cell large granular lymphocytic leukemia	Normocytic, normochromic anemia Decreased reticulocytes	Only rare erythroblasts evident Other hematopoietic lineages unremarkable Increased lymphocytes in some cases

***Often multiple inheritance patterns; predominant one listed*
**Transient red cell aplasia in immunocompetent patients secondary to parvovirus infection is clinically occult.*
†Unusual features such as increased erythroblasts and intact erythroid maturation noted in occasional immunosuppressed patient; AML=acute myeloid leukemia; PNH = paroxysmal nocturnal hemoglobinuria

i4.1 Acute parvovirus infection

Giant erythroblast with basophilic intranuclear inclusion in bone marrow aspirate of an immunosuppressed patient with acute parvovirus infection. *(Wright stain)*

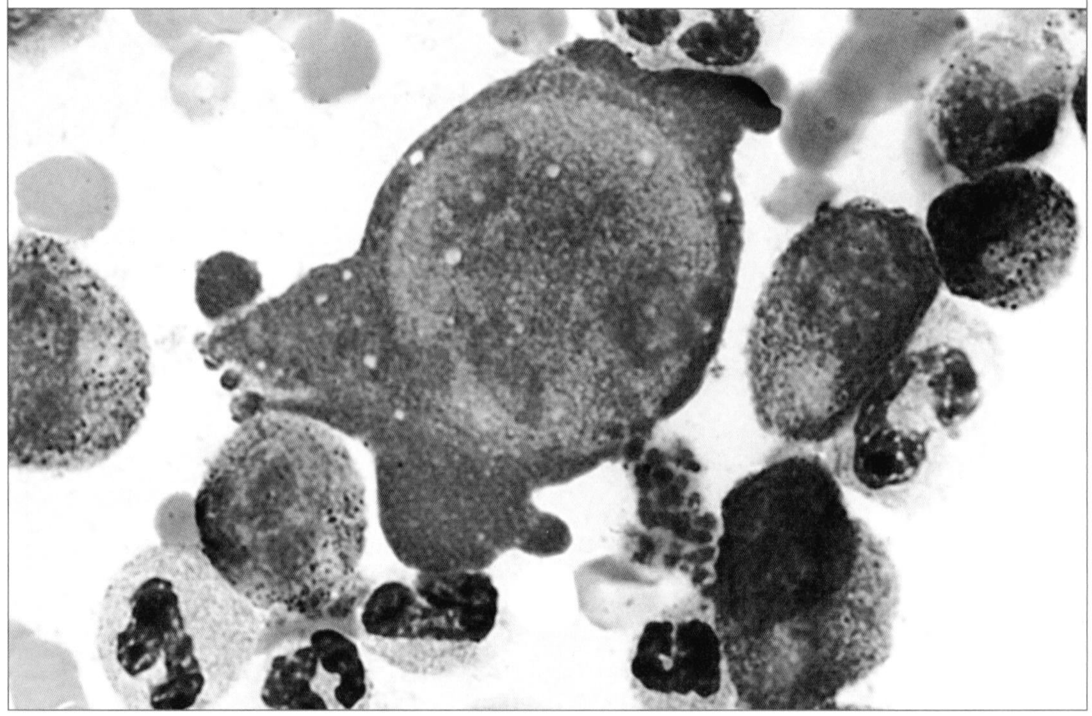

t4.3 Types of Acquired Sustained Pure Red Cell Aplasia

Type	Associated Disorders/Conditions
Primary (one-half of cases)	Idiopathic
Secondary (one-half of cases)	T-cell large granular lymphocytic leukemia
	Other hematopoietic neoplasms
	Drug treatments
	Thymoma
	Immune disorders
	Viral infections*

**Parvovirus excluded*

while faulty ribosome biogenesis occurs in dyskeratosis congenita, Shwachman-Diamond syndrome, and Diamond-Blackfan anemia.

Acquired anemias such as transient erythroblastopenia of childhood are probably caused by a self-limited, infection-induced immunoregulatory abnormality. Indeed immunoregulatory abnormalities are the likely cause of many other types of acquired pure red cell aplasia and aplastic anemia.

The most extensive pathophysiologic studies have been performed on patients with acquired aplastic anemia. Defects described in these patients include deficient or suppressed progenitor cells, humoral and cellular immunoregulatory defects, and microenvironmental abnormalities. The dominant abnormality is destruction of CD34+ progenitor cells through apoptotic mechanisms stimulated by cytokines released from activated bone marrow cytotoxic T cells. In addition, T cells produce inhibitory cytokines such as interferon-γ and tumor necrosis factor-α, which suppress hematopoiesis. Gene expression profile analyses of CD34+

t4.4 Causes of Acquired Aplastic Anemia*

Drugs	**Viruses**
Chloramphenicol	Hepatitis (non A, non B, non C, non G)
Phenylbutazone	Epstein-Barr virus
Anticonvulsants	Human immunodeficiency virus-1
Sulfonamides	
Gold	**Other conditions/exposures**
Chemotherapy†	Radiation exposure
Antithyroid medications	Immune disorders
Penicillamine	Paroxysmal nocturnal hemoglobinuria‡
Allopurinol	Chronic lymphocytic leukemia
Non-steroidal anti-inflammatory agents	Other neoplasms (thymoma, thymic carcinoma)
Phenothiazines	Pregnancy
Toxins	
Benzene	
Insecticides	
Solvents	

**Majority of aplastic anemia cases are idiopathic.*
†Predictable transient aplasia is associated with myeloablative therapy.
‡Acquired clonal disorder is both a cause and a consequence of aplastic anemia.

cells in aplastic anemia confirm increased expression of genes implicated in apoptosis and cell death. Studies also confirm markedly reduced numbers of CD34+ cells in aplastic marrows, compatible with destruction of these cells.

Several viral infections, notably hepatitis and Epstein-Barr viruses, have been linked to aplastic anemia. One theory regarding viral-induced aplasia states that stem cells are directly suppressed or damaged by these infectious agents. Another theory suggests that the viruses initiate an immune response that suppresses hematopoiesis. Finally, many drug treatments and some toxic exposures have been associated with acquired aplastic anemia caused either by a dose-related or an idiosyncratic host response to the drug, or by the production of a bone marrow toxic metabolite of the drug.

Acquired pure red cell aplasia is likewise thought to be immune-mediated based on studies implicating auto-antibodies, natural killer (NK)-cell mediated, or T-cell mediated effects impairing erythropoiesis. Furthermore, treatments for acquired pure red cell aplasia target immunologically-mediated disease.

4.1.2 Clinical Findings

Depending on its severity, patients with hypoplastic or aplastic anemia may present with weakness, fatigue, or tachycardia. If pancytopenia is present, additional findings can include petechiae and purpura secondary to thrombocytopenia, as well as fever from neutropenia-associated infections. Most constitutional types of hypoplastic anemias have associated phenotypic abnormalities, such as bony defects, mental retardation, or skin and nail abnormalities (see **t4.2**). Hepatosplenomegaly and lymphadenopathy are not evident in patients with uncomplicated hypoplastic or aplastic anemias.

4.1.3 Diagnostic Approach

The diagnosis of hypoplastic anemia requires an approach that both identifies the specific type of disorder and excludes bone marrow-effacing diseases, which also can be manifested by blood cytopenias. The approach to diagnosis generally follows these steps:

1. Determine the types and severity of the blood cytopenias.
2. Assess the patient for hepatosplenomegaly and lymphadenopathy on physical examination.
3. Evaluate infants and young children for other manifestations of hereditary hypoplastic disorders, including physical and radiographic defects and family history (see **t4.2**).
4. Document bone marrow hypocellularity and rule out an infiltrative or fibrotic process.
5. Use the clinical history and other clinical evidence of chronic hemolytic anemia to assess for a possible parvovirus-related aplastic crisis of an underlying RBC disorder such as hereditary spherocytosis or sickle cell anemia.
6. Evaluate adults with pure red cell aplasia for hematopoietic neoplasms, thymoma, other tumors, drug/toxin exposure, or infection (see **t4.2** and **t4.3**).
7. Evaluate patients with acquired aplastic anemia for evidence of neoplasm, immune disorders, toxin/drug exposure, or infection.

4.1.4 Hematologic Findings

In some types of hypoplastic anemia, only erythropoiesis is reduced; in others, all bone marrow cell lines are affected. Therefore, the hematologic manifestations of these conditions can range from isolated anemia to pancytopenia.

Blood Cell Measurements

Patients with hypoplastic anemias generally have a moderate to severe normochromic anemia, which may be normocytic or macrocytic. An elevated mean corpuscular volume (MCV) is characteristic of Diamond-Blackfan anemia and also may be present in some cases of acquired aplastic anemia. Except for patients with hereditary hemolytic anemia and secondary parvovirus-induced red cell aplasia, erythrocytes generally show little anisopoikilocytosis, as evidenced by a normal red cell distribution width (RDW). The reticulocyte count is markedly reduced. In patients with either acquired or constitutional aplastic anemia, thrombocytopenia and neutropenia are present also. The severity of aplastic anemia is often gauged by the absolute neutrophil count: <200/μL (very severe), 200-500/μL (severe), and >500/μL (non-severe).

Peripheral Blood Smear Morphology

Erythrocytes, neutrophils, and platelets are generally morphologically unremarkable in the various hypoplastic disorders **i4.2**. Parvovirus-induced red cell aplasia occurring in patients with underlying constitutional hemolytic anemias, however, is often associated with distinct erythrocyte-shape abnormalities. As a reflection of profound reticulocytopenia, polychromasia is markedly reduced to absent.

Bone Marrow Examination

Patients with Diamond-Blackfan anemia, transient erythroblastopenia of childhood, and acquired pure red cell aplasia show a marked decrease in erythroid precursors in the bone marrow with essentially normal granulopoiesis and megakaryocytopoiesis. Erythroid precursors may be totally absent, or only the earliest RBC precursors may be identified **i4.3**. Parvovirus inclusions may be evident in erythroblasts in patients with this type of acquired red cell aplasia **i4.1** and **i4.4**. A lymphocytosis with many hematogones may be present with all types of hypoplastic or aplastic anemias, especially in specimens from young children (see **i4.3**).

Early in their disease course, patients with Fanconi anemia may have a normal to hypercellular bone marrow with megaloblastic changes, followed by gradual aplasia. In acquired aplastic anemia and advanced Fanconi anemia, however, all three cell lines are usually markedly reduced **i4.5**, **i4.6**. There are no specific morphologic abnormalities of the rare residual hematopoietic elements in these patients.

i4.2 Diamond-Blackfan anemia

Peripheral blood smear demonstrating profound normocytic, normochromic anemia without significant polychromasia in a child with Diamond-Blackfan anemia. *(Wright stain) (courtesy Parvin Izadi, MD)*

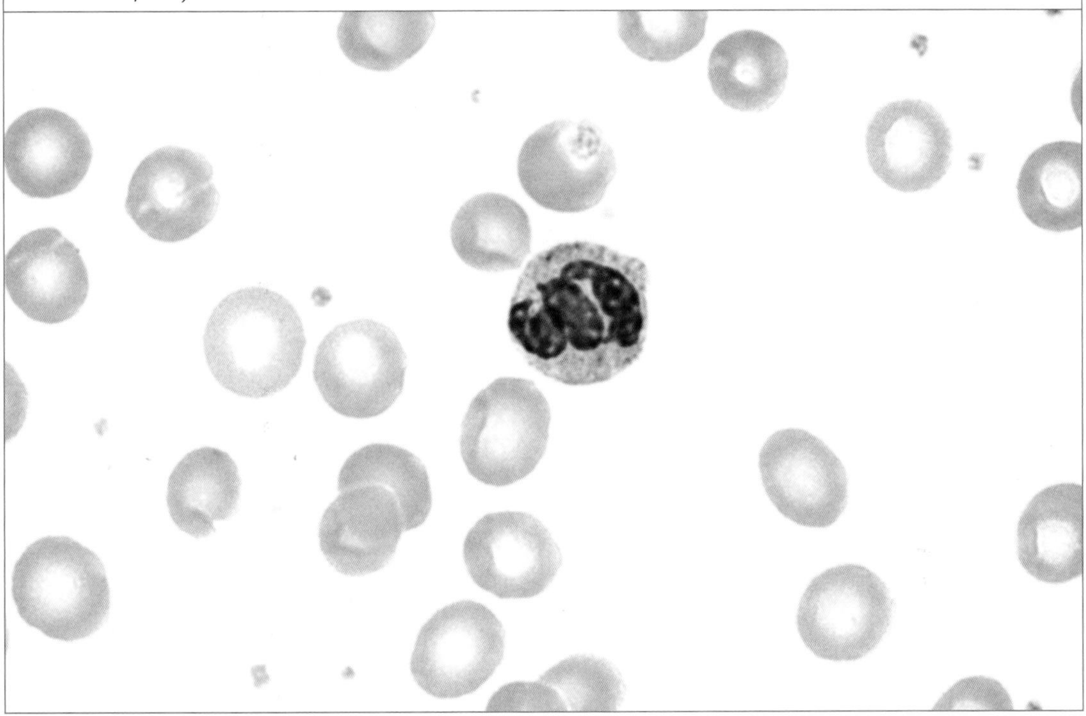

i4.3 Diamond-Blackfan anemia

Bone marrow aspirate smear from a child with Diamond-Blackfan anemia demonstrating only rare erythroblasts without evidence of erythroid maturation. Note predominance of hematogones. *(Wright stain) (courtesy Parvin Izadi, MD)*

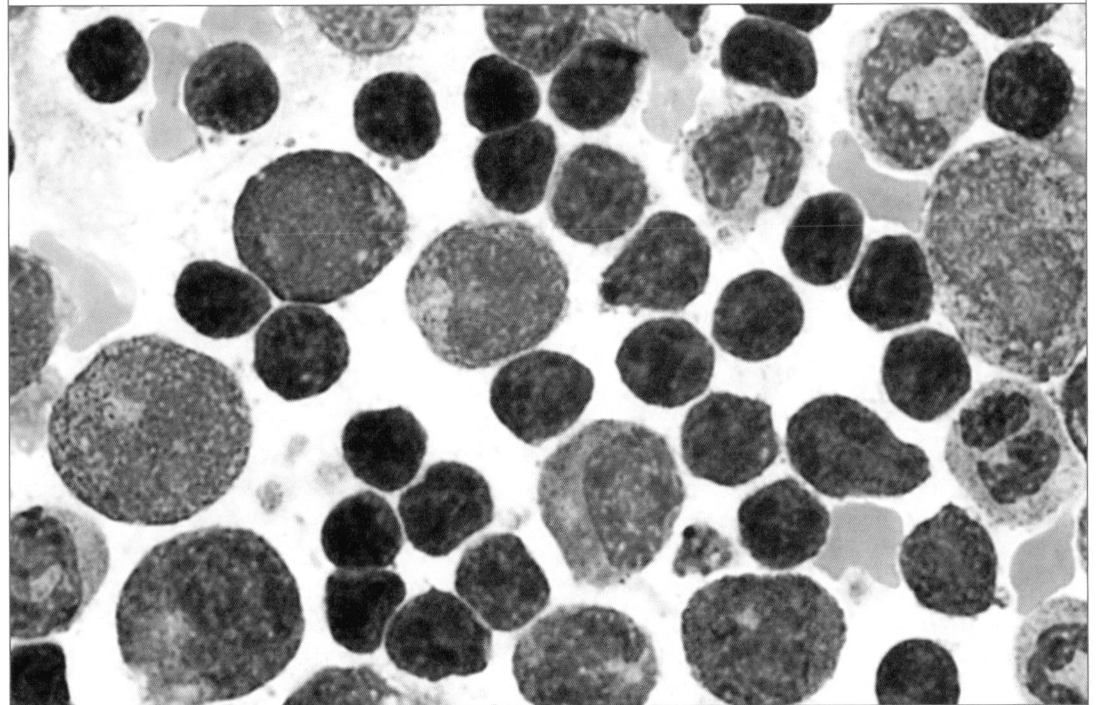

i4.4 Acute parvovirus infection

Giant erythroblast with intranuclear inclusion evident on bone marrow biopsy section in immunosuppressed patient with acute parvovirus infection. *(H&E)*

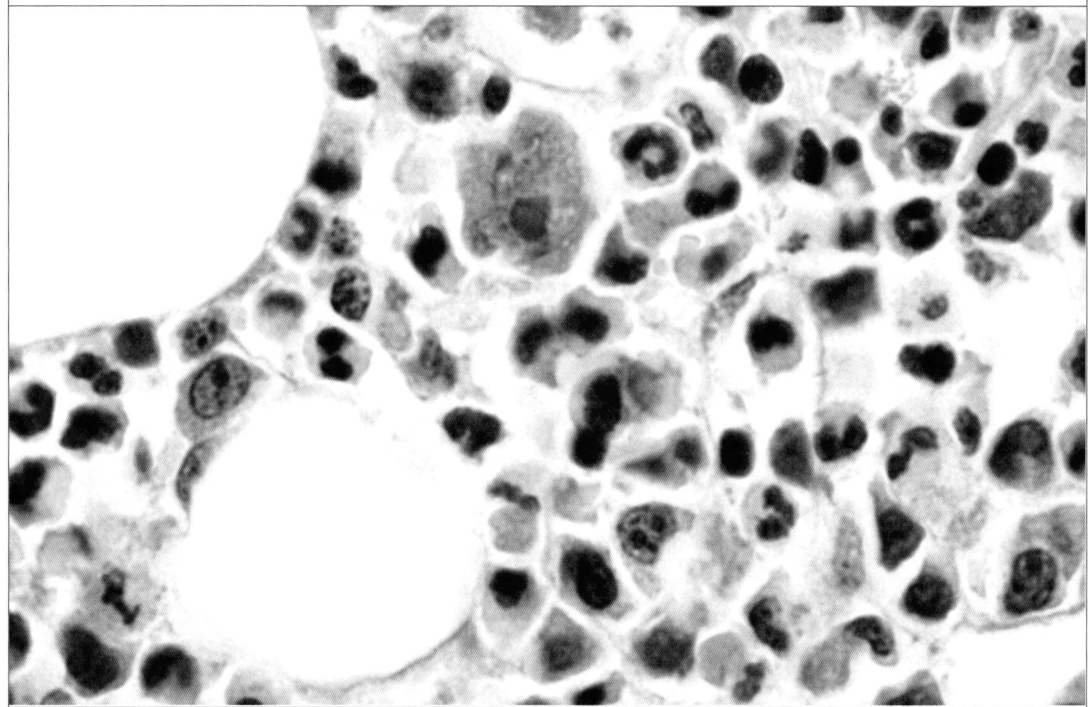

4.2 Other Laboratory Tests

Test 4.2.1 Automated Reticulocyte Count (see Test 1.5.2)

Purpose. Determination of reticulocyte numbers provides critical information in documenting an erythrocyte production defect (reduced reticulocyte count).

Principle. Specimen, Procedure, and Notes and Precautions. See Test 1.5.2.

Test 4.2.2 Fetal Hemoglobin Quantitation

Purpose. Fetal hemoglobin levels in erythrocytes can be used to distinguish between transient erythroblastopenia of childhood and constitutional disorders such as Diamond-Blackfan and Fanconi anemias.

Principle. Specimen, Procedure, and Notes and Precautions. See Test 10.5.3.

Interpretation. Erythrocyte fetal hemoglobin level is characteristically increased in Diamond-Blackfan and Fanconi anemias but normal in patients with transient erythroblastopenia of childhood. Erythrocyte fetal hemoglobin level also may be increased in some cases of acquired aplastic anemia.

4.3 Ancillary Tests

Because parvovirus infection can be sustained in immunocompromised patients, it is important to assess patients with acquired red cell aplasia for evidence of this infection. Tests include determination of serum IgM and IgG parvovirus titers, molecular tests for parvovirus using specific viral DNA probes, and in situ hybridization studies on bone marrow tissue sections. Other tests that can

i4.5 Acquired aplastic anemia

Virtually acellular bone marrow particle on aspirate smear in child with acquired aplastic anemia. *(Wright stain)*

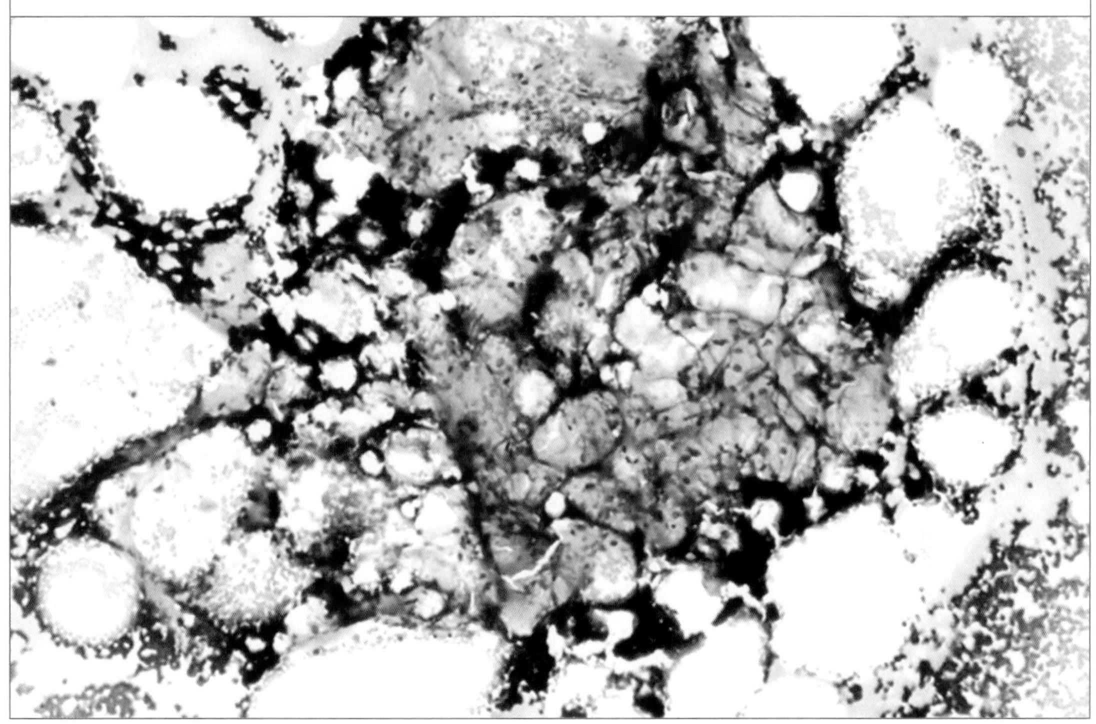

i4.6 Acquired aplastic anemia

Bone marrow core biopsy section exhibiting profound reduction in hematopoietic elements in child with acquired aplastic anemia. *(H&E)*

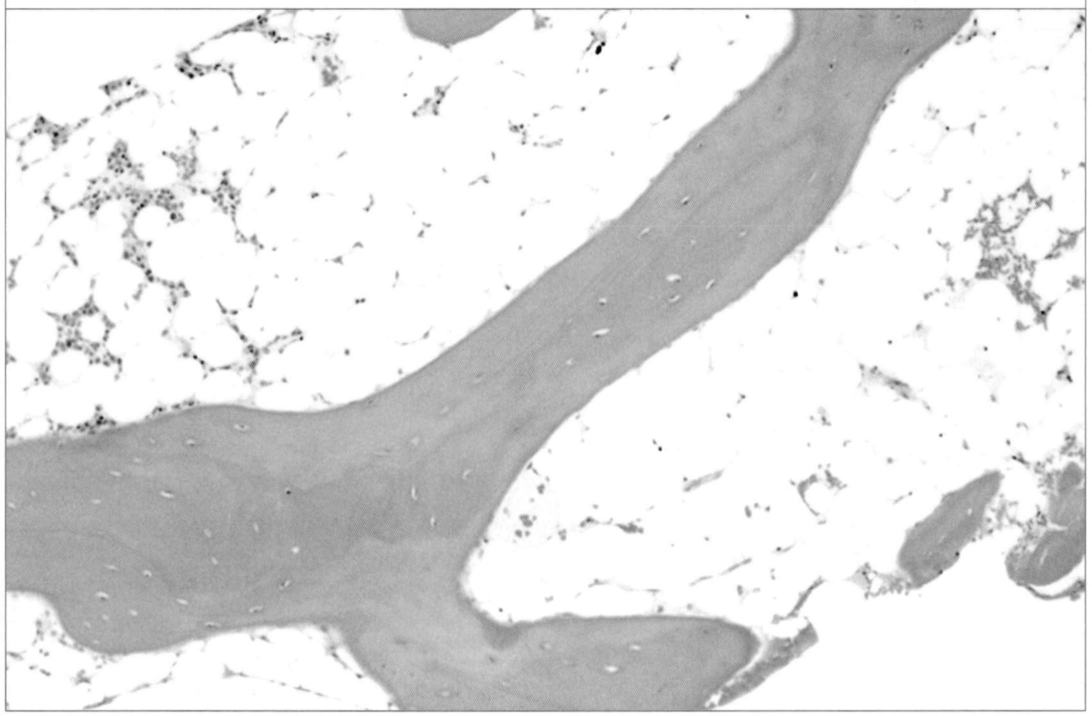

be used selectively to distinguish among the various types of aplastic and hypoplastic anemias include the RBC i antigen test and cytogenetic studies. Although not available in most laboratories, RBC i antigen can be detected in patients with Diamond-Blackfan and Fanconi anemia; i antigen is not present on erythrocytes in patients with either transient erythroblastopenia of childhood or other acquired hypoplastic disorders.

Cases of aplastic anemia associated with paroxysmal nocturnal hemoglobinuria can be detected by flow cytometric immunophenotyping to assess for reduced expression of neutrophil, monocyte, and erythrocyte antigens known to be attached to the cell membrane by GPI anchoring proteins. Antigens assessed include CD55, CD59, CD14, and CD16. In order for adequate interpretation, comparisons to antigen profiles on normal neutrophils, monocytes, and erythrocytes must always be performed.

In bone marrow cells of patients with Fanconi anemia, specialized cytogenetic studies generally reveal chromosomal defects including increased chromosomal breakage, translocations, sister chromatid exchange, and increased sensitivity to diepoxybutane, mitomycin C, and other agents. Karyotypic abnormalities are not usually found in the other types of hypoplastic and aplastic anemias. Family studies may help identify inheritance patterns associated with constitutional disorders. The use of routine standard karyotyping in aplastic anemia is controversial, although some authors report clonal cytogenetic abnormalities in approximately 10% of cases.

Because erythropoietin level is generally increased in all aplastic and hypoplastic anemias, it is not a useful test in distinguishing between these disorders.

4.4 Course and Treatment

The clinical course of patients with hypoplastic and aplastic anemias is diverse. Some patients with transient erythroblastopenia of childhood have brief, self-limited episodes of red cell aplasia that require no treatment. Likewise, spontaneous recovery generally occurs in immunocompetent patients with acute parvovirus-induced red cell aplasia, although transfusions may be necessary for exacerbations of the underlying hemolytic anemias.

Children and most adults with constitutional disorders, acquired aplastic anemia, or acquired sustained pure red cell aplasia generally require treatment that may include immune modulation, cytokine therapy, androgens, transfusion, or bone marrow transplantation. In patients with acquired disorders, any antecedent drug treatment should be discontinued, if possible. Suspected toxins should be removed from the patient's environment. In general, blood product transfusions should be reserved for life-threatening situations. Because these transfusions can have a negative effect on the outcome of subsequent bone marrow transplantation, they should be used very judiciously in patients with aplastic anemia who are likely to require such a transplant.

The bone marrow of patients with pure red cell aplasia often responds to corticosteroid therapy. If this fails, other interventions may include plasmapheresis, azathioprine, cyclosporin, antithymocyte globulin, or danazol treatment. Human recombinant erythropoietin also may be used to stimulate erythropoiesis. A careful search for underlying causes of acquired (sustained) pure red cell aplasia should be undertaken.

The clinical course of patients with acquired aplastic anemia depends on the severity of the pancytopenia, the patient's age, and the patient's response to treatment. These patients must be monitored carefully for evidence of infection or bleeding. Drugs that have been used successfully to treat acquired aplastic anemia include antithymocyte globulin, cyclosporin, and human recombinant colony-stimulating factors. However, use of recombinant granulocyte colony-stimulating factor is linked to an increased incidence of myelodysplasia in some studies. Stem cell/bone marrow transplantation is generally recommended for young patients with severe refractory acquired aplastic anemia who have an HLA-matched related donor.

Immunosuppressive regimens, generally antithymocyte globulin with cyclosporin, are utilized in older aplastic anemia patients and in those patients who do not have a related donor. Long-term survivors treated with immunosuppressive therapy, especially in conjunction with recombinant colony stimulating factor therapy, may develop myelodysplasia/acute myeloid leukemia. The risk of leukemia is highest in patients with constitutional DNA repair defects such as Fanconi anemia. The association of acquired aplastic anemia with both PNH and myelodysplasia is possible, since a significant number of aplastic anemia patients exhibit either a PNH-like defect by flow cytometric immunophenotype or, less commonly, a clonal cytogenetic abnormality. Furthermore, there is a proposed increase in PNH and myelodysplasia following successful immunosuppressive therapy for aplastic anemia with rates of clonal hematopoietic disorders over 25% in longterm survivors. Since some investigators regard aplastic anemia, PNH, and myelodysplasia as part of a spectrum of bone marrow failure disorders, these distinctive associations may not be random.

4.5 Bone Marrow Replacement Disorders

Patients with bone marrow replacement disorders suffer from a failure of hematopoiesis because the medullary portion of the bone marrow has been replaced by fibrosis, neoplastic cells, or non-neoplastic cells **t4.5**. Even if the neoplastic cells are of hematopoietic origin, they are incapable of producing normal peripheral blood elements. Therefore, patients with bone marrow replacement disorders generally present with cytopenias ranging from isolated anemia to pancytopenia.

t4.5 Causes of Bone Marrow Failure Secondary to Replacement

Neoplastic disorders replacing bone marrow parenchyma	
Acute and chronic leukemias, myeloproliferative neoplasms and myelodysplastic syndromes	Multiple myeloma
Malignant lymphoma (Hodgkin and non-Hodgkin lymphomas)	Metastatic carcinoma and sarcoma
Disorders/therapy causing bone marrow fibrosis	
Primary myelofibrosis	Chronic renal failure
Mastocytosis	Chronic infections
Other fibrosis-inducing neoplasms	Vitamin D deficiency
Metabolic bone disorders/endocrine abnormalities	Collagen vascular diseases
Following chemotherapy/toxin exposure/necrosis	Systemic crystal deposition disorders such as oxalosis and cystinosis
Miscellaneous disorders replacing bone marrow parenchyma	
Storage diseases	Osteopetrosis
Other histiocytic disorders	Abnormal deposition disorders/amyloid

4.5.1 Pathophysiology

Despite the bone marrow's ability to compensate, hematopoiesis fails once a significant portion of the active bone marrow medullary space is replaced by fibrous tissue, tumor, or other abnormal cells. This failure is the primary cause of cytopenias in patients with bone marrow replacement disorders. As described in Chapter 3, however, patients with neoplasms may develop other types of anemia. For example, these patients can suffer from chronic blood loss, anemia of chronic disease, bone marrow suppression by chemotherapy, hypersplenism, and even immune-mediated hemolysis (see **t3.3**).

4.5.2 Clinical Findings

The clinical findings in patients with bone marrow replacement disorders are as diverse as the types of disorders themselves. Most patients with significant bone marrow replacement disorders develop symptoms of cytopenia, notably malaise and fatigue secondary to anemia. Manifestations of leukopenia and thrombocytopenia, such as infection or bleeding, also may be present. Patients with acute and chronic leukemias, malignant lymphomas, storage diseases, and primary myelofibrosis often have significant splenomegaly, which can cause left upper quadrant pain and early satiety. Lymphadenopathy also may be present especially in patients with lymphomas.

4.5.3 Hematologic Findings

Although most patients with bone marrow replacement disorders have cytopenias, some also have specific morphologic abnormalities suggestive of a certain type of replacement disorder.

Blood Cell Measurements

A normocytic, normochromic anemia is the most common cytopenia in patients with bone marrow replacement disorders. Although these erythrocytes generally show little anisopoikilocytosis, as manifested by a normal RDW, some patients (such as those with primary myelofibrosis) exhibit marked anisopoikilocytosis. The reticulocyte count is typically reduced in these patients, but nucleated RBCs are fairly commonly seen. The WBC and platelet counts are more variable and may exhibit changes during the disease course. For example, thrombocytosis may be evident early in the disease course of primary myelofibrosis, but thrombocytopenia is characteristic of advanced bone marrow fibrosis.

Peripheral Blood Smear Morphology

Most secondary bone marrow replacement disorders have no specific morphologic abnormalities of RBCs, WBCs, or platelets. However, patients with primary hematopoietic neoplasms may have pronounced blood abnormalities such as anisopoikilocytosis with teardrop forms, a leukoerythroblastic blood picture, and large platelets. Leukemic or lymphoma cells may be identified in the peripheral blood in patients with primary hematolymphoid disorders replacing bone marrow. A leukoerythroblastic blood picture also may be seen in patients with bone marrow metastases by other neoplasms.

Bone Marrow Examination

There is a wide spectrum of potential morphologic abnormalities in patients with diverse primary and secondary bone marrow replacement disorders. In some patients, the bone marrow parenchyma is packed with infiltrating tumor cells, whereas in others it is replaced by collagen i4.7, i4.8. In histiocytic disorders, such as storage diseases, the bone marrow may be replaced by distinctive large, benign-appearing macrophages.

4.5.4 Other Laboratory Tests

Because this group of disorders is so diverse, many tests potentially may be used on a selective basis to help establish the diagnosis of specific bone marrow replacement disorders (see Volume II).

4.5.5 Course and Treatment

Fibrotic and benign histiocytic bone marrow replacement disorders tend to exhibit gradually progressive bone marrow infiltration, while neoplasms generally progress more rapidly. The treatment and disease course vary for each type of replacement disorder.

i4.7 Metastatic adenocarcinoma

Virtually complete effacement of bone marrow by metastatic adenocarcinoma is evident on this bone marrow core biopsy section. *(H&E)*

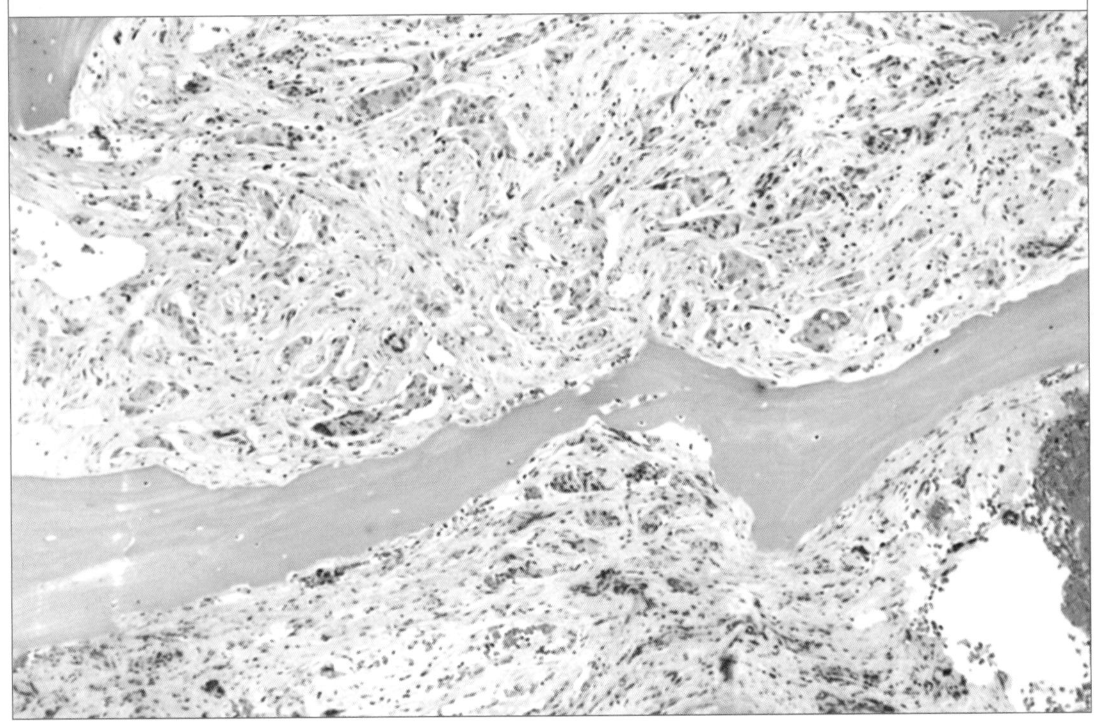

i4.8 Collagen fibrosis

Hematopoietic cavity is replaced by extensive collagen fibrosis in this bone marrow core biopsy specimen. *(H&E)*

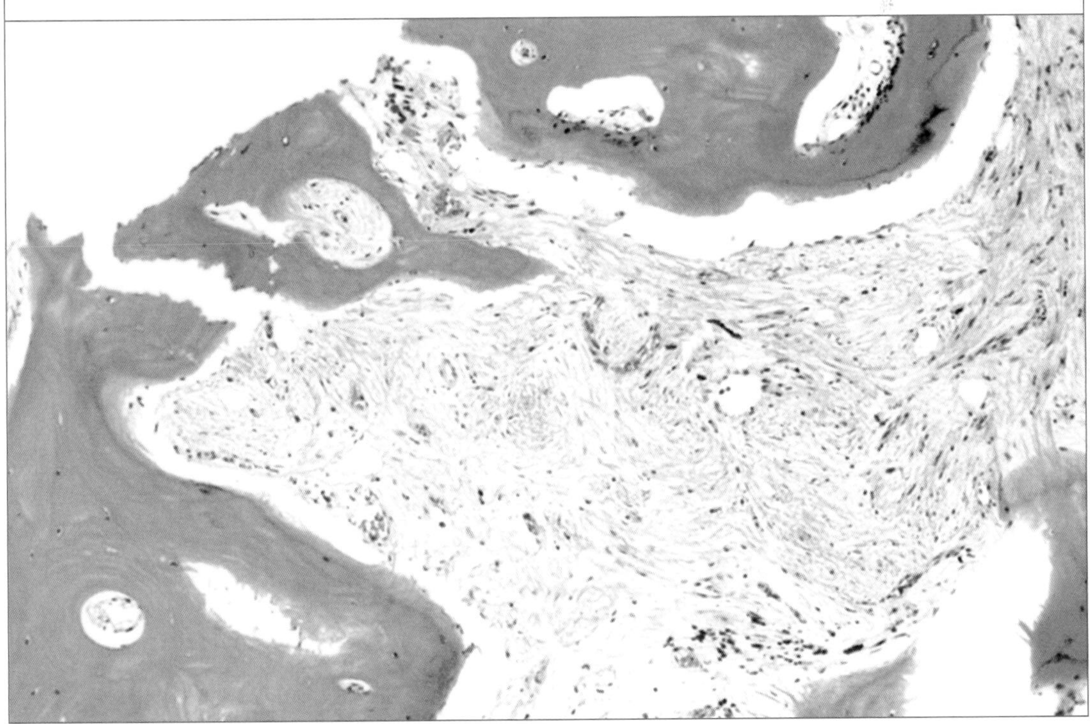

4.6 Congenital Dyserythropoietic Anemias

Congenital dyserythropoietic anemias (CDAs) are rare disorders initially described in 1951 and characterized by profound blood and bone marrow morphologic abnormalities of erythroid cells and ineffective erythropoiesis resulting primarily from mitotic defects. Other features common to this group of disorders include reticulocytopenia, a mildly elevated indirect bilirubin level, and an elevated lactate dehydrogenase level. Splenomegaly is variable. An autosomal recessive pattern of inheritance has been determined in some patients with CDA. Patients with CDA generally have a mild to moderate anemia, with variable anisopoikilocytosis, punctate basophilic stippling, and low reticulocyte count i4.9.

At least 3 types of CDA have been described based on specific morphologic features within the bone marrow t4.6. In type I, the erythroid cells within the bone marrow show megaloblastic changes with internuclear chromatin bridges i4.10. Type II CDA is characterized by binucleated and multinucleated erythroid precursors. In type III CDA, the multinucleation is pronounced with up to 12 nuclei present in some erythroid precursors i4.11, i4.12. Mature erythrocytes are often macrocytic in all types of CDA.

The bone marrow in patients with CDA shows erythroid hyperplasia with asynchronous nuclear-cytoplasmic maturation. Nuclear abnormalities include variations in size and structure as well as shape abnormalities described for the CDA subtypes. Other nuclear abnormalities, such as lobulation, budding, fragmentation, and karyorrhexis, also have been described. Cytoplasmic abnormalities include vacuolization, basophilic stippling, and excess iron within erythroid precursors.

The pathogenesis of CDA is uncertain, but theories include some primary defect in mitosis or a nuclear or cell membrane defect. Because this type of anemia is usually mild, affected patients are frequently asymptomatic and do not require treatment. However, some patients develop complications of iron overload.

i4.9 Congenital dyserythropoietic anemia type I

Moderate anisopoikilocytosis is evident on this peripheral blood smear from a patient with congenital dyserythropoietic anemia type I. *(Wright stain) (courtesy Parvin Izadi, MD)*

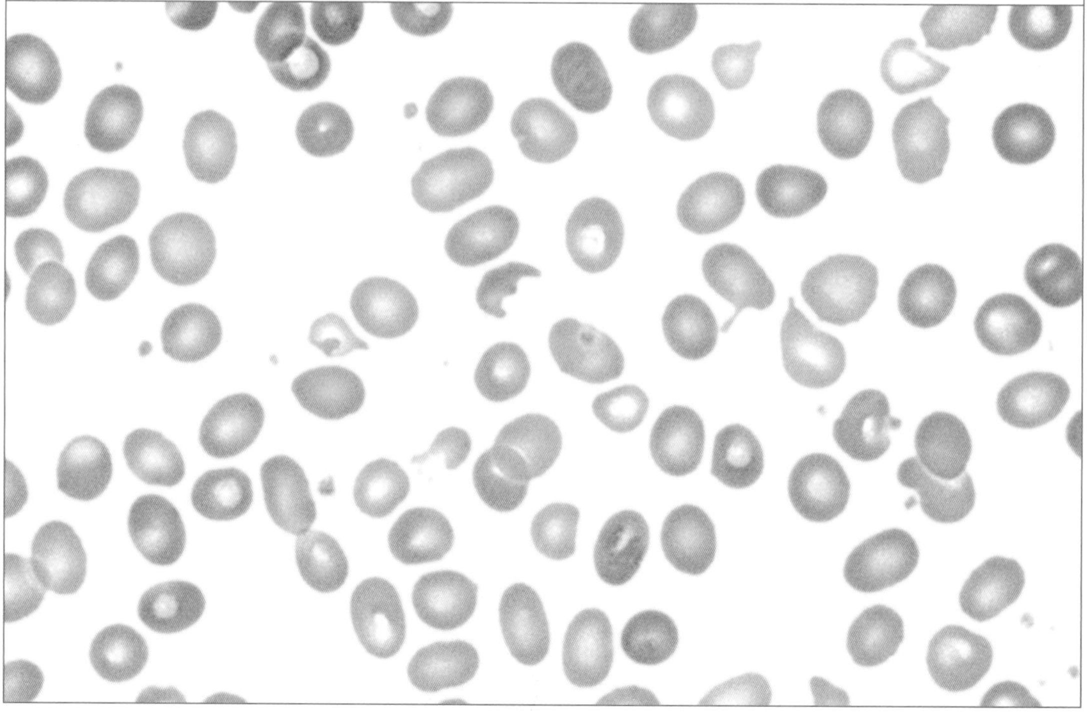

t4.6 Peripheral Blood and Bone Marrow Findings in Patients with Congenital Dyserythropoietic Anemias (CDAs)

	CDA I	CDA II*	CDA III
Blood			
Red blood cell size	Macrocytic	Normocytic	Normocytic to macrocytic
Red blood cell morphology	Anisopoikilocytosis	Anisopoikilocytosis	Anisopoikilocytosis
Anemia	Mild-moderate	Mild-severe	Mild
Bone marrow†			
Erythroid hyperplasia	Prominent	Prominent	Prominent
Erythroid morphology	Megaloblastic; internuclear chromatin bridging; nuclear budding; occasional binucleate forms	Normoblastic; bi/multinucleated normoblasts; nuclear karyorrhexis	Megaloblastic; "gigantoblasts" (up to 12 nuclei); nuclear karyorrhexis
Other laboratory tests			
Acidified-serum test	- (rare +)	+	-
Sugar water test	- (rare +)	-	-
Agglutination by anti-i and anti-I	Slight	+	+ (variable)
SDS-PAGE	Normal	Abnormal	Abnormal

**A designation HEMPAS (hereditary erythroblastic multinuclearity with positive acidified serum) (test) sometimes applied to patients with CDA II*
†Bone marrow examination generally required for diagnosis
SDS-PAGE = sodium dodecyl sulfate polyacrylamide gel electrophoresis; + = positive; - = negative

i4.10 Congenital dyserythropoietic anemia type I

Bone marrow aspirate smear shows erythroid hyperplasia with mild megaloblastic changes and intranuclear bridging in this case of congenital dyserythropoietic anemia type I. *(Wright stain)*

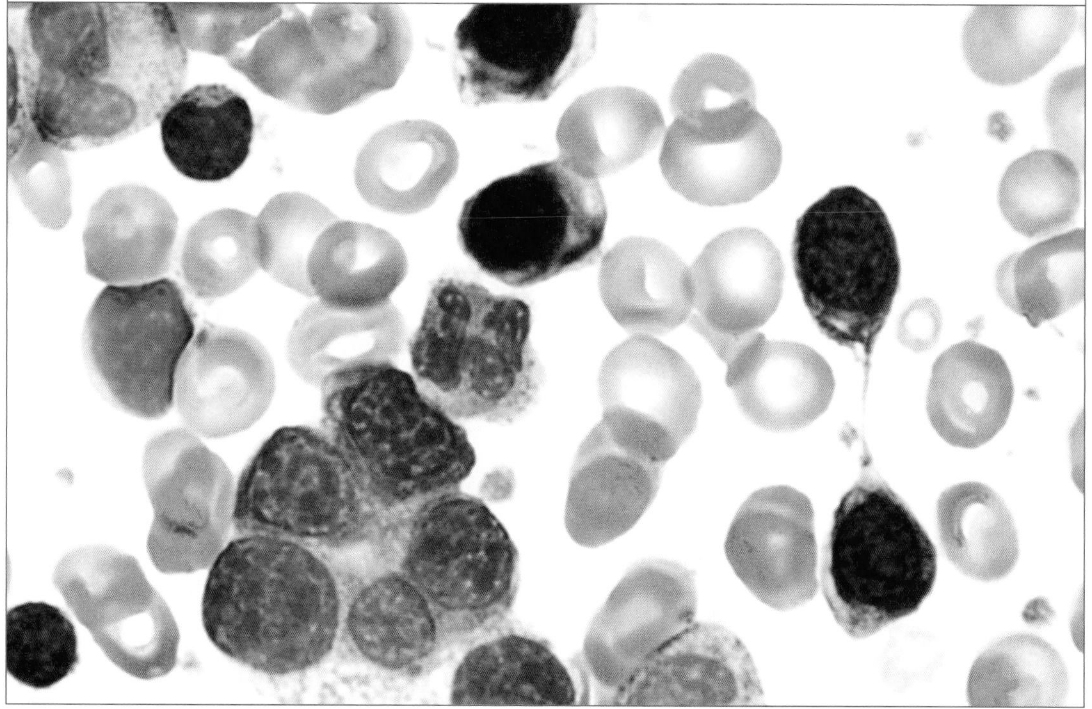

i4.11 Congenital dyserythropoietic anemia type III

Multinucleation is evident on this bone marrow aspirate smear from a patient with congenital dyserythropoietic anemia type III. *(Wright stain) (courtesy Richard Larson, MD)*

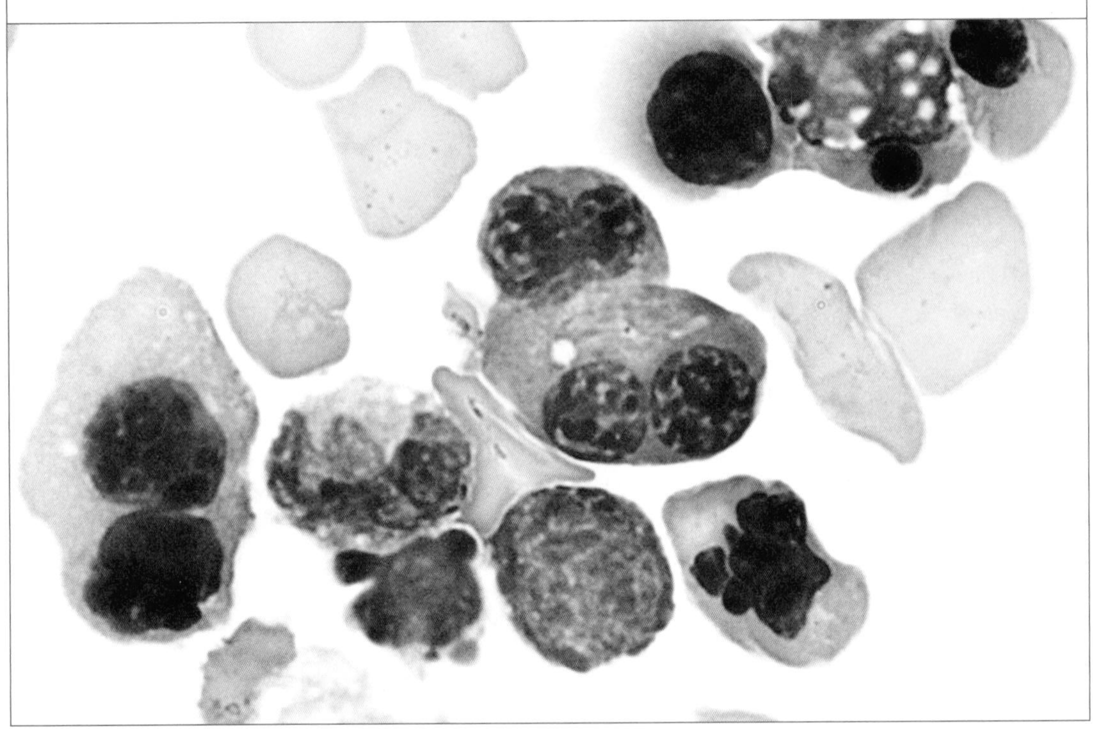

i4.12 Congenital dyserythropoietic anemia type III

Marked multinucleation characteristic of CDAIII on bone marrow aspirate smear. *(Wright stain) (courtesy Russell Brynes, MD)*

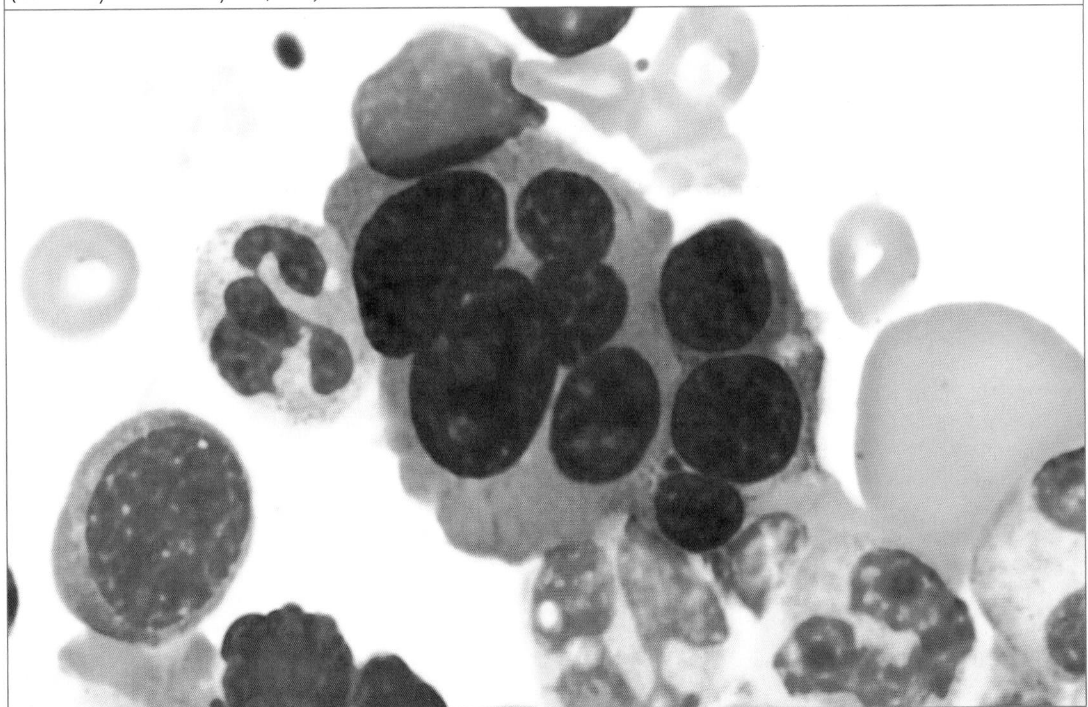

4.7 References

Bacigalupo A. Aplastic anemia: pathogenesis and treatment. *Hematology Am Soc Hematol Educ Program.* 2007;2007:23-28.

Bennett CL, Cournoyer D, Carson KR, et al. Long-term outcome of individuals with pure red cell aplasia and antierythropoietin antibodies in patients treated with recombinant epoetin: a follow-up report from the Research on Adverse Drug Events and Reports (RADAR) Project. *Blood.* 2005;106:3343-3347.

Brodsky RA. Advances in the diagnosis and therapy of paroxysmal nocturnal hemoglobinuria. *Blood Rev.* 2008;22:65-74.

Calado RT, Young NS. Telomere maintenance and human bone marrow failure. *Blood.* 2008;111:4446-4455.

Casadevall N, Nataf J, Viron B, et al. Pure red-cell aplasia and antierythropoietin antibodies in patients treated with recombinant erythropoietin. *N Engl J Med.* 2002;346:469-475.

Crook T, Barton-Rogers B, McFarland R, et al. Unusual bone marrow manifestations of parvovirus B19 infection in immunocompromised patients. *Hum Pathol.* 2000;31:161-168.

Dokal I, Vulliamy T. Inherited aplastic anaemias/bone marrow failure syndromes. *Blood Rev.* 2008;22:141-153.

Farhi DC, Luebbers EL, Rosenthal NS. Bone marrow biopsy findings in childhood anemia: prevalence of transient erythroblastopenia of childhood. *Arch Pathol Lab Med.* 1998;122:638-641.

Fisch P, Handgretinger R, Schaefer HE. Pure red cell aplasia. *Br J Haematol.* 2000;111:1010-1022.

Florea AV, Ionescu DN, Melhem MF. Parvovirus B19 infection in the immunocompromised host. *Arch Pathol Lab Med.* 2007;131:799-804.

Foucar K. Non-neoplastic erythroid lineage disorders. In: King D, Gardner W, Sobin L, et al., eds. *Non-Neoplastic Disorders of Bone Marrow* (AFIP fascicle). Washington, DC: American Registry of Pathology; 2008:75-124.

Frickhofen N, Heimpel H, Kaltwasser JP, et al. Antithymocyte globulin with or without cyclosporin A: 11-year follow-up of a randomized trial comparing treatments of aplastic anemia. *Blood.* 2003;101:1236-1242.

Fujishima N, Sawada K, Hirokawa M, et al. Long-term responses and outcomes following immunosuppressive therapy in large granular lymphocyte leukemia-associated pure red cell aplasia: a Nationwide Cohort Study in Japan for the PRCA Collaborative Study Group. *Haematologica.* 2008;93:1555-1559.

Ganapathi KA, Shimamura A. Ribosomal dysfunction and inherited marrow failure. *Br J Haematol.* 2008;141:376-387.

Gazda HT, Sieff CA. Recent insights into the pathogenesis of Diamond-Blackfan anaemia. *Br J Haematol.* 2006;135:149-157.

Gupta V, Brooker C, Tooze JA, et al. Clinical relevance of cytogenetic abnormalities at diagnosis of acquired aplastic anaemia in adults. *Br J Haematol.* 2006;134:95-99.

Heimpel H, Anselstetter V, Chrobak L, et al. Congenital dyserythropoietic anemia type II: epidemiology, clinical appearance, and prognosis based on long-term observation. *Blood.* 2003;102:4576-4581.

Heimpel H, Schwarz K, Ebnother M, et al. Congenital dyserythropoietic anemia type I (CDA I): molecular genetics, clinical appearance, and prognosis based on long-term observation. *Blood.* 2006;107:334-340.

Hill A, Richards SJ, Hillmen P. Recent developments in the understanding and management of paroxysmal nocturnal haemoglobinuria. *Br J Haematol.* 2007;137:181-192.

Iolascon A, Delaunay J, Wickramasinghe SN, et al. Natural history of congenital dyserythropoietic anemia type II. *Blood.* 2001;98:1258-1260.

Kaufman DW, Kelly JP, Issaragrisil S, et al. Relative incidence of agranulocytosis and aplastic anemia. *Am J Hematol.* 2006;81:65-67.

Koduri PR. Novel cytomorphology of the giant proerythroblasts of parvovirus B19 infection. *Am J Hematol.* 1998;58:95-99.

Kojima S, Ohara A, Tsuchida M, et al. Risk factors for evolution of acquired aplastic anemia into myelodysplastic syndrome and acute myeloid leukemia after immunosuppressive therapy in children. *Blood.* 2002;100:786-790.

Lipton JM. Diamond blackfan anemia: New paradigms for a "not so pure" inherited red cell aplasia. *Semin Hematol.* 2006;43:167-177.

Lu J, Basu A, Melenhorst JJ, et al. Analysis of T-cell repertoire in hepatitis-associated aplastic anemia. *Blood.* 2004;103:4588-4593.

Maciejewski JP, Rivera C, Kook H, et al. Relationship between bone marrow failure syndromes and the presence of glycophosphatidyl inositol-anchored protein-deficient clones. *Br J Haematol.* 2001;115:1015-1022.

Maciejewski JP, Risitano A, Sloand EM, et al. Distinct clinical outcomes for cytogenetic abnormalities evolving from aplastic anemia. *Blood.* 2002;99:3129-3135.

Matsui WH, Brodsky RA, Smith BD, et al. Quantitative analysis of bone marrow CD34 cells in aplastic anemia and hypoplastic myelodysplastic syndromes. *Leukemia.* 2006;20:458-462.

McKoy JM, Stonecash RE, Cournoyer D, et al. Epoetin-associated pure red cell aplasia: past, present, and future considerations. *Transfusion.* 2008;48:1754-1762.

Mochizuki K, Sugimori C, Qi Z, et al. Expansion of donor-derived hematopoietic stem cells with PIGA mutation associated with late graft failure after allogeneic stem cell transplantation. *Blood.* 2008;112:2160-2162.

Mori KL, Furukawa H, Hayashi K, et al. Pure red cell aplasia associated with expansion of CD3+ CD8+ granular lymphocytes expressing cytotoxicity against HLA-E+ cells. *Br J Haematol.* 2003;123:147-153.

Olteanu H, Karandikar NJ, McKenna RW, Xu Y. Differential usefulness of various markers in the flow cytometric detection of paroxysmal nocturnal hemoglobinuria in blood and bone marrow. *Am J Clin Pathol.* 2006;126:781-788.

Oosterkamp HM, Brand A, Kluin-Nelemans JC, et al. Pregnancy and severe aplastic anaemia: causal relation or coincidence? *Br J Haematol.* 1998;103:315-316.

Perkins SL. Pediatric red cell disorders and pure red cell aplasia. *Am J Clin Pathol.* 2004;122 Suppl:S70-86.

Prassouli A, Papadakis V, Tsakris A, et al. Classic transient erythroblastopenia of childhood with human parvovirus B19 genome detection in the blood and bone marrow. *J Pediatr Hematol Oncol.* 2005;27:333-336.

Sawada K, Fujishima N, Hirokawa M. Acquired pure red cell aplasia: updated review of treatment. *Br J Haematol.* 2008;142:505-514.

Shalev H, Kapelushnik J, Moser A, et al. A comprehensive study of the neonatal manifestations of congenital dyserythropoietic anemia type I. *J Pediatr Hematol Oncol.* 2004;26:746-748.

Skeppner G, Kreuger A, Elinder G. Transient erythroblastopenia of childhood: prospective study of 10 patients with special reference to viral infections. *J Pediatr Hematol Oncol.* 2002;24:294-298.

Socie G, Mary JY, Schrezenmeier H, et al. Granulocyte-stimulating factor and severe aplastic anemia: a survey by the European Group for Blood and Marrow Transplantation (EBMT). *Blood.* 2007;109:2794-2796.

Thompson CA, Steensma DP. Pure red cell aplasia associated with thymoma: clinical insights from a 50-year single-institution experience. *Br J Haematol.* 2006;135:405-407.

Tiu R, Gondek L, O'Keefe C, Maciejewski JP. Clonality of the stem cell compartment during evolution of myelodysplastic syndromes and other bone marrow failure syndromes. *Leukemia.* 2007;21:1648-1657.

Viswanatha D. Bone marrow failure disorders. In: King D, Gardner W, Sobin L, et al., eds. *Non-Neoplastic Disorders of Bone Marrow* (AFIP fascicle). Washington, DC: American Registry of Pathology; 2008 221-248.

Wang H, Chuhjo T, Yasue S, et al. Clinical significance of a minor population of paroxysmal nocturnal hemoglobinuria-type cells in bone marrow failure syndrome. *Blood.* 2002;100:3897-3902.

Wickramasinghe SN, Wood WG. Advances in the understanding of the congenital dyserythropoietic anaemias. *Br J Haematol.* 2005;131:431-446.

Young NS. Hematopoietic cell destruction by immune mechanisms in acquired aplastic anemia. *Semin Hematol.* 2000;37:3-14.

Young NS, Brown KE. Parvovirus B19. *N Engl J Med.* 2004;350:586-597.

Young NS, Calado RT, Scheinberg P. Current concepts in the pathophysiology and treatment of aplastic anemia. *Blood.* 2006;108:2509-2519.

Zdebska E, Wozniewicz B, Adamowicz-Salach A, et al. Short report: erythrocyte membranes from a patient with congenital dyserythropoietic anaemia type I (CDA-I) show identical, although less pronounced, glycoconjugate abnormalities to those from patients with CDA-II (HEMPAS). *Br J Haematol.* 2000;110:998-1001.

Zeng W, Chen G, Kajigaya S, et al. Gene expression profiling in CD34 cells to identify differences between aplastic anemia patients and healthy volunteers. *Blood.* 2004;103:325-332.

Chapter 5
Megaloblastic Anemia

Kathryn Foucar, MD

Megaloblastic anemia is a distinctive type of anemia which develops as a result of deficiencies in the coenzyme forms of folate or vitamin B_{12} (cobalamin). As a result, the ability of all proliferating cells to synthesize enough DNA per unit of time to allow for mitosis is impaired and more cells are in the DNA synthesis phase of the cell cycle. Because RNA synthesis is not dependent on these coenzymes, an asynchrony between nuclear and cytoplasmic maturation occurs, resulting both in giantism of all proliferating cells and in cell nuclei that appear less mature than the cytoplasm. Ineffective hematopoiesis results from high rates of intramedullary cell death in a setting of bone marrow hypercellularity. Although impaired proliferation of hematopoietic cells is the major clinical manifestation of vitamin B_{12} (cobalamin) and folate deficiency, other disorders, especially neuropsychiatric, can precede, occur simultaneously with, or occur independently of hematologic manifestations. Although constitutional megaloblastic anemias are well-described, these disorders are exceedingly rare. Consequently, this chapter will focus on acquired megaloblastic anemia.

Characteristics of vitamin B_{12} (cobalamin) and folate, including dietary sources, recommended daily requirements, normal blood levels, and amounts of stored vitamins, are shown

t5.1 Characteristics of Vitamin B_{12} (Cobalamin) and Folate

	Vitamin B_{12} (Cobalamin)	Folate
Origin	Synthesized exclusively by bacteria	Synthesized by plants and microorganisms
Dietary source	Meat, fish, dairy products (heat stabile)	Vegetables (especially green leafy) and fruits (heat labile)
Parent compound	Cyanocobalamin	Pteroglutamic acid
Recommended daily requirements		
Infants	0.3 µg	25 µg-35 µg
Children	0.7 µg-1.4 µg	50 µg-100 µg
Adults	2.0 µg	180 µg-200 µg
Pregnant women	2.2 µg	400 µg
Lactating women	2.6 µg	280 µg
Normal blood levels	150-1,000 pg/mL	>3.7 ng/mL (red blood cell: 130-640 ng/mL)
Normal total stores* (major storage site)	3,000-5,000 mg (liver)	20-70 mg (liver)
Storage duration on deficient diet	2-5 years	3-5 months

**Total stores are much smaller in infants.*

in **t5.1**. Vitamin B_{12} circulates in the peripheral blood bound to various proteins. Except in infants, total body stores of vitamin B_{12} are abundant and are sufficient to adequately supply the host for 2 to 5 years. Folate is very heat labile and is destroyed readily in the cooking process. Small amounts of folate derivatives circulate largely unbound in the blood; greater concentrations of these derivatives are present intracellularly. Except in infants, total body stores of folate are moderate and are sufficient to maintain normal cellular proliferation for approximately 3 to 5 months. Because of the relatively short time that folate stores will meet host needs, the incidence of folate deficiency secondary to inadequate intake is substantially greater than that of dietary vitamin B_{12} deficiency. Because of lower stores, deficiency of either vitamin B_{12} or folate develops more rapidly in children, especially infants. Maternal dietary restrictions are often the cause of infantile megaloblastic anemia.

5.1 Pathophysiology

The physiology and biochemistry of vitamin B_{12} (cobalamin) and folate are detailed in **t5.2** and **t5.3**, respectively. In patients with vitamin B_{12} deficiency, both the megaloblastic anemia and the neurologic complications appear to be secondary to the defective formation of methionine (see **t5.3**). The rate-limiting step in DNA (pyrimidine) synthesis that requires folate is the conversion of deoxyuridine monophosphate to deoxythymidine monophosphate.

The sequence of events in the development of vitamin B_{12} and folate deficiency is listed in **t5.4** and **t5.5**, respectively. Although folate stores are depleted much more rapidly than vita-

t5.2 Physiology of Vitamin B_{12} (Cobalamin) and Folate

	Vitamin B_{12} (Cobalamin)	Folate
Compounds in food	Several cobalamin forms	Several polyglutamate forms
Physiology of absorption	Vitamin B_{12} released from food by gastric acid, gastric enzymes, and small bowel enzymes ® free vitamin B12 bound to R-binders primarily; some also binds to IF ® pancreatic enzymes degrade R-binder–B12 complexes ® released B_{12} is then bound to IF	Polyglutamate deconjugated by conjugase enzymes in bile and small bowel lumen
Site of absorption	Vitamin B12–IF complex adheres to receptors on brush border of ileum (pH and calcium-dependent process)	Deconjugated folate absorbed in jejunum
Physiology of circulation	30% of vitamin B12 binds to TCII, which delivers it to liver, bone marrow, and other sites 70% of vitamin B12 binds to TCI, TCIII, and R-binders, which deliver it exclusively to liver	Folate circulates unbound in blood as 5-methyl THF
Entry into cells	TCII-B12 attaches to specific membrane receptors Vitamin B12 transferred across plasma membrane (TCII degraded in this process)	Vitamin B_{12} necessary for folate (THF form) to pass across plasma membranes and be retained in cell
Function	Two active forms, methylcobalamin and 5-deoxyadenosyl cobalamin, which facilitate formation of methionine and succinate, respectively	THF essential for all one-carbon transfer reactions in mammalian cells THF required for both purine and pyrimidine synthesis
Excretion	Bile, urine	Urine, sweat, saliva, feces

IF = intrinsic factor; TC = transcobalamin; R-binder = found in every tissue in body, named for rapid mobility on electrophoresis; THF = tetrahydrofolate

t5.3 Biochemistry of Vitamin B_{12} (Cobalamin) and Folate Activity

	Vitamin B_{12} (Cobalamin)	Folate
Biologically active form(s)	Coenzyme B_{12} (5-deoxyadenosyl cobalamin) and methylcobalamin	5-methyl THF
Reactions requiring vitamin B_{12} and/or folate cofactors	I. Homocysteine → Methionine (methylcobalamin; 5-methyl THF → THF) Failure in this pathway results in megaloblastosis; reaction also important in central nervous system methylation, and for incorporation of folate into cells II. Methylmalonate → Succinate (Coenzyme B_{12} (adenosylcobalamin mutase)) Failure of this reaction not involved in neurologic disease or megaloblastosis	I. Required for both purine and pyrimidine synthesis II. Rate limiting step in DNA synthesis (pyrimidine synthesis) dUMP → dTMP (THF → DHF) III. Required for methionine synthesis (see I), vitamin B_{12} IV. Folate also essential in amino acid synthesis

THF = tetrahydrofolate; dUMP = deoxyuridine monophosphate; dTMP = deoxythymidine monophosphate; DHF = dihydrofolate

min B_{12} stores, the sequence of events in the development of blood and bone marrow abnormalities as deficiency evolves is similar for both. Hypersegmentation of neutrophils appears early in the development of megaloblastic anemia, whereas actual anemia is a late event associated with florid megaloblastic morphologic changes. Damage to myelin in peripheral nerves and eventual axonal degeneration occur progressively throughout the evolution of vitamin B_{12} deficiency.

t5.4 Probable Sequence in Development of Vitamin B_{12} (Cobalamin) Deficiency*

Time Interval After Onset of Intake Failure	Pathologic Abnormality
1-2 years	Vitamin B_{12} level in serum decreased Early blood and bone marrow abnormalities, including hypersegmentation and macrocytosis Early myelin damage of nerves
2-3 years	Vitamin B_{12} level markedly decreased Vitamin B_{12} binders < 10% saturated Florid megaloblastosis in blood and bone marrow Decreased RBC folate, normal to increased serum folate Severe damage to myelin, axonal degeneration

**Deficiency arises much faster in infants due to lower stores; increased numbers of cases of infantile megaloblastic anemia in conjunction with mothers following restricted diets or other causes of poor maternal nutrition.*

t5.5 Sequence in Development of Folate Deficiency*

Time Interval After Onset of Intake Failure	Pathologic Abnormality
3 weeks	Decreased serum folate
5-7 weeks	Hypersegmentation of neutrophils in bone marrow and blood
10 weeks	Mild megaloblastic changes in bone marrow
17-18 weeks	Macro-ovalocytes, decreased RBC folate
19-20 weeks	Florid megaloblastosis with anemia

**Deficiency arises much faster in infants due to lower stores; cases of infantile megaloblastic anemia linked to maternal factors such as restricted diets or other causes of poor nutrition.*

There are five basic mechanisms leading to vitamin B_{12} deficiency including inadequate intake, increased requirement, defective absorption, defective transport, and disorders of B_{12} metabolism **t5.6**. By far, the most common mechanism for vitamin B_{12} deficiency is defective absorption. For vitamin B_{12} absorption to occur, there must be normal amounts of intrinsic factor, sufficient pancreatic enzymes to degrade the vitamin B_{12}-R-binder complexes, appropriate calcium and hydrogen ion concentrations to facilitate the transfer of vitamin B_{12} across plasma membranes, an intact ileal mucosal surface, and lack of competing parasites or bacteria for the ingested vitamin B_{12} (see **t5.2**). Although abnormalities in any of these components can result in defective absorption, the one most commonly encountered in clinical practice is decreased intrinsic factor in patients with pernicious anemia, an autoimmune disorder associ-

t5.6 Mechanisms of Vitamin B_{12} (Cobalamin) Deficiency

	Example	Condition/Disorder
Inadequate intake	Dietary deficiency	Strict vegetarianism
Increased requirement	Growth, development	Pregnancy*, lactation
Defective absorption	Decreased IF	Pernicious anemia, congenital IF deficiency
	Gastritis with atrophy of gastric glands	Helicobacter pylori infection
	Decreased pancreatic enzymes	Pancreatitis
	Lack of calcium or abnormal pH	Zollinger-Ellison syndrome
	Defective ileal mucosa	Sprue, regional enteritis, surgical resection
	Parasitic or bacterial overgrowth	Tapeworm, blind loop, Helicobacter
	Drug interference with absorption	Alcoholism, colchicine treatment, PAS treatment
	Selective intestinal malabsorption of IF-cobalamin complex	Rare hereditary disorder caused by mutation in IF-cobalamin receptor, cubilin (Imerslund-Gräsbeck syndrome)
Defective transport	Decreased TCII	Congenital deficiency of TCII, rare
Disorders of metabolism	Suppression or inhibition of metabolic enzymes	Nitrous oxide administration, enzyme deficiencies; inborn errors of metabolism, rare

**Deficiency in infants can result from inadequate maternal intake.*
IF = intrinsic factor; TC = transcobalamin; PAS = para-amino salicylic acid

ated with chronic atrophic gastritis and autoantibody production. Intrinsic factor is secreted by gastric parietal cells stimulated by gastrin and histamine. The antibodies directed against intrinsic factor and parietal cells commonly detected in patients with pernicious anemia may cause the decreased intrinsic factor. Other disorders associated with defective absorption are listed in **t5.6**. Recent studies suggest an association between Helicobacter pylori infection and vitamin B_{12} deficiency.

Although vitamin B_{12} deficiency may occur secondary to insufficient dietary intake, a stringent diet deficient in all meat, egg, and milk products must be followed for a sustained period. Because vitamin B_{12} stores are so abundant, the increased requirement for this vitamin during pregnancy and lactation is rarely associated with megaloblastic anemia unless the mother is following a restricted diet or other causes of poor nutrition. In this situation both mother and the newborn infant may be vitamin B_{12} deficient. If the mother's deficiency is subclinical, vitamin B_{12} deficiency may not be suspected in the infant, especially since the symptoms in the infant are non-specific failure to thrive. Vitamin B_{12} deficiency secondary to either transport or metabolic defects is extremely rare and not generally encountered in clinical practice.

The major causes of folate deficiency include dietary deficiency and increased requirement, although defective absorption and disorders of metabolism are occasionally responsible for folate deficiency **t5.7**. Dietary deficiency of folate is common in chronic alcoholics, drug addicts, and patients in low socioeconomic conditions who consume inadequate diets. Excessive cooking destroys folate. Increased folate is required by infants, pregnant and lactating women, and patients with either malignancies or chronic hemolytic anemias. Premature infants have very low folate stores and are highly susceptible to folate deficiency. Infants of mothers on restricted diets are also highly susceptible to folate deficiency, which typically manifests as failure to thrive in these infants. Disorders and drug treatments associated with defective absorption of folate and abnormal folate metabolism are listed in **t5.7**.

t5.7 Mechanisms of Folate Deficiency

	Example	Condition/Disorder
Inadequate intake	Dietary deficiency Inactivation of folate	Alcoholism, drug addiction, poverty Overcooking of food
Increased requirement	Growth, development States of increased cell turnover	Pregnancy*, lactation, infancy Chronic hemolytic anemias, malignancies
Defective absorption	Defective jejunal mucosa Drug-induced malabsorption	Sprue, amyloidosis, lymphoma, surgical resection Anticonvulsant, antituberculous, oral contraceptive drug therapy, alcoholism
Disorders of metabolism	Suppression or inhibition of metabolic enzymes	Methotrexate, pyrimethamine treatment, alcoholism Congenital disorders of folate metabolism, rare

**Deficiency in infants can result from inadequate maternal intake.*

5.2 Clinical Findings

Patients with megaloblastic anemia characteristically present with moderate to severe fatigue and malaise of several months' duration. Their skin may be lemon-yellow because of the combined effects of a moderately increased bilirubin level and the marked pallor of the underlying anemia. Because the defective DNA synthesis affects all proliferating cells, such patients experience atrophy of the mucosal surfaces of the tongue, gastrointestinal tract, and vagina. This can cause pain in the mouth and vagina and can lead to secondary malabsorption in the gastrointestinal tract. Clinical manifestations of megaloblastic anemia are much more nonspecific in infants; either vitamin B_{12} or folate deficiency should be considered in infants with failure to thrive.

Although the neurologic manifestations of pernicious anemia have been well described, patients with folate deficiency also may rarely develop neuropsychiatric disorders, including irritability, forgetfulness, sleepiness, and depression. Occasionally, patients with folate deficiency manifest peripheral neuropathy similar to that described in patients with vitamin B_{12} deficiency. In pernicious anemia, this peripheral neuropathy is secondary to defective myelin synthesis followed by axonal disruption or degeneration and is insidious in onset, beginning first in peripheral nerves and gradually progressing to involve the posterior and lateral columns of the spinal cord. The clinical manifestations of peripheral nerve involvement include paresthesias, such as numbness and tingling in the hands and feet; decreased vibration sense; and decreased position sense. With progression to spinal cord involvement, the patient may experience ataxia and eventually symmetrical paralysis. If the megaloblastic anemia is untreated, the patient may eventually develop cerebral involvement, which has been called "megaloblastic madness" and is manifested by mental changes, paranoia, and depression.

5.3 Diagnostic Approach

The approach to the diagnosis of megaloblastic anemia includes the following elements:

1. Establishing the presence of a macrocytic anemia
2. Distinguishing between the various causes of macrocytic anemia; other causes of macrocytosis include reticulocytosis, chemotherapeutic agents, antiretroviral agents, liver disease, alcohol, myelodysplastic syndromes, other medications, post splenectomy, and hypothyroidism
3. Determining whether the patient is deficient in vitamin B_{12}, folate, or both vitamins
4. Identifying and treating the underlying disease responsible for the megaloblastic anemia
5. Knowing that neurologic manifestations may predominate in some patients with vitamin B12 deficiency in the absence of any hematologic finding; infants with vitamin B_{12} or folate deficiency typically manifest with failure to thrive and may have a normal MCV

Clinical history and a review of the blood smear help exclude these alternate diagnoses. The clinical history should include questions regarding family history (some rare types of megaloblastic anemia are secondary to hereditary disorders), drug ingestion, intestinal function, diet, occupational exposures, and prior surgical procedures. Evidence of peripheral neuropathy and other neurologic manifestations of vitamin B_{12} or, rarely, folate deficiency should be assessed by physical examination. Once the diagnosis of megaloblastic anemia has been established, the specific vitamin deficiency causing the anemia must be determined via the laboratory tests discussed in this chapter. Finally, the cause of the vitamin deficiency must be identified and treated appropriately.

5.4 Hematologic Findings

The hematologic findings can be virtually diagnostic in many patients with megaloblastic anemia in whom characteristic abnormalities of erythrocytes and neutrophils can be identified readily. However, in rare cases, the blood of patients with severe vitamin B_{12} deficiency may fail to exhibit substantial erythrocyte or neutrophil abnormalities. In addition, features of megaloblastic anemia may be masked in patients suffering from either concurrent iron deficiency anemia or constitutional microcytic anemia.

5.4.1 Blood Cell Measurements

A patient with megaloblastic anemia typically has a moderate to severe normochromic macrocytic anemia with mean corpuscular volumes (MCVs) ranging from 100 to 150 µm3 (100 to 150 fL), while the mean corpuscular hemoglobin concentration (MCHC) is normal. Although MCVs at the lower end of this size range can be seen in a variety of disorders, a patient with an MCV exceeding 120 µm3 (120 fL) who is not receiving specific medications such as sulfasalazine is likely to have megaloblastic anemia. Some patients with vitamin B_{12} or folate deficiency have normal MCVs because they also have iron deficiency, inflammatory disorders, or renal failure. Characteristically, the red cell distribution width (RDW) is markedly elevated in megaloblastic anemia because of extreme anisocytosis. Circulating macrocytes are often disrupted, producing minute RBC fragments. The reticulocyte count is very low; in severe cases, the neutrophil and platelet counts also are decreased.

5.4.2 Peripheral Blood Smear Morphology

The peripheral blood smear characteristically contains numerous oval macrocytes as well as schistocytes of various sizes, broken erythrocytes, and spherocytes i5.1, i5.2. RBC fragmentation occurs because of the increased fragility of these large erythrocytes, which probably are damaged during their passage through the spleen. Basophilic stippling and Howell-Jolly bodies also have been seen in RBCs. When the hematocrit value drops below 20% (0.20), nucleated RBCs may be found in the blood. Although challenged by some authors, hypersegmentation of mature neutrophils is considered a characteristic feature that appears very early in the development of megaloblastic anemia and is a likely reflection of the nuclear maturation defect i5.3. Hypersegmentation can be manifested by cells with six or more nuclear lobes or by an elevation in the mean neutrophil lobe count.

5.4.3 Bone Marrow Examination

The bone marrow in patients with megaloblastic anemia is characteristically hypercellular with erythroid and granulocytic hyperplasia i5.4. Mitotic activity is abundant, but there is significant intramedullary cell death secondary to the nuclear maturation defect. The proliferating erythroid and myeloid cell lines show megaloblastic changes i5.5, i5.6, i5.7, i5.8. In the erythroid elements, the major morphologic manifestation is nuclear-cytoplasmic asynchrony, in which the nuclei are large with finely dispersed chromatin, whereas the cytoplasm is more mature with effective hemoglobinization. The dominant myeloid abnormality is giantism of bands and metamyelocytes and nuclear hypersegmentation of mature granulocytes. Large megakaryocytes also have been described.

Erythroid megaloblastosis can be masked because of concomitant iron deficiency or other confounding causes of anemia. In patients with such conditions, the peripheral blood and bone marrow erythroid picture may be intermediate between those described for iron deficiency and megaloblastic anemia, although the megaloblastic changes in the granulocytic cell line persist.

i5.1 Severe megaloblastic anemia

Oval macrocyte along with fragmented red blood cells is evident in this peripheral blood smear from an adult with severe megaloblastic anemia. *(Wright stain)*

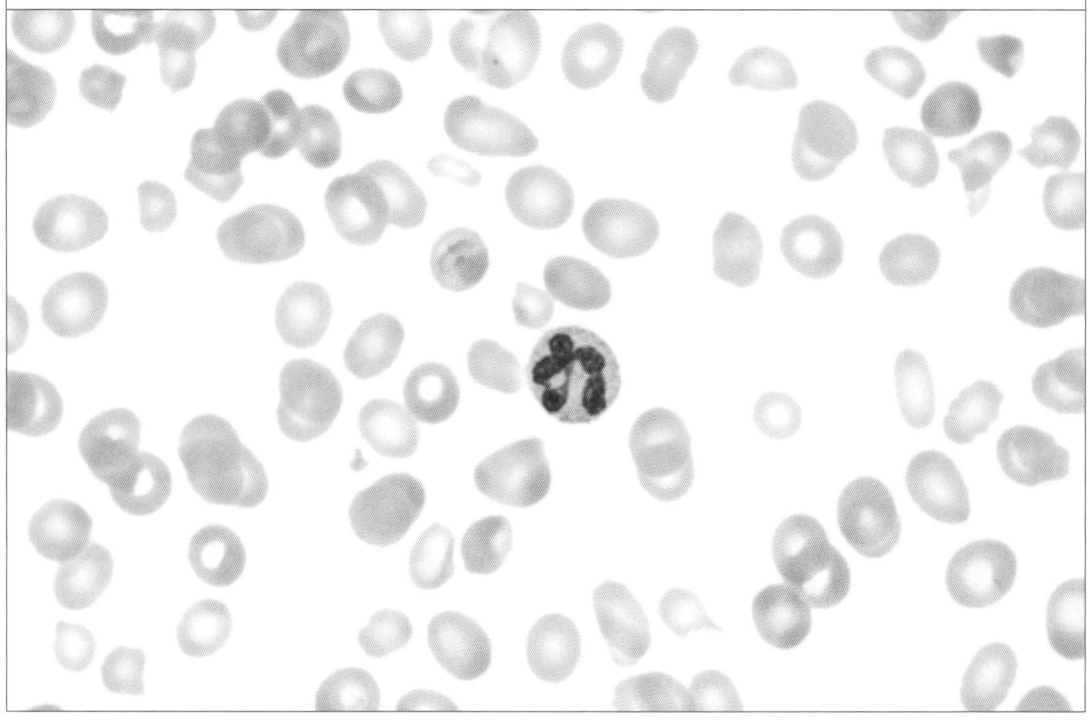

i5.2 Severe megaloblastic anemia

This peripheral blood smear from a 7-month-old baby shows circulating erythroblasts with megaloblastic features in this infant with megaloblastic anemia. Note red blood cell fragmentation (MCV normal). *(Wright stain)*

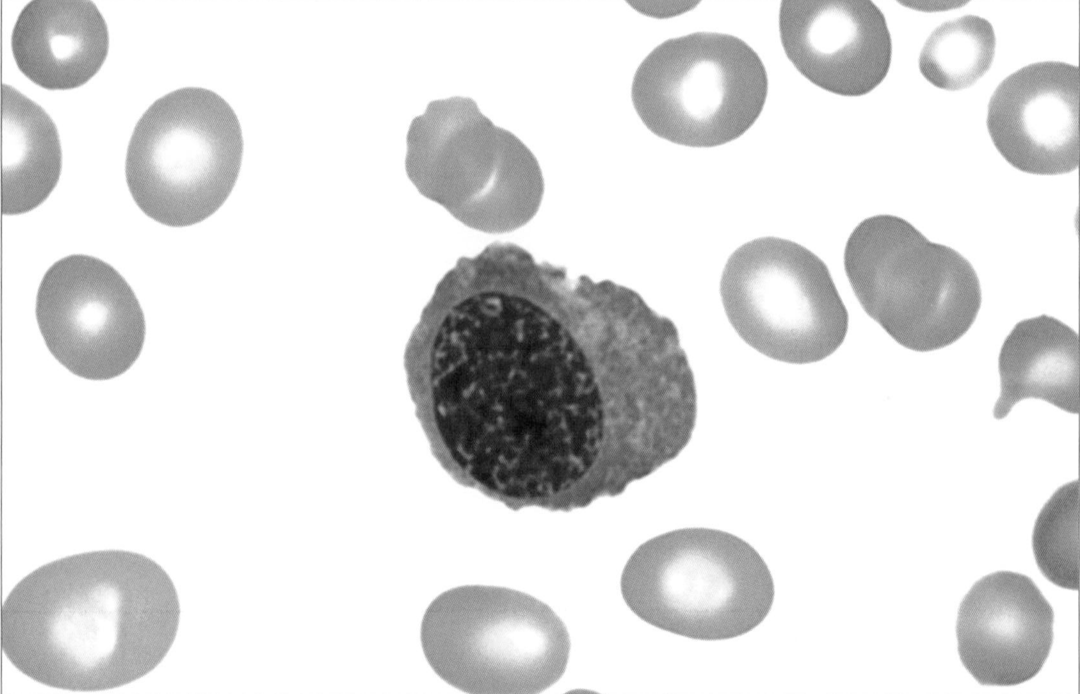

i5.3 Neutrophil hypersegmentation

Nuclear hypersegmentation of neutrophil in patient with severe megaloblastic anemia. *(Wright stain)*

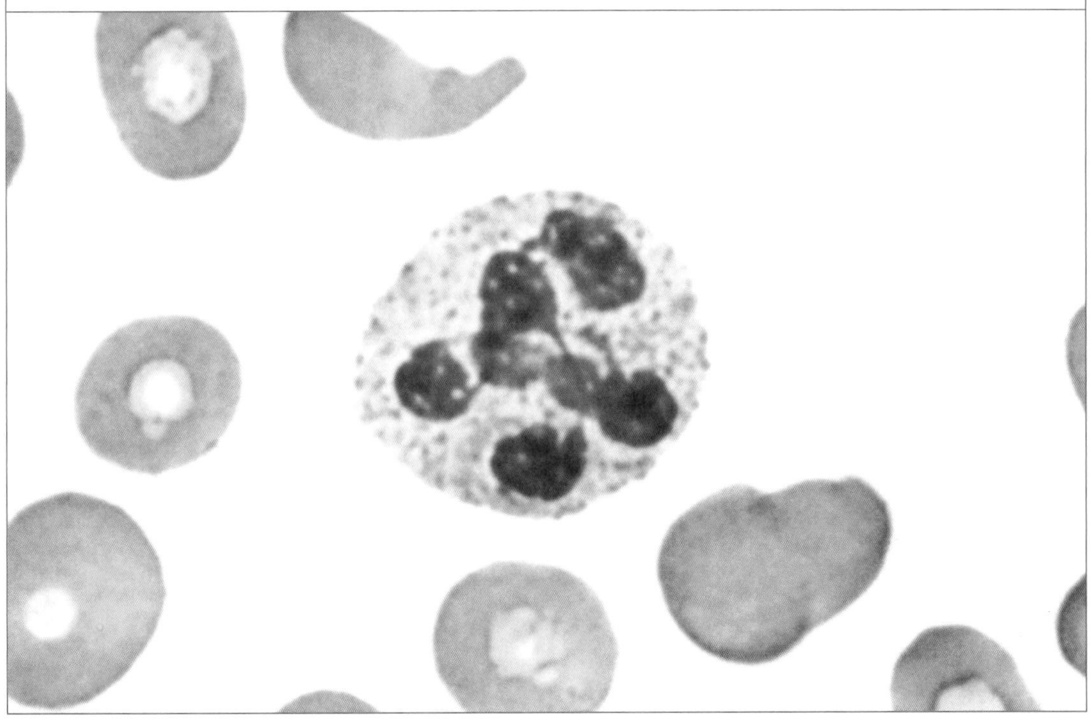

i5.4 Hypercellularity in megalobastic anemia

Markedly hypercellular bone marrow core biopsy specimen in patient with florid megaloblastic anemia. *(H&E)*

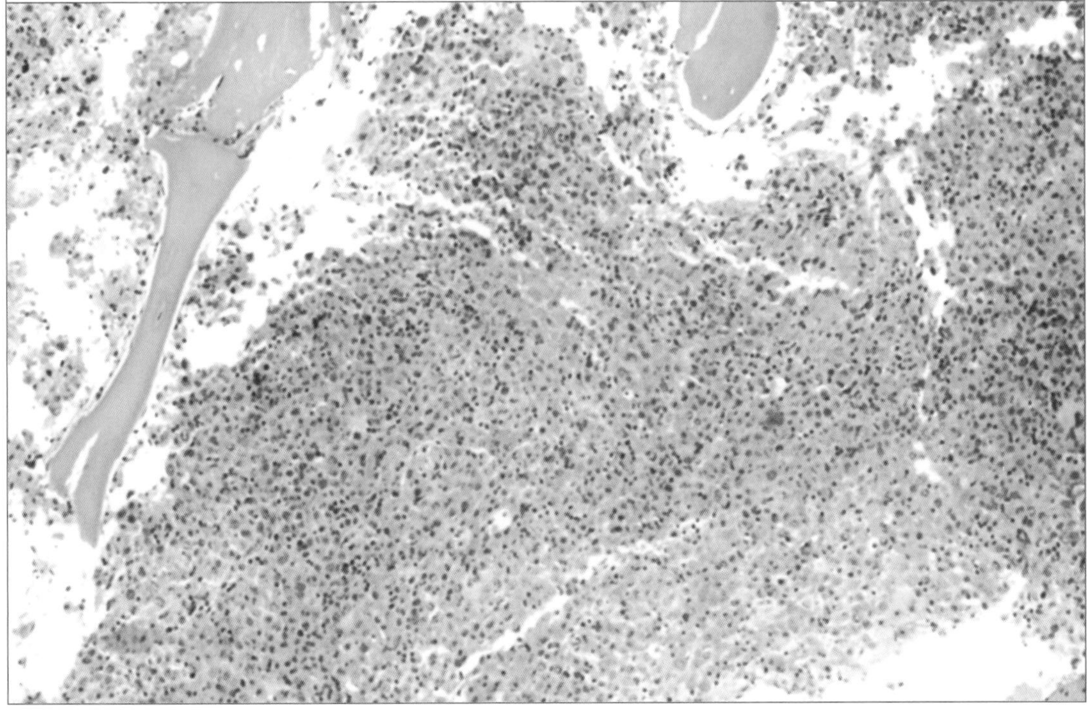

i5.5 Florid megaloblastic anemia

Erythroid hyperplasia with marked megaloblastic changes in adult with florid megaloblastic anemia. *(Wright stain)*

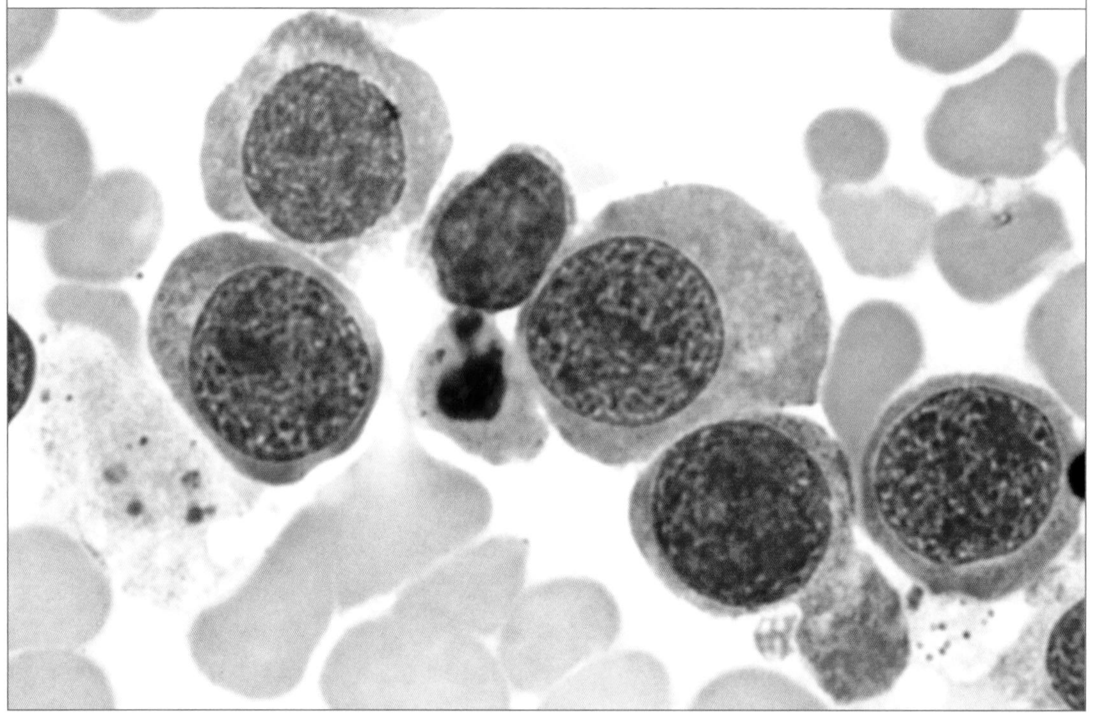

i5.6 Florid megaloblastic anemia

Myeloid hyperplasia with marked megaloblastic changes including giant bands in bone marrow aspirate smear from 7-month-old baby with florid megaloblastic anemia. *(Wright stain)*

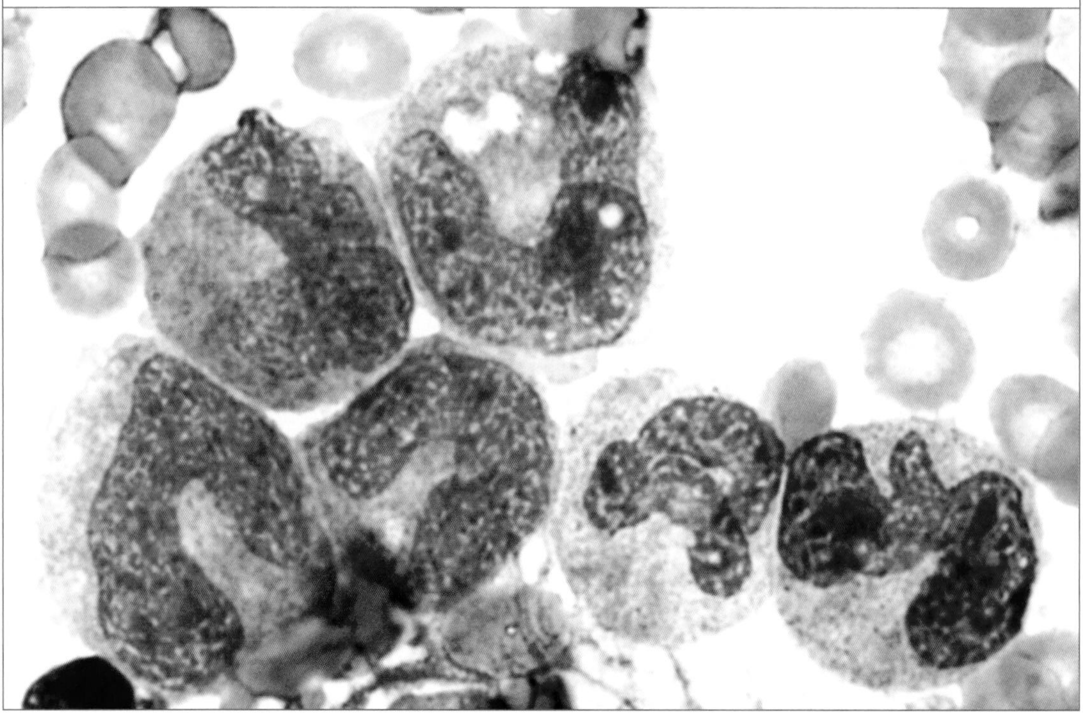

i5.7 Florid megaloblastic anemia

Hypercellular bone marrow with increased immature erythroid elements and myeloid hyperplasia with giant band (center) in patient with florid megaloblastic anemia. *(H&E)*

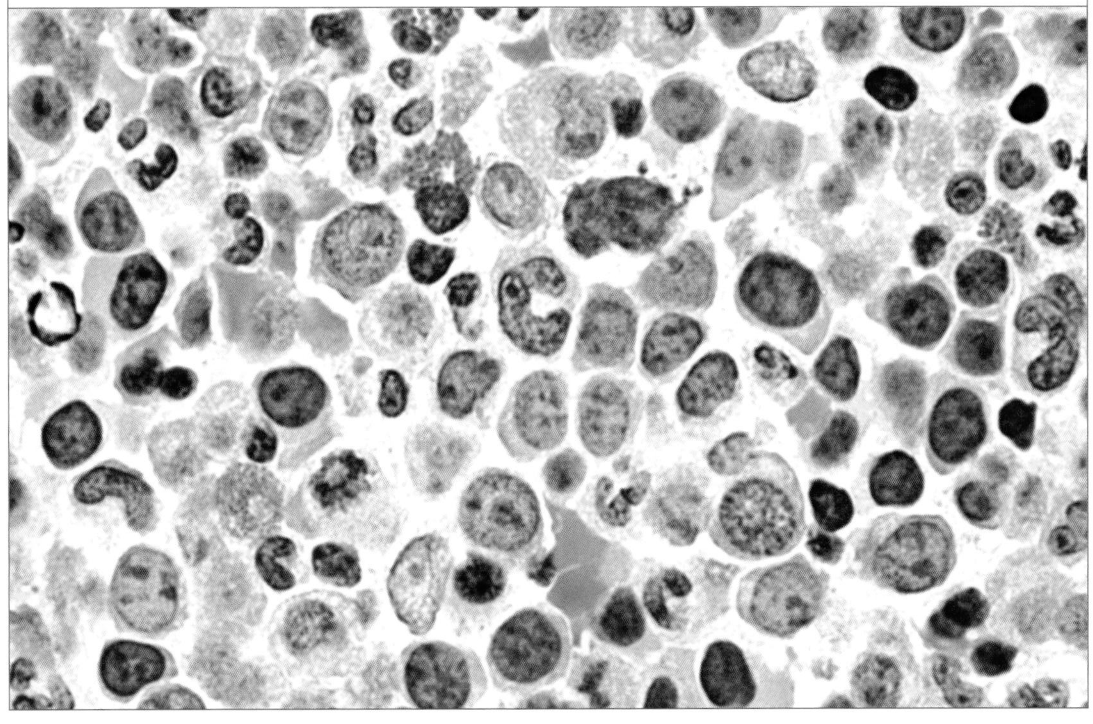

i5.8 Florid megaloblastic anemia

Immunoperoxidase staining for HgbA shows confluent erythroid hyperplasia in this 7-month-old infant with florid megaloblastic anemia. *(Immunoperoxidase for HgbA)*

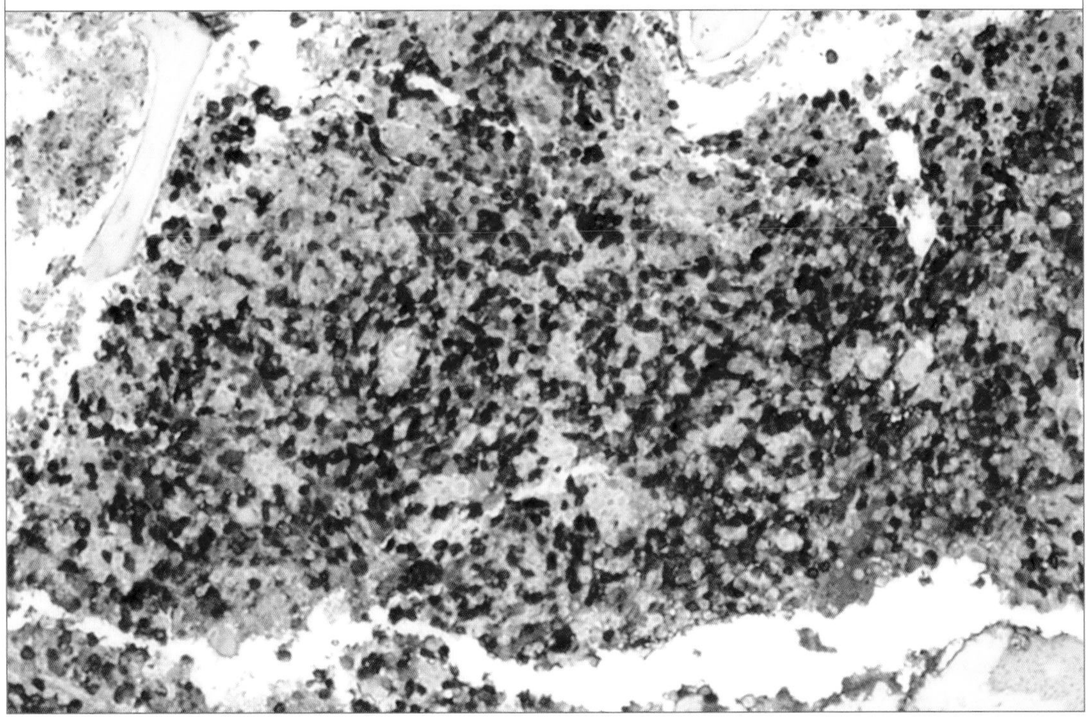

5.5 Other Laboratory Tests

The primary laboratory tests used in the diagnosis of megaloblastic anemias include measurements of serum vitamin B_{12}, fasting serum folate, and RBC folate. A variety of additional tests enhance sensitivity and specificity in the diagnosis of either vitamin B_{12} or folate deficiency, as well as in determining the likely cause of vitamin B_{12} deficiency, such as pernicious anemia. Some features of primary and ancillary laboratory tests are shown in **t5.8**.

t5.8 Laboratory Tests for Diagnosis of Megaloblastic Anemia

Test*	Specimen	Procedure
Vitamin B_{12}* (cobalamin)	Serum/plasma	Competitive binding assay
Folate*	Serum/plasma	Competitive binding assay
RBC folate*	Lysed RBCs	Similar to serum folate assay except lysed erythrocytes used; competitive binding assay
LDH	Serum/heparinized plasma	LDH catalyzes oxidation of lactate to pyruvate with reduction of NAD to NADH; absorbance of NADH measured
Iron, IBC	Serum/heparinized plasma	See Chapter 2
IF antibodies	Serum	Competitive protein-binding assay
Parietal cell antibodies	Serum	Immunofluorescent test using sections of mouse stomach and appropriate control tissues
Indirect bilirubin	Serum	See Chapter 6
Gastrin	Serum	Competitive protein-binding assay
Methylmalonic acid	Serum/plasma/urine	Gas chromatography-mass spectrometry or high pressure liquid chromatography
Total homocysteine	Serum/plasma/urine	Gas chromatography-mass spectrometry or high pressure liquid chromatography

**Tests should be performed in all cases of suspected megaloblastic anemia; other tests are helpful in selected clinical settings.*

Test 5.5.1 Serum Vitamin B12 Quantitation

Purpose. The level of vitamin B_{12} in the blood is a useful measure of the patient's vitamin B_{12} stores.

Principle. Most laboratories currently use a competitive protein binding assay for the determination of serum B_{12} levels. In this assay, a patient's vitamin B_{12} competes with vitamin B_{12}-coated polystyrene beads for intrinsic factor. Antibodies specific for intrinsic factor detect immobilized intrinsic factor bound to the polystyrene beads. The amount of bound intrinsic factor is inversely proportional to the patient's vitamin B_{12} levels.

Interpretation	Notes and Precautions
Decreased in PA and other anemias secondary to vitamin B_{12} deficiency; may see moderate decrease in patient with severe folate deficiency Level < 100 pg/mL deficient; level < 300 pg/mL indeterminate, level Δ 300 pg/mL not deficient	Low values common in HIV-1 infected patients, may not reflect true deficiency
Decreased in anemias due to folate deficiency; normal or increased in PA	False normal results in some patients with concurrent severe iron deficiency Levels fluctuate with diet; fasting specimen more stable Falsely elevated level with hemolyzed specimen
Since RBCs are metabolically inactive, RBC folate level reflects patient folate status at time these cells formed; level is decreased in folate and vitamin B_{12} deficiency	Because vitamin B_{12} is required for folate to enter cell, level is decreased in either B_{12} or folate deficiency, or in combined deficiency
Markedly elevated LDH in megaloblastic anemia due to intramedullary destruction of cells	Hemolysis falsely elevates results
Increased serum iron, storage iron, and IBC in megaloblastic anemias due to decreased iron utilization in erythropoiesis	See Chapter 2
Present in 50%-70% of cases of PA	Very specific for PA, but present in only 50%-70% of cases
Fluorescence of parietal cells in stomach sections (with negative controls) indicates that patient has parietal cell antibodies	Sensitive for PA (positive in 90% of cases) but also found in other disorders
Mildly increased in megaloblastic anemia due to hemolysis of some abnormal RBCs and intramedullary destruction Markedly increased in PA	See Chapter 6
Increased in vitamin B_{12} deficiency; normal in folate deficiency	Highly sensitive and specific; useful in early detection of vitamin B_{12} deficiency May be useful when serum cobalamin level indeterminate
Increased in both vitamin B_{12} and folate deficiency; also increased in some constitutional enzyme deficiencies or constitutional transport protein defects	Highly sensitive; useful in early detection of deficiency May be useful when serum cobalamin level indeterminate

IF = intrinsic factor; PA = pernicious anemia; IBC = iron-binding capacity; LDH = lactate dehydrogenase; NAD = nicotinamide adenine dinucleotide; NADH = reduced nicotinamide adenine dinucleotide.; HIV-1 = human immunodeficiency-1 virus

Specimen. Serum or plasma can be used for this test. The serum specimen must be separated and the test performed within 8 hours of collection; specimen should be frozen if analysis cannot be performed within this time frame.

Procedure. The sample is treated with alkaline potassium cyanide and dithiothreitol to denature B_{12} binding proteins and to convert all forms of vitamin B_{12} to cyanocobalamin. In a second reaction tube, patient vitamin B_{12} competes with vitamin B_{12}-coated polystyrene beads for hog intrinsic factor. An alkaline phosphatase-labeled antibody to hog intrinsic factor is used to quantitate immobilized hog intrinsic factor (ie, the intrinsic factor that has bound to the vitamin B_{12}-coated beads).

Interpretation. Decreased vitamin B_{12} levels are seen in patients with pernicious anemia and all other types of megaloblastic anemia caused by vitamin B_{12} deficiency. Recent studies document that patients within the "low normal" range may exhibit neurologic manifestations and respond to cobalamin therapy. Consequently, the lower limit of normal range may vary among patients.

Notes and Precautions. In patients with pernicious anemia and coexisting diseases such as iron deficiency, liver disease, hemoglobinopathy, or myeloproliferative disorders, the vitamin B_{12} level may be normal or even increased. Falsely low levels may be seen in patients with severe folate deficiency, pregnant women, patients with multiple myeloma, women taking oral contraceptives, and patients with transcobalamin deficiency. Serum vitamin B_{12} levels are often low in patients with HIV-1, although only a small proportion of these patients appear to have a true deficiency. Documentation of a concurrently low RBC folate level enhances the likelihood of true vitamin B_{12} deficiency in this population. Recent dietary supplementation can affect test accuracy. EDTA can interfere with results so specimens collected with this anticoagulant should not be used. Delays in specimen transport may result in falsely low values due to degradation of cobalamin. If serum folate levels are to be simultaneously measured, the patient should be fasting.

Test 5.5.2 Serum Folate Quantitation

Purpose. Assays of serum folate, in conjunction with RBC folate, are useful in determining the status of the patient's folate stores.

Principle. Serum folate is currently measured using a competitive protein binding assay analogous to that used for vitamin B_{12}. The amount of folate binding proteins that bind to anti-folate binding protein antibody-coated polystyrene beads is inversely proportional to the patient's folate level.

Specimen. Serum or plasma can be used for this test. The serum specimen must be separated and the test performed within 8 hours of collection; the specimen should be frozen if analysis cannot be performed within this time frame. Excessive exposure to direct light should be avoided.

Procedure. The specimen is first treated to release folate from binding proteins. In a second tube the folate released from binding proteins competes with ligand-labeled folate (polystyrene beads coated with anti-folate protein binding antibody) for FBP (folate binding proteins). The bead is washed and alkaline phosphatase-labeled anti-ligand is added. The amount of FBP bound to the bead is inversely proportional to the patient folate level.

Interpretation. Decreased serum folate levels are detected in patients with megaloblastic anemia secondary to folate deficiency, whereas normal or increased levels of serum folate are found in patients with pernicious anemia.

Notes and Precautions. Because serum folate shows significant fluctuation with diet, a patient can have a normal serum folate level and actually be folate deficient. Fasting serum folate levels more reliably reflect folate stores and, consequently, fasting samples are required. Folate deficiency also can be masked by a concurrent, more severe iron deficiency in which the serum and RBC folate levels may be within normal limits. The reason for this phenomenon is unknown. Hemolyzed samples give markedly elevated serum folate levels because of the large amounts of folate normally present in erythrocytes; even a small amount of RBC hemolysis will skew results.

Test 5.5.3 Red Blood Cell Folate Quantitation

Purpose. RBC folate determination is a more reliable measurement of the status of the patient's folate stores than is serum folate. Because RBCs are metabolically inactive, the RBC folate levels reflect the patient's folate status at the time these cells were produced.

Principle. RBC folate is measured analogously to that used for measuring serum folate.

Specimen. Whole blood is collected in ethylenediaminetetraacetic acid (EDTA), which can be frozen or processed immediately. RBCs are lysed with ascorbic acid.

Procedure. The procedure for the quantitation of RBC folate is similar to that used for serum folate (see Test 5.5.2).

Interpretation. Because vitamin B_{12} cofactor is necessary for folate to enter and be retained within RBCs, decreased RBC folate is found in patients with either folate or vitamin B_{12} deficiency. **t5.9** compares the serum vitamin B_{12}, serum folate, and RBC folate levels in patients with vitamin B_{12} deficiency, folate deficiency, or both. Fasting serum folate levels may supplant the need to routinely assess RBC folate levels.

t5.9 Serum Vitamin B_{12} (Cobalamin), Serum Folate, RBC Folate, Methylmalonic Acid, and Homocysteine Levels in Megaloblastic Anemia

Disorder	Serum Vitamin B_{12}	Serum Folate*	RBC Folate	Methylmalonic acid (serum)	Homocysteine (total, serum)
Vitamin B_{12} deficiency	Decreased	Normal or increased	Decreased	Elevated	Elevated
Folate deficiency	Normal or mildly decreased	Decreased	Decreased	Normal	Elevated
Deficiency of both vitamin B_{12} and folate	Decreased	Decreased	Decreased	Elevated	Elevated

5.6 Ancillary Tests

Several additional laboratory tests, including measurements of serum lactate dehydrogenase, bilirubin, serum and storage iron, intrinsic factor antibodies, parietal cell antibodies, gastrin, and deoxyuridine suppression tests can be useful in evaluating patients with megaloblastic anemia. Because of both their high sensitivity in detecting early deficiency and their utility in accurately distinguishing vitamin B_{12} from folate deficiency, measurement of metabolites such as methylmalonic acid and total homocysteine are being more commonly utilized in routine clinical practice. The expected values for these tests, along with the reason they are abnormal in megaloblastic anemia, are detailed in **t5.8** and **t5.9**.

5.6.1 Methylmalonic Acid

Increased methylmalonic acid concentration is a highly sensitive and specific indicator of cobalamin deficiency. Increased methylmalonic acid concentration is especially useful in cases in which the vitamin B_{12} levels are indeterminate. However, testing for methylmalonic acid is currently substantially more costly than the more routine tests for megaloblastic anemia. In addition, this assay is generally performed by reference laboratories. Methylmalonic acid levels are normal in patients with folate deficiency.

5.6.2 Parietal Cell and Intrinsic Factor Antibodies

Most patients with pernicious anemia have parietal cell and intrinsic factor antibodies. Although parietal cell antibodies are more sensitive for pernicious anemia, they also are seen fairly frequently in patients with chronic gastritis. Antibodies to intrinsic factor are substantially more specific for pernicious anemia and are present in the majority of patients.

5.6.3 Gastrin Test

Gastrin stimulates parietal cells to secrete intrinsic factor and hydrochloric acid; typically, serum gastrin levels are markedly elevated in patients with pernicious anemia. Recent evidence suggests that some parietal cell antibodies may be directed against the gastrin receptor on these cells, which explains the failure of parietal cells to respond to gastrin. The achlorhydria in gastric juices is secondary to the failure of parietal cells to produce hydrochloric acid; achlorhydria is a further stimulus for gastrin secretion.

5.6.4 Schilling Test

Due to testing complexity, expense, difficulties with 24-hour urine collection, and availability of alternate tests, the Schilling test is no longer a frontline test in the workup of a patient for cobalamin deficiency. However, in highly selected circumstances the three-part Schilling may provide useful information when other tests yield ambiguous results. The first part of this test measures only the patient's ability to absorb vitamin B_{12}. Intrinsic factor and vitamin B_{12} are given to the patient in the second part of the test; the third part uses antibiotics to destroy bacteria and is designed to detect patients with intestinal bacterial overgrowth disorders. The patient ingests radio labeled vitamin B_{12}, followed by an injection of a loading dose of unlabeled vitamin B_{12}. A 24-hour urine sample is collected and the amount of radioactivity in this sample is measured. In patients with pernicious anemia, the urinary excretion of labeled vitamin B_{12} is normal only when intrinsic factor is given.

Several problems are common in performing the Schilling test. First, the collection of a 24-hour urine sample is cumbersome, and often an incomplete sample is submitted for evaluation. The patient must have normal renal function and normal intestinal mucosa for the test to be valid. In addition, some patients who cannot absorb dietary vitamin B_{12} are able to absorb the crystalline vitamin B_{12} that is used, giving a falsely normal result. Due to these complexities, the routine use of the Schilling test in the assessment of patients for megaloblastic anemia is discouraged, especially since there are many other testing options that require only serum/plasma samples.

5.7 Course and Treatment

Correction of the vitamin deficiency results in prompt improvement of the patient's hematologic abnormalities, with normalization of the hemogram within 4 to 8 weeks. Although parenteral injections of vitamin B_{12} have been used most frequently for pernicious anemia patients, recent studies document efficacy with oral dosing (high dose), sublingual dosing, and even intranasal administration. Oral therapy is effective for folate supplementation; occasional patients with folate deficiency need parenteral therapy until the gastrointestinal tract epithelium has regenerated. Patients with megaloblastic anemia should be evaluated carefully to determine the underlying cause of the vitamin deficiency.

Because the slow development of the anemia allows for some compensation, patients with megaloblastic anemia usually do not require transfusion; however, rare patients may present with cardiovascular decompensation requiring immediate treatment. Transfusion in this clinical situation must be considered carefully owing to the possibility of further cardiac decompensation and death secondary to volume overload. Plasmapheresis with RBC infusions may prevent volume overload. Another cardiac complication that occurs in small numbers of patients receiving treatment for megaloblastic anemia is cardiac arrhythmia, which may result in sudden death. The postulated mechanism for this catastrophic complication is the precipitous decrease in potassium level that occurs following vitamin B_{12} therapy. Patients with megaloblastic anemia undergoing therapy also may develop thrombotic complications because of changes in platelet activity associated with restoration of normal vitamin B_{12} or folate levels in platelets.

Following vitamin therapy, there is a rapid and marked decline in the lactate dehydrogenase and plasma iron levels, as well as a normalization of the serum bilirubin level. The megaloblastic changes in bone marrow erythroid precursors revert to normal within several days of treatment, followed by reversal of the megaloblastic changes within myeloid precursors a few days later. Reticulocytes can be identified in the peripheral blood within 3-5 days after treatment is begun, and they generally peak within 7-10 days. The height of the reticulocyte count is inversely proportional to the degree of anemia. All peripheral blood parameters return to normal within 1-2 months.

In patients with pernicious anemia, the neurologic manifestations of this disorder generally improve substantially with vitamin B_{12} therapy, although they may not resolve entirely. There should be no progression of these neurologic defects, however, while the patient continues to receive vitamin B_{12} therapy. In patients with pernicious anemia, large doses of folate can reduce the hematologic abnormalities, but the neurologic disease still progresses.

Prognosis is good for patients with megaloblastic anemia, provided the vitamin deficiency is adequately treated and the underlying disorder that led to the vitamin deficiency is identified and managed appropriately.

5.8 Acknowledgments

The author is grateful to Michael Crossey, MD, PhD, of TriCore References Laboratories for advice on the laboratory testing methodologies in this chapter.

5.9 References

Andres E, Affenberger S, Zimmer J, et al. Current hematological findings in cobalamin deficiency. A study of 201 consecutive patients with documented cobalamin deficiency. *Clin Lab Haematol.* 2006;28:50-56.

Carmel R, Green R, Jacobsen DW, et al. Neutrophil nuclear segmentation in mild cobalamin deficiency: relation to metabolic tests of cobalamin status and observations on ethnic differences in neutrophil segmentation. *Am J Clin Pathol.* 1996;106:57-63.

Carmel R. Nutritional anemias and the elderly. *Semin Hematol.* 2008;45:225-234.

Carmel R. How I treat cobalamin (vitamin B12) deficiency. *Blood.* 2008;112:2214-2221.

Chan CW, Liu SY, Kho CS, et al. Diagnostic clues to megaloblastic anaemia without macrocytosis. *Int J Lab Hematol.* 2007;29:163-171.

Chanarin I. Historical review: a history of pernicious anaemia. *Br J Haematol.* 2000;111:407-415.

Dharmarajan TS, Adiga GU, Norkus EP. Vitamin B12 deficiency: recognizing subtle symptoms in older adults. *Geriatrics.* 2003;58:30-34, 37-38.

Foucar K. Non-neoplastic erythroid lineage disorders. In: King D, Gardner W, Sobin L, et al., eds. *Non-Neoplastic Disorders of Bone Marrow* (AFIP fascicle). Washington, DC: American Registry of Pathology; 2008:75-124.

Foucar K. Non-neoplastic erythroid lineage disorders. In: King D, Gardner W, Sobin L, et al., eds. *Non-Neoplastic Disorders of Bone Marrow* (AFIP fascicle). Washington, DC: American Registry of Pathology; 2008:75-124.

Fyfe J, Madsen M, Hojrup P, et al. The functional cobalamin (vitamin B12)–intrinsic factor receptor is a novel complex of cubilin and amnionless. *Blood.* 2004;103:1573-1579.

Kaptan K, Beyan C, Ural AU, et al. Helicobacter pylori–is it a novel causative agent in vitamin B_{12} deficiency? *Arch Intern Med.* 2000;160:1349-1353.

Katar S, Nuri Ozbek M, Yaramis A, Ecer S. Nutritional megaloblastic anemia in young Turkish children is associated with vitamin B-12 deficiency and psychomotor retardation. *J Pediatr Hematol Oncol.* 2006;28:559-562.

Koury MJ, Price JO, Hicks GG. Apoptosis in megaloblastic anemia occurs during DNA synthesis by a p53-independent, nucleoside-reversible mechanism. *Blood.* 2000;96:3249-3255.

Kristiansen M, Aminoff M, Jacobsen C, et al. Cubilin P1297L mutation associated with hereditary megaloblastic anemia 1 causes impaired recognition of intrinsic factor-vitamin B(12) by cubilin. *Blood.* 2000;96:405-409.

Moridani M, Ben-Poorat S. Laboratory investigation of vitamin B_{12} deficiency. *Labmedicine.* 2006;37:166-174.

Solomon LR. Cobalamin-responsive disorders in the ambulatory care setting: unreliability of cobalamin, methylmalonic acid, and homocysteine testing. *Blood.* 2005;105:978-985.

Solomon LR. Disorders of cobalamin (vitamin B12) metabolism: emerging concepts in pathophysiology, diagnosis and treatment. *Blood Rev.* 2007;21:113-130.

Weiss R, Fogelman Y, Bennett M. Severe vitamin B12 deficiency in an infant associated with a maternal deficiency and a strict vegetarian diet. *J Pediatr Hematol Oncol.* 2004;26:270-271.

Whitehead VM. Acquired and inherited disorders of cobalamin and folate in children. *Br J Haematol.* 2006;134:125-136.

Wickramasinghe S. Bone marrow. In: Mills S, ed. *Histology for Pathologists. 3rd ed.* Philadelphia: Lippincott Williams & Wilkins; 2007:799-836.

Wickramasinghe SN. Diagnosis of megaloblastic anaemias. *Blood Rev.* 2006;20:299-318.

Zhao R, Min SH, Qiu A, et al. The spectrum of mutations in the PCFT gene, coding for an intestinal folate transporter, that are the basis for hereditary folate malabsorption. *Blood.* 2007;110:1147-1152.

Part II

Hemolytic Anemias

Chapter 6

Accelerated Erythrocyte Turnover

Sherrie Perkins, MD, PhD

Hemolysis is characterized by premature removal of circulating red blood cells due to lysis within the circulatory system (intravascular hemolysis) or premature removal by the reticuloendothelial system of the spleen, liver, and bone marrow (extravascular hemolysis). The hemolytic state is accompanied by increased bone marrow production of replacement erythroid cells, attempting to compensate for the shortened life span of the red blood cell in the circulation. Anemia develops when the bone marrow cannot adequately compensate for the shortened red blood cell lifespan. This pattern of accelerated erythrocyte turnover is associated with various hereditary and acquired hemolytic disorders.

6.1 Pathophysiology

Accelerated red blood cell destruction or hemolysis, leading to development of anemia, may be on the classified basis of the defect (inherited versus acquired defects) **t6.1**. Similarly,

t6.1 Hemolytic Disorders

Hereditary disorders	
Membrane defects	Hereditary spherocytosis Hereditary elliptocytosis
Abnormalities in red cell enzymes	G6PD deficiency Glycolytic pathway enzyme deficiencies (eg, pyruvate kinase deficiency) Glutathione pathway deficiency
Hemoglobin synthesis abnormalities	
Quantitative (decreased production)	Thalassemias
Qualitative (abnormal production)	Hemoglobin S, hemoglobin C hemoglobin E
Acquired disorders	
Immune	
Infections	*Mycoplasma*, malaria, *Clostridium perfringens*
Alloantibodies	Maternal fetal incompatibilities, transfusions
Autoantibodies	Collagen vascular diseases, lymphomas, drugs, idiopathic
Non-immune	
Mechanical damage	Heart valves, DIC, TTP, HUS
Physiochemical damage	Burns, oxidative damage
Membrane abnormalities	Paroxysmal nocturnal hemoglobinuria

G6PD = glucose-6-phosphate dehydrogenase; DIC = disseminated intravascular coagulation; TTP = thrombotic thrombocytopenia purpura; HUS = hemolytic uremic syndrome

hemolytic processes may be classified based on the pathophysiology of the underlying hemolysis including intrinsic defects of the red blood cell (intracorpuscular defects) or processes that are external to the cell (extracorpuscular defects) **t6.2**. Intracorpuscular defects include inherited or acquired abnormalities in red blood cell shape or size, abnormal membrane characteristics, and hemoglobinopathies. Extracorpuscular defects include immune or other physiochemical processes that interact with or secondarily damage red blood cells. Use of a combination of these classification approaches usually is the most effective in identifying pertinent clinical information and laboratory testing that will lead to the specific pathophysiologic process giving rise to hemolysis.

t6.2 Pathophysiologic Classification of Hemolytic Disorders

Intrinsic (intracorpuscular) defects

Red blood cell membrane defects
Red blood cell enzyme defects
Hemoglobinopathies

Extrinsic (extracorpuscular) defects

Immune mediated hemolysis
Physical damage to red blood cells
  Toxins
  Thermal injury
  Mechanical disruption

Hemolysis may be further subclassified as extravascular (mediated by the spleen and other components of the reticuloendothelial system) or intravascular (direct cell lysis within the circulation). Although less useful in determining the etiology of the hemolytic process, this classification provides insights into red blood cell destruction. Most hemolytic anemia arises secondary to extravascular hemolysis occurring when mononuclear phagocytic cells remove abnormal red blood cells and fragments from the circulation. The spleen removes marginally damaged erythrocytes and the liver or bone marrow macrophages remove more severely damaged red blood cells. Intravascular hemolysis occurs with the most severe cell damage and is associated with extracorpuscular defects arising from mechanical trauma to cells or cellular damage by toxins, thermal stress, or immune mechanisms.

In general, the life span of the red blood cell has three distinct phases: bone marrow production, circulation, and removal and breakdown of senescent or damaged cells. A diagnosis of hemolysis requires evaluation of the three phases of the erythrocyte life cycle to demonstrate accelerated red blood cell turnover and a shortened life span. Various laboratory tests provide insights into each red blood cell phase **t6.3**.

Red blood cells arise from a multipotential bone marrow stem cell that is stimulated to proliferate and differentiate under the influence of the growth factor erythropoietin. Erythroid precursors require approximately 6 days to differentiate from an erythroblast to a marrow reticulocyte to be released into peripheral circulation. Each erythroblast can give rise to approximately eight reticulocytes. Marrow reticulocytes expel their nuclei before passing through marrow sinusoids into the peripheral blood as circulating (peripheral) reticulocytes. The reticulocytes shed all remaining reticular network (ribosomal RNA) in the circulation over 1 to 2 days to become mature erythrocytes. Mature red blood cells circulate for about 120 days and are finally removed from the circulation by reticuloendothelial system activity in the spleen, liver, and bone marrow. The daily production of red blood cells is estimated at 3×10^9

t6.3 Laboratory Evaluation of Red Blood Cell Production and Breakdown*

Phase of Life Cycle	Laboratory Test or Findings
Bone marrow production	**Reticulocyte count**, bone marrow cellularity, ^{59}Fe uptake
Red blood cell circulation	**Hemoglobin/hematocrit**, ^{51}Cr red blood cell survival studies
Red blood cell sequestration	^{51}Cr red cell sequestration
Red blood cell breakdown	**Haptoglobin, bilirubin, lactate dehydrogenase**, hemoglobinemia, methemalbumin, bone marrow iron
Excretion	**Hemosiderinuria, hemoglobinuria**

**Boldface indicates the most useful tests*

cells per kilogram of body weight. This level of red blood cell production normally equals the rate of red blood cell destruction (approximately 1% per day), creating homeostasis.

Red blood cell destruction releases heme, globin, and iron. Heme is broken down into biliverdin, reduced to bilirubin by biliverdin reductase in the reticuloendothelial system, conjugated to soluble monoglucuronides and diglucuronides in the liver, and excreted in the feces as urobilin, urobilinogen, and stercobilinogen. Minimal amounts of the soluble urobilinogen are reabsorbed from the portal circulation and excreted in the urine. Iron released from heme is taken up by reticuloendothelial cells and is recycled for bone marrow synthesis of new red blood cells or is stored in the reticuloendothelial cells as ferritin or hemosiderin. The globin peptide chains are degraded to component amino acids that return to metabolic pools. Enzymes such as lactate dehydrogenase (LDH), that are normally present within red blood cells, also are released with hemolysis. Accelerated red blood cell turnover results in increased accumulation of all the breakdown products, many of which can be measured in the clinical laboratory, providing insights into the degree of hemolysis.

When intravascular hemolysis occurs, free hemoglobin is released into the plasma where it is bound by the α2-globulin, haptoglobin. The haptoglobin-hemoglobin complex is then metabolized directly by the reticuloendothelial system. If the binding capacity of haptoglobin is exceeded, free hemoglobin may be seen, resulting in hemoglobinemia and hemoglobinuria. Free hemoglobin also may be bound by transferrin and albumin. Oxidation of the ferrous ion of albumin-heme complexes produces the brown pigment, methemalbumin. Increases in free hemoglobin are less common in extravascular hemolysis, unless very high levels of cell destruction occurs.

6.2 Clinical Findings

A detailed and complete history including drug ingestion, transfusions, medical conditions, operations (such as insertion of heart valves), or a family history of hemolysis or jaundice is extremely important in determining the cause(s) of accelerated red blood cell turnover. This information helps to narrow the differential diagnosis of hemolysis, facilitating laboratory testing for the patient.

Clinical findings depend on the rate of hemolysis and the ability of the bone marrow to compensate for red blood cell destruction by increased production. If the bone marrow responds by increasing erythropoiesis so the hematocrit remains normal or near normal, the patient has a well-compensated hemolytic anemia and symptoms may be minimal. However, in severe hemolysis when the bone marrow synthesis is unable to compensate for the rapid loss of red blood cells, severe anemia may occur. The most common symptoms of anemia are pallor and fatigue. Fever, chills, and headache may be associated with extensive acute hemolytic episodes. If extensive hemolysis occurs, there is increased evidence of hemoglobin catabolism. As normal metabolic pathways are overwhelmed, hemoglobinemia or hemoglobinuria as well as jaundice may occur. With long-standing hemolysis, pigment gallstones may be formed.

Mild to moderate splenomegaly is variable but is common. Hepatomegaly is less common but is usually associated with long-standing hemolysis, reticuloendothelial hyperplasia, and iron deposition. Lymphadenopathy is not characteristic of hemolytic anemia unless there is an underlying lymphoproliferative disorder. In severe hemolytic anemia, extramedullary hematopoiesis may lead to enlargement of the spleen, liver, and lymph nodes. Bone pain and deformities may arise in cases of severe congenital hemolytic anemias secondary to bone marrow erythroid hyperplasia and resultant thinning of the cortical bone.

6.3 Diagnostic Approach

Diagnosis of accelerated red blood cell turnover requires establishing that hemolysis is occurring and then determining the underlying cause of the shortened red blood cell lifespan. When hemolysis is suspected, several laboratory tests can help confirm the diagnosis of accelerated red blood cell turnover by documenting decreased red blood cell lifespan and increased bone marrow erythroid production. Decreased red blood cell lifespan is documented by demonstration of increased levels of red blood cell breakdown products, most frequently serum bilirubin and serum haptoglobin levels. Additional testing for other breakdown products including demonstration of hemoglobinemia, hemoglobinuria, and hemosiderinuria and increases in lactate dehydrogenase may be useful. Increased bone marrow erythroid production is usually documented by an increased reticulocyte count. If a bone marrow aspiration is performed, erythroid hyperplasia will be seen.

The following approach provides laboratory information that allows a diagnosis of accelerated red blood cell turnover:

1. Peripheral blood smear morphology and red blood cell indices characterize the anemia, which is usually normochromic and normocytic, although it may be macrocytic if there are sufficient increases in reticulocytes. Morphologic changes in red blood cells, including red blood cell fragmentation and spherocytes or abnormal shapes in hemoglobinopathies may also provide insights into the basis of the hemolytic process. An elevated reticulocyte count indicates accelerated release of new red blood cells to the peripheral blood, and nucleated red blood cells may occasionally be seen.
2. Hemoglobin breakdown products in the plasma and urine increase with rapid destruction of red blood cells, and may help red blood cell destruction. Tests for these products and their relative usefulness are summarized in **t6.4**. In episodes of acute hemolysis, bilirubin (total and fractionated) and plasma or urine hemoglobin are most commonly measured. In less acute or chronic compensated hemolysis, urine hemosiderin may be a more sensitive indicator of long-term occult red blood cell degradation. Determination of bilirubin in compensated hemolytic anemia is of limited usefulness. Tests for urobilin and fecal and urine urobilinogen are unsatisfactory and unnecessary.
3. Serum haptoglobin is consumed by the binding of free hemoglobin released from hemolyzed cells. Thus, falls in haptoglobin levels are indicative of hemolysis.
4. Lactate dehydrogenase (LDH) is released into the plasma as red blood cells are rapidly destroyed. LDH1 is the isoenzyme found predominantly in red blood cells and myocardium. Isoenzyme determinations of LDH are useful if the source of total LDH elevation is not clearly from red blood cells.

t6.4 Urine and Serum Testing in Hemolysis

Pigment	Normal Range	Comments
Bilirubin, serum	0.5-2.0 mg/dL (8-34 μmol/L)	Limited significance; jaundice seen >3.0 mg/dL (52 μmol/L); fractionation may not be diagnostic in jaundiced patients
Indirect bilirubin, serum	<0.5 mg/dL (8 μmol/L)	Increased early in hemolysis; physiologic evaluation in hereditary conjugation disorders (Crigler-Najjar syndrome, Gilbert disease)
Haptoglobin, plasma	10 mg/dL (1.6 μmol/L)	Significant above 50 mg/dL (8 μmol/L), cherry-red plasma >150 mg/dL (24 μmol/L), binds to haptoglobin, transferrin, or albumin
Hemoglobin, urine	None present	Appears after haptoglobin saturation, hematuria must be excluded, myoglobinuria gives false-positive result on dipstick test
Methemalbumin,	None present	Qualitative determination by electrophoresis or serum spectrophotometric measurement

5. Bone marrow aspiration, including stains for iron, is useful in documenting accelerated marrow erythroid production. When the cause of anemia is clearly hemolysis rather than insufficient marrow production of red blood cells (eg, in hemoglobinopathies, red blood cell membrane defects or immune mediated hemolysis), bone marrow aspiration is unnecessary.
6. Radioisotope tracer studies usually are unnecessary and are rarely used unless other laboratory tests fail to document accelerated red blood cell turnover in the face of strong clinical suspicion. Radioisotope studies are usually limited to chromium 51 (^{51}Cr)-labeled red blood cell studies, which estimate survival half-life of circulating red blood cells and identify sites of cellular sequestration and destruction. Ferrokinetic studies with iron 59 (^{59}Fe) are also rarely performed. The radiolabeled iron is incorporated into precursor erythrocytes and is useful in evaluating rates and sites of erythroid production, rate of red blood cell release, and site of sequestration.
7. Ancillary screening tests, as summarized in **t6.5**, are used to document the pathophysiologic cause of accelerated erythrocyte turnover once its presence has been established. These tests are discussed at greater length in subsequent chapters with reference to specific causes of hemolysis.

t6.5 Common Screening Tests for Causes of Hemolysis

Inherent Case of Hemolysis	Test
Hereditary	
Membrane defects	Red blood cell morphology, osmotic fragility, flow cytometry with EMA staining
Enzyme defects	G6PD screening, pyruvate kinase screening
Hemoglobin defects	Red blood cell morphology, hemoglobin analysis, Heinz body test, hemoglobin A_2 and hemoglobin F quantitation
Acquired or extrinsic	
Infection	Malarial smears, blood cultures
Physiochemical-burns	Red blood cell morphology-microspherocytes
Mechanical-intravascular fibrin, prosthetic valves	Red blood cell morphology-schistocytes
Drugs-enzyme defect	G6PD screening
Drug-induced antibody	Antibody screening with drug-treated cells
PNH	Acid hemolysis test, sucrose lysis test, flow cytometry for CD55 and CD59 expression

EMA = eosin-5-maleimide, G6PD = glucose-6-phosphate dehydrogenase; PNH = paroxysmal nocturnal hemoglobinuria

6.4 Hematologic Findings

Accelerated red blood cell destruction or loss stimulates increased bone marrow production. This results in premature release of bone marrow reticulocytes, which appear on Wright-stained blood smears as polychromatophilic macrocytes. Nucleated RBCs also may be seen in prolonged or severe hemolytic anemia, but are usually <1% of nucleated cells. With increased cellular destruction and a competent bone marrow, the reticulocyte count is persistently elevated. Reticulocytosis varies with severity and duration of hemolysis but is usually proportional to the degree of the anemia. In acute blood loss, the reticulocytosis is of brief duration and usually less than 5%. Bone marrow erythroid production in chronic hemolysis may increase four- to six-fold, permitting reticulocyte counts as high as 60% to 70%, although reticuloctye counts of 5%-20% are more common.

Patients with hemolysis may have sufficient bone marrow erythropoiesis to compensate for accelerated red blood cell turnover and not be anemic. However, if red blood cell destruction exceeds the bone marrow ability to produce red blood cells, an anemia will develop. Anemia is more likely in cases of acute hemolysis or red blood cell defects that lead to marked decreased in red blood cell lifespan. Patients who were previously compensated for a hemolytic process may have an acute exacerbation of anemia due to an increase in red blood cell turnover, usually following an infection that activates or increases activity of the macrophages in the reticuloendothelial system so that red blood cells are removed more rapidly than normal (hemolytic crisis) or impairment of bone marrow red blood cell production (aplastic crisis). Viral infections, in particular with parvovirus B19, are the most common cause of an aplastic crisis. Chronic hemolysis may deplete bone marrow levels of folic acid or other nutrients, decreasing the ability of the bone marrow to mount a reticulocyte response adequate to compensate for the degree of anemia (marrow exhaustion).

6.4.1 Blood Cell Measurements

Anemia can be mild (hemoglobin, 11.5 g/dL [115 g/L]) to severe (hemoglobin, 2 g/dL [20 g/L]). The anemia is usually normochromic and normocytic, although mean corpuscular volume (MCV) may range from 80 to 110 μm^3 (80 to 110 fL) because reticulocytes may produce a mild macrocytosis. An MCV greater than 115 μm^3 (115 fL) suggests macrocytic anemia or (rarely) secondary folate depletion. An MCV less than 70 μm^3 (70 fL) in a normochromic anemia suggests hemolysis is due to a hemoglobinopathy or paroxysmal nocturnal hemoglobinuria (PNH). Reticulocytes, which may be enumerated with most modern hematology analyzers automatically or by cresyl blue staining (see **Test 1.5.1**), should be increased. Platelets and white blood cells are usually unaffected unless there is underlying infection or lymphoproliferative disorder that may result in a leukocytosis.

6.4.2 Peripheral Blood Smear Morphology

Morphologic characteristics generally include polychromatophilia, increased macrocytes, and nucleated red blood cells in severe cases. The blood smear may show red blood cell fragments or spherocytes, depending on the underlying mechanism of the hemolysis. Note that identification of red blood cell fragments or spherocytes is not required to make a diagnosis of hemolysis and some patients may demonstrate normal cell morphology The specific appearance of red blood cells is variable, depending on the etiology of the hemolysis. Morphologic findings associated with specific causes of hemolysis include:

1. **Spherocytes**—hereditary spherocytosis, autoimmune hemolytic anemia, ABO fetal-maternal incompatibility, burns or thermal injury (microspherocytes)
2. **Target cells**—hemoglobinopathies, liver disease, postsplenectomy
3. **Cell fragments**—hemolytic-uremic syndrome (HUS), thrombotic thrombocytopenic purpura (TTP), disseminated intravascular coagulation (DIC), prosthetic valves

Platelets and white blood cells are usually unremarkable in hemolysis, but may show reactive changes if hemolysis is occurring secondary to infection. Similarly, if hemolysis is occurring secondary to a lymphoproliferative disorder, circulating malignant lymphoid cells may be seen in the blood smear.

6.4.3 Bone Marrow Examination

The bone marrow is usually hypercellular with normoblastic erythroid hyperplasia. Dyssynchronous nuclear and cytoplasmic maturation due to rapid cell turnover may cause mild dyserythropoiesis or megaloblastoid cells without giant metamyelocytes or other stigmata of vitamin deficiency. If folic acid or vitamin B_{12} are relatively depleted by prolonged rapid turnover, a true megaloblastic cell population may appear. Bone marrow exhaustion with resultant aplasia may eventually result. Special staining of particle smears with acid potassium ferricyanide (Prussian blue) shows increased reticuloendothelial iron. If normoblasts contain stainable iron granules, they are often larger than usual and cover the nucleus. Sideroblastic iron is often increased and may form occasional ring sideroblasts when extensive ineffective erythropoiesis is present. Absence of stainable bone marrow iron in the clinical setting of hemolysis suggests paraoxysmal nocturnal hemoglobinuria (PNH) with extensive urinary iron losses or superimposed iron deficiency.

6.5 Other Laboratory Tests

Test 6.5.1 Serum Bilirubin, Total and Fractionated

Purpose. Increases in indirect bilirubin concurrent with clinical jaundice support the diagnosis of hemolysis.

Principle. Hyperbilirubinemia indicates increased red blood cell destruction, failure of liver conjugation, or blockage of excretory pathways. In hemolysis, an increased bilirubin load is presented to the liver faster than conjugation can proceed, so non-water-soluble (indirect) fraction of bilirubin is increased. In liver failure or obstructive jaundice, conjugation results in direct hyperbilirubinemia.

Specimen. Serum specimens, which are stable for days when refrigerated, are used for this test.

Procedure. Bilirubin levels are measured with an internationally standardized test, generally using the Evelyn-Malloy method or a modification. Bilirubin is coupled with a diazo dye, and the color is quantitated spectrophotometrically at 450 nm at 1 minute. The quick-reacting fraction is considered to be direct (or conjugated) bilirubin. The total bilirubin is measured after the addition of alcohol, and the indirect fraction is calculated by subtracting the amount of direct bilirubin from the total.

Interpretation. Normal ranges for total bilirubin are 0 to 1.5 mg/dL (0 to 25.65 μmol/L) and less than 0.3 mg/dL (5.13 μmol/L) for indirect bilirubin. Total bilirubin levels greater than 2.5 mg/dL (42.75 μmol/L) are usually associated with clinical jaundice. Bilirubin levels depend on the ability of the liver to compensate for increased levels of heme breakdown products. Initially, more than half the bilirubin is in the indirect or unconjugated fraction. If liver function is adequate, after several days the hepatic rate of glucuronide conjugation increases so direct and indirect fractions are nearly equal, and bilirubin fractionation is no longer diagnostic.

Notes and Precautions. In well-compensated hemolytic anemia, levels of total bilirubin may be less than 3 mg/dL (51.3 μmol/L), and no clinical jaundice is seen. Thus, bilirubin levels should not be used to exclude the diagnosis of accelerated red blood cell turnover.

In hemolytic disease of the newborn, the lipid-soluble, indirect fraction bilirubin is deposited in the striate nucleus of the brain, producing kernicterus. In the newborn, a shift in conjugation from indirect to direct bilirubin usually occurs at 7 to 10 days as liver function matures. Misleading elevations of indirect bilirubin can be seen in hereditary disorders of conjugation (Crigler-Najjar syndrome, Gilbert disease) and secondary to steroids found in breast milk that interfere with conjugation of bilirubin (breast milk jaundice).

Test 6.5.2 Plasma Hemoglobin Quantitation

Purpose. Increased plasma hemoglobin indicates acute intravascular hemolysis. Quantitation is useful in sera where other pigments (eg, bilirubin) make interpretation of plasma color uncertain.

Principle. Massive red blood cell injury results in intravascular hemolysis and release of hemoglobin into the plasma. This is detected macroscopically as pink to cherry-red plasma. Free hemoglobin can be quantitated with a modified benzidine reaction that measures oxidation of benzidine by hydrogen peroxide.

Specimen. Five milliliters of blood is collected in heparin or ethylenediaminetetraacetic acid (EDTA). A clot is not a desirable specimen because mechanical hemolysis of red blood cells during clot formation does not allow for the most accurate measurement. Blood must be drawn atraumatically, and plasma should be separated within 1-2 hours.

Procedure. Visual inspection of the plasma fraction shows a qualitative pink to red tint. Quantification uses a modified benzidine reaction (see Notes and Precautions) that oxidizes a colorless benzidine dye to violet-blue in the presence of hemoglobin and hydrogen peroxide. The color is measured spectrophotometrically at 515 nm or with a photoelectric colorimeter. Quantitation often requires a reference laboratory.

Interpretation. The normal level of plasma hemoglobin is less than 10 mg/dL (1.6 μmol/L). At low levels, test variability is great, and thus the test is only reliable above 50 mg/dL (8 μmol/L), which is the threshold for visual detection of pink coloration of the plasma. Free hemoglobin levels less than 30 mg/dL (4.8 μmol/L) are technically inaccurate and may be seen with difficult venipuncture, with mechanical destruction of RBCs by Vacutainer™ AE tubes, or during clotting of the specimen. Hemoglobinemia greater than 150 mg/dL (24 μmol/L) results in hemoglobinuria. At levels above 200 mg/dL (32 μmol/L), the plasma becomes clear cherry red.

Notes and Precautions. Benzidine may not be available as a result of federal regulations limiting potentially carcinogenic agents in the environment. Ortholidine (o-toluidine) may be substituted. Spectrophotometric results may be falsely high if the serum contains peroxidases or other oxidants that increase the development of color in the benzidine reaction.

Test 6.5.3 Serum Haptoglobin Quantitation

Purpose. Decreased or absent serum haptoglobin indicates hemolysis. Decreased haptoglobin also may be seen in liver failure or (rarely) as a genetic variant.

Principle. Haptoglobin is an α2-globulin produced in the liver that binds free hemoglobin on a molecule-for-molecule basis. The haptoglobin-hemoglobin complex is metabolized in the reticuloendothelial system, maintaining serum hemoglobin levels below renal thresholds. During intravascular hemolysis, haptoglobin binding is completely saturated. The excess hemoglobin is then bound by other serum proteins (hemopexin, transferrin, and albumin) before spilling into the urine as hemoglobinuria. Absence of haptoglobin implies binding saturation and degradation. Decreased haptoglobin reflects active hemolysis or, alternatively, failure of production due to liver failure. Rare abnormal haptoglobins (such as Hp–) are genetic variants that do not bind hemoglobin but are of little clinical significance.

Specimen. Fresh serum is obtained atraumatically. To avoid extraneous hemolysis, serum should not be allowed to remain on red blood cells. Testing specimens with macroscopic hemoglobinemia is superfluous, as it is easily detected by sight.

Procedure. The haptoglobin molecule has separate sites for antibody and hemoglobin binding. Haptoglobin is quantitated with turbidimetric methods using a nephelometer. Antihaptoglobin is added to the patient's serum, forming immune complexes with serum haptoglobin (1:1). These immune complexes scatter light proportionate to their concentration. Most larger hospitals have nephelometers.

Interpretation. The normal range for haptoglobin is 40-180 mg/dL (0.4-1.8 g/L). Less than 25 mg/dL (0.25 g/L) of haptoglobin is consistent with active hemolysis. Haptoglobin is an acute phase reactant, increasing three to four times in inflammation, infection, or tissue necrosis (eg, pneumonia or myocardial infarction). Such increases may mask changes in haptoglobin levels secondary to hemolysis. Haptoglobin levels greater than 200 mg/dL (2.0 g/L) are consistent with inflammation and not helpful in the diagnosis of hemolysis.

Notes and Precautions. Molecular sites for hemoglobin binding are not the same as those for antibody binding by antihaptoglobin. With radial immunodiffusion testing, elevations of haptoglobin may be falsely interpreted due to measurement of saturated haptoglobin-hemoglobin complexes that have not been removed by the reticuloendothelial system. Haptoglobin is decreased or absent in patients with liver failure, after recent massive transfusion due to removal of senescent transfused red blood cells, and in some abnormally functioning haptoglobin molecules (eg, Hp–).

Test 6.5.4 Direct Antiglobulin Test (DAT) (Direct Coombs' Test)

Purpose. Detection of globulin adsorbed to the patient's red blood cells indicates immune mechanisms may be an underlying cause of hemolysis.

Principle. Rabbit antihuman globulin reagent agglutinates human red blood cells that are coated with human globulin. Broad-spectrum reagents agglutinate cells coated with IgG, IgM, and/or complement. Monospecific sera agglutinate only red blood cells coated with the specific globulin (ie, IgG, IgM, or complement) to which the reagent is directed.

Specimen. Use of the red blood cells from EDTA specimens prevents non-specific absorption of complement in specimens. Specimens must be maintained at 37°C until cells and serum have been separated.

Procedure. The patient's red blood cells are washed with saline and centrifuged with antiglobulin reagent. Agglutination is graded from 0 to 4+. The adsorbed globulin must be eluted and tested for activity against control red blood cells before it is classified as an antibody.

Interpretation. Weakly positive results (+/–) usually are not clinically significant and eluates are generally unsuccessful. Strongly positive tests (2 to 4+) due to antibody may not correlate with the degree of hemolysis. Common causes of positive direct antiglobulin tests not associated with hemolysis include multiple myeloma, systemic lupus erythematosus (SLE), human immune-deficiency virus (HIV) infection, and cephalosporin therapy. A negative DAT result does not exclude hemolysis if red blood cell destruction has been massive and complete, as in incompatible transfusions.

Notes and Precautions. Refrigeration of blood specimens containing cold agglutinins may cause false-positive results or exaggerated positive results by non-specific cold adsorption of the agglutinin and complement.

6.6 Ancillary Tests

6.6.1 Urine Hemoglobin and Hemosiderin

Hemoglobinuria indicates concurrent or recent hemoglobinemia above the renal excretion threshold of 150 mg/dL (1.5 g/L). It usually appears as cloudy, smoky, dark-red, or cola-colored urine. It may be detected qualitatively by peroxidase reaction of o-toluidine or benzidine, which produces a blue color. In the absence of detectable hemoglobin, urine hemosiderin indicates ongoing hemolysis. Even in occult hemolysis, heme is deposited in renal epithelial cells and oxidized to hemosiderin.

In a healthy patient, no urinary hemoglobin or hemosiderin is detectable. Urinary sediments that contain significant numbers of red blood cells usually produce some free hemoglobin in hypotonic or alkaline urines. False-positive results may be seen with hematuria or myoglobinuria. Hemosiderin granules must be intracellular to have significance.

6.6.2 Total Lactate Dehydrogenase (LDH)

LDH increases with either normal or pathologic cell destruction as red blood cell glycolytic pathway enzymes, including LDH, are released to the plasma. Total LDH is usually measured with spectrophotometric kinetic analysis of the reduced form of nicotinamide adenine dinucleotide (NADH) production. Serum LDH catalyzes the reaction:

$$\text{Lactate} + \text{NAD} \longrightarrow \text{Pyruvate} + \text{NADH}$$

Because NADH absorbs light at 340 nm, LDH activity can be detected spectrophotometrically by increasing absorbance.

6.6.3 Other Serum Pigments

For the most part, measurement of methemalbumin is unnecessary for documentation of hemolysis; however, it may be useful in specialized cases. The presence of methemalbumin indicates chronic or continuing hemolysis and may be used as a marker of hemolysis. This is particularly true in patients with hemolysis induced by overconsumption of oxidizing agents. Free hemoglobin dissociates into α- and β-dimers and binds to plasma proteins, including haptoglobin, transferrin, and albumin. The ferrous iron of hemoglobin bound to albumin oxidizes to ferric iron, forming methemalbumin, which gives a distinctive rusty appearance to serum. Free hemoglobin in the presence of chloride ion produces hematin, which is bound by the protein hemopexin. Tests for methemalbumin are available in reference laboratories. Methemalbumin is not present in a healthy patient and clears within 4 or 5 days of the cessation of hemolysis. Tests for hemopexin are not generally available. Hemopexin has a normal range of 80-100 mg/dL (0.8-1.0 g/L). Levels <40 mg/dL (0.4 g/L) indicate hemolysis.

6.7 Laboratory Test Selection

Documentation of accelerated red blood cell turnover usually may be made on the basis of peripheral blood smear morphology, red blood cell indices, reticulocyte count, serum haptoglobin, and demonstration of elevation of hemoglobin breakdown products such as serum bilirubin, plasma or urine hemoglobin, or urine hemosiderin. Additional testing including bone marrow examination and LDH levels may provide useful information. Other tests, such as radioisotopic studies, are rarely required.

Evaluation of the mechanism underlying accelerated red blood cell turnover may make use of many different laboratory tests, depending on the etiology of the process. By obtaining a good clinical history and physical examination, test selection can be streamlined and directed to document the cause of hemolysis in a cost-efficient and logical manner. Thus, patients with a family history of hemolysis may undergo workup for heritable disorders of the red blood cell membrane, enzyme deficiencies, or hemoglobin synthesis, whereas these tests may not be chosen in an elderly patient with acute onset of hemolysis, no family history, and recent onset of generalized lymphadenopathy and splenomegaly.

6.8 Course and Treatment

The course and treatment of hemolysis varies, depending on the underlying etiology of the hemolysis. Patients with an intrinsic red blood cell defect (hemoglobinopathy, red blood cell membrane, or enzymatic defect) will have normal survival of transfused red blood cells, allowing for effective transfusion therapy when severe anemia develops. In contrast, those processes associated with antibody mediated destruction or physical destruction will have increased destruction of both patient and transfused cells, rendering transfusion therapy relatively ineffective. Treatment of an underlying infection (eg, malaria or *Mycoplasma*) or secondary process (eg, lymphoproliferative disorder or collagen vascular disorder) may decrease or alleviate hemolysis associated with these disorders. Patients receiving recurrent blood transfusions or with marked erythroid hyperplasia may develop iron overload.

6.9 References

An X, Mohandas N. Disorders of red cell membrane. *Br J Haematol.* 2008:141:367-375.
Bain BJ. Neonatal/newborn haemoglobinopathy screening in Europe and Africa. *J Clin Pathol.* 2009;62:53-56.
Franco RS. The measurement and importance of red cell survival. *Am J Hematol.* 2009;84:109-114.
Pierre RV. Red blood cell morphology and the peripheral blood film. *Clin Lab Med.* 2002;22:25-61.
Provan D, Weatherall, J. Red blood cells II: acquired anaemias and polycythaemia. *Lancet.* 2000;355:1260-1268.
Sahai I, Marseden D. Newborn screening. *Crit Rev Clin Lab Sci.* 2009; 46:55-82.
Segel GB, Hirsh MG, Feig SA. Managing anemia in pediatric office practice: part 1. *Pediatr Rev.* 2002;23:75-84.
Tavazzi D, Taher A, Cappellini MD. Red blood cell enzyme disorders: an overview. *Pediatr Ann.* 2008;37:303-310.
Existing Tefferi A. Anemia in adults: a contemporary approach to diagnosis. *Mayo Clin Proc.* 2003;78:1274-1280.

CHAPTER 7

Hereditary Erythrocyte Membrane Defects

Sherrie Perkins, MD, PhD

Hereditary abnormalities in red blood cell shape include hereditary spherocytosis (HS) and hereditary elliptocytosis (HE). These disorders arise secondary to inheritance of abnormal integral proteins underlying the red blood cell membrane that maintain cellular shape, membrane stability, and cellular flexibility. Abnormalities in these proteins may lead to premature hemolysis, as in HS, or may have little effect on red blood cell life span, as in most cases of HE.

7.1 Pathophysiology

The red blood cell membrane is composed of a lipid bilayer with associated proteins overlying and linked to a protein network, called the "membrane cytoskeleton." This structural configuration gives the red blood cell enough flexibility to squeeze through capillaries without fragmentation, yet retain the ability to regain a stable biconcave shape in larger vessels without loss of cellular integrity. The membrane cytoskeleton is formed by interactions of numerous proteins, including spectrin (α and β chains), actin, ankyrin, protein 4.1, protein 4.2, and a transmembrane protein, AE1 (also called band 3). Long, linear arrays of spectrin proteins form a meshwork that is anchored to the red blood cell lipid bilayer by interactions with ankyrin (binding to protein 4.2 on the inner aspect of the membrane) and to AE1 (spanning the membrane) as well as direct binding to protein 4.1 **f7.1**. The abnormalities observed in red blood cell shape are postulated to arise due to the disconnection of the protein framework underlying the lipid bilayer. In HS, this results in formation of microscopic vesicles of unsupported membrane. These vesicles are removed during transit through the spleen, leading to a progressive reduction in membrane surface area and formation of spherocytes. In HE, this leads to destabilization of the protein network so that the cells lose their characteristic biconcave shape after transit through small capillaries.

Hereditary spherocytosis is the most common hereditary hemolytic anemia among individuals of northern European origin, but it occurs in all races throughout the world. It is observed in about 1 in 5000 individuals in the United States and northern Europe. Various mutations affecting different proteins of the membrane cytoskeleton may give rise to the HS phenotype **t7.1**. The inheritance pattern is mixed, with over 65% of cases inherited as an autosomal dominant trait with evidence of other family members being affected (most often associated with mutations in ankyrin, spectrin β-chain and AE1, or band 3 genes) and the remainder being inherited as a recessive phenotype (including rare cases of HS arising due to spectrin α-chain mutations or protein 4.2 mutations) or as sporadic mutations with both parents being normal. In the Caucasian population the most common mutations are in the ankyrin gene (ANK1)

f7.1 Erythrocyte membrane structure

Schematic representation of the relationships between proteins in the red blood cell cytoskeleton and lipid bilayer of the cellular membrane. Defects in the proteins of the cytoskeleton or anchoring proteins give rise to the hereditary disorders of red blood cell shape including hereditary spherocytosis, hereditary elliptocytosis, and hereditary poikilocytosis.

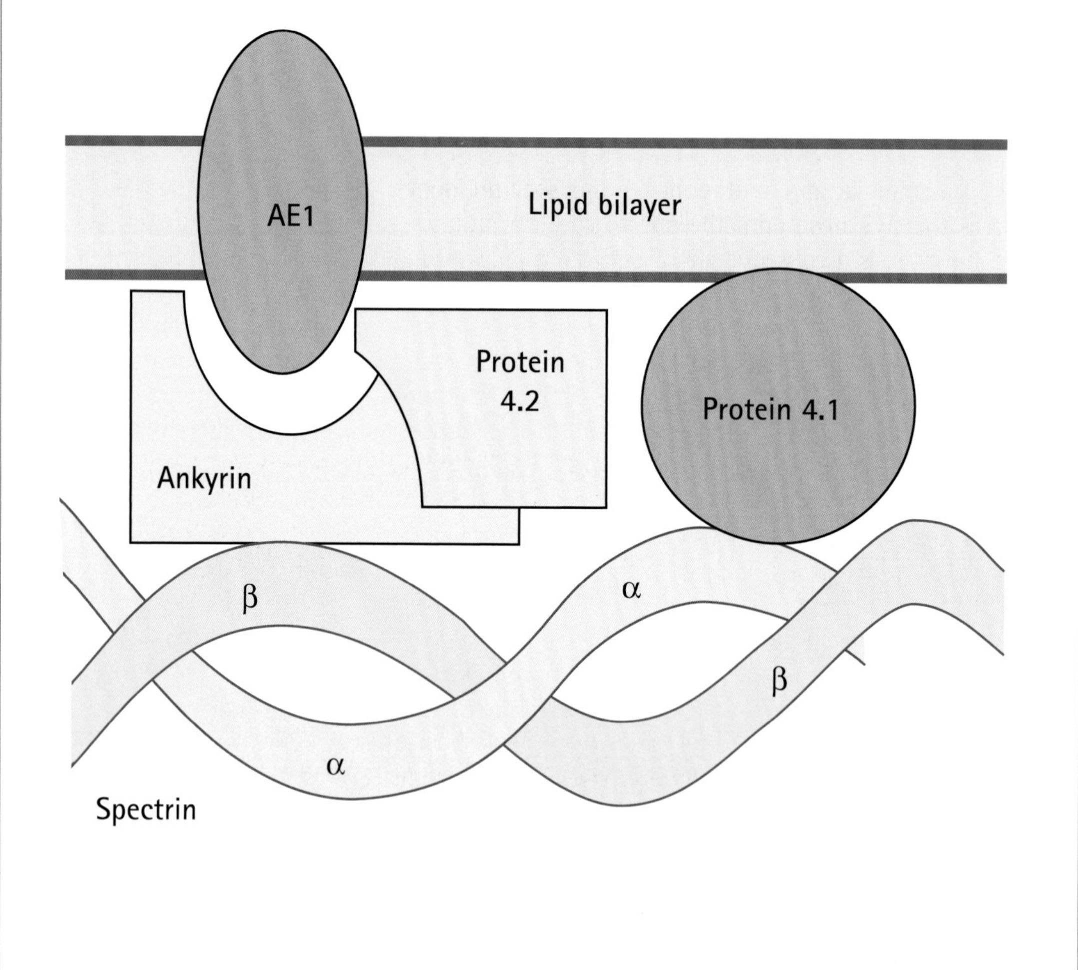

t7.1 Heterogeneity of Hereditary Spherocytosis

Protein defect	Hemolysis	Inheritance pattern	Frequency
Spectrin α-chain	Severe	Autosomal recessive	Rare
Spectrin β-chain	Mild to moderate	Autosomal dominant	Common, often associated ankyrin deficiency ~20% of cases
Ankyrin deficiency	Mild to severe	Autosomal dominant	Common ~60% of cases
AE1 (band 3) deficiency	Mild to moderate	Autosomal dominant	Common ~20% of cases
Protein 4.1 deficiency	Mild	Autosomal dominant	Most common in North Africa
Protein 4.2 deficiency	Moderate to severe (not responsive to splenectomy)	Autosomal recessive	Most common in Japan, rare in European population

located on chromosome 8p11, accounting for up to 60% of cases. Other frequently seen mutations in this population include mutations in the gene encoding AE1 (approximately 20% of cases) and spectrin β-chains (approximately 20% of cases). Most of these mutations are unique to a specific affected family and are most often nonsense or frameshift types that lead to decreased production of the affected protein rather than synthesis of an abnormal protein. Mutations in spectrin α-chains and protein 4.2 are rare, although the incidence of protein 4.2 mutations may be higher in the Japanese populations, where it gives rise to an atypical form of HS where splenectomy is only partially effective at relieving hemolysis.

The disease phenotype in HS is caused by a primary defect in membrane stability due to a decrease in the amounts of membrane proteins or in formation of atypical proteins that do not interact in the normal manners. Most patients with HS will have decreased amounts of spectrin heterodimers, despite lacking mutations in the spectrin genes, an observation that led to early hypotheses that HS arose primarily due to spectrin mutations. The observed decrease in spectrin content, however, is a consequence of deficits in ankyrin and other cytoskeletal protein synthesis and not a mutation in the spectrin gene. The lack of these proteins leads to a secondary decrease in spectrin content due to an inability of the spectrin protein to anchor to ankyrin or other proteins. Often the spectrin or ankyrin content deficiencies correlate with the degree of spherocytosis and hemolysis. The abnormal protein content and interactions maintaining the integrity of the red blood cell cytoskeleton leads to abnormal membrane micovesiculation and loss of membrane surface area by membrane removal in the spleen. In addition, spherocytes are less flexible than normal red blood cells, leading to increased retention or transit time within the spleen. This further accelerates loss of cellular membrane and premature cellular destruction by hemolysis.

Hereditary elliptocytosis is a heterogeneous group of disorders characterized by elliptocytes in the peripheral blood smear. These represent red blood cells that have failed to regain their normal biconcave shape following passage through the microcirculation. HE is usually a mild disorder without clinically significant hemolysis, although the spectrum of disease includes rare patients with transfusion dependent hemolysis. HE is seen in all populations with an overall incidence of 1 in 5000. There is an increased incidence of disease in African and Mediterranean populations where it may have conferred some resistance against malarial infection. In the United States the incidence of HE is estimated to be 1 in 2000 to 4000, although it may be higher as many patients are asymptomatic and not identified (silent carriers). Various red blood cell membrane skeletal defects have been associated with HE, including mutations in spectrin α-chains (comprising about 60% of cases) as well as mutations in spectrin β-chains, glycophorin C, and protein 4.1 genes (see **t7.2**). Defects in protein 4.1 account for about 20%-30% of HE in Caucasians and gives rise to asymptomatic disease with numerous long elliptocytes. The genetic defects associated with HE include point

t7.2 Heterogeneity in Hereditary Elliptocytosis and Hereditary Poikilocytosis

Protein defect	Red cell features	Clinical presentations	Inheritance
Spectrin α-chain binding site	Elliptocytes with variable poikilocytosis and cell fragments	Most common, variable hemolysis dependent on mutation	Usually autosomal dominant
Protein 4.1 deficiency	Smooth elongated elliptocytes with few poikilocytes	Caucasian patients, often asymptomatic	Autosomal dominant
Spectrin β-chain binding site	Elliptocytes that may appear rounder, may have increased spherocytes	Rare, usually mild hemolysis	Autosomal dominant

mutations, gene deletions, gene insertions and mRNA processing defects, all of which lead to mechanical weakness of the red blood cell cytoskeletal structure. This weakness leads to an inability of the red blood cell to tolerate shear stress and makes the cells more likely to undergo permanent deformation to an elliptocyte or fragmentation to form poikilocytes. HE is usually inherited as an autosomal dominant trait.

Creating part of the disease spectrum in HE is hereditary poikilocytosis (HP), representing the extreme range of HE that is often highly symptomatic with significant hemolysis. The mutations that give rise to HP are the same as seen in HE, but represent more severe impairment of the red blood cell cytoskeleton leading to increased red blood cell fragmentation. Patients will have elliptocytes as well as increased numbers of poikilocytes (and in severe cases, almost all poikilocytes), due to a loss of red blood cell elasticity.

7.2 Clinical Findings

The chronic hemolytic state in HS varies widely in severity, ranging from an asymptomatic compensated hemolysis to a moderately severe chronic anemia (see **t7.1**, **t7.3**). Approximately one-third of patients have mild disease, about 60% have moderate disease and 10% or less have moderately severe to severe HS. The age at which the diagnosis is made usually reflects the severity of the hemolytic process, with the more severe forms of the disease being diagnosed in early childhood. Clinical manifestations usually are first noted in children or adolescents. Typical

t7.3 Laboratory Features of Hereditary Spherocytosis
Blood
RBC
Variable normochromic, normocytic anemia (9-15 g/dL)
Variably increased reticulocytes
MCV lower than expected for number of reticulocytes
MCHC increased
Spherocytes present
WBC
Normal
Platelets
Normal
Bone Marrow
Variable cellularity (normocellular to hypercellular)
Variable erythroid hyperplasia
Laboratory
Evidence of hemolysis
Increased LDH
Elevated direct bilirubin
Specific testing
Increased osmotic fragility
Decreased fluorescence intensity for eosin-maleimide by flow cytometry

LDH = lactate dehydrogenase; MCHC = mean corpuscular hemoglobin concentration; MCV = mean corpuscular volume; RBC= red blood cell; WBC = white blood cell

complaints include mild jaundice and non-specific manifestations of anemia, such as weakness. Because of an increased bilirubin turnover, patients with this condition have a high incidence of gallstones or biliary obstruction. Usually patients can maintain normal hemoglobin levels owing to increased red blood cell production by the bone marrow. However, infection or other stress may lead to acute anemic episodes due to increased splenic activity (hemolytic crisis) or decreased bone marrow production (aplastic crisis). The most consistently positive physical finding is splenomegaly, which may be marked. Variable degrees of jaundice and scleral icterus are frequently seen. A therapeutically important feature of HS is the clinical cure of hemolytic anemia by splenectomy. The red blood cell life span after this procedure is usually restored to normal or near normal.

HE may present either as a primary cosmetic disorder with little or no hemolysis or, much more rarely, with a moderately severe hemolytic anemia (see **t7.2**). Patients with the usual form of HE have no anemia or splenomegaly. The hemolytic forms of the disease, comprising about 10% of cases, may have splenomegaly and often show spherocytes, fragmented red blood cells, and numerous poikilocytes in addition to elliptocytes. In some cases poikilocytes are the predominant red blood cell form seen in the blood smear, leading to classification as HP.

7.3 Diagnostic Approach

A diagnosis of HS should be suspected in patients with chronic hemolytic anemia, especially when spherocytes are seen in the peripheral blood smear f7.1. Because of the common autosomal dominant inheritance pattern of the disorder, family studies are important. Sometimes examination of the blood of family members reveals spherocytosis, even when there is no history of anemia, jaundice, or gallstones. This reflects the clinical spectrum of disease observed in HS, with variable hemolysis and symptomatology in the affected individuals. On rare occasions, the disorder may arise as a new mutation without a positive family history or be inherited in an autosomal recessive pattern. Since autoimmune hemolytic anemia may also have significant numbers of spherocytes in the blood smear, it must be excluded by appropriate testing (such as direct antiglobulin testing).

Splenectomy usually abolishes the hemolysis in HS. If significant hemolysis persists after splenectomy in a patient presumed to have HS, the presumptive diagnosis is incorrect, there is incomplete removal of splenic tissue or the patient may have one of the rarer forms that are not responsive to splenectomy (such as protein 4.2 mutation). Evaluation of a patient presumed to have HS includes the following:

1. Evaluation of the peripheral blood smear with attention to red blood cell morphology to identify the presence of spherocytes. A complete blood count (CBC) to determine the mean corpuscular hemoglobin concentration (MCHC), and the reticulocyte count should be performed.
2. An osmotic fragility test (see Test 7.5.1) or flow cytometric testing using eosin-5-maleimide staining (see Test 7.5.2) to confirm the presence of spherocytes. In most cases an osmotic fragility test will provide adequate information for diagnosis. When the osmotic fragility test is indeterminant or there is concern about the presence of spherocytes from another process, such as autoimmune hemolytic anemia, flow cytometry may provide more specific information. The flow cytometry testing is a specialized test that is offered in limited reference laboratories.
3. A direct antiglobulin test (see Test 6.5.4) may be performed to rule out autoimmune hemolytic anemia as a cause for spherocytosis.

4. If the diagnosis is uncertain, studies of red blood cell glycolytic or hexose monophosphate shunt enzyme activities (see Chapters 8 and 9) to rule out enzymatic disorders (usually non-spherocytic hemolytic anemia) may be performed.
5. In very unusual cases, additional testing for red cell membrane protein composition by radioimmunoassay, enzyme-linked immunoabsorbent assays (ELISA), or gel electrophoresis analysis for specific quantification of membrane cytoskeletal proteins may be performed. In most cases this type of testing is done for research purposes only and is not required for diagnosis or clinical management. This testing requires a specialty research laboratory.

Elliptocytes are readily identified on the stained blood smear i7.2. Because this generally represents a benign anomaly, clinically significant HE should only be considered as the cause of anemia when evidence for hemolysis, such as an elevated reticulocyte count, is found. Patients with significant anemia often have HP with increased numbers of pokilocytes in the blood smear.

7.4 Hematologic Findings

7.4.1 Blood Cell Measurements

Hemoglobin levels in patients with HS and HP frequently range between 9 and 15 g/dL (90 and 150 g/L) (see **t7.3**), and the mean corpuscular volume (MCV) is usually normal but may be elevated in the presence of prominent reticulocytosis. Hemoglobin levels in HE may be normal or slightly decreased. The MCHC in HS is characteristically elevated as high as 37 g/dL (370 g/L) (normal, 26 to 34 g/dL [260 to 340 g/L]), due to membrane loss without attendant loss of cellular hemoglobin. The reticulocyte count usually ranges between 5% and 15% (0.05 and 0.15). The degree of reticulocytosis in HS is characteristically greater than that in other types of hemolytic anemia with similar hemoglobin levels.

7.4.2 Peripheral Blood Smear Morphology

The central morphologic finding in HS is the presence of spherocytes on the peripheral blood smear. Spherocytes appear as densely staining red blood cells that are slightly smaller than normal with an absence of central pallor (i7.1). The increased intensity of staining is partially caused by increased cellular thickness due to the spherical shape and the increased MCHC. In mild forms of the disease, spherocytes may not be present in large numbers. The appearance of red blood cells varies in different parts of the blood smear. Improper technique in preparing the smear or looking in an area of the blood film at the edge where the blood is spread too thinly may result in artifactual spherocytes that may be over-interpreted by an inexperienced observer (see i7.3). Care should be taken to look for spherocytes in an appropriately thick area of the blood smear. Prominent macrocytosis and polychromasia may be present in association with very high reticulocyte counts.

Elliptocytosis is diagnosed when most or all of the cells on the smear have an oval shape with a long diameter that is two or more times the short diameter (see i7.2), although some cases may have relatively few elliptocytes. Other causes of elliptocytosis including iron deficiency anemia, megaloblastic anemia, or myelodysplasia should be excluded. HE and HP will have variable numbers of poikilocytes or irregularly shaped or fragmented cells admixed with the elliptocytes, and one form of HE may have prominent numbers of spherocytes present.

i7.1 Hereditary spherocytosis

Numerous densely staining spherocytes lacking central pallor are present (arrows). *(Wright stain)*

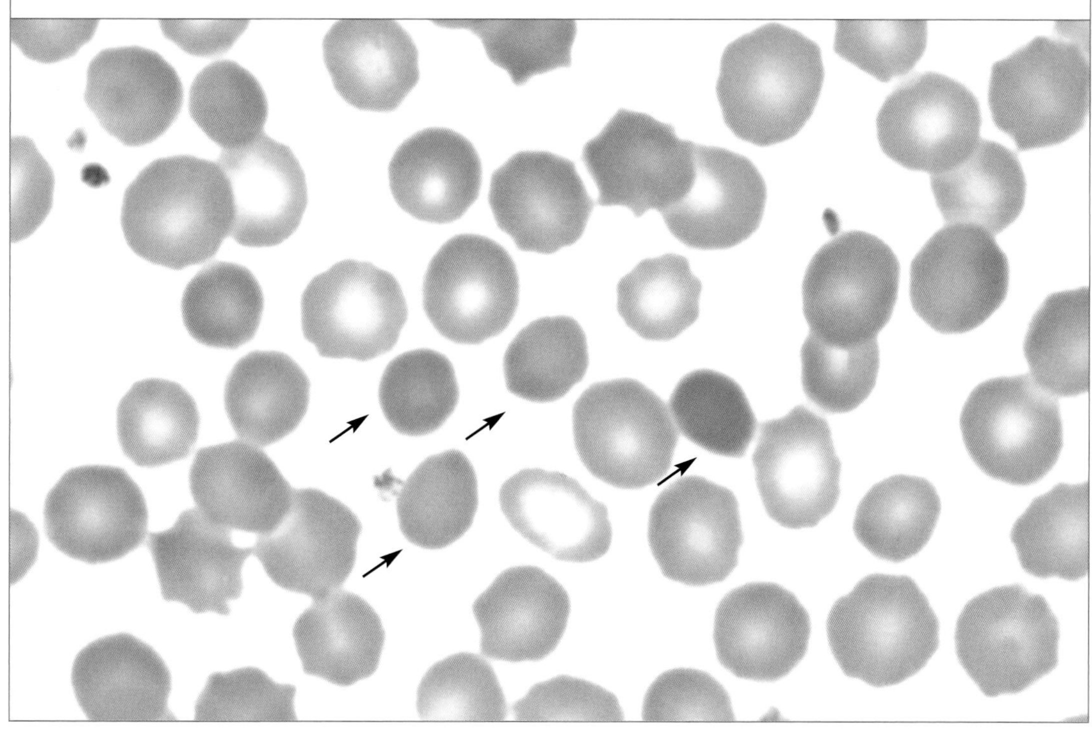

i7.2 Hereditary elliptocytosis

Hereditary elliptocytosis. *(Wright stain)*

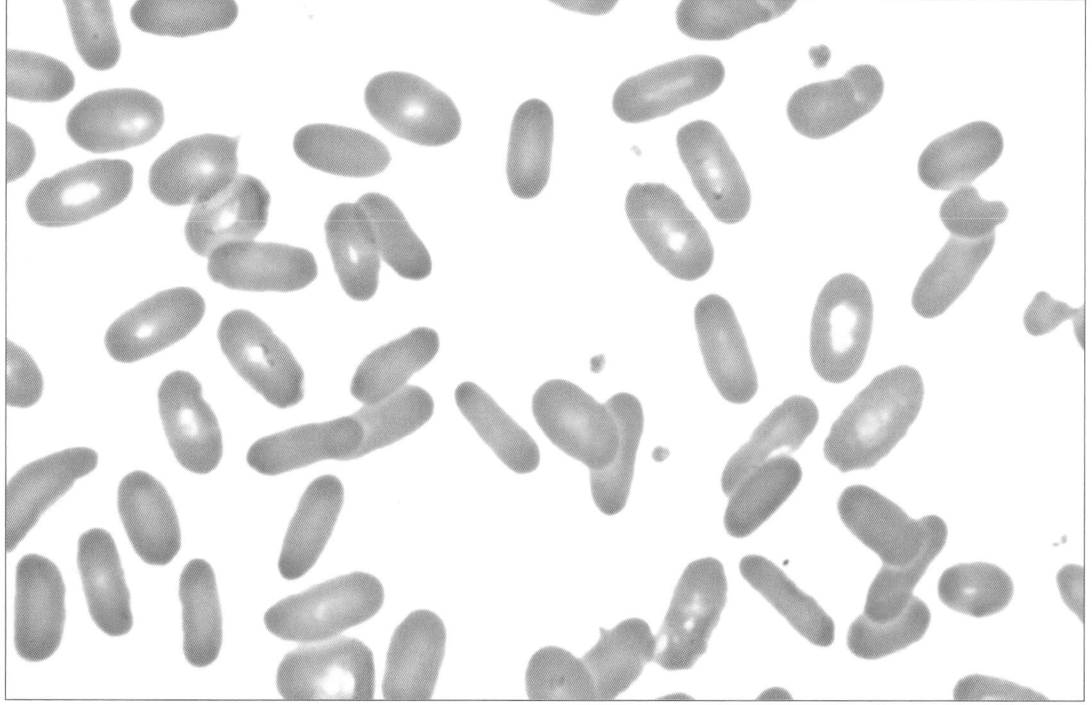

i7.3 Artifact

Artifactual spherocytes seen in area of the blood film that is too thinly distributed. *(Wright stain)*

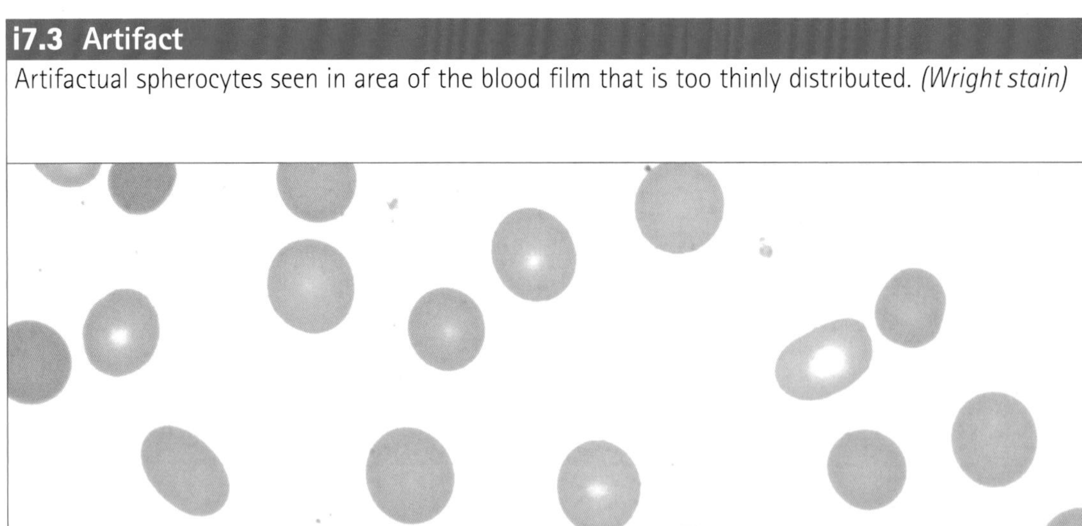

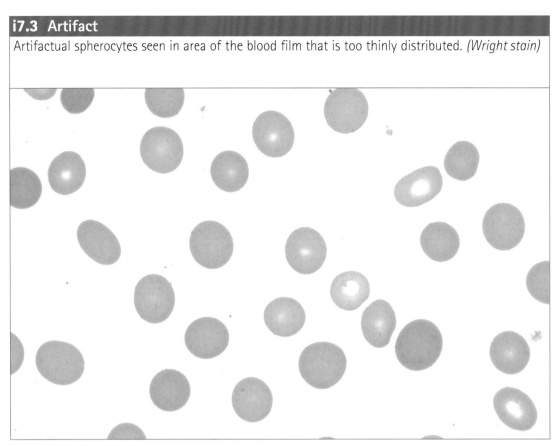

7.4.3 Bone Marrow Examination

The bone marrow characteristically shows normoblastic erythroid hyperplasia when significant hemolysis is occurring. Depending on the degree of stress on erythropoiesis to maintain the hematocrit, there may be variable degrees of dyserythropoiesis seen. The dyserythropoiesis may be exacerbated if there is insufficient intake of nutrients (including iron, folate, and B_{12}) to support the increased requirements of hematopoiesis. During aplastic crises, erythroid precursors are diminished and evidence of viral infection, such as parvovirus B19 inclusions, may be seen.

7.5 Other Laboratory Tests

Test 7.5.1 Osmotic Fragility Test

Purpose. The osmotic fragility test indirectly measures the presence of spherocytes.

Principle. This test measures the ability of the red blood cell to swell, a property that reflects the cellular surface-to-volume ratio. In a hypotonic medium, red blood cells take up water until the osmotic pressure inside the cell is reduced to that outside the cell. The red cell membrane normally has enough redundancy so the volume of the cell can increase to about 1.8 times the resting volume before reaching the critical hemolytic volume where further entry of water produces lysis. A cell that is spherocytic in the resting state has less membrane redundancy than a normal biconcave cell, so less water can enter before cellular rupture occurs.

Specimen. Blood freshly drawn into heparin or ethylenediaminetetraacetic acid (EDTA) is used. Samples older than 48 hours may show an artifactual shift toward increased fragility.

Procedure. The osmotic fragility test is performed by adding small volumes of blood to a series of tubes containing buffered salt solutions with an osmolarity equivalent to that of a 0.2% to 0.9% sodium chloride (NaCl) solution. A control tube contains distilled water. After standing at room temperature for 1 hour, the tubes are centrifuged, and the percentage of hemolyzed cells is estimated by measuring the amount of hemoglobin released into the supernatant solution by absorbance at 540 nm.

t7.4 Normal Values for Osmotic Fragility Tests

	Lysis (%)	
NaCl (%)	**Fresh**	**Incubated**
0.20	97-100	95-100
0.30	97-100	85-100
0.35	90-99	75-100
0.40	50-90	65-100
0.45	5-45	55-95
0.50	0-5	40-85
0.55	0	15-70
0.60	0	0-40
0.65	0	0-10
0.70	0	0-5
0.75	0	0

NaCl = sodium chloride

Testing should be carried out on freshly drawn blood and, if necessary, on blood that has been incubated at 37°C for 24 hours. Incubated osmotic fragility tests are more sensitive for detecting low levels of hemolysis. This may be useful when hereditary spherocytosis is suspected clinically but the levels of hemolysis seen with fresh blood are within normal ranges. However, the increase in sensitivity for detection of osmotic fragility is offset by a loss of specificity in the incubated test.

Interpretation. The normal range of values for the osmotic fragility test is seen in **t7.4** and **f7.2**. Increased osmotic fragility is an essential diagnostic feature of hereditary spherocytosis. In mild

f7.2 Osmotic fragility testing

Osmotic fragility of normal RBCs and those from a patient with hereditary spherocytosis. Normal areas are shown in the shaded areas for fresh RBCs (**a** and **b**) and for RBCs incubated at 37°C for 24 hours (**c** and **d**). The hemolysis curve for control or normal RBCs is shown in panels **a** and **c**. The hemolysis curve for a patient with hereditary spherocytosis is represented in panels **b** and **c**.

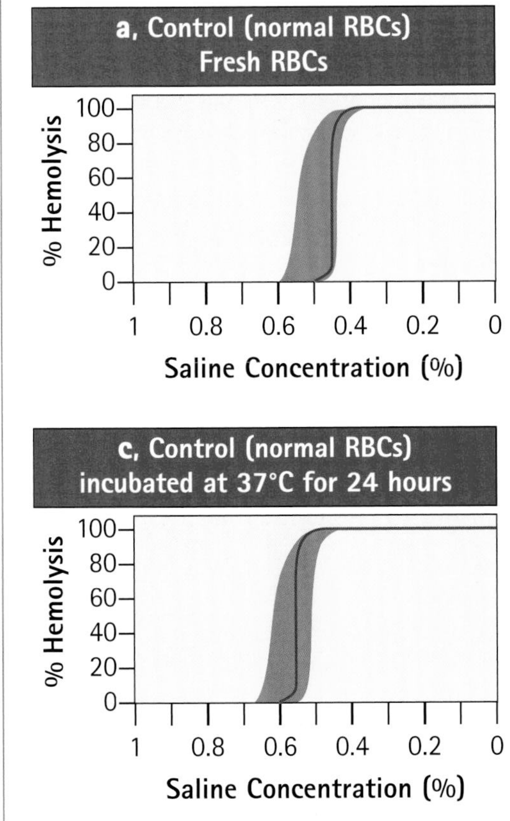

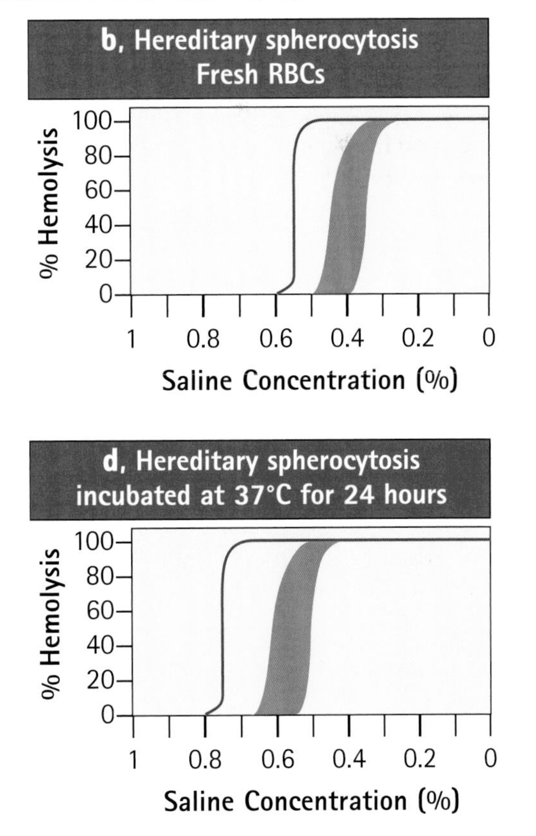

forms of the disease, it is common to find only a minimal increase in osmotic fragility on freshly drawn blood; however, incubated osmotic fragility tests are almost always abnormal in such cases. Decreases in hemolysis or decreased osmotic fragility are seen in thalassemia, iron deficiency, and other conditions where there is an increase in the surface area-to-volume ratio for the red blood cell.

Notes and Precautions. Because increased osmotic fragility merely reflects the presence of spherocytes, this finding does not distinguish HS from autoimmune hemolytic disease with spherocytosis, in which the osmotic fragility of red blood cells is also increased, although usually to a lesser degree. Reporting osmotic fragility as percent saline concentrations for beginning and completion of hemolysis is an inadequate representation of test results. Osmotic fragility is best appreciated when reported graphically (see f7.2).

Test 7.5.2 Flow Cytometric Detection of Band 3 Staining

Principle. This test studies the levels of the AE1 (band 3) protein utilizing flow cytometry methods. The AE1 protein is an essential component of the red blood cell cytoskeleton that is decreased in spherocytes. AE1 binds the fluorescent dye eosin-maleimide (EMA) at a protein site in an extracellular loop domain at a lysine-430 residue. The EMA dye emits a fluorescent signal that may be detected using the green fluorescence channel. Gating on the red blood cell population using single channel data collection, the mean fluorescence intensity is determined for 15,000-20,000 events and compared to normal controls.

Purpose. This test detects most cases of HS as defects in any of the cytoskeletal proteins (including spectrin and ankyrin) leads to a relative decrease in levels of AE1 and decreased fluorescence.

Specimen. 5.0 mL of freshly drawn blood in ethylenediaminetetraacetic acid (EDTA) must be tested within 72 hours of collection. The procedure is appropriate for testing of neonates and children due to small blood volumes required for testing.

Procedure. The red blood cells are washed and 5 µL of washed packed red blood cells are incubated with 25 µL of eosin-5-maleimide (0.5 mg/mL in phosphate buffered saline) for 1 hour in the dark. The cells are centrifuged and unbound dye removed, followed by three washes in phosphate buffered saline containing 0.5% bovine serum albumin (PBS/BSA). The cell suspension is resuspended into 500 µL, and a 100 µL aliquot of this suspension is diluted into 1.4 mLs of PBS/BSA. This suspension is analyzed by flow cytometry using the green fluorescence channel and gating on the red blood cell population. Control samples of normal blood are run at the same time as patient samples for comparison.

Interpretation. Patients with HS will show a decrease of mean fluorescence intensity compared to normal controls, forming a second peak at lower mean channel fluorescence. The test is highly specific for HS, and spherocytes in patients with other forms of hemolytic anemia will not have a significant decrease in fluorescence intensity. Patients with HE will have fluorescent intensities in the normal range, although some patients with a significant spherocytic component and HE, or patients with HP may have decreased fluorescence with this test. The test is very specific and sensitive, and may be useful in mild cases of HS where osmotic fragility testing is not conclusive. Note that decreases in mean channel fluorescence are not correlated with clinical severity.

Notes and Precautions. Recent transfusions may impact the interpretation by shifting the mean channel fluorescence towards normal values. Patients with iron deficiency may have a higher than expected mean channel fluorescence for the size of the cell. Macrocytosis (including significant reticulocytosis) will demonstrate an increase in mean fluorescence intensity that may impact on interpretation (forming broad normal red cell peaks). Patients on oral contraceptives or H2 blockers may have interference with the dye binding. Patients with mean fluorescence values that are indeterminant (falling between normal and definitely decreased) may require ELISA, radioimmunoassay, or electrophoretic analysis of red blood cell membrane proteins if HS is still suspected clinically, although this would be a very rare situation with combination of osmotic fragility and flow cytometric approaches.

7.6 Course and Treatment

Both HS and HE/HP have symptoms dependent on the degree of hemolysis caused by the alterations in the red blood cell cytoskeletal stability that impact on the maintenance of the red blood cell shape. Although hemolysis may be severe in some cases, many patients have a benign clinical course, particularly following splenectomy in cases with significant hemolysis. Complications that may occur include the development of cholelithiasis and cholecystitis and the occurrence of aplastic or hemolytic crises, particularly after viral infection. Splenectomy prolongs red blood cell survival in HS and hemolytic forms of HE or HP. However, this procedure may not be required if the bone marrow can adequately compensate for the anemia by increasing red blood cell production.

7.7 References

An X, Mohandas N. Disorders of red cell membrane. *Br J Haematol.* 2008;141:367-375.

Bennett V, Healy J. Organizing the fluid membrane bilayer: diseases linked to spectrin and ankyrin. *Trends Mol Med.* 2008;14:28-36.

Ebner S, Lux SE. Hereditary spherocytosis-defects in proteins that connect the membrane skeleton to the lipid bilayer. *Semin Hematol.* 2004;41:118-141.

Gallagher PG. Update on the clinical spectrum and genetics of red cell membrane disorders. *Curr Hematol Rep.* 2004;3:85-91.

Gallagher PG. Hereditary elliptocytosis: spectrin and protein 4.1. *Semin Hematol.* 2004;41:142-164.

Gallagher PG, Glader B. Hereditary spherocytosis, hereditary elliptocytosis, and other disorders associated with abnormalities of the erythrocyte membrane in: Greer JP, Foerster J, Rodger GM, et al eds. *Wintrobe's Clinical Hematology. 12th ed.* Philadelphia: Lippincott Williams & Wilkins; 2009:911-932.

Iolascon A, Perrotta S. Stewart GW. Red cell membrane defects. *Rev Clin Exp Hematol.* 2003;7:22-56.

King MJ, Smythe JS, Mushens R. Eosin-t-maleimide binding to band 3 and Rh-related proteins forms the basis of a screening test for hereditary spherocytosis. *Br J Haematol.* 2004;124:206-213.

Miraglia del Guidice E, Nobili B, Francese M. et al. Clinical and molecular evaluation of non-dominant hereditary spherocytosis. *Br J Haematol.* 2001;112:42-47.

Tracy ET, Rice HE. Partial splenectomy for hereditary spherocytosis. Pediatr Clin North Am. 2008;55:503-519.

Williamson RC, Toye AM. Glycophorin A: Band 3 aid. *Blood Cells Mol Dis.* 2008;41:35-43.

Chapter 8

Hereditary Erythrocyte Disorders Due to Deficiencies of the Glycolytic Pathway

Sherrie Perkins, MD, PhD

Mature red blood cells, lacking in mitochondria, have the capacity for a limited number of enzymatic reactions. In order to maintain both functional and structural integrity, most red blood cell energy requirements are met by metabolism of glucose to lactate via the glycolytic, or Embden-Meyerhof, pathway with subsequent production of adenosine triphosphate (ATP). Hereditary deficiencies of some of the glycolytic enzymes have been documented, and several of these deficiencies predominantly cause a congenital non-spherocytic hemolytic anemia (CNSHA), whereas others cause multisystemic disease in addition to non-spherocytic hemolytic anemia. Most glycolytic pathway enzymatic deficiencies are rare, with less than a hundred to a few hundred cases documented in the literature for any specific enzyme.

8.1 Pathophysiology

Glucose is the main metabolic substrate of red blood cells. Because the mature erythrocyte does not contain mitochondria, it must depend entirely on anaerobic glycolysis to produce energy. About 90% of glucose metabolism occurs by way of the main glycolytic pathway (Embden-Meyerhof pathway), in which glucose is metabolized to lactate by a series of enzymatic reactions that give rise to adenosine triphosphate (ATP) and reduced nicotinamide-adenine dinucleotide (NADH) **f8.1**. There is a net generation of 2 moles of ATP for each mole of glucose that is metabolized. ATP is essential to cellular function, allowing active cationic transport across the cellular membrane and membrane protein phosphorylation. One mole of NADH is generated, that is required for methemoglobin reduction reactions. 2,3-Diphosphoglycerate (2,3-DPG), which alters the hemoglobin oxygen affinity and regulates oxygen delivery to tissues, is another important intermediate formed during glycolysis.

The remaining 10% of glucose is metabolized via the hexose monophosphate (HMP) shunt, bypassing the early steps of the main glycolytic pathway and generating reduced nicotinamide adenine dinucleotide phosphate (NADPH). This coenzyme is required for reduction of glutathione, which protects hemoglobin and red blood cell enzymes from oxidative damage (see Chapter 9).

Deficiencies in glycolytic pathway enzymes give rise to congenital non-spherocytic hemolytic anemia (CNSHA), which is first observed during infancy or childhood, lacks significant numbers of spherocytes, and exhibits normal osmotic fragility. CNSHA may result from a heterogeneous group of disorders; however the most clinically important disorders are the glycolytic pathway enzyme deficiencies **t8.1**. The exact cause of hemolysis in glycolytic defects is unknown; however, it is postulated to be secondary to abnormal membrane function and

f8.1 Glycolytic pathway

The glycolytic pathway (Embden-Meyerhof pathway). The enzymes in which a deficiency may lead to a hereditary non-spherocytic hemolytic anemia are shown in magenta.

ADP = adenosine diphosphate; ATP = adenosine triphosphate; G6PD = glucose-6-phosphate dehydrogenase; NAD = nicotinamide-adenine dinucleotide; NADH = reduced form of NAD

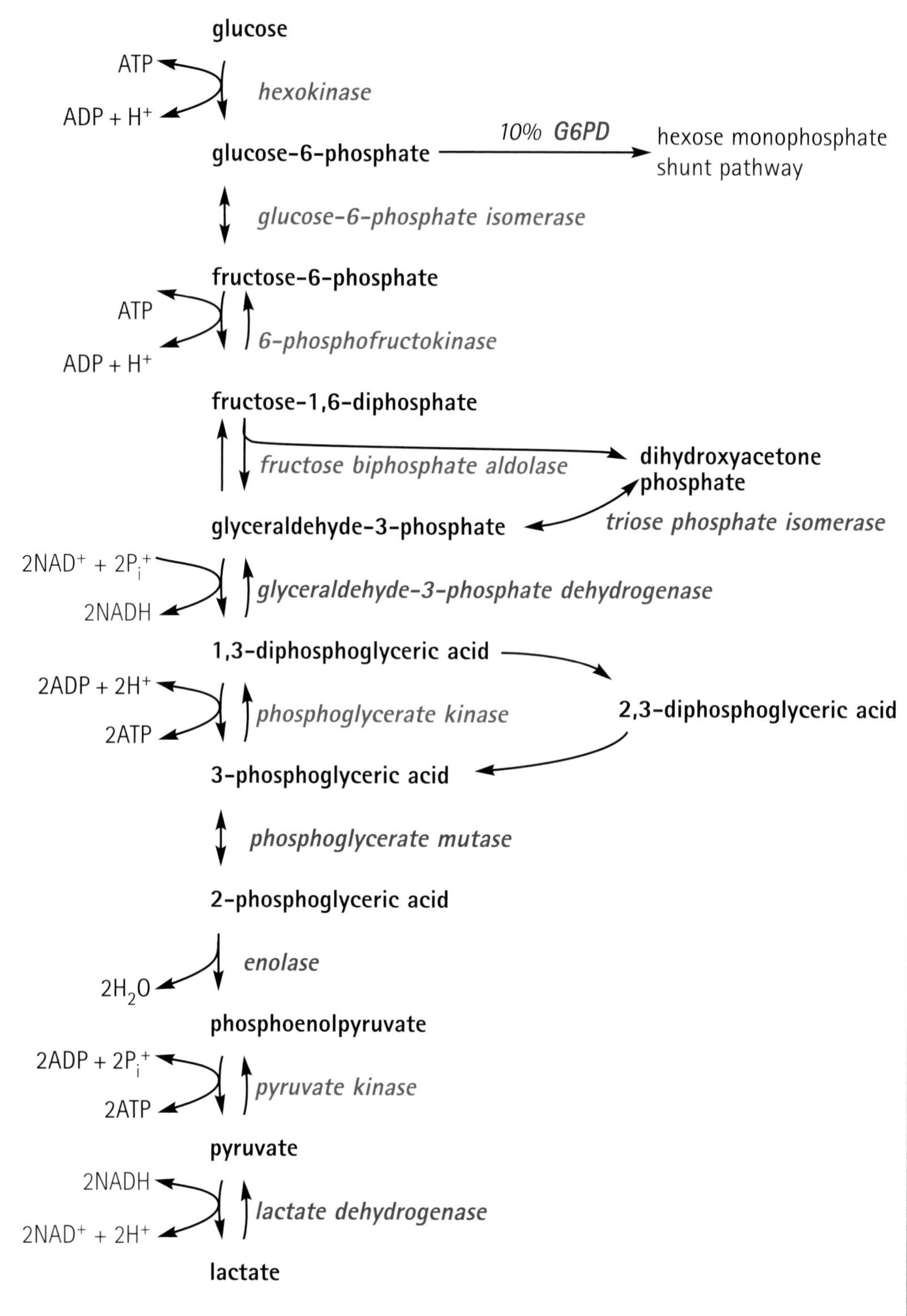

t8.1 Red Blood Cell Glycolytic Pathway Enzyme Deficiencies Associated with Hemolysis

Glycolytic enzymes	Clinical	Inheritance	Frequency
Hexokinase	CNSHA	Autosomal recessive	<100 cases reported
Glucose-6-isomerase	CNSHA, rare myopathy and neuropathy, recurrent infections. May have fetal hydrops	Autosomal recessive	~100 cases reported
Phosphofructokinase	CNSHA, may have glycogen storage, muscle disorder, myoglobinuria	Autosomal recessive	<100 cases reported
Aldolase	CNSHA and liver glycogen storage defect	Autosomal recessive	<10 cases reported
Triosephosphate isomerase	CNSHA and severe neuromuscular disease, recurrent infections	Autosomal recessive	<100 cases reported
Phosphoglucerate kinase	CNSHA, myoglobinuria, behavioral abnormalities	X-linked	<100 cases reported
Diphosphoglycerate mutase	CNSHA, polycythemia	Autosomal recessive	<100 cases reported
Pyruvate kinase	CNSHA, may have fetal hydrops	Autosomal recessive, rarely autosomal dominant	~500 cases reported

CNSHA = congenital non-spherocytic hemolytic anemia

development of irreversible membrane damage. Because reticulocytes retain some mitochondria, they are relatively resistant to hemolysis. Depending on the intracellular levels of ATP, RBC life span may range from near normal to markedly shortened. Other observed causes of CNSHA that should be considered in the differential diagnosis include unstable hemoglobins as well as disorders of the enzymes of the HMP shunt and glutathione metabolism **t8.2**.

t8.2 Defects Associated With Congenital Nonspherocytic Hemolytic Anemia (CNSHA)

Enzymatic deficiencies
- Glycolytic pathway: most common
- Hexose monophosphate shunt pathway: rare variants
- Glutathione pathway: rare variants
- Hemoglobinopathies

Unstable hemoglobins

Deficiencies in red blood cell enzymes may arise from different genetic changes that can decrease or change the properties of the enzyme. Usually this results in the accumulation of metabolites proximal to the enzyme and depletion of distal intermediates. However, as many of the intermediate metabolites from the glycolytic pathway act as secondary regulators of enzymatic activity, studies of pathway intermediate metabolite concentrations may be difficult to interpret when attempting to define a specific abnormality. Often screening for metabolites (ATP or NADH) is more useful as screening tests.

Most of the defects are associated with mutations that are specific to a particular patient or family and include genetic deletions, insertions or substitutions giving rise to missense or nonsense mutations in a variety of different coding exons for a specific enzymatic gene. This wide diversity of genetic changes makes development of specific genetic screening tests difficult. Most of the described abnormalities arise from a single or limited base pair substitutions.

The genetic changes may affect enzymatic synthesis, enzyme stability, or activity. A wide array of clinical manifestations observed with these disorders probably arises due to the wide variety of defects and their associated spectrum of impact on enzymatic function.

8.2 Clinical Findings

Nearly all deficiencies of the glycolytic pathway are extremely rare (see **t8.1**). Pyruvate kinase deficiency, although seen infrequently, is the most prevalent, accounting for about 90% of cases of glycolytic pathway deficiency-associated CNSHA. Pyruvate kinase and most other glycolytic pathway deficiencies are most often inherited as autosomal recessive traits. Thus, a patient must be homozygous for the trait to be fully expressed. An exception to the autosomal recessive inheritance pattern is phosphoglycerate kinase (PGK) deficiency, which is inherited as an X-linked disorder (see **t8.1**).

Pyruvate kinase or other glycolytic pathway deficiencies usually are first detected in infancy or later in childhood because of chronic anemia, jaundice, development of pigment gallstones, and slight to moderate splenomegaly due to red blood cell sequestration. The severity of the anemia and other clinical manifestations is widely variable. Often hemolysis is worsened by infection or other stresses. Severely affected individuals are often jaundiced and anemic at birth, requiring repeated transfusions. In some cases of pyruvate kinase or glucose-6-isomerase deficiency, the hemolytic anemia may be so severe during fetal development as to give rise to fetal hydrops. Individuals affected to a lesser degree may have mild to moderate hemolysis that may or may not require transfusions. Patients are susceptible to hemolytic crises secondary to increased red blood cell turnover during infections, leading to worsening of their anemia. Similarly, anemia may be temporarily worsened due to an aplastic crisis when viruses, such as parvovirus B19, inhibit erythropoiesis by infecting red blood cell precursors in the marrow.

Most cases of CNSHA manifest in childhood or infancy with anemia secondary to chronic hemolysis, often associated with splenomegaly, some degree of hyperbilirubinemia, and increased reticulocytes. In contrast to deficiencies of the HMP shunt, there is no association of anemia with drug ingestion or oxidative stress. Patients with phosphoglycerate kinase (PGK) deficiency may have CNSHA associated with behavioral or muscle abnormalities. Similarly, patients with glucose-6-isomerase or triosephosphate isomerase deficiency also may have neuromuscular disease-associated manifestations. Often patients with severe forms of these diseases die from neuromuscular dysfunction at an early age.

8.3 Diagnostic Approach

A CNSHA is often suspected when there is chronic hemolysis in a patient with normal red blood cell morphology and normal osmotic fragility testing. In the most frequently observed autosomal recessive forms of CNSHA, the family history is usually negative unless other siblings are affected. Biochemical studies of family members, however, reveal the hereditary nature of the disorder by demonstrating subnormal levels of an enzyme, although usually this deficit is not sufficient to cause significant anemia. A child or infant presenting with a chronic hemolytic anemia must first be evaluated for possible non-congenital causes. This usually involves a direct antiglobulin test (Coombs' test; see **Test 6.5.4**) to rule out an autoimmune hemolytic process and a sucrose lysis test (see **Test 11.5.1**) to rule out paroxysmal nocturnal hemoglobinuria.

If the anemia is thought to be a hereditary process, it is usually next classified as either a non-spherocytic or spherocytic process. This is usually accomplished by morphologic evaluation of the peripheral blood smear to look for spherocytes. An osmotic fragility test (see Test 7.5.1) will also help rule out hereditary spherocytosis. If the anemia is thought to be a CNSHA, hemoglobin electrophoresis (see Test 10.5.1) to rule out a hemoglobinopathy and an isopropanol stability test (see Test 10.5.9) to identify unstable hemoglobins may be performed. Finally, screening tests for deficiencies of specific red blood cell enzymes such as glucose-6-phosphate dehydrogenase (G6PD; see Tests 9.5.1 and 9.5.2) and pyruvate kinase (Test 8.5.1) may be performed, followed by appropriate quantitative RBC enzyme assays to determine the specific nature of the enzymatic defect.

8.4 Hematologic Findings

There are varying degrees of anemia, with hemoglobin levels ranging from 5-12 g/dL (50-120 g/L). Reticulocytosis proportional to the severity of the anemia is present (up to 25% or higher) but may be increased to more than 50% after splenectomy. Mean corpuscular volume (MCV) may be moderately increased when reticulocytosis is present. In most cases the morphologic characteristics of the red blood cells are unremarkable. Cells are normocytic and normochromic, but when there is extensive hemolysis, the increase in reticulocytes may give rise to red cell indices that are macrocytic with extensive polychromatophilia seen within the blood smear. Rare spicular and densely staining red blood cells or nucleated RBCs may be present, and are more commonly seen following splenectomy (see i8.1). Heinz bodies and spherocytes are notably absent.

i8.1 Severe pyruvate kinase deficiency

Blood smear in a patient with severe pyruvate kinase deficiency showing predominantly normochromic, normocytic cells with occasional spicular and densely staining cells reflecting red blood cell damage due to insufficient ability to meet red blood cell metabolic demands. The marked polychromasia reflects ongoing hemolysis. *(Wright stain)*

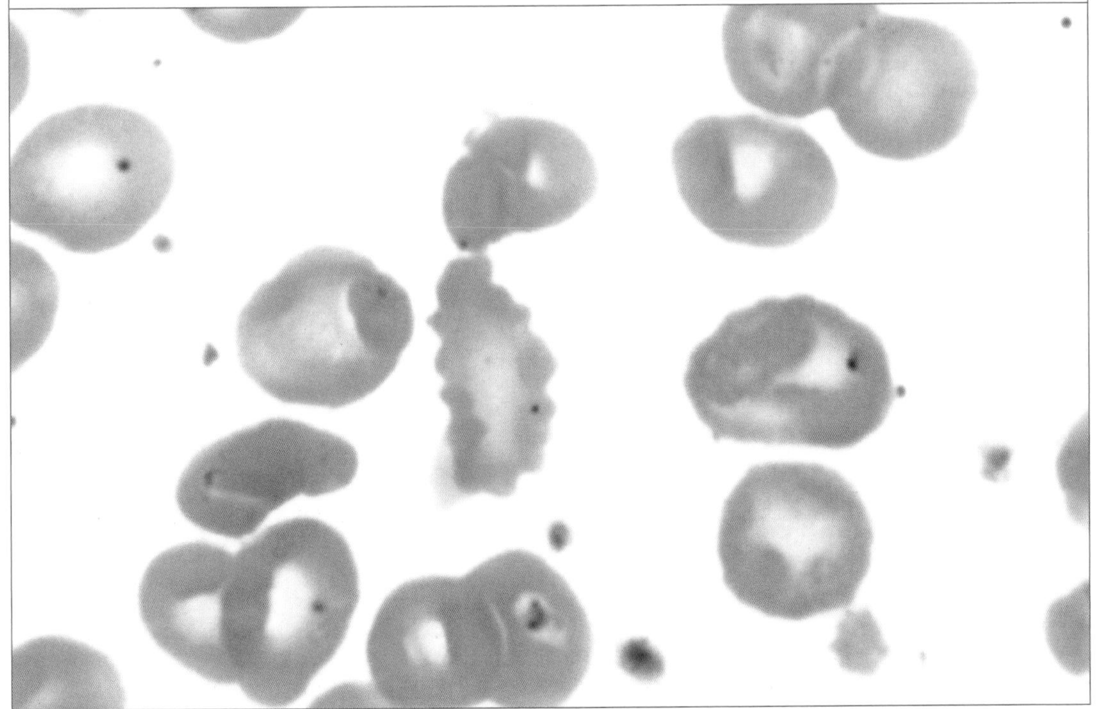

8.5 Other Laboratory Tests

Test 8.5.1 Fluorescent Screening Test for Pyruvate Kinase Deficiency

Purpose. Fluorescence of NADH acts as a useful screening test for the detection of RBC enzyme deficiencies. In practice, it is often enough to know whether the activity of the enzyme in question is markedly deficient. Slight deviations from normal are unlikely to be of clinical importance.

Principle. Reduced pyridine nucleotides (NADH) fluoresce when illuminated with long-wave ultraviolet light, whereas no fluorescence occurs with oxidized pyridine nucleotides, providing an indicator of enzymatic activity. Screening procedures are available for pyruvate kinase, glucose-phosphate isomerase, NADH diaphorase triosephosphate isomerase, and G6PD (see Chapter 9). Pyruvate kinase screening is the most common screening test for a glycolytic pathway deficiency.

Pyruvate kinase catalyzes the phosphorylation of adenosine diphosphate (ADP) to ATP by phosphoenolpyruvate (PEP). This reaction is coupled with the NADH-dependent conversion of pyruvate to lactate:

$$\text{phosphoenolpyruvate} + \text{ADP} + P_i^+ \xrightarrow{\textit{pyruvate kinase}} \text{pyruvate} + \text{ATP}$$

$$\text{pyruvate} + \text{NADH} + H^+ \xrightarrow{\textit{lactate dehydrogenase}} \text{lactate} + \text{NAD}^+$$

Because lactate dehydrogenase (LDH) is present in excess amounts when compared to pyruvate kinase, NAD^+ production is limited by pyruvate kinase levels. Thus, there should be a time-dependent loss of fluorescence as NADH is oxidized to NAD^+ when normal levels of pyruvate kinase activity are present.

Specimen. Whole blood collected in heparin or ethylenediaminetetraacetic acid (EDTA) is suitable for several days at 4°C and for about 1 day at room temperature.

Procedure. The blood sample is centrifuged; the plasma and buffy coat are aspirated. The red blood cell suspension is lysed in a buffered hypotonic screening solution. The screening mixture provides PEP, ADP, NADH, and magnesium chloride ($MgCl_2$). It is spotted on filter paper immediately after mixing and every 15 minutes thereafter. After the spots are thoroughly dry, the paper is examined under long-wave ultraviolet light. The patient's sample is compared with that of a healthy control subject.

Interpretation. The first spot should fluoresce brightly. With the normal sample, fluorescence disappears after 15 minutes of incubation. In contrast, in pyruvate kinase–deficient samples, fluorescence fails to disappear even after 45 or 60 minutes of incubation as there is no oxidation of the fluorescent NADH molecule.

Notes and Precautions. False-negative results may be observed if the patient has recently received a transfusion and large numbers of transfused cells containing normal levels of pyruvate kinase are still circulating. There may be little relationship between the severity of hemolysis and the measured level of pyruvate kinase activity to different stabilities of the pyruvate kinase variants or the degree of reticulocytes. Some patients with high reticulocyte counts may have normal screening tests.

Test 8.5.2 Red Blood Cell Enzyme Activity Assays

Purpose. Quantitative red blood cell enzyme assays give definitive confirmation of the results of screening tests and allow detection of heterozygotes for possible genetic counseling.

Principle. Most of the quantitative assays of RBC enzyme activity use spectrophotometric techniques that depend on the absorption of light of the reduced pyridine nucleotide, NADPH, or NADH at 340 nm. Reduction results in the formation of NADPH or NADH, with an increase in absorbance at 340 nm, and oxidation results in the formation of NADP or NAD with a decrease in absorbance. The change in absorbance may be used to calculate enzyme activity.

Specimen. Blood is collected in EDTA, heparin, or acid-citrate-dextrose (ACD). Most red blood cell enzymes are stable for several days at 4°C under these conditions. The blood should not be allowed to freeze, because washed red blood cells are used for the enzyme assays, and the stability of red blood cell enzymes is usually lower in hemolysates than in intact cells.

Procedure. The procedure for each enzyme measurement is different, and all procedures usually require specialized reference laboratories.

Interpretation. Interpretation differs for each enzyme. In general, only very severe enzyme deficiencies cause hemolytic anemia. Even relatively severe deficiencies of some enzymes, such as LDH, glutathione peroxidase, and inosine triphosphate, are without known clinical effect.

Test 8.5.3 Molecular Identification of Enzymatic Defects

Purpose. Molecular analysis provides definitive evidence of an enzymatic defect and may provide information useful in genetic counseling.

Principle. Analysis of DNA sequences may identify the specific molecular defect giving rise to an enzyme deficiency.

Specimen. Bone marrow is collected in heparin, and DNA is isolated for molecular detection of enzyme deficiencies. This methodology is best used for pyruvate kinase defects.

Procedure. DNA is analyzed by Southern blot testing and mutational analysis gels to identify structural mutations in the pyruvate kinase gene.

Interpretation. Pyruvate kinase is encoded for two genes that give rise to four distinct isoforms of the enzyme. More than 50 different mutations have been identified as causes of hemolytic anemia. Most are missense mutations that give rise to abnormal proteins. Some nonsense or splicing mutations also have been identified. The mutated DNA will demonstrate different electrophoreretic mobility than wild-type enzyme.

Notes and Precautions. The molecular tests for glycolytic pathway enzymopathies are highly specialized and require laboratories that have experience with this testing methodology and interpretation. Many are still considered investigational rather than diagnostic tools.

8.6 Ancillary Tests

Osmotic fragility testing (see **Test 7.5.1**) may serve as a useful screen for identifying hereditary spherocytosis and autoimmune hemolytic anemia with spherocytosis, whereas no increase in osmotic fragility is seen in CNSHA, helping to differentiate between these types of hemolytic anemia. The isopropanol stability test (see **Test 10.5.9**) is used to screen for and exclude unstable hemoglobins as a cause of CNSHA.

8.7 Course and Treatment

The course of red blood cell enzyme deficiency associated CNSHA varies widely. Severe pyruvate kinase deficiency may require splenectomy early in life; response to such treatment is variable. Other patients have a mild, benign course. Some severe cases may have unrelenting, transfusion-dependent anemia. In disorders with associated neuromuscular deficits, severely affected patients may die at an early age from the neuromuscular disease. Genetic counseling and prenatal diagnosis is possible for most defects.

8.8 References

Biachi P, Zanella A. Hematologically important mutations: red cell pyruvate kinase (third update). *Blood Cells Mol Dis.* 2000;47-53.

Fujii H, Miwa S. Red blood cell enzymes and their clinical application. *Adv Clin Chem.* 1998;33:1-54.

Glader B. Herditary hemolytic anemias due to red blood cell enzyme disorders. In: Greer JP, Foerster J, Rodger GM, et al eds. *Wintrobe's Clinical Hematology. 12th ed.* Philadelphia: Lippincott Williams & Wilkins; 2009: 933-955.

Jacobasch G, Rapoport SM. Hemolytic anemias due to erythrocyte enzyme deficiencies. *Mol Aspects Med.* 1996;17:143-170.

Larochelle A, Magny P, Tremblay S, et al. Erythropoiesis: pyruvate kinase deficiency which cause nonspherocytic hemolytic anemia–the gene and its mutations. *Hematology.* 1999;4:77-87.

Lakomek M, Winkler H. Erythrocytic pyruvate kinase and glucose phosphate isomerase deficiency: perturbation of glycolysis by structural defects and functional alterations of defective enzymes and its relation to the clinical severity of chronic hemolytic anemia. *Biophys Chem.* 1997;66:269-284.

Martinov MV, Plotnikov AG, Vitvitsk VM, et al. Deficiencies of glycolytic pathways as a possible cause of hemolytic anemia. *Biochim Biophys Acta.* 2000;1474:75-87.

McMullin MF. The molecular basis of disorders of red cell enzymes. *J Clin Pathol.* 1999;52:241-244.

Steiner LA, Gallagher PG. Erythrocyte disorders in the perinatal period. *Semin Perinatol.* 2007;31:254-261.

Tavazzi D, Taher A, Cappellini MD. Red blood cell enzyme disorders: an overview. *Pediatr Ann.* 2008;37:303-310.

Weatherall DJ. ABC of clinical hematology: the hereditary anaemias. *Br Med J.* 1997;314:492-496.

Chapter 9

Glucose-6-Phosphate Dehydrogenase Deficiency

Sherrie Perkins, MD, PhD

About 10% of the red blood cell's glucose is metabolized by the hexose monophosphate (HMP) oxidative shunt. This pathway protects the cell against oxidative injury and uses glutathione as an oxidation substrate to regenerate nicotinamideadenine dinucleotide phosphate (NADP) from its reduced form of NADPH. NADPH is an essential reducing agent in circulating red blood cells, allowing for detoxification of oxidated metabolic intermediates and maintenance of the red blood cell membrane. Glucose-6-phosphate dehydrogenase (G6PD) catalyzes the first step of the pathway. Deficiency of this enzyme is the most prevalent inborn metabolic disorder affecting red blood cells, afflicting more than 400 million people worldwide. Compared to other red blood cell enzymatic hemolytic anemias, most people with G6PD deficiency are not anemic and have minimal intrinsic hemolysis—hemolysis is only caused by exposure to extrinsic agents that induce oxidative damage to the red blood cell. Glutathione deficiency and mutations of the glutathione regeneration pathway are other, much more rare, causes of acute hemolytic anemia that are caused by oxidative damage to the red blood cell.

9.1 Pathophysiology

The HMP shunt produces NADPH by a series of enzymatic reactions that generate reducing equivalents f9.1. In turn, NADPH is used as a cofactor for glutathione reductase to regenerate oxidized glutathione (GS-SG) to reduced glutathione (GSH). Normally, red blood cells use GSH to bind and detoxify low levels of oxygen radicals that form spontaneously or as a result of drug administration. GSH also reduces oxidized sulfhydryl groups of hemoglobin, membrane proteins, or cellular enzymes. Red blood cells deficient in G6PD are unable to maintain sufficient levels of GSH, and thereby are at high risk for cellular oxidative damage by formation of reactive oxygen radicals or hydrogen peroxide. The ability to deal with oxidative stress leads to integral membrane damage and the accumulation of oxidized cellular products in the form of Heinz bodies. This will ultimately lead to premature red blood cell lysis in the spleen and possible hemolytic anemia. Most patients with G6PD deficiency have episodic hemolytic anemia induced by oxidative stress following infection or administration of specific drugs **t9.1**. A minority of patients may have a chronic non-spherocytic hemolytic anemia.

Deficiency of G6PD results from the inheritance of an abnormal G6PD gene located on the X chromosome, leading to a sex-linked inheritance pattern. Thus, the effect is fully expressed in affected men, who carry only one X chromosome, and inheritance is from the mother. In women, only one of the two X chromosomes in each cell is active. Consequently, women who are heterozygous for G6PD deficiency may have two populations of red blood cells: deficient and normal cells. The ratio of deficient to normal cells may vary greatly as a

f9.1 Hexose monophosphate shunt

The hexose monophosphate shunt and glutathione pathway. The enzyme glucose-6-phosphate dehydrogenase (G6PD) responsible for sex-linked inherited hemolytic anemia is shown in magenta.

G6PD = glucose-6-phosphate dehydrogenase; NADP = nicotinamide-adenine dinucleotide phosphate

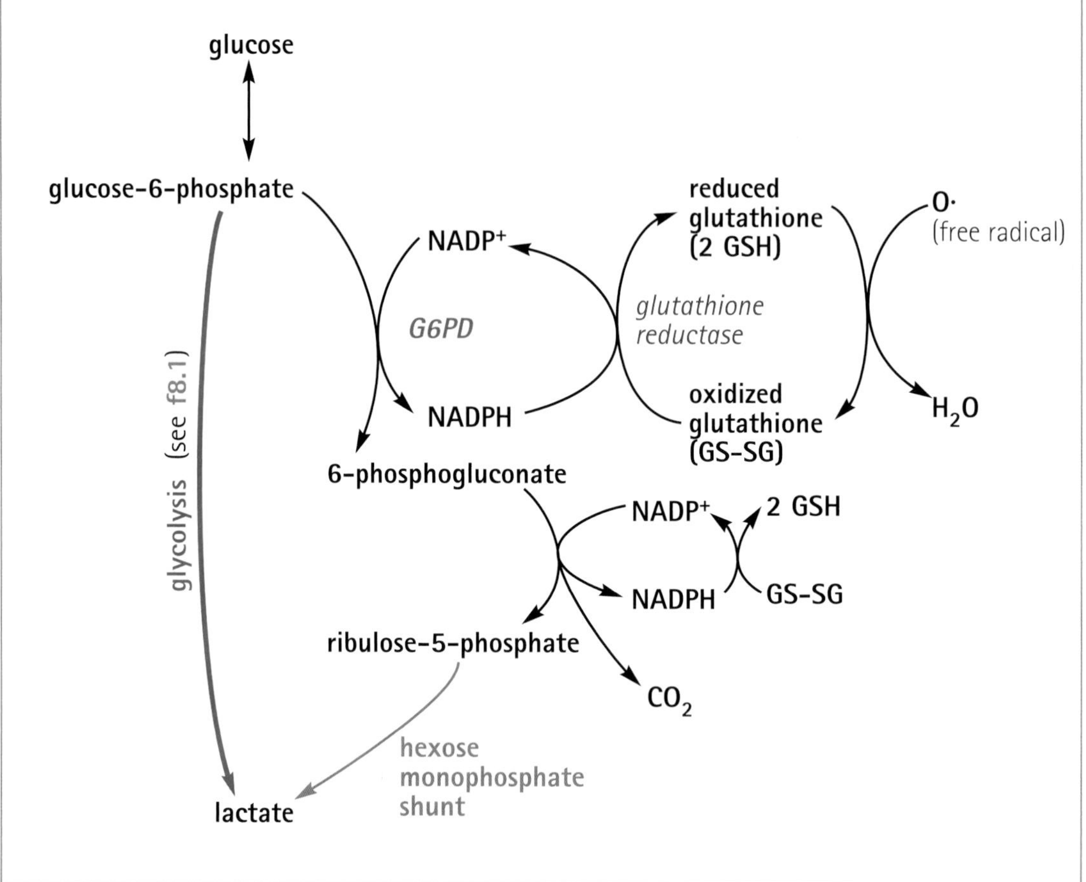

t9.1 Drugs Commonly Associated With Hemolysis in Glucose-6-Phosphate Dehydrogenase Deficiency

Antimalarial agents
Primaquine
Quinacrine

Sulfonamides
Sulfanilamide
Salicylazosulfapyridine
Sulfacetamide

Other antibacterial agents
Nitrofurantoin
Nitrofurazone
Para-aminosalicylic acid
Nalidixic acid

Analgesics
Acetanilid

Sulfones
Diaminodiphenyl sulfone
Thiazolsulfone

Miscellaneous agents
Dimercaprol
Naphthalene (mothballs)
Methylene blue
Trinitrotoluene (TNT)

result of the intrinsic variability of X-chromosome inactivation. Some women who are heterozygous for the disease appear to be completely healthy, whereas others are fully affected. More than 30 different G6PD mutations with variable clinical manifestations have been described.

Two main normal or wild type enzyme isotypes of G6PD, termed A and B, can be distinguished by their electrophoretic mobilities. The G6PD B isoform is the most common type of enzyme and is found in all population groups. The G6PD A isoform, found in about 20% of black men in the United States, migrates more rapidly on electrophoretic gels than does the normal B enzyme. However, both the A and B isoforms have full enzymatic activity and neither enzyme is associated with clinical disease. Mutations of the G6PD gene has led to identification of more than 400 other G6PD protein variants **t9.2**. Up to 11% of black men in the United States have a G6PD variant (G6PD A^-) that has the same electrophoretic mobility as G6PD A, but it is unstable, resulting in rapid enzyme degradation and resultant enzyme deficiency as the red blood cell ages. Thus, older circulating red blood cells from individuals with this variant may contain only 5% to 15% of the normal amount of enzymatic activity. G6PD A^- is the most common, clinically significant, type of G6PD deficiency among the U.S. black population. Other G6PD variants predominate in other racial groups. G6PD Mediterranean (G6PD^{MED}) is found frequently in Sicilians, Greeks, Sephardic Jews, and Arabs. Several other variants, such as G6PD^{CANTON} or G6PD^{MAHIDOL}, are common in Asian populations. The population distribution of G6PD deficiency reflects its probable origins in tropical and subtropical areas, and a possible selection for the mutation based on increased resistance to malarial infection.

t9.2 Common G6PD Variants

G6PD Variant	Association with Hemolysis	Population Distribution
G6PD A	No: normal variant	Blacks
G6PD B	No: normal variant	All
G6PD A^-	Yes: moderate	Blacks
G6PD^{MED}	Yes: severe	Whites
G6PD^{CANTON}	Yes: moderate	Asians
G6PD^{MAHIDOL}	Yes: moderate	Asians
G6PD^{IOWA}	Yes: severe, chronic	Sporadic mutation

G6PD = glucose-6-phosphate dehydrogenase

Mutational and biochemical analysis of G6PD variants have identified predominantly amino acid substitutions caused by substitutions of a single DNA base pair or small deletions. These mutations have wide ranging effects on enzymatic function with effects on enzymatic activity, synthesis, and structure. Even in severely deficient cells, some small amount of G6PD activity is present, suggesting that large deletions or nonsense mutations are probably incompatible with life. Most of the genetic abnormalities appear to lead to structural changes in the enzyme rather than changes in the overall amount of the enzyme synthesized, resulting in changes in catalytic activity, protein stability, or both. Most mutations appear to be sporadic, but there does appear to be genetic selection as similar mutations may be seen in divergent population groups.

Other enzyme deficiencies in the HMP shunt and glutathione metabolism are comparatively rare **t9.3**. Hereditary red blood cell GSH deficiency results from a lack of either of two enzymes of GSH synthesis: γ-glutamylcysteine synthetase or GSH synthetase. In some patients, the clinical manifestation of these deficiencies is similar to that of G6PD defi-

t9.3 Enzyme Deficiencies of Hexose Monophosphate Shunt Pathway Associated With Hemolytic Anemia

Enzyme Deficiency	Occurrence
G6PD	Common
γ-Glutamylcysteine synthetase	Rare
GSH synthetase	Rare
Glutathione reductase (total deficiency only)	Rare

G6PD = glucose-6-phosphate dehydrogenase; GSH = reduced glutathione

ciency with episodic hemolysis associated with oxidative stress, whereas other patients will present with a chronic hemolytic anemia. Dietary deficiencies of flavin adenine dinucleotide (FAD), which is a cofactor for glutathione reductase, may cause a decrease in enzymatic activity that mimics glutathione reductase deficiency but may be remedied by dietary manipulation. Actual glutathione reductase deficiency is rare and only total enzyme deficiency is associated with hemolytic anemia. Other HMP shunt deficiencies are rarely or never associated with hemolytic anemia.

9.2 Clinical Findings

All patients with G6PD deficiency have some degree of decreased red blood cell survival, although it is usually well compensated and many patients appear normal without significant anemia in the steady state. G6PD deficiency usually manifests as an episode of acute hemolytic anemia following infection or ingestion of an oxidant drug in an otherwise apparently healthy person. Hemolysis begins acutely in the case of infection or within 1 to 3 days after administration of an oxidant drug (**t9.1**) or ingestion of fava beans. Hemolysis is often severe, leading to plasma hemoglobinemia (pink to brown plasma), hemoglobinuria (dark or black urine), and jaundice. Rare patients may have a clinical picture of chronic hemolysis or be asymptomatic. Presentation as a congenital non-spherocytic hemolytic anemia (CNSHA) is rare, although G6PD deficiency is associated with neonatal jaundice without anemia in males, particularly in areas of Africa where there is high incidence of G6PD deficiency.

The length of the hemolytic episode and its severity depend on the degree of the stress as well as the G6PD variant **t9.4**. In patients with G6PD A^- deficiency, the hemolytic anemia

t9.4 Clinical Features of G6PD Variants

Clinical Feature	G6PD A^-	G6PD^{MED}	G6PD^{CANTON}
Drug-induced hemolysis	Common	Common	Common
Infection-induced hemolysis	Common	Common	Common
Favism	Not seen	Common	Not usually seen
Neonatal icterus	Rare	Observed	Observed
Hereditary non-spherocytic hemolytic anemia	Not seen	Occasionally	Not seen
Degree of anemia	Moderate	Severe	Moderate
Chronic hemolysis	Not seen	Not seen	Not seen

G6PD = glucose-6-phosphate dehydrogenase

is usually self-limited because the reticulocytes produced in response to hemolysis have nearly normal G6PD levels and are relatively resistant to hemolysis. In contrast, in other types of G6PD deficiency, such as G6PD^{MED}, where there are decreased levels of enzyme activity in all red blood cells (including reticulocytes), an oxidative stress may cause severe, prolonged hemolysis, requiring transfusion therapy.

Due to the polymorphic nature of the enzyme mutations and resultant effects on enzymatic activity, the World Health Organization (WHO) has classified different G6PD variants based on the degree of enzyme deficiency and severity of hemolysis or clinical features **t9.5**. Only the Class I, II, and III variant groups are clinically significant, with Classes II and III being most common and Class I disease (CNSHA) being very rare. Class IV and V disease groups have no significant clinical expression and are associated with normal to supranormal enzymatic activity levels.

t9.5 Clinical Classification of G6PD Deficiency

Class	Enzyme Levels	Clinical Presentation
I	Very severe deficiency (<10% normal)	Chronic hemolytic anemia
II	Severe deficiency	Intermittent hemolysis associated with drugs or infection
III	Moderate deficiency (10%-60% normal)	Intermittent hemolysis associated with drugs or infection
IV	Very mild or no enzyme deficiency	No hemolysis
V	Increased enzyme levels	No hemolysis

G6PD = glucose-6-phosphate dehydrogenase

9.3 Diagnostic Approach

The occurrence of episodic hemolysis suggests a hereditary deficiency of one of the HMP enzymes. Patients with the most common types of G6PD deficiency present with acute hemolytic anemia or neonatal jaundice. In cases with acute hemolytic anemia a careful history regarding ingestion of drugs or infections is important. Other causes of episodic anemia include paroxysmal nocturnal hemoglobinuria (see Chapter 11), parasitic infections such as malaria, and unstable hemoglobins (see Chapter 10). When the hemolytic nature of the episodes is less apparent, particularly in cases associated with infection, differential diagnosis includes an aplastic crisis that may occur in any of the severe hereditary anemias. In neonatal icterus, fetal-maternal Rh or ABO incompatibility must be ruled out (see Chapter 13).

Testing for G6PD deficiency is easily carried out by quantitative measurement of NADPH production (see **Test 9.5.2** below) or by use of several screening tests including the dye decolorization test, the methemoglobin reduction test, and the fluorescent spot test (**Test 9.5.1** below). The screening tests are used in population studies and may not be useful in the post-hemolytic period when reticulocyte counts are high or in heterozygous females. G6PD deficient patients identified by screening tests should be confirmed with the more precise quantitative NADPH production testing **Test 9.5.2**.

Deficiencies of glutathione synthesis or regeneration are rare causes of episodic hemolytic anemia with oxidative stress and may be considered if no evidence of G6PD deficiency or other cause of episodic hemolysis is identified. Patients will have low levels of glutathione that may be determined by measurements of reduced glutathione levels (see **Test 9.5.4**). Marked decreases in glutathione reflect deficiencies in either γ-glutamylcysteine synthetase or glutathione synthetase.

9.4 Hematologic Findings

The severity of the anemia is extremely variable. The hemoglobin concentration in the blood may be near normal or as low as 5 g/dL (50 g/L). Examination of the peripheral blood smear usually does not show a distinctive red blood cell appearance. Heinz bodies, particles of denatured hemoglobin, and membrane proteins that adhere to the membrane, may be seen in supravitally stained preparations used for the enumeration of reticulocytes or with crystal violet staining. They are not seen on Wright- or Giemsa-stained smears. As hemolysis progresses, Heinz bodies disappear, presumably due to splenic removal or hemolysis. Bite cells and red blood cells with irregularly contracted hemoglobin on one side (eccentrocytes) may be seen (see i9.1). At the beginning of the hemolytic episode, the reticulocyte count may be normal, but if the episode has been underway for several days, the reticulocyte count is usually elevated corresponding to the degree of anemia. Slight macrocytosis may be seen if many reticulocytes are present; otherwise, RBC indices are normocytic and normochromic. The WBC count may be low, normal, or elevated because of neutrophilia secondary to infection.

Similar findings of variable anemia with increased reticulocytes, polychromasia, and macrocytosis as well as eccentrocytes and bite cells may also be seen with abnormalities in the glutathione synthesis or regeneration pathways. Usually the blood findings are usually not as severe as seen with G6PD associated hemolysis. Infants may have a transient neonatal hemolysis that is self-limited that arises due to a deficiency of selenium, a necessary cofactor for glutathione peroxidase, that causes a functional deficiency of the enzyme. Supplementation of selenium will correct the transient defect.

i9.1 Glucose-6-phosphate dehydrogenase deficiency

Blood film from patient with G6PD deficiency showing red blood cells with asymmetrically distributed hemoglobin and bite cells following an oxidative challenge. *(Wright stain)*

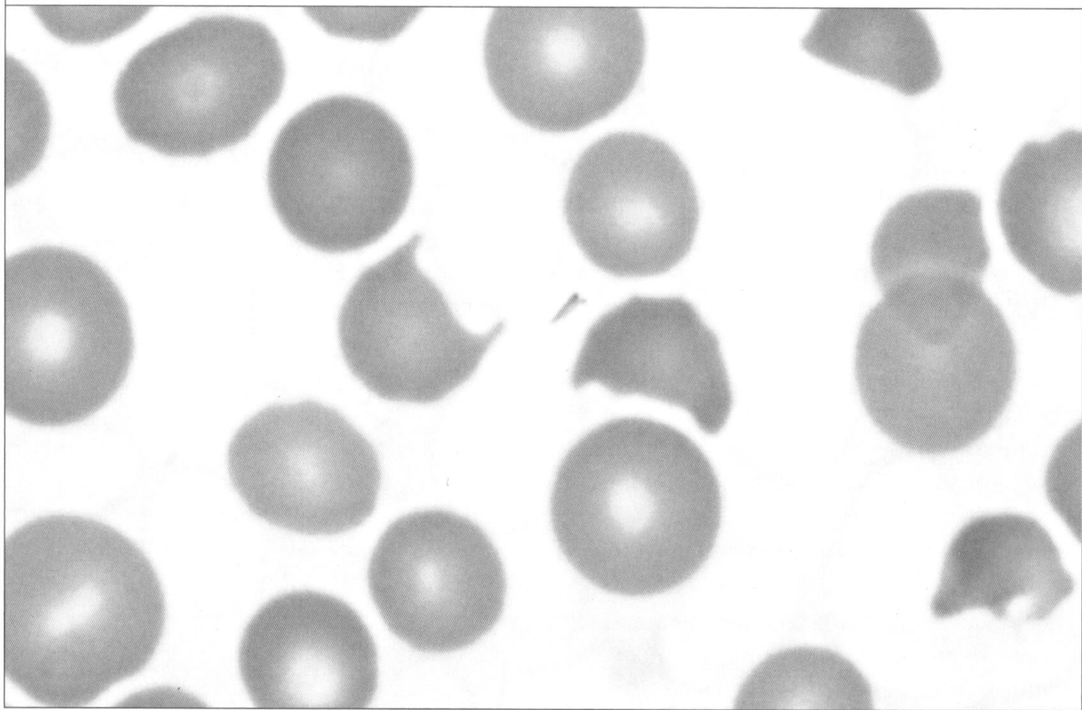

9.5 Other Laboratory Tests

Test 9.5.1 Fluorescent Screening Test for G6PD Activity

Purpose. The fluorescent screening test that detects formation of NADPH, which fluoresces under UV light, is highly reliable for the detection of both severe and mild types of G6PD deficiency in men who are not experiencing an active episode of hemolysis. It is best used as an initial screening mechanism. Because blood may be collected and spotted onto filter paper, this is an approapriate test for population screening or screening of neonates.

Principle. Whole blood or blood hemolysates contain the enzymes of the HMP shunt. In the presence of $NADP^+$, G6PD is oxidized to form 6-phosphogluconate and NADPH. 6-Phosphogluconate dehydrogenase (6-PGD) gives rise to additional NADPH by the following reaction:

$$\text{6-Phosphogluconate} + NADP^+ \xrightarrow{\text{6-PGD}} \text{Ribulose-5-phosphate} + NADPH + H^+ + CO_2$$

When G6PD activity is low, only a small amount of NADPH is formed. In the presence of GS-SG, provided in the screening mixture, NADPH is reoxidized in the glutathione reductase reaction to $NADP^+$.

Whereas NAPDH may be detected fluorescently, $NAPD^+$ does not fluoresce. The screening test measures the difference between G6PD and 6-PGD activity (which forms NADPH) and glutathione reductase activity (which consumes NADPH).

Specimen. Blood collected in heparin, ethylenediaminetetraacetic acid (EDTA), acid-citrate-dextrose (ACD), or citrate-phosphate-dextrose (CPD) anticoagulants is satisfactory. Blood stored at 4°C for 1 week, or even spots of blood collected on filter paper and dried, may be used.

Procedure. Whole blood is added to a buffered screening solution containing saponin, glucose-6-phosphate, NAPD+, and GS-SG. After incubation for 5 or 10 minutes at room temperature, the mixture is spotted on filter paper, allowed to dry, and observed for NADPH fluorescence under long-wave UV light. In patients with G6PD A^- who have had a recent episode of hemolysis, the test may be modified by centrifuging the blood sample in a microhematocrit tube and using the bottom 10% of the red cell column (representing the reticulocyte-poor, enzyme-deficient cell fraction) for the test.

Interpretation. Normal samples show a bright fluorescence after 5 or 10 minutes of incubation, whereas deficient samples show no fluorescence. No false-positive or false-negative test results are observed. In severe $G6PD^{MED}$ or a similar type deficiency in which even young cells have very low levels of G6PD, a screening test suffices for diagnosis, even in the presence of a severe hemolytic reaction. In patients with G6PD A^- and ongoing or acute hemolysis, however, the remaining young cells and reticulocytes have normal or near-normal G6PD activity, and most of the enzyme-deficient cells may have been removed from the circulation. Diagnosis of G6PD deficiency under these circumstances can be accomplished either by repeating the test in 2 or 3 weeks or by modifying the test using reticulocyte-poor fractions, as previously noted. Heterozygotes may not be detected with the latter method. Recent blood transfusions also may invalidate the results.

Notes and Precautions. Because G6PD is sex-linked, women who are heterozygous for G6PD deficiency have two red cell populations in which some red cells are grossly deficient and others are normal. Although the deficient cells are susceptible to hemolysis, the enzymatic activity, as measured on hemolysates, may be normal, intermediate, or low. The extent of deficiency is a function of the proportion of normal and deficient cells in the particular patient. Special methods for the detection of individual cell G6PD activity may be used to help detect heterozygosity. Leukocytosis ($>12 ˘ 10^9$ cells/L) may cause spuriously normal results due to leukocyte G6PD activity. In such cases, the use of washed, leukocyte-poor red cells may be warranted.

Test 9.5.2 Quantitative G6PD Assay

Purpose. Quantitative enzyme assays may be useful in identifying deficiencies in patients who have had an episode of hemolysis, women with heterozygous disease, or in confirming a screening test result.

Principle. Formation of NADPH from $NADP^+$ is measurable by a change in absorbance created by formation of NADPH. The rate of increase of optical density that occurs with the formation of NADPH from $NADP^+$ in blood hemolysates is measured at 340 nm in a spectrophotometer.

Specimen. Blood collected in EDTA or ACD solution is satisfactory. The G6PD activity is stable for several weeks at 4°C and for several days at room temperature. The blood should not be allowed to freeze, because enzymatic activity is rapidly lost when red cells are lysed.

Procedure. The final assay mixture contains 100 mmol/L tris(hydroxymethyl)aminomethane (TRIS) with 0.5 mmol/L EDTA buffer (pH 8.0); 10 mmol/L $MgCl_2$; 0.2 mmol/L NADP; and 0.6 mmol/L G6P. The reaction is started by the addition of the G6P, with water being substituted for G6P in the blank cuvette. The change in fluorescence at 340 nm is used with the hemoglobin concentration to calculate the G6PD activity by the following formula:

$$\text{G6PD units}/10^{10}\ \text{RBC} = \frac{\Delta\ \text{Absorbance 340 nm/min}}{\text{RBC (in millions)}} \times 482$$

Interpretation. Normal levels of G6PD are 2.5 ± 0.5 units per 1×10^{10} RBCs. The quantitative assay for G6PD activity may reveal the presence of G6PD deficiency even in patients who have had a recent episode of hemolysis. Because G6PD levels may vary with red cell age, activity should be increased in a patient with reticulocytosis. Normal or slightly lower than normal G6PD activity in such a patient implies that G6PD deficiency is present. Enzyme activity in women with heterozygous disease may be below the normal range.

Notes and Precautions. This assay measures the activity of both G6PD and 6-PGD, because the product of the G6PD reaction, 6-phosphogluconolactone, is converted rapidly to the substrate for the 6-PGD reaction. In practice, this causes no difficulty because no hemolytic anemia has been associated with deficiency of 6-phosphogluconic acid and normal levels of this enzyme do not mask G6PD deficiency. Note the precaution in the diagnosis of heterozygosity discussed under Test 9.5.1.

Test 9.5.3 Heinz Body Test

Purpose. Deficiency of G6PD, as well as other rarer enzyme deficiencies, or unstable hemoglobin types are associated with increased formation of Heinz bodies. This finding in association with episodic hemolysis supports the diagnosis of drug-induced hemolysis due to G6PD deficiency. The Heinz body test may be used as a screening test, but is not diagnostically specific.

Principle. The oxidative pathway of glycolytic red blood cell enzymes maintain hemoglobin stability. In G6PD deficiency, as well as deficiencies of glutathione synthetic enzymes, or in the presence of unstable hemoglobins, oxidation leads to hemoglobin denaturation. The denatured hemoglobin precipitates on the red blood cell membrane, forming Heinz bodies. Normal red blood cells can be induced to form small numbers of Heinz bodies. In contrast, G6PD-deficient cells will produce three or four Heinz bodies per red blood cell in the presence of oxidative stress.

Specimen. Fresh whole blood is collected in EDTA.

Procedure. Crystal violet or brilliant cresyl blue is added to a few drops of blood. Wet mount smears are prepared from the mixture after 15 minutes, 30 minutes, or 1 hour of incubation at room temperature. Red blood cells also can be incubated with phenylhydrazine (acting as an oxidizing agent) before preparation of the smears to exaggerate the findings in G6PD deficiency.

Interpretation. Heinz bodies are seen as small purple to blue inclusions located close to the cellular membrane, ranging in size from 1-4 μm. Normal cells may produce a single Heinz body. After phenylhydrazine incubation, G6PD-deficient cells may have three to four Heinz bodies in every cell (see i9.2). If abrupt hemolysis has occurred, the test results may be negative because of hemolytic removal of the Heinz body–positive cells.

i9.2 Heinz bodies

Heinz body staining showing multiple deposits of precipitated, denatured hemoglobin in a patient with severe G6PD deficiency following an oxidative challenge. *(Brilliant cresyl blue stain)*

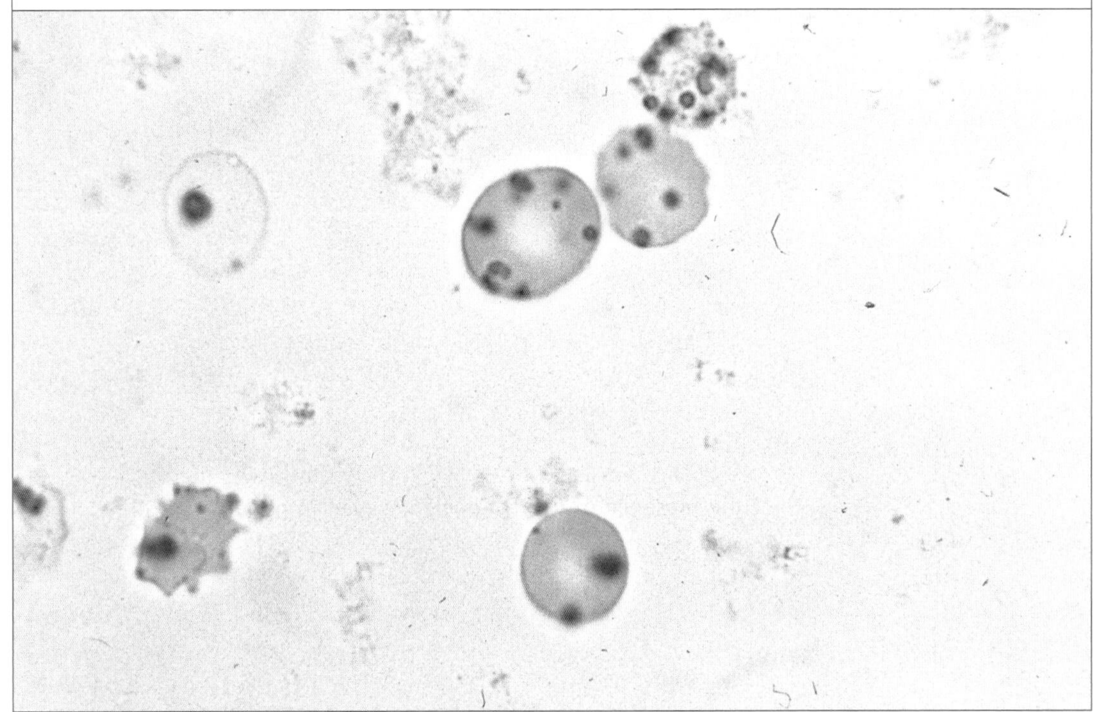

Notes and Precautions. This test may be used as a screening tool, but is not diagnostically specific. It requires interpretation by personnel familiar with the staining patterns and test performance for reproducible results. The ease of specific screening for G6PD activity or hemoglobin analysis by current methodologies makes this test less useful than in the past.

Test 9.5.4 Reduced Glutathione Determination

Purpose. Red cell GSH levels are often decreased in patients with HMP shunt or GSH synthetic pathway deficiencies.

Principle. The dithiol compound, dithio-bis-nitrobenzoic acid (DTNB), is reduced by GSH to form a yellow anion, the optical density of which is readily measured at 412 nm. The absorbance measurement is directly proportional to GSH concentration.

Specimen. Whole blood collected in heparin, EDTA, or ACD solution may be used. The GSH levels remain unaltered for 3 weeks in ACD solution or for 1 day in EDTA or heparin at 4°C.

Procedure. In this procedure, 0.2 mL of whole blood is added to 1.8 mL of distilled water. To lyse the cells, 3 mL of a metaphosphoric acid EDTA–sodium chloride precipitating solution is added, and the mixture is filtered. Then 2 mL of the filtrate is added to 8 mL of 0.3 mol/L Na_2HPO_4 solution, 1 mL of DTNB reagent is added, and the optical density is read at 412 nm.

Interpretation. The normal red blood cell glutathione concentration is 4.5 to 8.7 µmol/g (47-100 mg/dL) of hemoglobin. A severe deficiency of glutathione results from a genetic defect in one of the two enzymes of glutathione synthesis: γ-glutamylcysteine synthetase or glutathione synthetase. Modest reductions of GSH levels and marked instability to challenge by oxidative agents (such as that seen with incubation of 1-acetyl-1,2-phenylhydrazine in the incubation mix for 2 hours at 37°C) is found in G6PD-deficient red blood cells. Elevated levels of red blood cell glutathione are found in patients with myeloproliferative disorders and in those with pyrimidine-5'-nucleotidase deficiency.

Notes and Precautions. Virtually all of the protein-free DTNB reducing activity in RBCs is due to glutathione. Because DTNB is reduced readily by other sulfhydryl compounds, such as cysteine, the degree of specificity varies from tissue to tissue.

9.6 Ancillary Tests

In patients with severe glutathione deficiency, it is desirable to measure the activities of γ-glutamylcysteine synthetase and glutathione synthetase. Assay of these enzymes is a relatively difficult radiometric procedure that is best performed by specialized laboratories. Precise identification of the G6PD variants requires electrophoresis, kinetic studies, and other biochemical techniques that are also performed in specialized laboratories. Usually detailed characterization of the G6PD variant is not necessary for clinical management.

9.7 Course and Treatment

Infants with G6PD deficiency and neonatal icterus/kernicterus may require exchange transfusions. Adult patients with G6PD deficiency should avoid the ingestion of fava beans and oxidative drugs. Splenectomy is not usually useful in patients with G6PD deficiency associated with chronic hemolytic anemia, and patients with severe anemia may require periodic transfusions.

9.8 References

Cappellini MD, Fiorelli G. Glucose-6-phosphate dehydrogenase deficiency. *Lancet.* 2008;371:64-74.

Fibach E, Rachmilewitz E. The role of oxidative stress in hemolytic anemia. *Curr Mol Med.* 2008;8:609-619.

Hirono A, Ivori H, Sekine I, et al. Three cases of hereditary nonspherocytic hemolytic anemia associated with red blood cell glutathione deficiency. *Blood.* 1996;87:2071-2074.

Kohrl J, Brigelius-Flohe R, Bock A, et al. Selenium in biology: facts and medical perspectives. *Biol Chem.* 2000;381:849-864.

Mason PJ, Bautista JM, Gilsanz F. G6PD deficiency: the genotype-phenotype association. *Blood Rev.* 2007;21:267-283.

Minucci A, Giardina B, Zuppi C. Capoluongo E. Glucose-6-phosphate dehydrogenase laboratory assay: How, when, and why? *IUBMB Life.* 2009;61:27-34.

Miwa S, Fujji H. Molecular basis of erythroenzymopathies associated with hereditary hemolytic anemia. *Am J Hematol.* 1998;51:122-132.

Ristoff E, Larsson A. Patients with genetic defects in the gamma-glutamyl cycle. Chem. *Biol Interact.* 1998;112:113-121.

Steiner LA, Gallagher PG. Erythrocyte disorders in the perinatal period. *Semin Perinatol.* 2007;31:254-261.

Tavazzi D, Taher A, Cappellini MD. Red blood cell enzyme disorders: an overview. *Pediatr Ann.* 2008;37:303-310.

CHAPTER 10

Disorders of Hemoglobin Synthesis

Sherrie Perkins, MD, PhD

Hemoglobin is a tetrameric protein composed of 4 globin polypeptides complexed with four heme groups. As hemoglobin is responsible for the primary red blood cell function of binding and transport of oxygen and is the major red blood cell protein, abnormalities in hemoglobin synthesis may lead to significant disease. Clinically significant abnormalities in hemoglobin synthesis, termed hemoglobinopathies, may be qualitative or quantitative. Qualitative defects result in formation of an abnormal hemoglobin molecule at a normal or near-normal rate, but abnormal properties of that hemoglobin may lead to premature red blood cell hemolysis. Quantitative defects, or thalassemias, arise due to decreased synthesis of the globin proteins with resultant decreased hemoglobin formation, leading to diminished hemoglobin content in red blood cells.

10.1 Pathophysiology

Approximately 98% of the protein in a red blood cell is hemoglobin (Hb) that is formed from four protein globin chains and four iron containing heme molecules. A normal adult red blood cell contains predominantly HbA, composed of 2 α- and 2 β-globin chains ($\alpha_2\beta_2$). Two other minor hemoglobins found in adults are HbA_2, in which the β-chains are replaced by δ-chains to form $\alpha_2\delta_2$, and HbF, in which the β-chains are replaced by γ-chains ($\alpha_2\gamma_2$) **t10.1**. At birth, HbF is the predominant type of hemoglobin. Within the first year of life, it is largely replaced by HbA to reflect the adult proportions of approximately 97% HbA, 2% HbA_2, and 1% HbF. HbA_{1c} is a minor hemoglobin that is formed by posttranslational addition of glucose to the terminal of the HbA β-chains. HbA_{1c} is found in increased amounts in patients with diabetes mellitus with increased blood glucose levels, and provides a useful tool for monitoring glucose control.

t10.1 Hemoglobin Types Found in Healthy Adults

Hemoglobin Type	Globin Chains	% Total Hemoglobin
HbA	$\alpha_2\beta_2$	>95
HbA2	$\alpha_2\delta_2$	<3.5
HbF	$\alpha_2\gamma_2$	1

Each globin chain (α, β, γ, and δ) has its own autosomal genetic locus. Qualitative alterations in these globin chains occur via genetic mutations of one of these genes. Most often this is a point mutation that results in substitution of a single amino acid within the globin chain. The abnormal hemoglobin that is formed may or may not exhibit altered functional characteristics. If the hemoglobin structural abnormality gives rise to clinical manifestations, the patient is said to have a hemoglobinopathy. The most common hemoglobinopathies are mutations of the globin beta chain and include HbS, HbC, and HbE **t10.2**. Hemoglobinopathies include both heterozygous or homozygous genetic defects.

t10.2 Amino Acid Substitutions in the Beta Chains of Common Hemoglobin Variants

Hemoglobin	Position	Amino Acid Substitution
HbS	6	Glutamic acid → valine
HbC	6	Glutamic acid → lysine
HbE	26	Glutamic acid → lysine

Hemoglobin variants were initially differentiated by their electrophoretic mobility and were assigned names (ie, HbC, HbE). As other hemoglobin variants with the same mobility were discovered, the new variant was distinguished by following the letter previously ascribed to that mobility with the place of discovery of the new variant (ie, HbC_{Harlem}). More recently, with the advent of hemoglobin sequencing, when the exact amino acid structure of a hemoglobin variant is determined it is given a designation that characterizes the amino acid substitution (eg, for HbS, $\alpha_2\beta_2^{6\text{-glutamic acid}\rightarrow\text{valine}}$ indicates a mutation changing the glutamic acid at position six in the beta chain to a valine).

Clinical manifestations are often determined by the amount of variant Hb present. The amount of variant Hb is determined by whether the abnormal hemoglobin is inherited as a heterozygous or homozygous trait. Homozygous inheritance is associated with more severe manifestations due to increased amounts of the abnormal Hb. Sickle cell anemia or sickle cell disease refers to the homozygote for HbS, whereas the clinically less severe sickle cell trait reflects a heterozygous state. The word "disease" is used for homozygotes for a hemoglobin variant (eg, homozygous HbC disease or HbCC), whereas "trait" refers to the heterozygotes (eg, HbC trait or HbAC). The descriptor "disease" is also applied to the HbS heterozygous state in association with other hemoglobin mutations when significant clinical findings are associated with the heterozygous combination of two abnormal hemoglobins (eg, HbSC disease where patients have both HbS and HbC). When letter designations are used for the hemoglobins in heterozygous hemoglobinopathies, the first letter refers to the preponderant hemoglobin found in the red blood cell. Thus, "HbAS" indicates that the concentration of HbA exceeds that of HbS in the red blood cells of that particular heterozygote.

Mutations that decrease or prevent the synthesis of one of the globin chains cause quantitative decreases in structurally normal hemoglobin production. This gives rise to thalassemia syndromes. Thalassemias are classified according to the chain affected, the most common being α-thalassemia and β-thalassemia. The α-thalassemias are most commonly caused by the deletion of one or more of the four alpha globin genes. The β-thalassemic disorders are usually due to genetic mutations that affect RNA synthesis, processing, or stability so that decreased levels of beta globin protein are formed. β-Thalassemias are classified as either minor (heterozygous) or major (homozygous). Combined disorders involving the structural variants and thalassemia also are seen, the most common being sickle β-thalassemia disease.

10.2 Clinical Findings

10.2.1 Qualitative Hemoglobin Disorders Caused by Abnormal (Mutated) Globin Chains

Mutations involving the globin protein genes are usually amino acid substitutions. These lead to changes in protein folding and structure that may produce pronounced changes in the functional properties of hemoglobin, including solubility and oxygen affinity **t10.3**. Most are inherited as autosomal recessive traits.

t10.3 Functional Classification of Abnormal Hemoglobins

Type of Abnormality	Functional Effect	Clinical Disorder	Examples
Qualitative disorders			
Solubility	Aggregation of hemoglobin	Hemolytic anemia	Hemoglobin S, hemoglobin C
Oxidative susceptibility	Oxidative denaturation	Hemolytic anemia	Unstable hemoglobin
Increased oxygen affinity	Decreased oxygen to tissues	Erythrocytosis	Unstable hemoglobin
Decreased oxygen affinity	Premature oxygen release	Cyanosis/anemia	Unstable hemoglobin
Abnormal heme reduction	Inability to carry oxygen	Cyanosis	Methemoglobin
Quantitative disorders (thalassemias)			
α-chains	Decreased α-chains	Range from mild anemia to hydrops fetalis	α-thalassemia
β-chains	Decreased β-chains	Mild to severe hemolytic anemia	β-thalassemia
β- and δ-chains	Decreased β- and δ-chains	Thalassemia-like syndrome	δ-β-thalassemia
Combined disorders			
Abnormal hemoglobin and thalassemia	Decreased chain production with altered solubility	Often milder than homozygous structural disorder	Hemoglobin S-thalassemia

The most common clinically significant hemoglobinopathy is HbS where the mutation causes changes in hemoglobin solubility. The heterozygous sickle trait is an entirely benign disorder, although hematuria may occur on rare occasions. The homozygous disorder, sickle cell anemia or HbSS, is characterized by moderately severe hemolysis and painful crises resulting from occlusion of blood vessels by the abnormal red blood cells that sickle due to abnormal hemoglobin polymerization into linear arrays. When the gene for HbS is inherited with the gene for certain other abnormal hemoglobins, particularly for HbC (causing HbSC disease) or β-thalassemia (HbS-thalassemia), sickle cell diseases similar to sickle cell anemia result even in the heterozygous state. Within the African-American population, the HbS gene has a frequency of approximately 9%; the HbC gene, 3%; and the β-thalassemia gene, 1%. Thus, these mixed disorders are relatively common collectively, affecting approximately 1 in 260 African Americans.

Two other hemoglobinopathies that affect hemoglobin solubility are seen relatively frequently in the heterozygous state: HbD in African Americans and HbE in Asian populations. Both of these conditions result in mild hemolytic anemia in the homozygous state. In HbE disease, the anemia is hypochromic and associated with splenomegaly. Hypochromia with little or no anemia is a uniform finding in HbE trait.

The remaining hemoglobinopathies are much less common. Those caused by formation of unstable hemoglobins are usually inherited as autosomal dominant disorders and are characteristically associated with chronic hemolysis. The anemia is often hypochromic. Some unstable hemoglobins are associated with increased oxygen affinity, leading to erythrocytosis and reticulocytosis more severe than that usually observed for the degree of anemia. Other rarely seen hemoglobins have decreased oxygen affinity and produce anemia with cyanosis. A mutant hemoglobin, designated HbM, that is unable to maintain heme iron in the reduced state or to bind oxygen, results in hereditary methemoglobinemia. Methemoglobin is brownish, and patients who inherit this type of hemoglobin have cyanosis. HbM is inherited as an autosomal dominant disorder.

10.2.2 Thalassemias

The thalassemic syndromes arise from an impairment in the synthesis of globin chains, leading to a quantitative decrease in the amount of structurally normal hemoglobin within the cell. Thalassemias are divided into two main categories—α-thalassemia and β-thalassemia—on the basis of which globin chain is affected.

α-Thalassemia is a common disorder in many parts of the world. Severe forms of α-thalassemia are found in Southeast Asia, but milder disease forms are prevalent among those of African descent. Because of gene duplication of the alpha globin chain genetic locus, there are normally four alpha chain genes, with two on each chromosome. α-Thalassemia usually results from the deletion of one or more of these genes (see **t10.4**). The severity of disease is directly correlated with the number of genes deleted. The spectrum of α-thalassemic syndromes ranges from deletion of one gene (causing no clinical disease) to the deletion of all four alpha chain genes that is fatal, and is a frequent cause of stillbirth in Southeast Asia. The fetal red blood cell hemoglobin in this situation is composed entirely of gamma chain tetramers, a condition designated "Bart's hemoglobin." Because Bart's hemoglobin avidly binds oxygen, it is unable to release oxygen to the fetal tissues. This results in fetal death from hydrops fetalis, as manifested by severe intrauterine hypoxia, edema, pallor, and hepatosplenomegaly. If one functional alpha chain gene is present, a less severe disorder, termed HbH disease, occurs. At birth, both fetal hemoglobin and Bart's hemoglobin are present. From later infancy to adulthood, as beta globin synthesis replaces fetal hemoglobin, HbH may be detected by hemoglobin electrophoresis or high performance liquid chromatography (HPLC). This syndrome is associated with a moderately severe, chronic hemolytic anemia. If two normal alpha chain genes are present,

t10.4 α-Thalassemias

Phenotype	α Globin Output (%)	No. of Functional α Chain Genes and Genotype	Hematologic Findings
Normal	100	4: αα/αα	Normal
Silent carrier	75	3: -α/αα	Normal
α-Thalassemia trait	50	2:–α/–α or ––/αα	Mild microcytic, hypochromic anemia
HbH disease	25	1: –α/––	Hemolytic anemia
Hydrops fetalis	0	0: ––/––	Stillborn, severe anemia

– =deleted or absent α chain; –– = both genes on the locus deleted

a mild microcytic anemia designated α-thalassemia minor or α-thalassemia trait is observed. In α-thalassemia minor, no abnormalities are found on hemoglobin electrophoresis, and the diagnosis is often one of exclusion of other causes of anemia. The presence of three normal alpha chains does not result in any clinically detectable abnormality, creating an asymptomatic carrier state.

β-Thalassemia, common among those of Mediterranean descent, may arise from gene deletion or, more commonly, from point mutations leading to impaired or absent beta chain synthesis. Mutations leading to complete suppression of beta chain synthesis are designated as β^0 variants. Other mutations, where diminished synthesis of normal synthesis beta chains occurs, are designated as β^+ variants and may result in milder clinical syndromes than the β^0 variants.

As with the α-thalassemias, the degree of disease severity is dependent on the number of abnormal genes inherited. When only one β-thalassemic gene has been inherited (heterozygote), the patient has a benign, hypochromic microcytic anemia designated β-thalassemia minor. This anemia is characterized by microcytosis, with a mean corpuscular volume (MCV) of 60-70 μm^3 (60-70 fL), a hemoglobin of 10-13 g/dL (100-130 g/L), and an elevated or normal RBC count. Hemoglobin electrophoresis usually shows increased amounts of HbA_2 due to excess unpaired alpha chains combining with delta chains. Slightly elevated levels of HbF are also present in about 30% of patients with β-thalassemia minor. Often, patients with β-thalassemia minor are mistakenly diagnosed as having iron deficiency, because they have a hypochromic microcytic anemia (see Chapter 2).

When two β-thalassemic genes have been inherited (homozygote), a very serious disorder termed β-thalassemia major is manifested in infancy and early childhood. It is characterized by massive hepatosplenomegaly, extreme erythroid hyperplasia in the bone marrow leading to bony deformities, severe hemolytic anemia, and failure to grow or thrive. Hemoglobin electrophoresis shows prominent elevation of the HbF level (ranging from 30% to 100%). At the lower end of the spectrum of HbF values, the fetal hemoglobin is distributed heterogeneously among the red blood cell population. This allows β-thalassemia major to be distinguished from the benign condition termed hereditary persistence of fetal hemoglobin (HPFH), in which a homogeneous distribution is seen.

Another form of thalassemia, called δ-thalassemia, is associated with suppression of both delta and beta chain synthesis. These disorders are clinically similar to the β-thalassemias. Patients with heterozygous disease present with thalassemia minor, often with prominent elevation of the HbF level. Patients with homozygous disease, however, present with a clinically milder disease than that usually seen in β-thalassemia major. The Lepore syndromes, which are often classified in this category, are caused by a mutant hemoglobin called Hb Lepore. This hemoglobin results from a crossover mutation leading to a hybrid globin chain consisting of partial delta and beta chains. Hemoglobin Lepore can be detected with electrophoresis or high pressure liquid chromatography (HPLC) due to its abnormal physical characteristics.

10.3 Diagnostic Approach

Clinical evaluation and family history play a particularly important role in evaluating laboratory data in these disorders. Many of the tests can be performed easily. Evaluation of the hemoglobin disorders proceeds with the following steps f10.1:

1. Hematologic evaluation, with attention to red blood cell morphology and indices. Supravital stains may detect inclusion bodies (such as HbH).

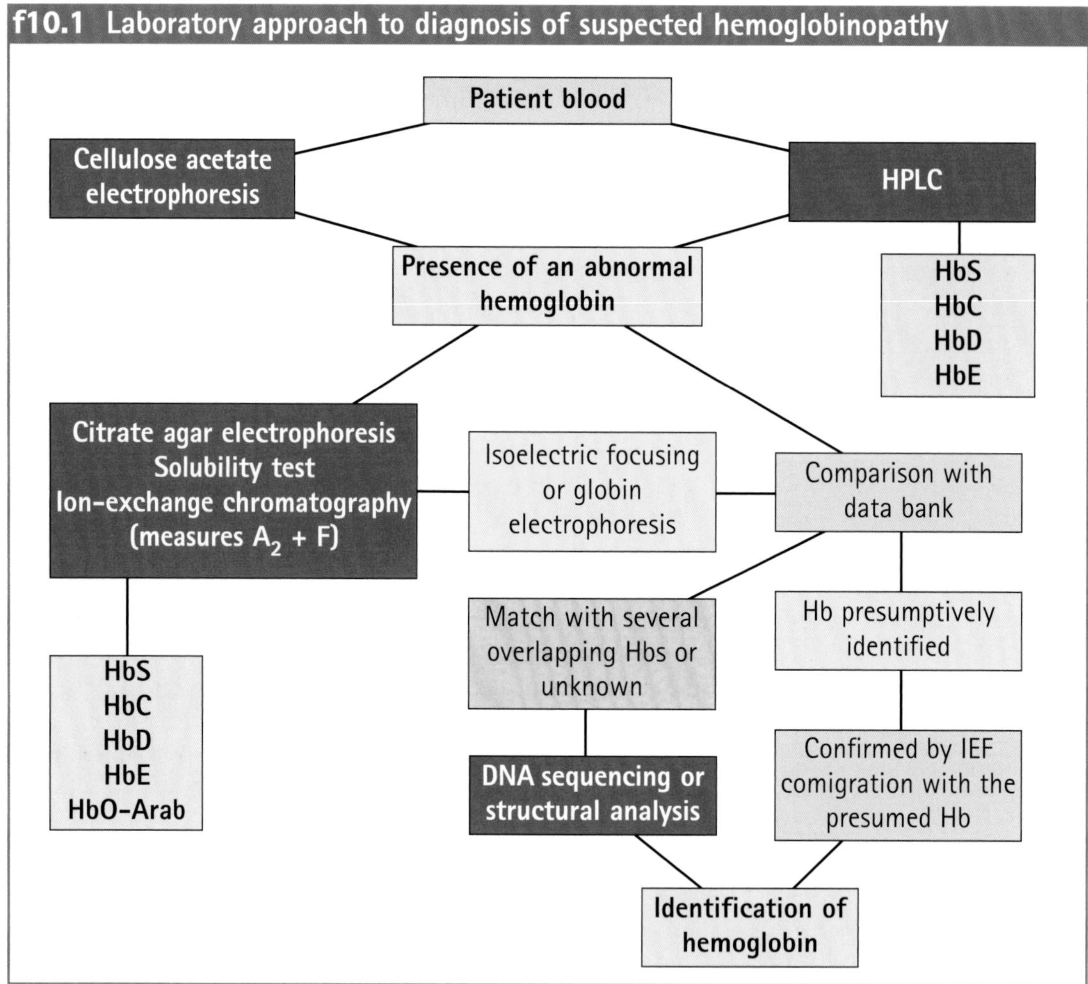

2. Hemoglobin analysis by electrophoresis or HPLC for the detection of globin chain variants with altered electrophoretic mobility or physical characteristics. Measurement of HbA_2 also may be determined chromatographically.
3. Tests of hemoglobin solubility as a means of distinguishing HbS from HbD and less frequent variants with overlapping electrophoretic mobilities. Solubility tests may also be used to screen for sickle cell trait prior to hemoglobin analysis.
4. Alkali denaturation test, acid elution test (Kleihauer and Betke method), or flow cytometric determination of fetal hemoglobin levels.
5. The isopropanol stability test for detecting unstable hemoglobins.

The following tests may be performed in specialized laboratories, but are rarely required:

1. When indicated, spectrophotometric determinations for methemoglobinemia seen with HbMs and measurement of oxyhemoglobin dissociation or $P_{50}O_2$ for detecting hemoglobins with altered oxygen affinity (see Chapter 12).
2. Globin chain synthetic studies when thalassemia is suspected but cannot be confirmed by simpler methods, and Southern blotting of alpha globin genes when additional genetic data are needed.
3. Detailed structural analysis of globin chains using "fingerprinting" of tryptic digests by electrophoresis, amino acid sequencing, or nucleic acid mutational analysis.

10.4 Hematologic Findings

The most severe anemia and the most striking morphologic changes are seen in the homozygous disorders, whereas heterozygous states may be hematologically normal or show minimal abnormalities. Common hematologic changes associated with hemoglobinopathies may be divided into three categories:

1. Findings associated with chronic hemolysis including increased reticulocytes, circulating nucleated red blood cells, and fragmented red blood cells.
2. Changes characteristic of a particular disorder, such as sickled cells in HbSS.
3. Findings seen after splenectomy or (in the case of sickle cell disease) findings related to splenic infarction/autosplenectomy.

Patients may demonstrate one or all of the above types of changes, depending on their specific disorder.

As patients with hemoglobinopathies have accelerated red blood cell turnover secondary to hemolysis, they are susceptible to episodic decreases in red blood cell numbers and more severe anemia due to increased activity of the reticuloendothelial system associated with infection (hemolytic crisis) or decreased marrow production (aplastic crisis).

10.4.1 Blood Cell Measurements

Anemia may be severe, with hemoglobin levels of 5-9 g/dL (50-90 g/L) in HbSS and 2.5-6.5 g/dL (25-65 g/L) in thalassemia major. Findings in heterozygotes may be normal or near normal, as in sickle cell trait, or they may demonstrate mild anemia, as in β-thalassemia minor. Often the thalassemia syndromes are characterized by decreased hemoglobin levels with normal to slightly increased red blood cell counts and microcytosis out of proportion to the anemia (MCV of 60-70 μm^3 [60-75 fL]).

10.4.2 Peripheral Blood Smear Morphology

A wide variety of characteristic red blood cell changes are associated with the disorders of hemoglobin synthesis and are summarized in **t10.5**. i10.1, i10.2, and i10.3 demonstrate the characteristic morphology seen in β-thalassemia minor, HbC disease, and HbSS, respectively. Careful examination of the blood smear with attention to red blood cell shape and hemoglobin distribution often provides information suggesting a specific type of hemoglobinopathy. Other findings, such as target cells, suggest that a hemoglobinopathy may be present but are relatively non-specific for a particular type of abnormality.

t10.5 Red Blood Cell Appearance in Disorders of Hemoglobin Synthesis

Disorder	Morphologic Findings
HbS	Sickle cells
HbC	Target cells, HbC crystals after splenectomy
HbE	Microcytosis, hypochromia, target cells
Unstable Hb	Red blood cell inclusions with supravital dyes
Thalassemia	Microcytosis, target cells, basophilic stippling
Changes due to splenectomy or splenic atrophy	Basophilic stippling, Howell-Jolly bodies, target cells, Pappenheimer bodies, poikilocytosis
Changes associated with hemolysis	Polychromatophilia, fine basophilic stippling, macrocytosis

i10.1 β-thalassemia

Blood film demonstrating microcytic hypochromic anemia with numerous target cells in a patient with β-thalassemia. *(Wright stain)*

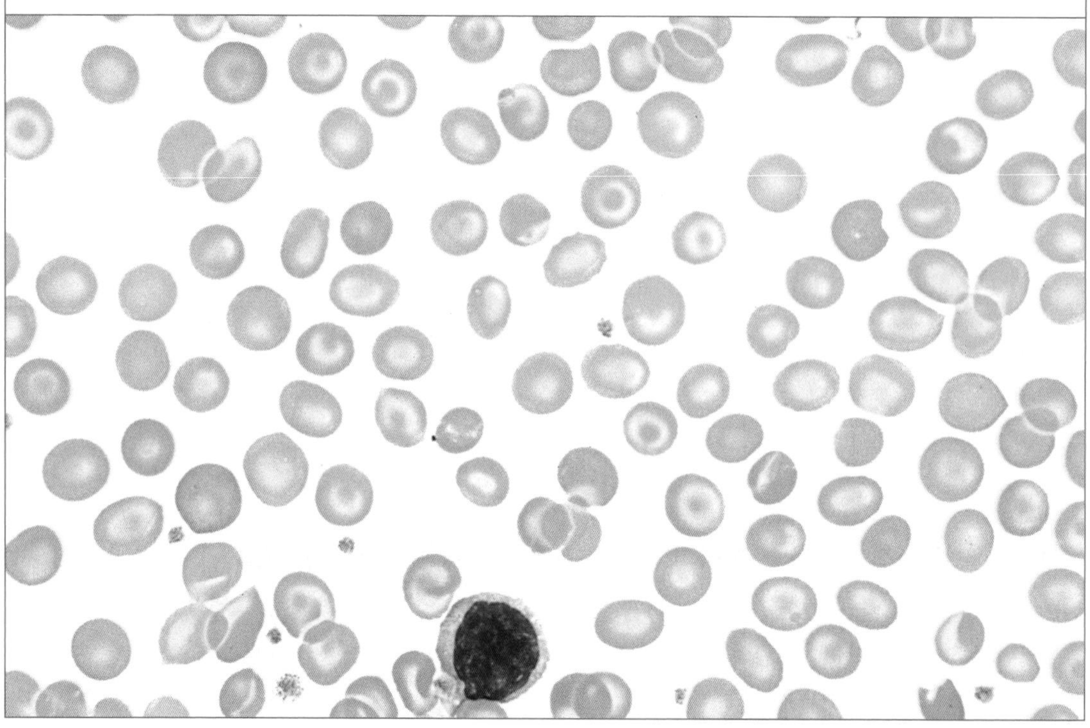

i10.2 Hemoglobin C disease post-splenectomy

Blood smear showing changes associated with hemoglobin C disease after patient splenectomy including target cells, folded red blood cells, and a hemoglobin C crystalline inclusion (center). *(Wright stain)*

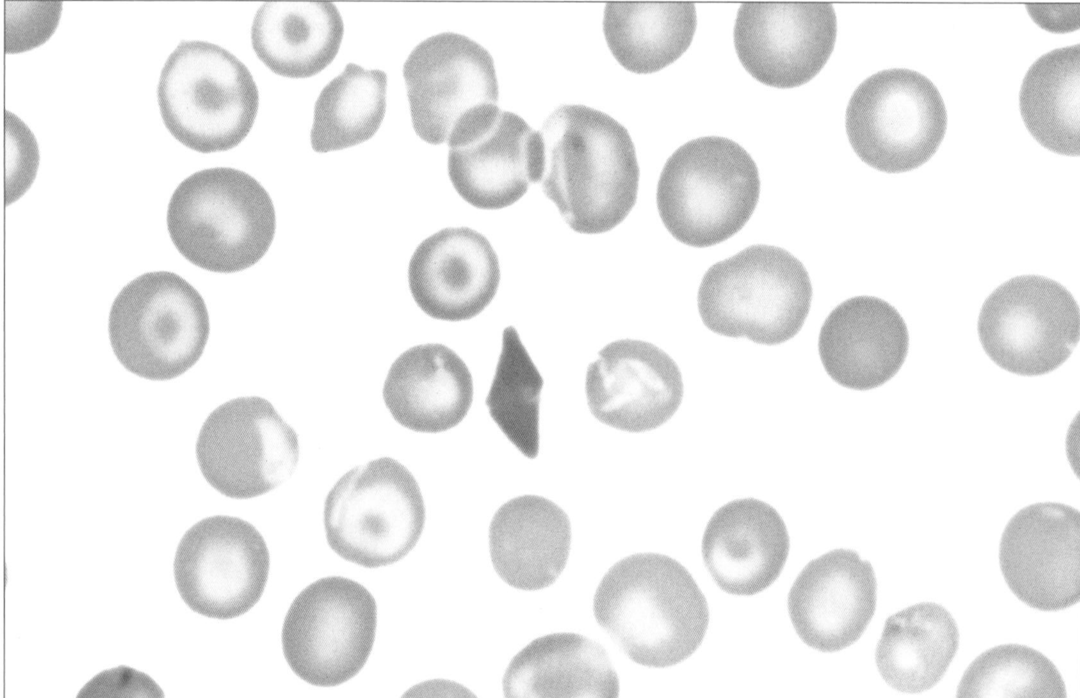

i10.3 Sickle cell disease

Blood smear showing sickled red blood cells, target cells, and polychromasia in a patient with sickle cell disease (HbSS). *(Wright stain)*

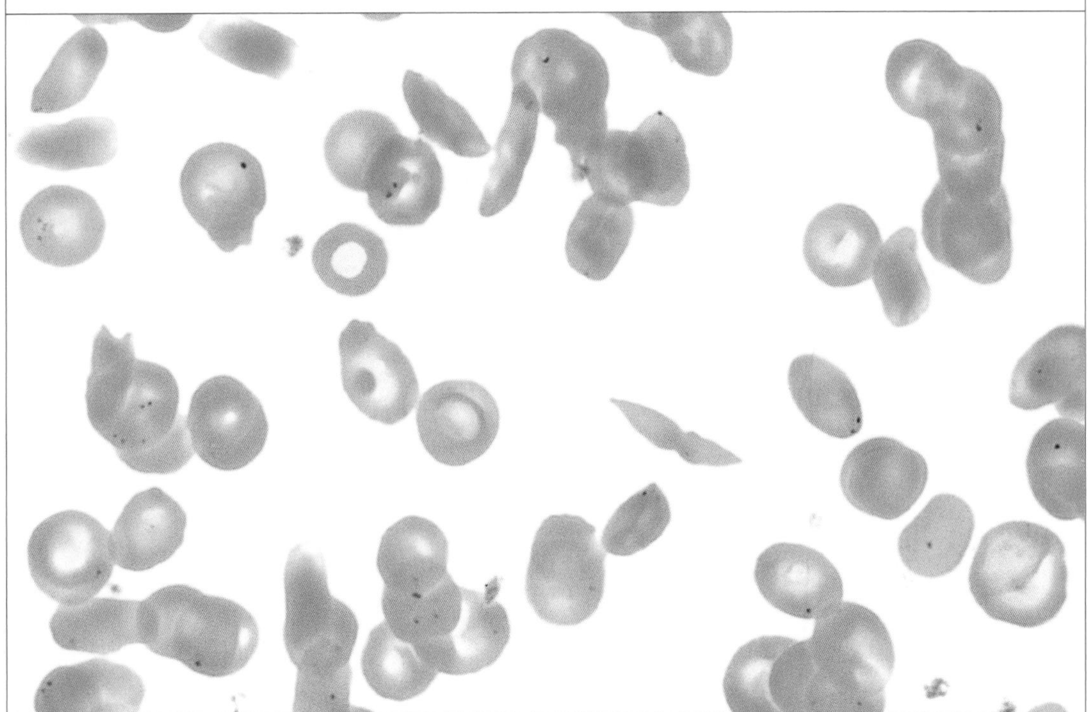

10.4.3 Bone Marrow Examination

Nearly all cases of hemoglobinopathy with associated anemia will demonstrate marrow erythroid hyperplasia. The degree of erythroid hyperplasia is proportional to the severity of the anemia, hemolysis, or ineffective erythropoiesis that results due to the abnormal hemoglobin. A prominent increase in iron deposition is often seen.

10.5 Other Laboratory Tests

Test 10.5.1 Hemoglobin Electrophoresis

Purpose. Hemoglobin electrophoresis separates, detects, and identifies abnormal hemoglobins. In some laboratories this is supplemented by HPLC analysis (see **Test 10.5.2**). There has been recent development of capillary isoelectric focusing methodologies that would allow for fine electrophoretic discrimination on small samples, although this method is not widely available.

Principle. Electrophoresis is the differential movement of charged protein molecules in an electric field. In a basic solution (pH >8) hemoglobins have a negative charge and migrate toward the anode with a mobility proportional to their net negative charges. Because HbS contains valine in place of the glutamic acid of HbA, it has a smaller negative charge and a slower anodal mobility than HbA in an alkaline medium. At an acid pH, hemoglobins are positively charged, and their relative mobilities in relation to the anode are the reverse of that seen in an alkaline medium.

Specimen. Anticoagulated whole blood or washed red blood cells are used for this test.

Procedure. Electrophoresis on cellulose acetate at pH 8.4 to 8.8 is the method of choice for initial electrophoretic testing in the general clinical laboratory (**f10.2**). Patient and control red blood cells are hemolyzed and subjected to electrophoresis for 15 to 30 minutes. Hemoglobins A, A_2, F, S, and C are most often included in controls. On completion of electrophoresis, the membrane is stained and the hemoglobins are identified by their relative positions on the gel. They can then be quantitated by elution and spectrophotometric assay or by densitometry scanning.

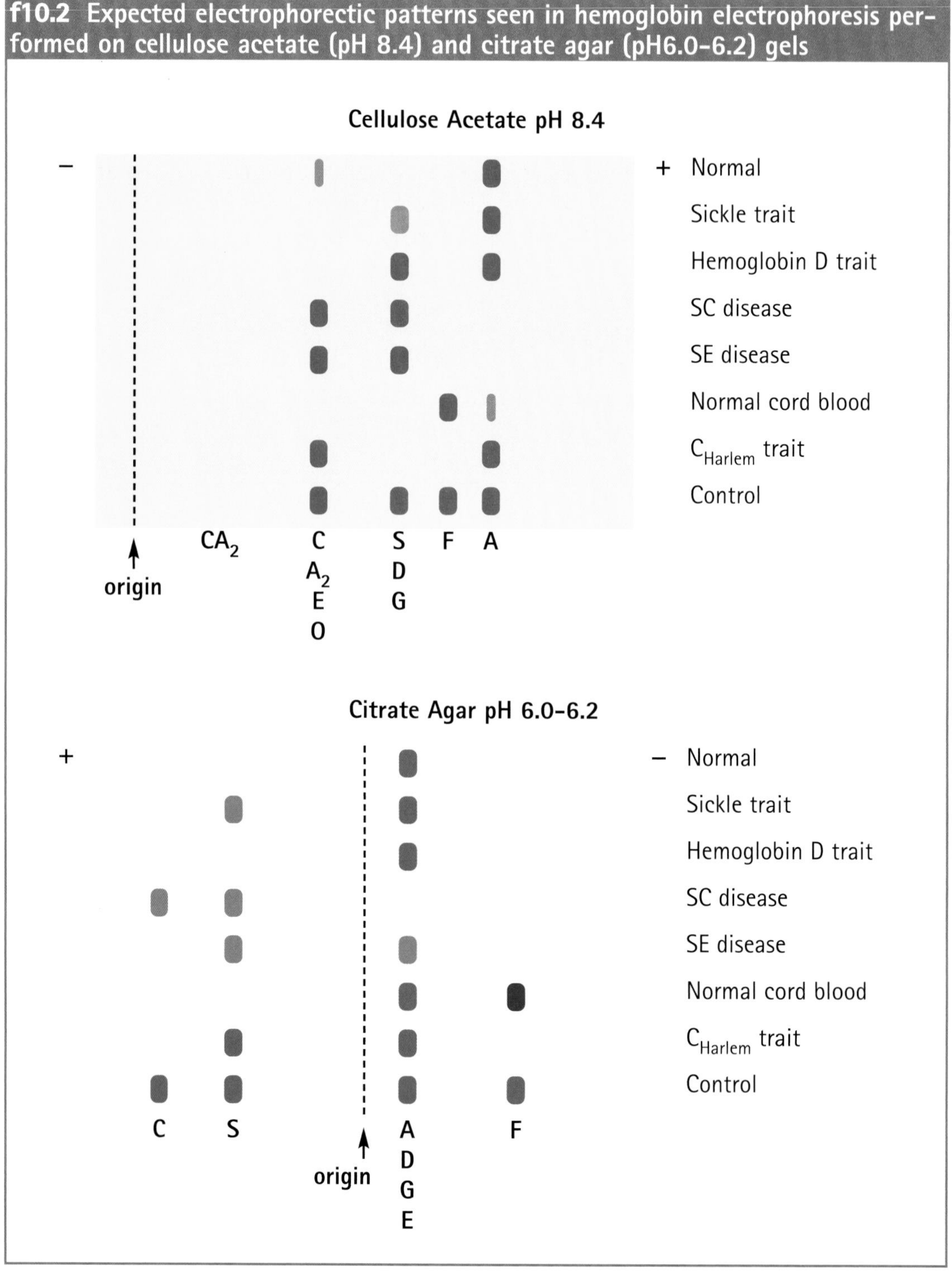

f10.2 Expected electrophorectic patterns seen in hemoglobin electrophoresis performed on cellulose acetate (pH 8.4) and citrate agar (pH6.0-6.2) gels

Electrophoresis in citrate agar at pH 6.2 can be used to complement conventional cellulose acetate electrophoresis (see Interpretation and f10.1). The procedure is basically the same as that described for cellulose acetate but requires electrophoresis for 45 to 90 minutes.

Interpretation. The electrophoresis patterns of some hemoglobin variants on cellulose acetate are shown in f10.3. At an alkaline pH, slow-moving hemoglobins include C, E, A_2, and O; intermediate hemoglobins include D, G, S, and Lepore; hemoglobins A and F are the most anodal. Among the fast-moving hemoglobins are I, and Hb Bart's. When a prominent band is found in the HbS region on cellulose acetate electrophoresis at pH 8.6, its identity can be confirmed with electrophoresis on citrate agar at pH 6.2. This separates HbS from HbD and HbG. Citrate agar also differentiates HbC from HbS, HbO, HbE, and HbA_2 and provides sharp separation of hemoglobins F and A.

Notes and Precautions. The main limitation of hemoglobin electrophoresis is its inability to detect amino acid substitutions that do not affect charge. Such variants are seen among the unstable hemoglobins and with hemoglobins associated with altered oxygen affinity. As noted previously, different amino acid substitutions may lead to identical or overlapping changes in elecrophoretic mobility, and these variants cannot be reliably distinguished by electrophoresis.

f10.3 Electophoretic mobilities seen during hemoglobin electrophoresis performed on cellulose acetate (pH 8.4) gels

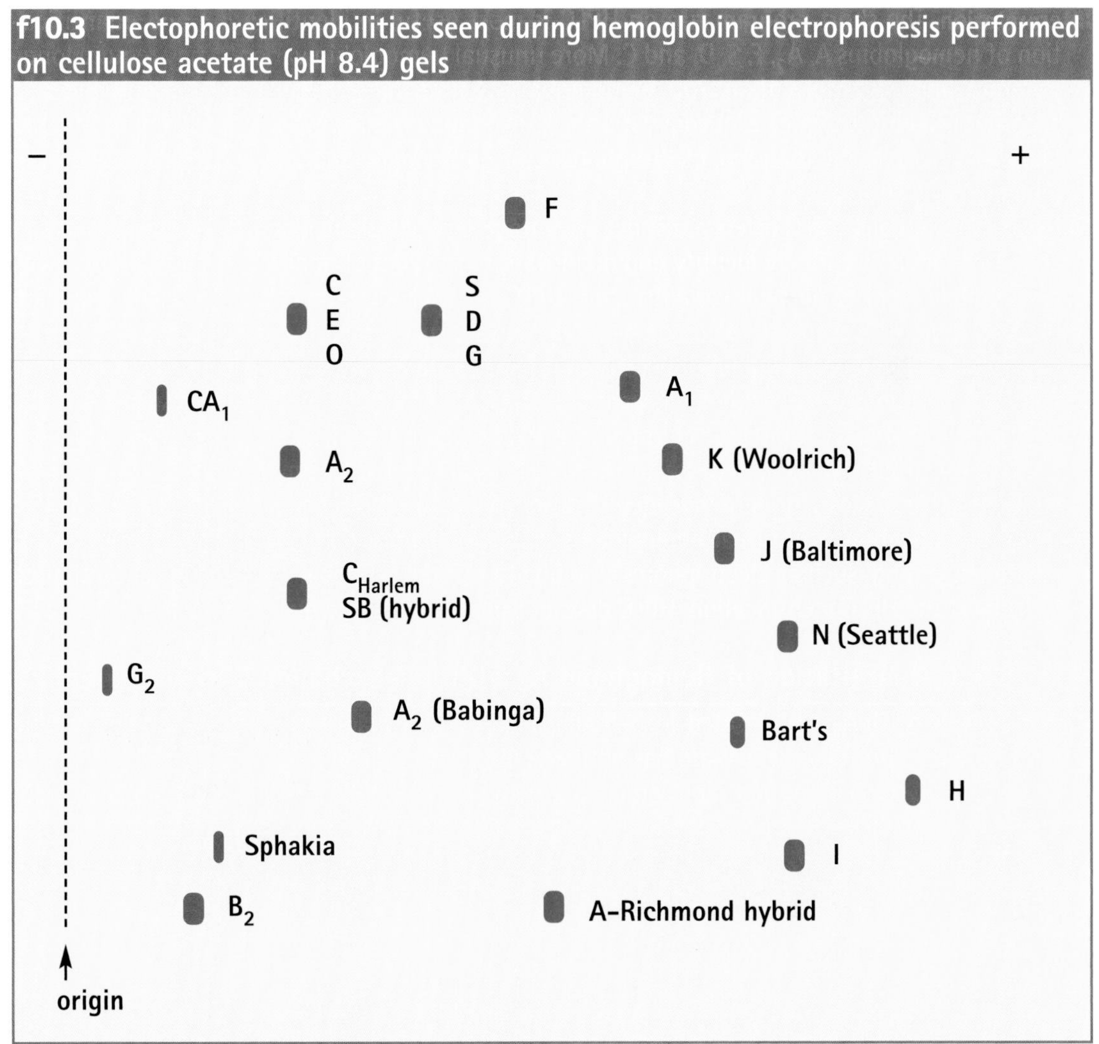

Test 10.5.2 High-Performance Liquid Chromatography Analysis of Hemoglobin

Purpose. Charge changes in hemoglobin variants allows chromatographic separation of different hemoglobin types based on column retention time, allowing rapid identification and quantification. This technology is approved by the Food and Drug Administration (FDA) for preliminary identification of unusual hemoglobins but will also identify and quantify more common hemoglobin variants.

Principle. Differences in charge allow separation of hemoglobin subtypes by column chromatography under high pressure. Hemoglobins are eluted in order of increasing charge, thus giving a unique retention time for each hemoglobin variant. The elution profile and column retention time allow for presumptive identification and qualification of hemoglobin variants.

Specimen. Anticoagulated blood is used.

Procedure. A sample of red blood cell hemolysate is loaded onto an HPLC non-porous cation-exchange column specific for hemoglobin analysis. The sample is eluted with two phosphate buffers that form an ionic gradient at a rate of 2 mL/min. An analysis of each sample can be run on two programs, which provide complementary data. The short program, which runs in about 6.5 minutes, provides elution profiles that give the retention time and approximate quantification for each hemoglobin variant present. The retention time is compared with known standards and a data bank to provide presumptive identification of the hemoglobin variant. The sample may then be run on a long program (approximately 20 minutes) that provides more accurate retention time data but is not as accurate for quantification.

Interpretation. The short program run on HPLC is most useful in identification and quantification of hemoglobins A, A_2, F, S, D, and C. More unusual hemoglobin variants may require long-program analysis. More than 700 hemoglobin variants have been analyzed and indexed according to elution times. Unusual variants of overlapping elution times may require further analysis by isoelectric focusing, electrophoresis, or globin gene analysis to definitively identify a hemoglobin subtype.

Notes and Precautions. HPLC offers a distinct advantage over classic hemoglobin electrophoresis in that it can more accurately identify and quantitate most types of abnormal hemoglobin as well as definitely identify unusual variants. Thus, HPLC is a very cost- and time-efficient screening methodology for a suspected hemoglobinopathy and forms the basis for most neonatal hemoglobinopathy screening programs. Specialized reference laboratories are usually required for this procedure. Hemoglobin E cannot be separated from HbA_2 by this method, and suspected HbE should be analyzed by standard electrophoresis. Hemoglobin H and Bart's hemoglobin may elute too quickly to be analyzed. Because of overlap, hemoglobins with similar retention times may require further analysis for definitive identification. Although this technology is FDA approved for initial identification of unusual hemoglobins, it is not approved for final identification. Thus, additional testing (such as electrophoresis, solubility testing, or globin chain analysis) is required to support the HPLC identification. HPLC does not provide accurate quantification.

Test 10.5.3 Quantitation of Hemoglobin A_2 with Ion-Exchange Chromatography

Purpose. Levels of HbA_2 are elevated in β-thalassemia minor. Quantitation of HbA_2 with routine electrophoresis on cellulose acetate has not been uniformly reliable.

Principle. The most accurate and rapid procedure generally available for measuring HbA_2 is chromatography using an anion exchange column to separate HbA_2 from HbA. HPLC (as described above) also may be used.

Specimen. Anticoagulated whole blood is used.

Procedure. Hemoglobin A_2 is separated from HbA by use of a microcolumn consisting of diethylaminoethyl cellulose (DEAE-cellulose) as the ion exchange resin. The resin is equilibrated with a tris(hydroxymethyl)aminomethane (TRIS) phosphate buffer, and the hemoglobin solution is applied. The more strongly charged HbA adheres to the ion exchange resin. Hemoglobin A_2 passes through and is quantitated spectrophotometrically at 415 nm. Commercial kits with disposable columns are available.

Interpretation. The normal range of values for HbA_2 is 1.6% to 3.5% (see **t10.6**). In β-thalassemia, the range is 3.5% to 8%.

t10.6 Hemoglobin Analysis in β-Thalassemic Disorders

Classification	Hemoglobin A	Hemoglobin A2	Hemoglobin F
Normal	Normal (97%)	Normal	Normal (<1%) (1.6% - 3.5%)
HPFH			Increased (15%-100%)
Heterozygous β-thalassemia (thalassemia minor)	Decreased (usually >90%)	Increased* (3.5%-8%)	Normal or slightly elevated
Homozygous β^+–thalassemia	Present, decreased	Variably increased*	Increased (<100%)
β^0-Thalassemia	Absent	Mildly increased	Increased (nearly 100%)
δ-β-Thalassemia	Absent	Absent	Increased (100%)

**Hemoglobin A_2 levels may be normal or decreased in patients with coexisting iron deficiency.*
HPFH = hereditary persistence of fetal hemoglobin; β^+ = reduced production of beta chains; β^0 = absence of beta chain production

Notes and Precautions. A number of hemoglobin variants are copurified under the usual test conditions. These include hemoglobins C, E, O, D, and (to a lesser extent) S. When a HbA_2value greater than 8% is found, the presence of such a variant is likely. Hemoglobin A_2 may be separated and quantitated in the presence of HbS by eluting the two hemoglobins separately, using buffers with different pH for elution. Hemoglobin A_2 levels may not be elevated in the presence of coexisting iron deficiency.

Test 10.5.4 Solubility Test for Hemoglobin S

Purpose. Solubility tests have been used most widely to screen for sickle cell trait and as a means of differentiating HbS from HbD, which are identical by electrophoresis at an alkaline pH.

Principle. The solubility test is based on the relative insolubility of reduced HbS compared with that of other hemoglobin variants and HbA in a high-phosphate buffer solution.

Specimen. Whole blood is used.

Procedure. A solution of 1.24 mol/L potassium dihydrogen phosphate (KH_2PO_4) containing saponin to lyse the red blood cells and sodium hydrosulfite (dithionite) to reduce the hemoglobin is used. Blood is added, and the solution is observed for turbidity by reading black lines held behind the test tubes. Commercial kits are available.

Interpretation. Positive test results are indicated by a turbid suspension; the ruled lines behind the test tube cannot be seen. Test results are positive for sickle cell trait and disorders with rare exceptions (eg, HbC_{Harlem}). Results are negative with all other hemoglobins. The differentiation of sickle cell trait from sickle cell disease may not always be clear because it is based on a quantitative difference in turbidity.

Notes and Precautions. In the presence of severe anemia, the blood sample used normally does not contain sufficient HbS to yield turbid solution. With a hemoglobin level less than 7 g/dL (70 g/L), the sample size should be doubled. False-positive results may be seen with lipemic plasma. The solubility test is inadequate as a sole means of screening for genetic counseling because it fails to detect the important carriers of HbC and β-thalassemia. In general, hemoglobin analysis by electrophoresis or HPLC is required for diagnosis of sickle cell disease, and the sickle cell test and solubility test for HbS are most useful as screening tests.

Test 10.5.5 Sickle Cell Test

Purpose. In most cases of sickle cell disease or the heterozygous sickle cell disorders (HbSC disease or the S-thalassemias), a few sickled red blood cells are readily seen on the routinely prepared blood smears. In sickle cell trait and some sickle cell disorders with a lesser propensity for sickling, manipulation is required to induce in vitro sickling to identify the presence of HbS.

Principle. When red blood cells containing HbS are deoxygenated, hemoglobin crystallizes to form the characteristic sickle shape. Deoxygenation can be accomplished by mixing a drop of blood with a reducing agent on a slide.

Specimen. Venous or capillary blood is used.

Procedure. The sickle cell test is performed by mixing the amount of blood that adheres to the end of an applicator stick with a drop of freshly prepared 2% sodium metabisulfite solution and covering the suspension with a cover slip. When sickle hemoglobin is present, cells begin to deform within 10 minutes, assuming crescent and holly leaf shapes. The preparation is observed on the microscope within 30 minutes with high-dry objective.

Interpretation. The test results are positive for sickle cell traits and all sickle cell disorders when HbS is present in a concentration of 25% or greater. Sickling has been described in other relatively rare variants, such as HbC_{Harlem}.

Notes and Precautions. The most frequently encountered technical problem resulting in a false-negative test result is outdated metabisulfite reagent that has lost its reducing power. With HbS disorders, test results may not be positive until an infant is 1 or 2 months of age because of the relatively high percentage of HbF during infancy that moderates the sickling properties of HbS.

Test 10.5.6 Alkali Denaturation Test for Fetal Hemoglobin

Purpose. Measurement of fetal hemoglobin helps in the diagnosis and differentiation of thalassemias, double heterozygotes with combined thalassemia and a structural hemoglobin variant, as well as in the diagnosis of HPFH. Because the mobility of HbF is close to that of HbA on routine electrophoresis, measurement of HbF based on electrophoretic techniques has not been reliable.

Principle. Hemoglobin F is relatively more resistant to denaturation by a strong alkali than other hemoglobins.

Specimen. Anticoagulated whole blood is used.

Procedure. Fresh alkali (1.2 N sodium hydroxide) is added to a hemolysate. After 1 minute, denatured hemoglobin is precipitated by the addition of ammonium sulfate. The filtrate contains HbF, which is quantitated spectrophotometrically at 415 nm.

Interpretation. The normal value for HbF is less than 2% (**t10.6**). Patients with β-thalassemia minor may have elevated HbF levels of 2% to 5%. Those with less common δ-β-thalassemia minor may show much higher levels. Patients with homozygous β-thalassemia show levels of HbF ranging from 30% to 100%. Levels in patients with hereditary persistence of fetal hemoglobin (HPFH) range from 15% to 100%. Elevated HbF levels ranging from 2% to 5% have been reported in numerous hematologic conditions, including aplastic anemia, pernicious anemia, hereditary spherocytosis, myelofibrosis, leukemia, and metastatic disease with bone marrow involvement.

Notes and Precautions. The alkali denaturation test is very sensitive at low levels of HbF. At levels greater than 10%, however, the method underestimates HbF, and accurate measurement requires special chromatographic techniques such as HPLC.

Test 10.5.7 Acid Elution Test for Fetal Hemoglobin in Red Blood Cells

Purpose. The acid elution test is used to differentiate HPFH from other states associated with high fetal hemoglobin levels.

Principle. When hemoglobin is precipitated inside the red blood cell and fixed with alcohol, the precipitated HbA and most variants can be dissolved in a buffered solution of citric acid and eluted from the cell. HbF remains precipitated inside the cell.

Specimen. Whole blood is used.

Procedure. A blood smear is prepared in the usual manner and fixed at 80% ethanol. It is then treated with a citric acid–phosphate buffer (pH 3.3), which elutes HbA from red blood cells. The blood film is then stained with eosin, which stains any residual precipitate.

Interpretation. Smears from normal blood show little, if any, staining and appear as ghosts. A heterogeneous distribution of fetal hemoglobin is seen in newborn infants, from fetal-maternal transfusion, and in the thalassemias, with elevated HbF levels. Hereditary persistence of fetal hemoglobin is the only condition in which HbF is evenly distributed among nearly all the red blood cells.

Notes and Precautions. The intensity of the staining often differs markedly from one part of the blood film to another, and considerable experience may be required for interpretation.

Test 10.5.8 Flow Cytometric Analysis of Fetal Hemoglobin

Purpose. Flow cytometric testing for detection and quantification of fetal hemoglobin is most useful in detecting maternal-fetal hemorrhage, but may also indicate increased levels of fetal hemoglobin associated with hemoglobinopathies.

Principle. Fluorescently labeled murine monoclonal antibodies directed against fetal hemoglobin (HbF) are used in a multiparametric flow cytometry assay to identify red blood cells containing HbF.

Specimen. Whole blood collected in EDTA is used. Refrigerated samples may be up to 72 hours old, whereas samples held at ambient temperatures are acceptable up to 12 hours after collection.

Procedure. Fluorescently labeled antibodies against HbF are incubated with the patient samples, positive controls (human cord blood), and negative controls (normal adult blood) and washed to remove unbound antibody. The sample is analyzed on a flow cytometer using red blood cell gating parameters and adjusted using the positive and negative controls run at the same time as the patient samples.

Interpretation. Normal adult cells will have a small amount of HbF that will appear as a small "shoulder" peak adjacent to the negative peak. The cord blood provides a positive control that is shifted away from the normal negative peak. Patient samples are compared to positive and negative controls run concurrently. Increased HbF will cause a shift of the patient sample towards the positive control peak.

Notes and Precautions. This testing is best used for detection of rare events, such as seen in a fetal-maternal bleed. However, patients with increased HbF due to hemoglobinopathy (i.e. thalassemia or HPFH) will also show increased HbF in all the patient red blood cells. When a hemoglobinopathy pattern is seen, the sample should be further tested by hemoglobin electrophoresis or HPLC hemoglobin analysis to confirm and further subclassify the process.

Test 10.5.9 Isopropanol Stability Test

Purpose. The isopropanol stability test is used to detect unstable hemoglobins.

Principle. Unstable hemoglobins have reduced stability when exposed to alcohol denaturation, compared with the stability of normal hemoglobins.

Specimen. Whole blood is used.

Procedure. A hemolysate is added to buffered isopropanol and incubated at 37°C. The preparation is observed for precipitation at 5-minute intervals over 30 minutes.

Interpretation. Unstable hemoglobins generally show turbidity within 5-10 minutes, whereas normal hemoglobins should remain clear for 30 minutes. False-positive test results may be obtained with sickle hemoglobin, fetal hemoglobin, and methemoglobin.

Test 10.5.10 Test for Hemoglobin H Inclusion Bodies

Purpose. Hemoglobin H is unstable and may be difficult to detect on routine electrophoresis. This test allows detection of HbH and may suggest the presence of other unstable hemoglobins.

Principle. Incubation of whole blood with brilliant cresyl blue causes oxidation and precipitation of HbH, resulting in diffuse stippling.

Specimen. Fresh whole blood is used.

Procedure. Three or four drops of whole blood are incubated with 0.5 mL of a 1% solution of brilliant cresyl blue in citrate-saline solution. Blood films are made at 10 minutes, 1 hour, and 4 hours.

Interpretation. The 10-minute slide is a control that shows the number of reticulocytes. Positive cells show a diffusely clumped pattern staining, resembling a golf ball, throughout the cell, with the reticulum staining light blue (see **i10.4**). In HbH disease, 50% or more of the cells on the 1-hour slide may be positive. Results with other unstable hemoglobins are variable, with a longer period of incubation usually required for precipitation and fewer cells staining.

i10.4 Hemoglobin H disease

Hemoglobin H disease showing the pattern of supravital staining of hemoglobin H precipitates following incubation and staining with brilliant cresyl blue. The hemoglobin H or unstable hemoglobins appear as a diffusely distributed particulate pattern of staining in most cells. *(Brilliant cresyl blue stain)*

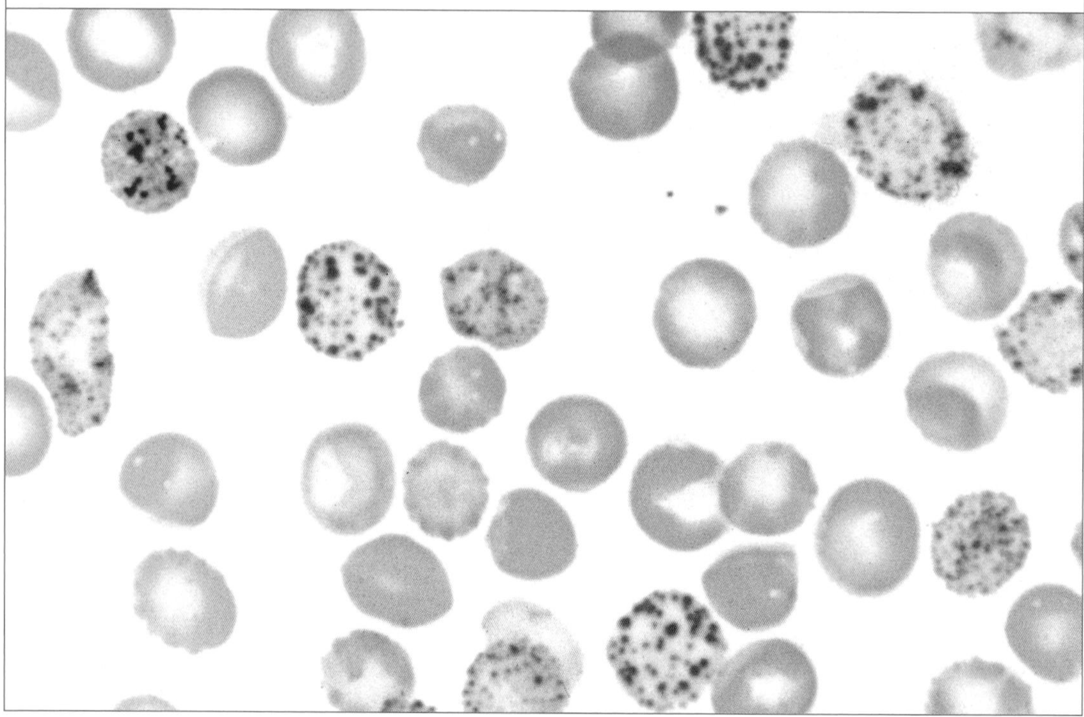

10.6 Ancillary Tests

10.6.1 Crystal Cells of Hemoglobin C Disease

Crystal cells of HbC disease (see i10.2) are present in as many as 10% of the circulating cells in affected patients who have undergone splenectomy, but these tetrahedral crystals are rare when a functional spleen is present. Crystal cells may be produced in vitro by hypertonic dehydration of red blood cells in a 3% sodium chloride buffer for up to 12 hours.

10.6.2 Globin Chain Analysis

Definitive diagnosis of a hemoglobin variant may require mutational analysis of the specific globin gene by polymerase chain reaction or electrophoretic gene analysis by Southern blot. Analysis is available at specialized laboratories and in the research setting. Clinical management is usually not dependent on this analysis, but it may be helpful in characterizing unusual or not previously described hemoglobinopathies.

10.7 Course and Treatment

The course and treatment of hemoglobin synthesis disorders varies greatly, depending on which mutation is present. Sickle cell disorders are characterized by disturbances in the microcirculation because sickle cells are so rigid and do not readily pass through capillaries, leading to microinfarction or vaso-occlusion. This may lead to pain or chronic, relentless organ damage due to infarction. In contrast, the clinical manifestations of HbC disease are minor, related almost entirely to the moderate hemolytic anemia that may be present. Patients with the disease may be asymptomatic or have a mild anemia with associated microcytosis.

The thalassemic syndromes also have a wide range of symptoms and clinical severity. The traits often have mild anemia. In β-thalassemia major, transfusions are required to maintain life. This often leads to iron overload, with attendant cardiac damage, requiring lifelong chelation therapy. Patients with hemoglobin H disease should avoid oxidative drugs, which could precipitate a hemolytic episode. Splenectomy may help to ameliorate the anemia in these patients.

10.8 References

Chui DH, Fucharoen S, Chan V. Hemoglobin H disease: not necessarily a benign disorder. *Blood.* 2003;101:791-800.

Clarke GM, Higgins TN. Laboratory investigation of hemoglobinopathies and thalassemias: review and update. *Clin Chem.* 2000;46(8 Pt 2):1284-1290.

Dorn-Beineke A, Frietsch T. Sickle cell disease—pathophysiology, clinical and diagnostic implications. *Clin Chem Lab Med.* 2002;40:1075-1084.

Fucharoen S, Winichagoon P. Thalassemia and abnormal hemoglobin. *Int J Hematol.* 2002;76(Suppl 2):83-89.

Fucharoen S, Winichagoon P. Clinical and hematologic aspects of hemoglobin E beta-thalassemia. *Curr Opin Hematol.* 2000;7:106-112.

Jenkins M, Ratnaike S. Capillary electrophoresis of hemoglobin. *Clin Chem Lab Med.* 2003;41:747-754.

Lo L, Singer ST. Thalassemia: current approach to an old disease. *Pediatr Clin North Am.* 2002;49:1165-1191.

Nagel RL, Fabry ME, Steinberg MH. The paradox of hemoglobin SC disease. *Blood Rev.* 2003;17:167-178.

Old JM. Screening and genetic diagnosis of haemoglobin disorders. *Blood Rev.* 2003;17:43-53.

Rubin LP, Hansen K. Testing for hematologic disorders and complications. *Clin Lab Med.* 2003;23:317-343.

Rund D, Rachmilewitz E. Pathophysiology of alpha- and beta-thalassemia: therapeutic implications. *Semin Hematol.* 2001;38:343-349.

Schrier SL. Pathophysiology of thalassemia. *Curr Opin Hematol.* 2002;9:123-126.

Thein SL. Genetic insights into the clinical diversity of beta thalassaemia. *Br J Haematol.* 2004;124:264-274.

Thein SL. Beta-thalassaemia prototype of a single gene disorder with multiple phenotypes. *Int J Hematol.* 2002;76(Suppl 2):96-104.

Waters HM, Seal LH. A systematic approach to the assessment of erythropoiesis. *Clin Lab Haematol.* 2001;23(5):271-283

Wethers DL. Sickle cell disease in childhood: Part I. Laboratory diagnosis, pathophysiology and health maintenance. *Am Fam Physician.* 2000;62:1013-1020.

Whitten CF, Whitten-Shurney W. Sickle cell. *Clin Perinatol.* 2001;28:435-48.

Weatherall DJ. The laboratory diagnosis of haemoglobinopathies. *Br J Haematol.* 1998;101:783-792.

Chapter 11

Paroxysmal Nocturnal Hemoglobinuria

Sherrie Perkins, MD, PhD

Paroxysmal nocturnal hemoglobinuria (PNH) is a rare acquired stem cell disorder characterized by recurrent, episodic intravascular hemolysis, hemoglobinuria, and venous thrombosis. The hemolysis occurs secondary to a mutation in the hematopoietic stem cell that causes a partial or complete loss of linkage of cell surface proteins to the membrane by glycophosphatidylinositol (GPI) anchor proteins. Clinically important proteins affected by this mutation include those regulating activity of the classic complement pathway. Although this defect is seen in all blood cells, the lack of complement regulatory proteins on the red blood cell results in the classic presentation of episodic hemolysis that is clinically seen in PNH. PNH may arise as a de novo disorder, termed hemolytic PNH. In addition, PNH is strongly associated with aplastic anemia (AA), where abnormal red blood cell clones may develop during the course of the aplastic anemia or hemolytic PNH may evolve into aplasia. This association has been termed AA/PNH.

11.1 Pathophysiology

PNH is an acquired RBC membrane disorder, arising secondary to a somatic mutation in the bone marrow pluripotential hematopoietic stem cell that gives rise to complete or partial deficiency of cell surface GPI anchoring of proteins. The affected gene is phosphatidylinositolglycan A (PIG-A), which is located on the X chromosome, and reintroduction of this gene into deficient PNH cells corrects the defect in GPI biosynthesis. The mutations associated with development of PNH may occur spontaneously or in patients with bone marrow injury associated with aplastic anemia or bone marrow hypoplasia. A spectrum of mutations have been described in association with hemolytic PNH that are usually small base pair deletions (1-14 base pairs) or insertions (1-8 base pairs) as well as base substitutions that lead to a DNA reading frameshift. These mutations may occur in many different sites throughout the PIG-A gene. PNH arising in association with AA often has similar types of mutations, although many cases will also contain mutations that include tandem duplications with insertions that are significantly larger than those described in hemolytic PNH as well as deletions of larger size. Patients with AA/PNH are also much more likely to have multiple mutations at different sites as well as several types of mutations. The mutated PIG-A deficient cell population may make up a minority of bone marrow cells, or may be expressed in nearly all hematopoietic cells. These mutations give rise to the intrinsic defect in the patient's red blood cells that make them susceptible to complement mediated hemolysis and give rise to the disease entity of PNH.

The GPI anchoring defect seen in PNH causes a variable deficiency in at least 17 cell surface proteins that may affect the functions of hematopoietic cells **t11.1**. Patients with PNH are deficient

t11.1 Hematopoietic Cell Surface Proteins Decreased or Absent in PNH Patients

Complement regulatory proteins
Decay accelerating factor (CD55)
Homologous restriction factor
Membrane inhibitor of reactive lysis (CD59)
Proteins associated with immune function
Lymphocyte function antigen-3 (LFA-3, CD58)
Fc receptor gamma III (CD16)
Endotoxin-binding protein receptor (CD14)
Other receptors
Urokinase receptor
Folate receptor
Enzymes
Alkaline phosphatase
Acetylcholinesterase
5'-ectonucleotidase
Other proteins
CD24
CD48
CD52 (campath-1)
CD66c
CD67
JMH-bearing protein

in two to three membrane glycoproteins that normally regulate complement activation. Proteins that have been found missing or deficient in affected patients include decay-accelerating factor (DAF or CD55), which regulates the activity of C3 convertase; homologous restriction factor (HRF), which regulates C9 activity and binding; and membrane inhibitor of reactive lysis (MIRL or CD59), which modulates terminal complement-mediated red blood cell lysis. Deficiency of one or more of these proteins leads to enhanced formation of the membrane complement lytic complex on the cell surface. Detection of decreased levels of CD55 and CD59 by flow cytometry on red blood cells or leukocytes forms the basis for diagnostic testing for PNH by flow cytometric methods (see below). Although WBCs and platelets also demonstrate abnormal cell-surface GPI anchoring proteins, it is the RBC deficiency that gives rise to the classic episodic intravascular hemolysis that is mediated by complement. Hemolysis is sometimes increased at night due to a slight fall in plasma pH that facilitates complement activation, and gives rise to the symptomatology of dark urine upon waking that may be seen in some patients.

A peculiar feature of PNH is the variable expression of the abnormal phenotype. This probably reflects genetic mosaicism in which some cells express normal levels of GPI-anchored proteins, others have intermediate expression, and still others are severely deficient. Three different subtypes of PNH cell types have been described based on the relative expression of complement regulatory proteins **t11.2**. It has been suggested that the relative numbers of each class of PNH cells seen in a particular patient will correlate with disease severity and may provide an indicator of disease progression. A patient may have some or all of the PNH cellular subtypes present, and the relative numbers of each cell type as well as disease phenotype may shift over time. Although red blood cells appear most susceptible to complement-mediated lysis, all hematopoietic cells are affected, which may lead to leukopenia and/or thrombocytopenia in some patients.

t11.2 Types of Cells Observed in PNH

PNH Cell Type	Sensitivity to Complement	Observed Complement Pathway Defects	GPI Protein Expression	Associated PIG-A Mutations
I	Normal to near normal	Near normal lytic behavior	Near normal to mild deficiency; partial lack of DAF (CD55) and/or MIRL (CD59)	None
II	Intermediate (10-15 times more sensitive)	Increased C3 binding to cell; increased C3/C5 convertase activity	Partial lack of DAF (CD55) and/or MIRL (CD59) (DAF deficiency appears most significant)	Missense (partial)
III	Highly sensitive (25 times more sensitive)	Increased binding of C3 to cell; increased C3/C5 convertase activity; increased binding of C5b67 complexes; increased C9 binding	Near total lack of DAF (CD55), MIRL (CD59), HRF	Nonsense, frameshift, deletion or insertion causing gene inactivation

PNH = paroxysmal nocturnal hemoglobinuria; GPI = glycophosphotidylinositol; PIG-A = phosphatidylinositolgycan A; DAF= decay accelerating factor; MIRL= membrane inhibitor of reactive lysis; HRF= homologous restriction factor

t11.3 Clinical Manifestations of PNH

Intravascular hemolysis—Anemia associated with dark urine, hemoglobinuria, hemosiderinuria and possible iron deficiency. May develop chronic renal failure.

Increased thrombosis (1/3 of patients)

Hepatic vein, mesenteric vein or cerebral vein thrombosis

Thrombophlebitis and pulmonary embolism

Thrombocytopenia

Leukopenia—sinopulmonary and blood infections

Bone marrow failure or aplastic anemia

Transformation to acute myelogenous leukemia or myelodysplastic syndrome

11.2 Clinical Findings

PNH is an uncommon disease, with an estimated prevalence of 1 to 10 cases per million. It is seen primarily in adults, but has also been described in children and adolescents. There is a wide spectrum of disease and many clinical manifestations **t11.3**. PNH usually begins as an insidious onset of anemia. Virtually all patients are anemic, often severely. The classically described pattern of episodic hemolysis—increased at night, causing dark urine after awakening—is frequently not seen. More often, hemolysis occurs in an irregular fashion, apparently precipitated by events such as infection, surgery, and transfusions. Hemolysis also may occur chronically throughout the day. Hemoglobinuria or dark urine may be absent. Chronic urinary iron loss, or hemosiderinuria, is a constant feature and may result in the development of iron deficiency anemia. The chronic hemolysis may also lead to chronic renal failure due to renal tubular damage.

Abnormal platelet function in PNH patients is frequently associated with venous thrombosis, which is a major cause of death as it is often refractory to thrombolytic therapies. Clinically significant thrombosis is seen in about one-third of affected patients. Thrombotic events may cause severe episodes of abdominal or back pain or severe refractory headaches. Development of Budd-Chiari syndrome (hepatic vein thrombosis), mesenteric vein or cerebral vein thromboses is most common. Thrombophlebitis may occur in the legs or arms and may lead to pulmonary thromboembolism. Arterial thrombosis is rare. Occasionally, patients may experience bleeding due to poor platelet function.

Patients are often leukopenic at some stage of the disease, leading to increased susceptibility to infection, in particular sinopulmonary and blood-borne infections. In addition, neutrophils show a decrease in leukocyte alkaline phosphatase (LAP) activity. Patients frequently progress to severe cytopenias, requiring transfusions or other therapeutic interventions.

Patients with AA may develop abnormal hematopoietic cell clones. Most often these clones have a PNH phenotype and are associated with mutations in the PIG-A gene. Small numbers of abnormal PIG-A deficient clones have also been seen in normal marrows, suggesting that that this is a frequent site of mutation. For unknown reasons, the PNH clones have a significant survival advantage in AA, perhaps by allowing the precursor cells to escape immune-mediated destruction. The PIG-A deficient clones do not have a survival advantage in normal hematopoiesis, leading to the characteristic mosaicism of PNH cell types.

11.3 Diagnostic Approach

Depending on the predominant features of the presenting illness, PNH may need to be differentiated from other causes of chronic hemolytic anemia, pancytopenia, iron deficiency, or hemoglobinuria.

Laboratory evaluation of this disorder is performed using the following steps:

1. Hematologic evaluation with complete blood cell count, peripheral blood morphology, and bone marrow examination is conducted.
2. The sucrose lysis and urine hemosiderin (Rous) tests are used to screen for PNH.
3. The acidified serum (Ham's) test and flow cytometric analysis for decreased expression of the CD55 (DAF) or CD59 (MIRL) proteins are definitive diagnostic tests for PNH.

11.4 Hematologic Findings

11.4.1 Blood Cell Measurements

The degree of anemia associated with PNH varies widely, with hemoglobin levels ranging from less than 6 g/dL (60 g/L) to normal. The mean corpuscular volume (MCV) may be somewhat increased (with prominent reticulocytosis or superimposed folate or vitamin B_{12} deficiency due to chronic hemolysis), or decreased owing to coexistent iron deficiency anemia. Often, the observed reticulocytosis is lower than expected for the degree of anemia. This discrepancy is attributed to the bone marrow stem cell defect.

11.4.2 Peripheral Blood Smear Morphology

No characteristic morphologic changes are seen. Macrocytosis and polychromatophilia may accompany prominent reticulocytosis. Iron deficiency may result in microcytosis and hypochromia. Spherocytes are absent. Variable leukopenia and thrombocytopenia may be seen and is often moderate to severe.

11.4.3 Bone Marrow Examination

Bone marrow cellularity is variable. Bone marrows are often hypocellular or aplastic in patients with AA/PNH and some forms of hemolytic PNH. Most patients with hemolytic PNH will have a hypercellular marrow with normoblastic erythroid hyperplasia and adequate numbers of megakaryocytes and myeloid elements. Some patients may exhibit megaloblastic maturation or other evidence of dyserthropoiesis. Stainable storage iron is usually absent, even when clinical iron deficiency is not present. Mild to moderate dyserythropoiesis may be seen in some cases, but other patients may demonstrate relatively normal erythroid differentiation.

11.5 Other Laboratory Tests

Test 11.5.1 Sucrose Lysis Test (Sugar Water Test)

Purpose. The sucrose lysis test is the most commonly used screening test for PNH.

Principle. An isotonic sucrose solution of low ionic strength aggregates serum globulins onto the RBC surface. This promotes binding and activation of complement on the red cell membrane. When a small amount of serum (as a source of complement) is added, PNH cells are lysed, whereas normal cells are not.

Specimen. Whole defibrinated blood is used. The blood should be collected in heparin.

Procedure. A small amount of fresh, normal, type-compatible serum is added to the buffered 10% sucrose solution. Washed red blood cells from the patient are added, and the suspension is incubated for 60 minutes at room temperature.

Interpretation. Lysis of greater than 5% of the red blood cells, as detected by release of hemoglobin (which imparts a red color to the supernatant) that is detectable by the eye, is compatible with the diagnosis of PNH. Very mild hemolysis, usually amounting to less than 5% of the red blood cells, may be found in some megaloblastic anemias and autoimmune hemolytic disease. A positive sucrose lysis test must be confirmed by the acidified serum test (Test 11.5.2) or flow cytometric analysis (Test 11.5.3) for a definitive diagnosis.

Notes and Precautions. It was originally suggested that the sucrose lysis test should be carried out using unbuffered sucrose solutions, which may lead to false-negative results. Ethylenediaminetetraacetic acid (EDTA) anticoagulation blocks complement activation and invalidates the test results.

Test 11.5.2 Acidified Serum Test (Ham's Test)

Purpose. The acidified serum test may be used to make a definitive diagnosis of PNH.

Principle. Complement fixes to red blood cells at a slightly acidic pH. Cells from patients with PNH lyse under these conditions, whereas normal red blood cells are resistant to lysis.

Specimen. Whole defibrinated blood is used. The blood should be collected in heparin.

Procedure. The test uses type-compatible blood from a healthy control subject and blood from a patient with suspected PNH. Red bood cells from the patient and control subject are suspended in each of the following serum preparations (from both subjects):

1. Unaltered serum.
2. Serum with a pH adjusted to 6.8 as measured with a pH meter.
3. Serum at pH 6.8 that has been heat activated to 55°C for 3 minutes to destroy complement proteins.
4. Heated serum to which guinea pig complement has been added.

Interpretation. A definitive diagnosis of PNH depends on demonstration of all of the following characteristics of in vitro hemolysis:

1. Hemolysis occurs with patient cells but not with control cells.
2. Hemolysis is enhanced by slightly acidifying the serum used.
3. Hemolysis is abolished by heat inactivating the serum at 55°C to destroy complement proteins.
4. Hemolytic activity is not restored to the heated serum by addition of guinea pig complement.

Some hemolysis may be present in the unaltered serum, but it is generally less than that observed in acidified serum. No hemolysis of control blood cells should occur in any of the tubes.

Notes and Precautions. Ethylenediaminetetraacetic acid anticoagulation of blood may block complement activation. Erroneous test results may be obtained due to underacidification or overacidification of serum. In the original description of the test, the serum pH was not verified with a pH meter because such instruments were not available. Careful adjustment of the serum pH to 6.78 ± 0.1 is necessary for reliable results. The correct performance and interpretation of the test is necessary, and use of a reference laboratory that performs testing on a routine basis may be indicated.

Test 11.5.3 Flow Cytometric Analysis for Decreased CD55 and CD59 Expression

Purpose. Flow cytometric detection of decreased levels of CD55 and/or CD59 allows for a definitive diagnosis of PNH to be made and excludes other causes of hemolysis.

Principle. Deficiency of GPI anchored protein activity leads to decreased expression of proteins linked to the cell surface by GPI anchor. Two proteins, CD55 and CD59, that modulate complement activity are anchored to the red blood cell surface by this mechanism. Detection of decreased or absent expression of these proteins by flow cytometry analysis provides a sensitive and specific means for diagnosis of PNH.

Specimen. Blood should be collected in a heparin tube.

Procedure. CD59 is present in high levels on the RBC membrane, whereas CD55 is found at lower levels (6-8 times less). The patient's red blood cells are stained with either anti-CD59 or anti-CD55 and analyzed by flow cytometry to generate a histogram of protein expression, which is compared with that of normal control cells.

Interpretation. Patients with PNH show variably decreased to absent expression of CD59 and/or CD55 (ie, decreased or absent fluorescence as seen in f11.1). A population of normal cells is also commonly seen in the patient, reflecting characteristic phenotypic mosaicism. The degree of CD55 and/or CD59 deficiency is often associated with the severity of disease.

Notes and Precautions. Blood should be maintained at ambient temperature because refrigeration may cause shedding of antigens and falsely decrease expression of CD59 and CD55. Optimal testing requires blood that is less than 24 hours old, although testing may be performed on samples taken up to 72 hours earlier.

CD59 is expressed at levels six to eight times those of CD55; thus, analysis of CD59 usually demonstrates the clearest pattern of deficiency when compared with normal controls. The number of cells expressing normal, low, or intermediate levels of CD59 may be enumerated. This may provide some insights into disease severity as well as a means for monitoring disease progression. Due to lower levels of expression, CD55 may be more difficult to separate into discrete populations. Flow cytometric analysis also may be performed on granulocytes, but this process is technically more challenging. Flow cytometry is very sensitive and can detect small populations (1% to 5%) of deficient cells, allowing for detection of early PNH, emergence of PNH clones in aplastic anemia or residual abnormal cell populations after transfusion or recent hemolytic episode.

Test 11.5.4 Test for Urine Hemosiderin

Purpose. Urine hemosiderin is nearly always present in PNH and provides a valuable screening test.

Principle. Even in the absence of discernible hemoglobinuria, the chronic low-grade intravascular hemolysis associated with PNH is sufficient to deplete serum haptoglobin. Hemoglobin in the plasma is reabsorbed by renal tubules. As the renal tubules become heavily laden with iron, it is excreted in the urine as hemosiderin granules, which are demonstrable with a Prussian blue stain.

Specimen. A random urine specimen is used.

Procedure. The presence of hemosiderin in the urine is demonstrated by adding a drop of a mixture of equal parts of 4% hydrochloric acid and 4% potassium ferricyanide to the sediment of centrifuged urine specimen. The mixture is incubated at room temperature for 10 minutes and agitated frequently.

Interpretation. Hemosiderin appears as blue particles. Although considerable emphasis has been placed on intracellular location of hemosiderin in urine, cells containing hemosiderin may have disintegrated and free hemosiderin may be the predominant form. Urine from a healthy patient does not contain hemosiderin.

f11.1 Flow cytometric histograms showing decreased expression of CD55 and CD59, diagnostic of PNH

Flow cytometric histograms from a patient with PNH showing a population of RBCs with decreased expression levels of CD55 (a, arrow) and CD 59 (b, arrow). This patient also has a second population of relatively normal CD55 and CD59 expression in the M1 area, indicating a partial deletion. For comparison, RBC expression of CD55 (c) and CD59 (d) demonstrating a single population in the M1 area is seen in a normal control.

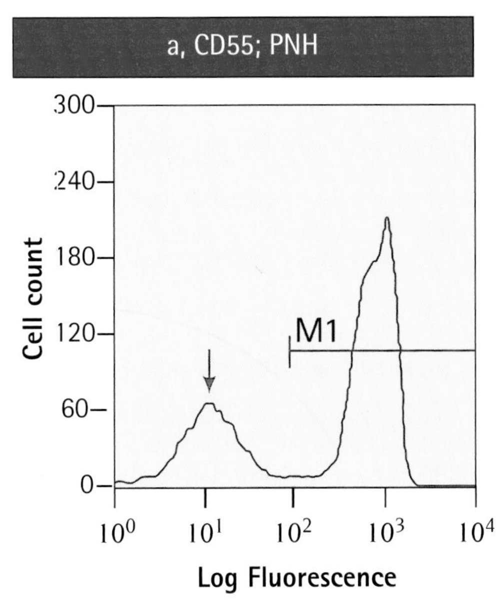

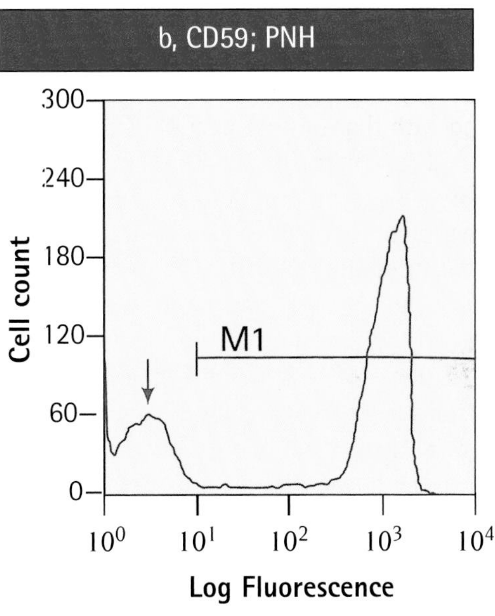

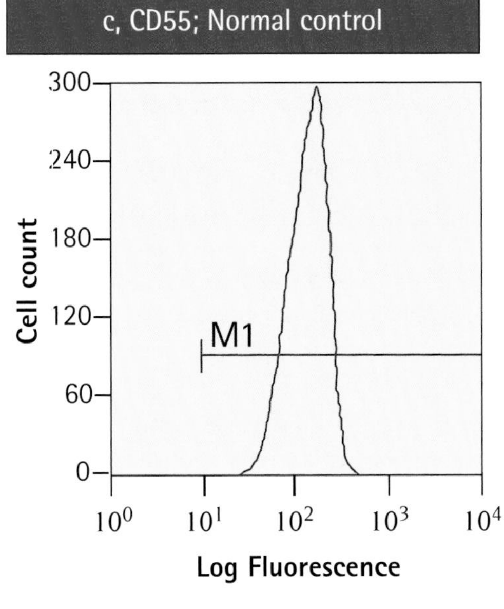

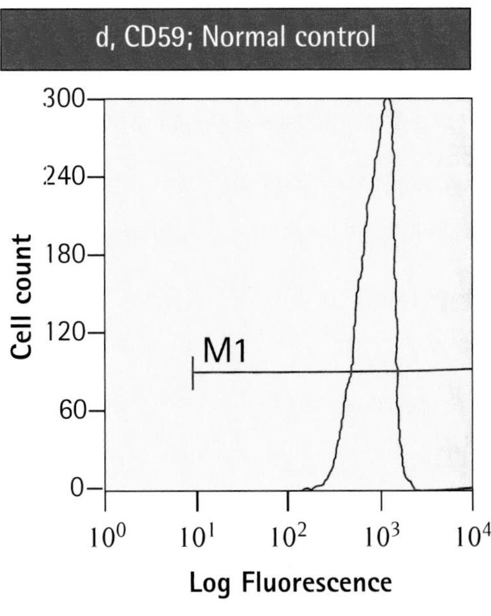

11.6 Ancillary Tests

Quantitative testing of complement sensitivity may give more precise information regarding the size of the complement-sensitive population; however, it is too complex for routine clinical use. Red blood cell acetylcholinesterase activity and leukocyte activity are diminished in PNH. Cytogenetic analysis may show abnormalities, including trisomy 9, loss of chromosome Y, and other deleted or lost chromosomes. No specific cytogenetic pattern has been identified. Molecular mutational analysis screening documenting mutations in the exons of the PIG-A gene (deletions, insertions, or substitutions) is definitive but is only offered for limited applications in some reference laboratories. Because of the wide diversity of mutational types and sites, typical screening will involve polymerase chain reaction based analysis and sequencing of specific mutational hot spots on the PIG-A gene.

11.7 Course and Treatment

The disease course of PNH may be fulminating or chronic. The median survival after diagnosis is 10 to 15 years, with 25% of patients surviving for more than 25 years. The major causes of morbidity and morality are thrombosis, bleeding, and infection. Rarely, acute myelogenous leukemia (1% to 5% of patients) or a myelodysplastic syndrome (5% of patients) may supervene. Thrombotic complications, particularly Budd-Chiari syndrome, may be rapidly fatal. Treatments include symptomatic blood transfusions, androgenic steroids to stimulate hematopoiesis, corticosteroids, thrombolytic or anticoagulant agents, and bone marrow transplant. Allogenic bone marrow transplant is curative. Gene therapies, such as transfection of normal PIG-A protein or retroviral transfer of CD59, are under investigation. Over a disease course of many years, about one third of patients may have a spontaneous remission or a decrease in disease severity, perhaps reflecting a decreased survival advantage for the abnormal clone in those patients.

11.8 References

Brodsky RA. Advances in the diagnosis and therapy of paroxysmal nocturnal hemoglobinuria. *Blood Rev.* 2008;22:65-74.

Brodsky RA, Hu R. PIG-A mutations in paroxysmal nocturnal hemoglobinuria and in normal hematopoiesis. *Leuk Lymphoma.* 2006;47:1215-1221.

Hall C, Richards SJ, Hillmen P. The glycosylphosphatidylinositol anchor and paroxysmal nocturnal hemoglobinuria/aplasia model. *Acta Haematol.* 2002;108:219-230.

Inoue N, Murakami Y, Kinoshita T. Molecular genetics of paroxysmal nocturnal hemoglobinuria. *Int J Hematol.* 2003;77:107-112.

Luzzatto L, Gianfaldoni G. Recent advances in biological and clinical aspects of paroxysmal nocturnal hemoglobinuria. *Int J Hematol.* 2006;84:104-112.

Mortazavi Y, Merk B, McIntosh J, et al. The spectrum of PIG-A gene mutations in aplastic anemia/paroxysmal nocturnal hemoglobinuria (AA/PNH): a high incidence of multiple mutations and evidence of a mutational hot spot. *Blood.* 2002;100:3897-3902

Nakao S, Sugimori C, Yamazaki H. Clinical significance of a small population of paroxysmal nocturnal hemoglobinuria-type cells in the management of bone marrow failure. *Int J Hematol.* 2006;84:118-122.

Parker CJ. Bone marrow failure syndromes: paroxysmal nocturnal hemoglobinuria. *Hematol Oncol Clin North Am.* 2009;23:333-346.

Richards SJ, Barnett D. The role of flow cytometry in the diagnosis of paroxysmal nocturnal hemoglobinuria in the clinical laboratory. *Clin Lab Med.* 2007;27:577-590.

Risitano AM, Maciejewski JP, Selleri C, Rotoli B. Function and malfunction of hematopoietic stem cells in primary bone marrow failure syndromes. *Curr Stem Cell Res Ther.* 2007;2:39-52.

Chapter 12

Extrinsic Hemolytic Anemia: General Concepts and Transfusion Reactions

Robert C. Blaylock, MD

The causes of extrinsic hemolytic anemia are some of the most feared and most common iatrogenic adverse outcomes encountered in medicine. Modern blood banking started around the middle of the last century with transfusion-associated death rates estimated near 1 per 1000 transfusions. By 1990, death rates declined to rates estimated at 1 per 800,000 per red blood cell units transfused with over half of the deaths due to hemolytic transfusion reactions.

The safety of the blood supply is improving yearly as new strategies for preventing transmission of infectious agents are implemented. Unfortunately, relatively little success has been seen regarding reduction of hemolytic transfusion reactions. This became apparent in an initial report in 1992, and a subsequent 10-year analysis of hemolytic reactions associated with transfusion in New York State. The 10-year report confirmed the low rate of deaths associated with transfusion at 1 in 1.8 million. The report identified 237 major ABO-incompatible transfusions, which occurred at a frequency of 1 in 38,000, and the statistic that 1 in 19,000 units of blood go to the wrong individual.

Hemolytic transfusion reactions are a large cause of morbidity in the United States, with approximately 300 ABO incompatible transfusions occurring annually. Very few result in death, but the etiology of these reactions is almost entirely due to errors. Over half of the errors occur outside of the blood bank with improper identification of the unit or recipient accounting for 37% of the mistakes, and phlebotomy errors at the time of procuring the sample for blood typing representing 13%. Errors isolated to the blood bank were responsible for 29% of the mistakes, and compound errors, which are errors made in the blood bank that should have been caught on the floor but were not, totaled 15% of the mistakes. When compared to the current risk of contracting HIV, which is approximately 1 in 2 million, it is clear why efforts to improve transfusion safety focus on preventing ABO incompatible transfusions.

Historically, medicine has blamed individuals for mistakes and moved on. The reality is that mistakes are made by bad systems and rarely by bad people. Hospitals must focus on improving systems involved in patient identification, electronic medical records, and standard operating procedures used in the administration of blood and medicine. The Food and Drug Administration and the Joint Commission on the Accreditation of Healthcare Organizations have recognized these system problems and recently mandated the use of barcoding to prevent mistakes. Further regulatory agency interventions will occur if the medical community does not take the initiative to prevent transfusion errors.

12.1 Pathophysiology

12.1.1 Acute Hemolytic Transfusion Reaction (AHTR)

Most hemolytic transfusion reactions result from the interaction of a major blood group antigen (A or B) and a naturally occurring isohemagglutinin. This most commonly occurs when antigens from a unit of blood react with antibodies found in a patient's plasma. The antigens are analogous to a lighted match tossed into a reservoir of gasoline, which is analogous to the antibodies. Isohemagglutinins are a combination of IgM and IgG antibodies **t12.1** capable of activating complement and causing intravascular hemolysis. The minority of intravascular reactions are caused by unexpected red blood cell alloantibodies directed at minor blood group antigens. Besides hemolysis, other complications include disseminated intravascular coagulation (DIC), vasomotor alterations, and renal failure.

t12.1 Properties of Immunoglobulins Acting in Alloimmune Hemolysis

Property	IgM	IgG
Size	900,000 d	160,000 d
Antigen binding sites	10	2
Agglutination	Yes	No
Optimal binding temperature	<37°C	37°C
Common antibodies	A, B blood group antigens	Antigens from previous transfusion or pregnancy
Mechanism of hemolysis	Complement-mediated lysis	Reticuloendothelial cell removal of Ig-coated cells
Type of transfusion reaction	Acute	Delayed

Infrequently, acute hemolytic transfusion reactions occur when incompatible antibodies are infused into a patient. In most cases, the amount of antibody infused is small and adsorbed onto other tissues that express blood group "A" and "B" antigen, such as endothelium. The incompatible plasma is also diluted so antibody titers remain low. Cases of acute hemolytic transfusion reactions due to incompatible plasma have been reported with platelet transfusions when the donor isohemagglutinin titer has been very high. Another clinical circumstance involves the infusion of incompatible plasma when blood type "O" trauma blood must be given in large quantities before the native blood type of the patient can be determined. Usually up to 800 mL of incompatible plasma can be given before hemolysis will occur, but again, this assumes donors have normal isohemagglutinin titers.

Intravenous immunoglobulin (IVIG) has also been associated with hemolysis. Since IVIG is pooled from many donors, the plasma pool may contain an unexpected red blood cell antibody.

DIC is caused by abnormal systemic thrombin generation. Old theories proposed the intrinsic coagulation pathway, via Hageman Factor activation, as the predominant source of thrombin; however, recent studies demonstrate the extrinsic coagulation pathway, via tissue factor activation, as the leading source of thrombin production through cytokine generation. Many cytokines multiply during the first few hours after a major hemolytic transfusion reaction. Included are cytokines responsible for thrombin generation: mainly tumor necrosis factor (TNF), and interleukin (IL)-1. The cytokine increase is dependent on the number of incompatible red blood cells transfused.

Cytokines increase thrombin generation by directly increasing tissue factor activity and by modulating effects on endothelial cells. TNF causes increased tissue factor activity. TNF and IL-1 are thought to act on endothelial cells in two ways. The first results in the increased expression of tissue factor on endothelial cells. The second involves a decrease in thrombomodulin activity. Thrombomodulin acts by binding circulating thrombin and activating protein C, which is critical for proper inactivation of the soluble coagulation system. Decreased activity of protein C leads to increased thrombosis.

Hypotension and shock are hemodynamic outcomes of acute hemolytic transfusion reactions, but hypertension can occur. In one study, 47% of patients involved in an acute hemolytic transfusion reaction had absolutely no signs or symptoms. Complement activation alone results in the production of C3a, C4a, and C5a, which are known anaphylatoxins. These can result in the release of histamine and serotonin, which cause vasodilatation and capillary leak.

Antigen/antibody complexes activate Hageman factor as discussed above. Hageman factor not only activates the intrinsic coagulation pathway, but also activates the kininogen system and ends in the production of bradykinin. Bradykinin in turns causes vasodilatation and hypotension.

Cytokines have already been implicated as a cause of DIC, but they also have a profound impact on blood pressure. IL-1, IL-6, IL-8 and TNF all increase in AHTR and all result in fever, capillary leak, and smooth muscle relaxation, which contribute to hypotension and shock.

Norepinephrine can be released from the adrenal gland as a direct effect of antigen/antibody complexes or as a sympathetic nervous systemic response to shock.

Renal failure is a common consequence of AHTR. Hemoglobin toxicity was believed to cause renal failure via direct toxicity to tubules and injury to renal epithelial cells, but this is not the case. However, the administration of hemoglobin preparations has revealed that the biggest problem with hemoglobin is not renal failure, but hypertension. There are two leading theories for the cause of the hypertension. The first involves the ability of hemoglobin to bind nitric oxide. Nitric oxide is a potent vasodilator and reduced levels leads to smooth muscle contraction in vascular walls. The second theory involves the increased delivery of oxygen to arterioles when pure hemoglobin is circulating. Some studies suggest that hemoglobin not contained in red blood cells may result in flooding arterioles with an excess of oxygen. The arterioles constrict in the rich oxygen environment, which results in systemic hypertension leading to decreased blood flow to end organs.

The major cause of renal failure is poor kidney perfusion which can be caused by mechanisms associated with AHTR that cause both hypertension and hypotension. Hypotension and shock associated with AHTR are an obvious cause of reduced renal blood flow. Thrombi caused by DIC obstruct renal vessels reducing perfusion.

Endothelin is a strong vasoconstrictor and may cause localized contraction of renal vascular supply. Endothelin is released from endothelium when vascular surfaces are exposed to substances like thrombin and bradykinin. These substances are circulating in abundance during AHTR.

12.1.2 Delayed Hemolytic Transfusion Reaction (DHTR)

DHTR is caused by red blood cell alloantibodies most commonly directed at antigens in the Rh, Kidd, Kell, or Duffy blood group systems. These antibodies are found in patients with a previous history of transfusion, pregnancy, or IV drug use. Most of the time these antibodies can be detected prior to transfusion and intravascular hemolytic reactions can be avoided. DHTR can occur 10-28 days after the initial exposure to the foreign alloantigen. Patients with a prior exposure to alloantigens can experience DHTR as early as 3 days after transfusion secondary to an anamnestic immune response. This only occurs when the initial foreign red blood cell antigen exposure was many years ago and the alloantibody titers have dropped below detectable levels prior to transfusion.

DHTR is rarely fatal and usually results in extravascular hemolysis, but intravascular hemolysis can occur. Typically DHTR causes a drop in hematocrit, which corresponds with the unit, or units of blood, that express the antigen specific for the antibody being produced. DHTR is often not noticed by clinicians and discovered when a specimen obtained 72 hours after transfusion is sent for an antibody screen.

12.1.3 Other Causes of Hemolysis

Many clinical situations arise which can be confused with an acute or delayed hemolytic transfusion reaction. Temperature extremes are common. Units of blood that have been unintentionally frozen will hemolyze. Freezing can occur if units are placed in refrigerators not approved for blood storage, or as units are shipped during cold weather. These obviously occur in vivo in burn patients, but can also occur in vitro due to improperly functioning blood warmers or intravenous normal saline solutions which have been heated inappropriately prior to mixing with packed red blood cells.

Red blood cells should only be mixed with normal saline. Other IV solutions can cause osmotic hemolysis of red blood cells (dextrose or albumin solutions improperly diluted with distilled water). The calcium contained in Lactated Ringer solutions can cause a unit of blood to clot and undergo subsequent hemolysis by reversing the citrate anticoagulant.

Mechanical destruction of red blood cells can occur during surgery when cell savers or cardiopulmonary bypass circuits are used secondary to poorly calibrated roller pump heads. Rapid infusers used in trauma or massive transfusion situations can be problematic if blood is forced through an IV line restriction. Mechanical destruction of red blood cells occurs with some prosthetic heart valves or in patients with vegetative endocarditis.

Units of red blood cells can be contaminated with bacteria. These units are infused with often catastrophic effects that include hemolysis. Hemolysis is also seen with malaria infections, red blood cell enzyme deficiencies, and in polyagglutination.

12.2 Clinical Findings

The signs and symptoms that can be associated with an AHTR are listed in **t12.2**. Up to 50% of patients experiencing an AHTR may be asymptomatic. Some patients will only demonstrate a fever, while others receiving the wrong unit of blood may have cardiovascular collapse and subsequent death.

t12.2 Acute Hemolytic Transfusion Reaction – Signs and Symptoms

Signs	Symptoms
Fever	Chills
Diaphoresis	Rigors
Hypertension	Flushing
Dyspnea	Anxiety
Tachycardia	Shortness of breath
Hemoglobinuria	Nausea
Hemoglobinemia	Vomiting
Urticaria	Diarrhea
Bleeding	Pain
Respiratory arrest	Infusion site
Cardiac arrest	Lumbar
	Chest
	Abdominal

In general, the clinical findings associated with hemolysis are related to subsequent anemia and include pallor, fatigue, malaise, weakness, shortness of breath, and jaundice.

12.3 Diagnostic Approach

Any sign or symptom during a transfusion must be investigated as a possible transfusion reaction. Unfortunately, the first indications of transfusion reaction may be subtle or seem insignificant. Too often they are ignored and the transfusion is not stopped. This is unfortunate because the severity of most reactions is dependent on the dose of red blood cells administered. Proper workup of a suspected transfusion reaction includes:

1. Stopping the transfusion
2. Maintaining venous access
3. Performing bedside clerical check for proper patient identification and unit label
4. Obtaining samples for blood bank workup of reaction
5. Returning the remaining blood product, tubing, and attached IV solutions to the blood bank
6. Contacting the patient's physician and blood bank physician to direct the workup and interpret the results

The blood bank physician will obtain a patient history, signs, and symptoms that led to the suspected reaction, and direct the laboratory workup of the reaction. Testing will include a direct antiglobulin test on the pre- and post-transfusion sample to look for the presence of antibody or complement on cells, and a check for free hemoglobin in plasma. Once haptoglobin is saturated and levels depleted, free hemoglobin will appear in the urine. Additional testing may include different methodologies for red blood cell antibody screening or crossmatch techniques.

12.4 Hematologic Findings

Often, hematologic tests for transfusion reactions are unrevealing unless a specimen is obtained during the transfusion. An abrupt fall in hemoglobin 3-28 days after transfusion, a failure to maintain hemoglobin levels, or the appearance of jaundice suggests an incompatible transfusion. Prolonged administration of incompatible blood can result in splenomegaly and lead to the mistaken diagnosis of autoimmune hemolytic anemia. Intravascular hemolysis may result from ABO-incompatible transfusion and with various other antibodies, including anti-Kell, anti-Duffy (anti-Fy^a), anti-Kidd (anti-Jk^a or anti-Jk^b), anti-E, anti-C, and anti-S.

12.4.1 Blood Cell Measurements

Variable anemia is present. One unit of packed RBCs should increase the hemoglobin (1.5 g/dL [15 g/L]) or the hematocrit (3% [0.03]) in an adult of average size. Acute hemolysis may be associated with leukocytosis and a left shift. In patients with thermal burns or ABO-incompatible transfusions with marked microspherocytosis, the mean corpuscular volume (MCV) may be decreased as low as 60-70 μm^3 (60-70 fL).

12.4.2 Peripheral Blood Smear Morphology

Usually, peripheral smear findings are non-specific. Transfusions that are ABO incompatible and IgG-mediated hemolysis are associated with the formation of microspherocytes. Patients with thermal burns have transient microspherocytosis lasting 24-48 hours. Disseminated intravascular coagulation can be associated with RBC fragmentation.

12.4.3 Bone Marrow Examination

Bone marrow examination usually is not helpful. Prolonged transfusions result in an increase in bone marrow iron. Prolonged hemolysis may lead to a compensatory erythroid hyperplasia.

12.5 Other Laboratory Tests

Test 12.5.1 Direct Antiglobulin Test (DAT)

Purpose. The DAT determines if immunoglobulin or complement is coating the surface of the patient's red blood cells.

Principle. Patient red blood cells are incubated with poly-specific IgM reagent with specificity for human IgG and complement.

Specimen. Red blood cells are collected in EDTA.

Procedure. Washed patient red blood cells are incubated with poly-specific IgM reagent and observed for agglutination. Reagents specific for human IgG or complement component C3d are used if the initial poly-specific test is positive.

Interpretation. Red blood cells coated with either IgG or C3d will clump in the presence of the poly-specific reagent. In most cases of acute or delayed hemolytic transfusion reactions the poly-specific DAT will be positive. Further characterization of the DAT can be performed using mono-specific reagents, which are IgM anti-IgG or IgM anti-C3d.

Notes and Precautions. It is important to determine if a mixed-field reaction is present. A mixed field reaction can be indicative of both AHTR and DHTR. Mixed-field reactions are evident when some cells clump when incubated with poly-specific DAT reagent, while others are free floating. This can occur when two cell populations are present, one of which is coated with antibody or complement, and the other population is not. Lack of a mixed field reaction may indicate the DAT was positive prior to transfusion and a pre-transfusion sample should be tested.

Test 12.5.2 Indirect Antiglobulin Test (IAT)

Purpose. The IAT detects unexpected alloantibodies in patient plasma or serum.

Principle. Commercially prepared screening cells are collected from 2-4 individuals, depending on the vendor, and methodology used in the test. The combination of cells is selected to ensure all commonly encountered, and problematic, minor red blood cell antigens are present on at least one of the screening cells. Key antigens are homozygous so that antigens are not missed due to reduced dosage.

Specimen. Serum or plasma is used.

Procedure. Patient plasma or serum is incubated with each individual screening cell. Most unexpected red blood cell alloantibodies are IgG class and will not clump red cells. IgM antiserum specific for human IgG and complement is added after the initial incubation. Agglutination with any of the screening cells determines a positive test.

Interpretation. Agglutination of one, or all screening cells, determines a positive test.

Notes and Precautions. IAT results must be negative before patients have invasive procedures which may require transfusion. If the IAT is positive, invasive procedures should be postponed until the alloantibodies have been identified and red blood cell units lacking the corresponding antigens have been crossmatched.

Test12.5.3 Antibody Identification

Purpose. This test determines the specificity of the alloantibody found after a positive IAT.

Principle. The availability and completeness of identification procedures vary in hospital laboratories and may be best handled by a reference laboratory. Simple antibodies may be identified in 4 hours; however, patients with multiple alloantibodies may require many days to complete testing.

Specimen. Serum or plasma is used.

Procedure. Serum or plasma is tested with commercially available panels of 9-12 RBC samples for which all antigens are known. Serum and cell samples are incubated at room temperature and at 37°C, and followed by the antiglobulin reaction. The presence of agglutination or hemolysis is noted and graded. Variability in the strength of agglutination, the temperature of reaction, or the medium of reaction may indicate the presence of more than one antibody. Once antibody specificity is known, the patient's RBCs are typed for the appropriate antigen.

Interpretation. Alloantibodies agglutinate specific cells of the panel, but not of the patient. The pattern of reactive cell samples is compared with the protocol sheet to determine specificity. The patient's cells should be negative for the particular antigen corresponding to the antibody identified by the panel; if they are not, the antibody specificity is not confirmed and must be reevaluated.

Notes and Precautions. IgG antibodies act at 37°C by indirect antiglobulin, enzyme, or LISS techniques. They usually follow previous transfusion or incompatible pregnancy. Unexpected red blood cell alloantibodies (eg, anti-Kell, anti-Fy^a, anti-Jk^a, or anti-Jk^b) are particularly dangerous because they cause AHTR. The Kidd antibodies may not be found during antibody screening if exposure to the antigen was years prior to current testing. However, titers increase rapidly with incompatible transfusions, causing initiation of DHTR.

Once identified, antibodies must be permanently recorded, because titers may decrease over time only to be re-induced with incompatible transfusions. Titers may be so weak that truly incompatible units appear compatible.

Test 12.5.4 Serum Haptoglobin

Purpose. An absence of haptoglobin indicates hemolysis, liver failure, or rare hereditary variants.

Principle. Haptoglobin is an a_2-globulin produced in the liver that binds free hemoglobin on a molecule-for-molecule basis. The haptoglobin-hemoglobin complex is metabolized in the reticuloendothelial system, maintaining serum hemoglobin levels below renal thresholds. During intravascular hemolysis, haptoglobin binding is completely saturated. Other serum proteins (hemopexin, transferrin, and albumin) then bind the excess hemoglobin before spilling into the urine. Absence of haptoglobin implies binding saturation and degradation. Decreased haptoglobin reflects active hemolysis or, alternatively, failure of production due to liver failure. Rare abnormal haptoglobins (such as Hp^-) are genetic variants that do not bind hemoglobin but are of little clinical significance.

Specimen. Fresh serum is obtained atraumatically. To avoid extraneous hemolysis, serum should not be allowed to remain on RBCs. Testing specimens with macroscopic hemoglobinemia is superfluous.

Procedure. The haptoglobin molecule has separate sites for antibody and hemoglobin binding. Haptoglobin is quantitated with turbidimetric methods using a nephelometer. Antihaptoglobin is added to the patient's serum, forming immune complexes with serum haptoglobin (1:1). These immune complexes scatter light proportionate to their concentration.

Interpretation. The normal range of haptoglobin is 40-180 mg/dL (0.4-1.8 g/L). Levels of less than 25 mg/dL (0.25 g/L) are consistent with hemolysis. Haptoglobin levels may be transiently decreased after massive transfusion as a result of destruction of senescent RBCs without hemolysis.

Notes and Precautions. Haptoglobin levels are rarely needed in the diagnosis of AHTR.

Test 12.5.5 Visual Check for Hemolysis

Purpose. This test checks patient plasma for free hemoglobin.

Principle. Free hemoglobin will turn plasma or serum red and is visible to the human eye.

Specimen. Serum or plasma is used. The blood sample should be obtained as soon as the reaction is suspected.

Procedure. A fresh sample is centrifuged to separate red blood cells from serum or plasma and inspected for color.

Interpretation. A pink hue is detectable with as little as 2.5 mL of lysed red blood cells in 3000 mL of plasma. This corresponds to a measured free hemoglobin level of 35 mg/dL.

Notes and Precautions. Measuring free hemoglobin levels after a suspected AHTR is unnecessary and a visual check for hemolysis is sufficient.

Test 12.5.6 Urine Hemoglobin

Purpose. Free plasma hemoglobin levels greater than 150 mg/dL (1.5 g/L) lead to spillover of hemoglobin into the urine. Urine hemoglobin confirms intravascular hemolysis, particularly when venous specimens have been difficult to obtain or collection is delayed.

Principle. Plasma proteins, haptoglobin, transferrin, and albumin bind free hemoglobin in normal metabolism. When the renal threshold is exceeded, free hemoglobin is detected in the urine. After incompatible transfusion, this is usually a transient occurrence, ending when the incompatible RBCs have been lysed.

Specimen. Random urine samples are collected within 2-3 hours of the clinical episode.

Procedure. Urine is tested with a dipstick that colorimetrically indicates the presence of hemoglobin.

Interpretation. Normally, no hemoglobin is present in the urine. Significant reactions are 1+ or greater (scale, 0 to 3+). The urine sediment should be examined for RBCs (hematuria), which may give rise to a false-positive test result. Urinary RBCs are not seen with hemolysis but usually result from bladder or prostate surgery and urinary instrumentation. Increased levels of myoglobin in the urine, secondary to muscle damage, also may cause false-positive results. If RBC destruction has occurred slowly over several days, urine hemosiderin may be present without overt hemoglobinuria.

Notes and Precautions. A visual change in urine color may be all that is necessary to evaluate acute hemolysis.

12.6 Course and Treatment

Prevention of AHTR is paramount. Most acute hemolytic transfusion reactions result from clerical error. Strict implementation and adherance to transfusion protocols, including proper patient identification, sample labeling, and unit checks prior to blood administration, must be followed.

Any change in signs or patient symptoms that develop during a transfusion must be addressed. Fever and chills are the most common findings during AHTR. Unfortunately, these are the most common findings in a non-hemolytic febrile transfusion reaction (NHFTR), which may be uncomfortable for the patient, but does not result in serious morbidity. NHFTR is common and sometimes desensitizes clinicians to what may be the first sign of a serious transfusion reaction. All serious transfusion reactions are dose dependent and transfusions must be stopped if a reaction is suspected.

The treatment of AHTR is supportive care, which may require intubation, blood pressure support, and dialysis. Cytokine levels will rise over the course of hours so patients with confirmed AHTR must be watched closely for a 24 hour period even if the initial clinical evaluation of the patient appears to be unremarkable.

Renal failure can be minimized if renal perfusion is maintained and may include renal dose dopamine. The use of heparin to prevent DIC is controversial and should be used in select situations by clinicians specializing in hemostasis/thrombosis. Blood component support may be required in moderate to severe DIC.

Future strategies for the treatment of AHTR may include the use of monoclonal antibodies to block the effect of cytokine either by neutralizing the cytokine or by blocking the cytokine receptor.

12.7 References

Angiolillo A, Luban NLC. Hemolysis following an out-of-group platelet transfusion in an 8-month-old with Langerhans cell histiocytosis. *J Pediatr Hematol Oncol.* 2004;26:267-269.

Anstall HB, Blaylock RC. Compatibility testing and pretransfusion screening. In: *Practical Aspects of the Transfusion Service.* Chicago, Ill: ASCP Press; 1996:33-56.

Arndt PA, Garratty G. A retrospective analysis of the value of monocyte monolayer assay results for predicting the clinical significance of blood group alloantibodies. *Transfusion.* 2004 Sep;44(9):1273-81.

Baumgarten R, van Gelder W, van Wintershoven J, Maaskant-Van Wijk PA, Beckers EA. Recurrent acute hemolytic transfusion reactions by antibodies against Doa antigens, not detected by cross-matching. *Transfusion.* 2006 Feb;46(2):244-9.

Beauregard P, Blajchman M. Hemolytic and pseudo-hemolytic transfusion reactions: an overview of the hemolytic transfusion reactions and the clinical conditions that mimic them. *Transfus Med Rev.* 1994;8:184-199.

Capon SM, Goldfinger D. Acute hemolytic transfusion reaction, a paradigm of the systemic inflammatory response: new insights into pathophysiology and treatment. *Transfusion.* 1995;35:513-520.

Callum JL, Kaplan HS, Merkley LL, et al. Reporting of near-miss events for transfusion medicine: improving transfusion safety. *Transfusion.* 2001;41:1204-1211.

Darabi K, Dzik S. Hyperhemolysis syndrome in anemia of chronic disease. *Transfusion.* 2005 Dec;45(12):1930-3.

Davenport RD. Pathophysiology of hemolytic transfusion reactions. *Semin Hematol.* 2005 Jul;42(3):165-8. Review.

Dutton RP, Shih D, Edelman BB, Hess J, Scalea TM. Safety of uncrossmatched type-O red cells for resuscitation from hemorrhagic shock. *J Trauma.* 2005 Dec;59(6):1445-9.

Elliott K, Sanders J, Brecher ME. Visualizing the hemolytic transfusion reaction. Transfusion. 2003;43:297.

Garratty G. The James Blundell Award Lecture 2007: do we really understand immune red cell destruction? *Transfus Med.* 2008 Dec;18(6):321-34.

Gauvin F, Lacroix J, Robillard P, Lapointe H, Hume H. Acute transfusion reactions in the pediatric intensive care unit. *Transfusion.* 2006 Nov;46(11):1899-908.

Goodnough LT, Brecher ME, Kanter MH, et al. Transfusion medicine, I: blood transfusion. *N Eng J Med.* 1999;349:438-447.

Harris SB, Josephson CD, Kost CB, Hillyer CD. Nonfatal intravascular hemolysis in a pediatric patient after transfusion of a platelet unit with high-titer anti-A. *Transfusion.* 2007 Aug;47(8):1412-7.

Janatpour K, Holland PV. Noninfectious serious hazards of transfusion. *Curr Hematol Reps.* 2002;1:149-155.

Jeter EK, Spivey MA. Noninfectious complications of blood transfusion. *Hematol Oncol Clin North Am.* 1995;9:187-201.

Kopko PM, Holland PV. Mechanisms of severe transfusion reactions. *Transfus Clin Biol.* 2001;8:278-81.

Larsson LLG, Welsh VJ, Ladd DJ. Acute intravascular hemolysis secondary to out-of-group platelet transfusion. *Transfusion.* 2000;40:902-906

Leape LL. From Robert E. Gross Lecture, Making health care safe: are we up to it? *J Pediatr Surg.* 2004;39:258-266.

Linden JV, Wagner K, Voytovich AE, Sheehan J. Transfusion errors in New York State: an analysis of 10 years' experience. *Transfusion.* 2000;40:1207-1213.

Linden JV, Kaplan HS. Transfusion errors: causes and effects. *Transfus Med Rev.* 1994;8:169-183.

Mollison PL, Engelfriet CP, Contreras M, eds. *Blood Transfusion in Clinical Medicine. 9th ed.* Oxford, England: Blackwell; 1993.

Pierce LR, Jain N. Risks associated with the use of intravenous immunoglobulin. *Transfus Med Rev.* 2003;17:241-251.

Sazama K. Reports of 355 transfusion-associated deaths: 1976 through 1985. *Transfusion.* 1990;30:583-590

Schroeder ML. Principles and practice of transfusion medicine. In: Lee GR, Foerster J, Lukens JN, et al, eds. *Wintrobe's Clinical Hematology. 10th ed.* Baltimore, MD: Williams & Wilkins; 1999:827-834.

Executive Summary. In: To Err is Human—Building a Safer Health System. Kohn LT, Corrigan JM, Donaldson MS, eds., Washington, DC: National Academies Press. 2000:1-16.Angiolillo A, Luban NLC. Hemolysis following an out-of-group platelet transfusion in an 8-month-old with Langerhans cell histiocytosis. *J Pediatr Hematol Oncol.* 2004;26:267-269.

Chapter 13

Extrinsic Hemolytic Anemia: Fetomaternal Incompatibility

Robert C. Blaylock, MD

Hemolytic disease of the newborn (HDN) was a significant cause of infant morbidity and mortality before the routine use of Rh immunoglobulin prophylaxis in the late 1960s. Prior to RhIG use, up to 16% of D negative mothers developed anti-D at some time in their reproductive years. Currently, anti-D is not the leading cause of HDN, but D sensitization still occurs in patients with poor healthcare.

13.1 Pathophysiology

HDN occurs when maternal antibodies cross the placenta, attach to fetal red blood cells, which causes hemolysis and subsequent anemia. The antibodies that cause in-utero hemolysis, or hemolytic disease of the fetus (HDF), are unexpected red blood cell alloantibodies. These antibodies are found in mothers with a prior history of pregnancy or exposure to alloantigens via transfusion. Antibodies must be IgG, since IgM antibodies do not cross the placenta. The infant must express the corresponding antigen, which is inherited from the father. Many alloantibodies can cause HDF, but severe anemia typically occurs with antibodies directed to D, c, K1, and Fy^a antigens. HDF is rare during a first pregnancy unless the mother has a prior exposure to allogeneic blood. The first pregnancy is spared because mothers are usually not exposed to fetal red blood cell until approximately the 28th week of pregnancy. Time is required to process the antigen and form antibodies. The first antibody produced, IgM, will not cross the placenta. IgG titers do not rise to significant levels before the baby is delivered. Future pregnancies will be complicated by HDF if the fetus inherits the same red blood cell antigen, since less blood is required to elicit an anamnestic response, and IgG titers will rise quickly.

HDN can develop during a first pregnancy secondary to ABO incompatibility, however, severe anemia in-utero is rare. Usually mothers must be blood group O, since anti-A,B has an IgG component that has access to the fetal circulation. Anemia is usually mild because fetal red blood cells weakly express major blood group antigens. Also, many other tissues in the fetus express A and B antigen and act as a reservoir for maternal antibody. A comparison of HDN caused by ABO incompatibility vs anti-D is shown in **t13.1**.

Increased red blood cell destruction stimulates release of premature red blood cell precursors from the bone marrow and extramedullary hematopoiesis. Blood smears from these infants demonstrate many nucleated red blood cells and thus the term "erythroblastosis fetalis." Nucleated red blood cells may not be seen in cases of HDF caused by anti-K1 since this antibody also suppresses red blood cell progenitor cells.

t13.1 Characteristics of Hemolytic Disease of the Newborn

Property	ABO	Rh_0
Clinical		
Pregnancy associated with disease	Any, including the first	After the first pregnancy
Clinical severity	Unpredictable	More severe with each antigen-positive pregnancy
Prenatal evaluation amniocentesis	None needed	Sequential anti-Rh_0 titers,
Onset of jaundice delivery	3-4 weeks after delivery	Intrauterine or immediately after
Treatment*	None; phototherapy or rare exchange therapy	None; early delivery, phototherapy, exchange transfusion, or intrauterine transfusion
Laboratory		
Direct Coombs' test	+/- to 1+	2+ to 4+
Fetal blood group	A, B, or AB	Rh_0 positive
Antibody causing hemolysis	Anti-A or anti-B	Anti-Rh_0 (anti-D)
Maternal blood group	O, A, B	Rh_0 or Du negative
Maternal antibody screening	Negative	Positive
Peripheral blood (newborn)	Microspherocytes	Not diagnostic

**Treatment options are listed by increasing severity of hemolysis*

13.2 Clinical Findings

Fetuses and infants with HDF/HDN have varying degrees of anemia and related signs and symptoms. The hemolysis is usually extravascular and occurs in the reticuloendothelial system. Increased hemolysis results in high levels of unconjugated bilirubin. In HDF, this unconjugated bilirubin crosses the placenta and is metabolized by the mother. However, once delivered, the immature infant's liver is not capable of conjugating the high bilirubin load. High levels of unconjugated bilirubin will cause permanent damage to the CNS, a condition termed kernicterus. Defining exact unconjugated bilirubin levels at which kernicterus occurs is controversial; however, pre-term infants are affected at lower levels compared to term infants.

Severe HDF results in fetal edema and is called "hydrops fetalis." The pathogenesis of the edema is not completely understood and probably multifaceted. The extramedullary hematopoiesis that occurs in the liver leads to hepatic congestion, poor albumin synthesis and reduced colloid oncotic pressure. Heart failure secondary to anemia also plays a role in the edema. Untreated, this condition will result in fetal demise.

13.3 Diagnostic Approach

Initial prenatal testing during the first trimester of pregnancy should include an ABO and D antigen typing of the mother, which should be repeated on a subsequent visit. During a first pregnancy mothers should have two blood types performed. The second type is important to ensure no woman is accidentally denied the necessary RhIG prophylaxis during the prenatal period. Mothers that type D negative can have a test for a weak D antigen, but this is optional. Some feel the odds of finding a weak D antigen does not justify the expense of weak D testing on every D negative individual, as the risks associated with RhIG administration are very low.

An indirect antiglobulin test (IAT) should also be performed with the initial blood type to screen for unexpected red blood cell alloantibodies. The test should be negative in mothers during their first pregnancy, unless they have been transfused. Repeating the antibody screen during the first pregnancy is not necessary. Antibody screens are sometimes ordered prior to the 28-week dose of RhIG to be sure no active anti-D has been formed. This is no longer required and left to the discretion of the obstetrician. Repeat IAT should be performed in any patient with a history of a clinically significant red blood cell antibody, after invasive procedures or if trauma occurs to the mother during pregnancy.

Any patient with a positive IAT should have the causative antibody identified. Even patients known to have received passive anti-D must be evaluated to be sure no other antibodies have formed. The exception would be antibodies known to be class IgM since they will not cross the placenta.

Once an antibody has been identified, it is not a certainty the fetus will be affected by HDF. This is especially true if the maternal alloantibody was produced in response to a blood transfusion. Paternal testing for red blood cell alloantigens can help predict what antigens the child may inherit. Polymerase chain amplification testing is available for antigens known to cause severe HDF. This testing is performed on amniotic fluid, which is not without risk to fetus or mother. Studies are underway which may allow routine Rh genotyping of a fetus using maternal plasma, which contains fetal DNA.

Titration of anti-D antibody is common in patients with actively forming antibodies. Titrations should only be used as a screening test and will not predict the severity of HDF. The titer is used to determine when to perform amniocentesis and quantify bilirubin levels, which are generally a good indication of hemolysis severity. Titrations should not be used to differentiate between passive and active anti-D, or for any other unexpected red blood cell antibody.

Spectrophotometric scanning of amniotic fluid can quantitate bilirubin by measuring peak absorbance at a wavelength of 450 nm. This is plotted against a predicted baseline based on gestational age of the fetus. Therapy can be directed depending on the severity of hemolysis. Bilirubin determinations will not predict fetal hemolysis in cases of HDF caused by anti-K1 and should not be used in this setting.

Cordocentesis is used to measure the actual hemoglobin concentration of the fetus. This is performed by cannulating an umbilical vessel using high-resolution ultrasound, and obtaining a sample for an automated hematology analyzer. The sample must be fetal in origin. This can be confirmed by comparing the mean corpuscular volume (MCV) of the sample to that of the mother—the fetal MCV will be larger. Other methods for confirming fetal blood include testing for blood group I (maternal) versus i (fetal) or performing a Kleihauer-Betke test, but these are time consuming and not practical.

Doppler studies of the middle cerebral artery are being evaluated as a non-invasive means of determining fetal anemia. Circulatory changes needed to compensate for fetal anemia increase blood flow through vessels supplying the brain. This relatively new methodology should only be used to support other traditional methods of determining anemia.

Serologic evaluation of alloantibodies that cause cytopenias in a fetus or newborn are always more accurate when maternal samples are used. (This is true for HFN/HDN or neonatal alloimmune thrombocytopenia.) Maternal titers of the offending antibody are always higher compared to the baby because antibody levels drop across the placenta and fetal antigens adsorb the alloantibody in the cell destruction process.

Unfortunately, tertiary care centers often have infants affected by HDN transported for care from remote locations and maternal samples are unavailable. In these cases, fetal blood can be used to identify the offending antibody. Testing should proceed with an ABO and D typing. A weak D test must be performed in infants if the initial D test is negative. The interpretation of ABO and D typing must be done cautiously until it is known if the baby received any in-utero transfusions. The blood bank must obtain the pregnancy history of the mother and sometimes the native blood type of the baby cannot be established until the infant is transfusion independent and the life span of transfused cells has passed.

An IAT must be performed to search for unexpected red blood cell antibodies. This may be negative in some cases of HDN, if antibody titers were sufficient to coat red cells and cause hemolysis, but not adequate to saturate red cells and spill into fetal plasma. A monospecific direct antiglobulin test (DAT) will detect IgG on the surface of fetal red cells. An eluate must be performed to remove the IgG from the cells, and the antibody in the eluate must be identified.

13.4 Hematologic Findings

Anemia may range from none to severe. HDN caused by ABO and less common RBC antibodies is usually mild. Rh-mediated HDN tends to be progressively more severe with each pregnancy. Persistent extramedullary hematopoiesis, in an attempt to compensate for hemolysis, results in increased circulating nucleated RBCs (erythroblastosis fetalis).

13.4.1 Blood Cell Measurements

Levels of hemoglobin in mild anemia are 14-16 g/dL (140-160 g/L). In moderate anemia, the levels are 10-14 g/dL (100-140 g/L); and in severe anemia, they are 8-10 g/dL (80-100 g/L). The reticulocyte count is often greater than 10% (0.10). The WBC count is normal to mildly elevated at 10-20 × $10^3/\mu L$ (10-20 × $10^9/L$). Platelets may be mildly to moderately decreased.

13.4.2 Peripheral Blood Smear Morphology

The peripheral blood smear shows polychromasia, correlating with the increased reticulocyte count, and nucleated RBCs greater than 10 per 100 WBCs (erythroblastosis). Microspherocytes usually indicate ABO hemolytic disease but are not typically prominent. Thrombocytopenia and leukocytosis are common. White blood cell counts must be corrected for the large number of nucleated red blood cells circulating in babies with HDN.

13.5 Other Laboratory Tests

Test 13.5.1 Determination of Blood Group

Purpose. Testing mother, father, and newborn blood groups determines possible fetal-maternal incompatibility.

Principle. Maternal and newborn RBC antigens are studied for ABO and Rh expression. Tests can be performed on father and for other antigens if indicated.

Specimen. RBCs from clots or anticoagulated specimens are washed well with saline. Specimens are stable for at least 7 days. Cord RBCs and plasma can be used if the RBCs are washed well to remove contaminants. Infant heelstick specimens also can be used.

Procedure. Standard typing procedures that detect direct agglutination of RBCs by anti-A, anti-B, and anti-D antibodies are used. Weak D testing is optimal for all mothers and must be performed on all infants.

Interpretation. In ABO hemolytic disease, the mother's blood is usually group O and the infant's blood is group A, B, or AB. Disease also may arise in a group A mother with a group B infant or a group B mother with a group A infant, but this is more rare since the majority of the isohemagglutinin in blood group A or B individuals is IgM unlike anti-A,B in group O mothers. In HDF caused by anti-D, the mother is D negative and the infant is D positive.

Where the serologic possibility of both ABO and Rh disease is possible (eg, an O-negative mother with an A- or B-positive child), hemolytic disease is more likely caused by the ABO incompatibility, because the major blood group incompatibility has usually lysed D incompatible cells throughout the pregnancy. However, the possibility of anti-D formation in the mother must be considered.

Mothers who are D positive are not excluded from having infants with hemolytic disease, because they may be negative for other antigens in the Rh system and their offspring may be positive.

Notes and Precautions. Weak D testing must be performed on all infants born to D negative mothers. Weak D testing is considered optional for mothers, but may lead to unnecessary RhIG administration if not performed.

Test 13.5.2 Maternal Antibody Screening and Identification

Purpose. A positive antibody screen may indicate the presence of unexpected red blood cell antibodies that can cause HDF/HDN.

Principle. Maternal serum is screened for antibody, usually early in pregnancy and sporadically thereafter, to detect the presence of IgG antibodies.

If necessary, the father's RBC antigens are tested as a predictive measure of fetal expression. Polymerase chain amplification methodology can be performed on amniotic fluid to determine fetal antigen typing. False negative results can occur and amniocentesis is not without risk to mother and baby.

Specimen. Serum or plasma obtained at the first obstetric visit is used. A specimen also should be obtained in the third trimester, and more frequently if the early specimen shows positive results or if an obstetric history of previous HDN, trauma to mother during pregnancy or invasive procedures (eg, amniocentesis) warrants more frequent testing (usually at 2-4 week intervals).

Procedure. Serum or plasma is incubated with test 2-4 reagent screening cells depending on vendor and methodology. Antiglobulin reagent (IgM anti-IgG) is added to detect IgG molecules attached to screening cells. All antibodies are identified with the same techniques, except 9-12 reagent red blood cells with known extended phenotypes are used. Patterns of reactivity are used to determine antibody specificity.

Interpretation. In ABO hemolytic disease, only the expected anti-A and/or anti-B antibodies are found in the group O mother, so the antibody screen is negative. In all other types of hemolytic disease, the maternal antibody screen is positive. The antibody must be identified to determine its significance to the newborn. Only IgG antibodies cross the placenta, and they must have sufficient affinity to coat the infant's RBCs to produce hemolysis. Common RBC antibodies found in pregnant women are anti-Lea and anti-Leb. These antibodies do not produce neonatal disease because they are IgM and cannot cross the placenta, and all infants are anti-Lea and anti-Leb negative.

Notes and Precautions. The current practice of administering RhIG at 28 weeks of gestation to prevent possible sensitization by the fetus results in a spurious positive maternal antibody screening due to weak anti-D. History of RhIG must be obtained and titers should not be used to differentiate active versus passive anti-D. Do not assume that anti-D is the only antibody; a search for the presence of other unexpected alloantibodies must follow.

Test 13.5.3 Direct Antiglobulin Test (DAT) in the Newborn

Purpose. The DAT detects antibodies coating the newborn's RBCs.

Principle. Fetal RBCs are coated with passively transmitted maternal IgG antibody specific for a RBC antigen.

Specimen. RBCs from either clotted or anticoagulated cord blood can be used but cells collected in ethylenediaminetetraacetic acid (EDTA) are preferred. Small capillary specimens from newborn heelsticks are also acceptable.

Procedure. Washed red blood cells are incubated with poly-specific IgM reagent and observed for agglutination. Reagents specific for human IgG or complement component C3d are used if the initial poly-specific test is positive.

Interpretation. Red blood cells coated with either IgG or C3d will clump in the presence of the poly-specific reagent. In most cases of HDN the poly-specific DAT will be positive. Further characterization of the DAT can be performed using mono-specific reagents, which are IgM anti-IgG or IgM anti-C3d. Red blood cells from infants with HDN typically demonstrate IgG on red blood cells.

Notes and Precautions. Positive DAT results on cord specimens without detectable antibody may indicate adsorption of antibody by Wharton's jelly, but the RBC control is usually positive. The test should be repeated on blood from a heel-stick or venous sample.

Test 13.5.4 Elution

Purpose. An elution removes IgG from patient red blood cells. The antibody is harvested and used in an IAT.

Principle. Antibodies are removed from red blood cells using various methods.

Sample. Red blood cells are collected in EDTA.

Procedure. Patient red blood cells are placed in an environment that disassociates the IgG from the red cell membrane. Heat or acid environments are commonly used.

Interpretation. Once the antibody has been eluted, it is reacted with screening cells to see if the antibody has specificity. Newborns with HDN have IgG with specificity for a blood group system.

Notes and Precautions. An elution is not necessary if the antibodies causing HDN have already been identified from a properly collected and identified maternal sample.

Test 13.5.5 Acid Elution (Kleihauer-Betke) Test

Purpose. Fetal-maternal hemorrhage of small amounts (0.1mL) of D-positive fetal RBCs may sensitize an Rh-negative mother, unless she is adequately immunized postpartum with RhIG. Doses are standardized to compensate for fetal hemorrhage volume of 15 mL of packed RBCs or less. The actual volume of hemorrhage can be calculated by staining a maternal peripheral blood smear for fetal cells. If the fetal hemorrhage exceeds 15 mL, an increased dosage of RhIG should be administered. Antepartum RhIG is administered at 26-28 weeks of gestation, but Kleihauer-Betke-stained peripheral smears usually are not useful at this time because the number of potentially positive cells is minimal.

Principle. Fetal hemoglobin is resistant to acid elution, whereas adult hemoglobin is not. A maternal peripheral blood smear is treated with dilute acid buffer for 10 minutes and then stained. The maternal erythrocyte adult hemoglobin is leached into the buffer, leaving RBC ghosts, whereas the fetal RBCs remain as dense red erythrocytes.

Specimen. Very thin peripheral blood smears fixed in 80% alcohol are prepared from maternal blood collected in EDTA.

Procedure. Dried smears are placed in McIlvaine's buffer (pH 3.2) for 10 minutes, followed by washing in distilled water. The smear is then stained with erythrosin and counterstained with hematoxylin. Two thousand cells are counted and the percentage of densely staining cells with fetal hemoglobin (presumably fetal in origin) is calculated. Control smears should be made from cord blood specimens (positive) mixed 1:10 with adult blood (negative), because questionably positive cells are sometimes seen even with the negative control. Tests kits are available, so small laboratories may perform this test.

Interpretation. Normal adult cells leak hemoglobin and appear as paler ghosts. Fetal cells are densely pink and refractile. The volume of fetal-maternal hemorrhage is calculated as milliliters of whole blood equal to the percentage of fetal cells multiplied by 50. Hemorrhage in excess of 15 mL packed cell volume requires a proportionate increase in Rh immune globulin administered. Because variability in the amount of acid hemoglobin elution may occur even within the same laboratory, it is important that appropriate controls of fetal (cord) blood and adult blood be done to aid in proper interpretation.

Flow cytometric tests to detect fetal cells, using staining for hemoglobin F in permeabilized RBCs are available in some laboratories. This technology allows detection of a very small number of fetal cells within a sample. Sending this test to a reference laboratory may be difficult if results cannot be obtained in time to administer RhIG within 72 hours of delivery.

Notes and Precautions. Adult hemoglobinopathies, such as persistence of fetal hemoglobin, may create a misleading picture. If the volume of fetal cells suggests significant blood loss from an otherwise healthy infant with normal hemoglobin, the possibility of a hemoglobinopathy in the mother should be considered.

Fetal screens are used in many blood banks to determine the need for quantification of fetal-maternal hemorrhage. Maternal blood is incubated with commercially modified anti-D, which will bind to circulating fetal D positive cells. Indicator D positive reagent cells are added to the mix, and will form rosettes around the fetal cells. The rosettes are counted. The manufacturer determines the number of rosettes, needed to call the test positive. A negative test indicates that one dose of RhIG is required after delivery. A positive fetal screen requires an acid elution be performed to quantify the bleed.

13.6 Ancillary Tests

Ultrasonography can demonstrate fetal hydrops and establishes location of the placenta prior to amniocentesis for bilirubin determination. Depending on the titer, obstetric history, and history of previous hemolytic disease, the first procedure is usually performed at 16-18 weeks of gestation. At least two sequential specimens are needed to verify an increase in optical density and to determine whether the differential absorption is increasing, decreasing, or stable, which provides insights into the clinical course of disease. Specimens are obtained every 1-2 weeks or, in borderline cases, every few days. If significant hemolysis is suspected based on increased levels of amniotic fluid bilirubin levels, fetal blood sampling or intrauterine transfusion may be required.

Amniotic fluid (5-10 mL) is withdrawn and immediately shielded from light, which degrades bilirubin and causes falsely decreased results. The specimen is centrifuged to separate vernix, and the supernatant is scanned in the ultraviolet spectrum from 350-700 nm. Bilirubin has a peak absorbance at 450 nm, although the curve is not linear. A tangent is constructed to create a straight line, and the difference in optical density from the tangent to the peak at 450 nm is the change in optical density. An optical density rise at 450 nm is common early in pregnancy, with peak levels at 23-24 weeks of gestation, but decreases after 26 weeks if no RBC sensitization is present.

Nomogram zones determined by Liley correlate the spectrophotometric data with week of gestation and probability of severe hemolytic disease. This may be verified in severe cases by direct fetal blood sampling via cordocentesis. If the anemia is severe and fetal lungs are markedly immature, intrauterine transfusion is considered. If fetal lung maturation is adequate, early delivery is undertaken, permitting extrauterine exchange transfusion.

13.6.1 Notes

False elevations in absorbance are seen when hemoglobin or meconium contaminate the specimen, because one of several hemoglobin A optical peaks occurs at 450 nm. Absorbance at 450 nm cannot be used to estimate fetal anemia when HDF is due to anti-K1 because red blood cell precursors are decreased.

13.7 Course and Treatment

The most notorious cause of HFN/HDN is maternal sensitization to the D antigen. Prevention is the mainstay of treatment in pregnant D negative women. The routine use of RhIG antepartum and postpartum has dropped the sensitization rate from double-digit percentages to approximately 0.1%. RhIG must also be used during pregnancy following procedures such as cordocentesis and amniocentesis. Other clinical scenarios where RhIG should be used include: termination of pregnancy, ectopic pregnancies, maternal abdominal trauma, abruptio placenta, placenta previa and fetal demise. RhIG should be given within 72 hours of delivery or another event which may expose a mother to fetal blood. However, if the 72 hour deadline is missed, RhIG should still be administered since it may have a beneficial effect as late as 13 days after delivery.

Strategies for monitoring mothers with red blood cell antibodies that can cause HFN/HDN should start with the least invasive testing possible and proceed to more invasive methods as indicated. The goal is to prevent severe fetal anemia and subsequent hydrops by administering intrauterine transfusions if fetal lungs are not developed, or by delivering the child if fetal lung maturity tests indicate delivery can be done safely.

Pregnancies are infrequently affected by HDF prior to 20 weeks of gestational age when cordocentesis becomes technically feasible. Intravenous immune globulin has been somewhat successful in treating severe HDF that occurs early in pregnancy. The mechanism of action is not completely understood but may involve the blocking of placenta receptors involved in antibody transfer into the fetus, or the traditional theory of reticuloendothelial blockade in the fetus, thereby reducing destruction of antibody coated red blood cells. Plasma exchange to reduce maternal antibody titers of the offending antibody has also been attempted, however, titers can rebound above pre-apheresis levels. Plasma exchange will also result in a dilutional coagulopathy (unless plasma is used) and this could lead to unwanted bleeding.

Intrauterine transfusions can be given after 20-22 weeks of gestational age in cases of severe anemia. Survival increases from 82% to 90% if intrauterine transfusions are initiated prior to the development of hydrops in the fetus. The offending antibody must be identified in the mother before red blood cell selection can proceed. Blood group O, D negative units of packed red blood cells lacking the corresponding antigen (compared to maternal antibody) are selected. The units must be washed to remove any isohemagglutinin that may exacerbate hemolysis in any fetus that is blood group A, B, or AB. Washing will also remove excess potassium that has leaked out of stored red cells and prevent fetal hyperkalemia and subsequent cardiac arrhythmias or arrest. The blood must also be irradiated to prevent transfusion associated graft-versus-host disease, which will be fatal. The blood should also be either sero-negative for CMV, or leukoreduced, which will remove CMV contained in leukocytes. Most institutions leukoreduce blood for these transfusions and they should be sickle cell negative as well.

Once the child is delivered, treatment focuses on symptomatic anemia and the prevention of kernicterus. Phototherapy is considered first line conservative therapy and should be initiated quickly in mild cases of hyperbilirubinemia. The light will permeate the skin and convert unconjugated bilirubin to a water-soluble form, which can be excreted in urine.

Exchange transfusion is required when unconjugated bilirubin levels cannot be controlled. Traditionally, a two-blood volume exchange is performed. Blood type O negative red blood cells are usually selected and modified (irradiated, washed, CMV negative, etc) as they would be for an intrauterine transfusion. Type specific blood can be used if it is not ABO incompatible with the mother. If the mother's sample is not available, the blood type of the infant must be checked using antiglobulin reagent to be sure no IgG isohemagglutinin is present. The washed, packed red cells must be reconstituted with plasma to the desired hematocrit of the neonatologist (usually 40% or greater). If type specific blood is chosen, try to match the unit of FFP that corresponds with the unit of red blood cells, since an additional donor exposure can be avoided. However, type AB plasma is often used to reconstitute type O negative red blood cells, since this combination provides the most inert combination of front type and back type possible. However, this requires an additional donor exposure. The use of plasma prevents a dilutional coagulopathy during, and after, the exchange transfusion, which could cause unwanted hemorrhage. A dilutional thrombocytopenia will occur after exchange transfusion so a post-procedure CBC is needed to check the platelet count and the final hematocrit in the newborn.

Exchange transfusion provides many benefits to the infant. Dilution of both bilirubin and the offending red blood cell antibody occur. Also, antibody coated red blood cells are removed and replaced with cells that will not react with maternal antibody. Usually only one procedure is needed, however, exchange transfusion only removes antibody and bilirubin contained in the intravascular space. Extravascular diffusion of offending agents, back into the vascular space, will start after the procedure ends. Infants with HDN must be followed closely for days after exchange transfusion is complete, to be sure bilirubin levels continue to normalize. Rarely, the effects of maternal antibody diffusing from extravascular to intravascular compartments cause hemolysis longer than 4-6 weeks after delivery.

13.8 References

American College of Obstetricians and Gynecologists. ACOG Practice Bulletin No. 75: management of alloimmunization. *Obstet Gynecol.* 2006 Aug;108(2):457-64.

Avent ND, Madgett TE, Maddocks DG, Soothill PW. Cell-free fetal DNA in the maternal serum and plasma: current and evolving applications. *Curr Opin Obstet Gynecol.* 2009 Apr;21(2):175-9.

Bowman J. The management of hemolytic disease in the fetus and newborn. *Semin Perinatol.* 1997;21:39-44

Bowman J. Assays to predict the clinical significance of blood group antibodies. *Semin Perinatol.* 1998;5:412-416.

Bowman JM. Alloimmune hemolytic disease of the fetus and newborn. In: Lee GR, Foerster J, Lukens JN, et al, eds. *Wintrobe's Clinical Hematology.* 10th ed. Baltimore, MD: Williams & Wilkins; 1999:1210-1232.

Chavez GF, Mulinare J, Edmonds LD. Epidemiology of Rh hemolytic disease of the newborn in the United States. *JAMA.* 1991;265:3270-3274.

Davis BH, Olsen S, Biglow NC, et al. Detection of fetal red cells in fetomaternal hemorrhage using a fetal hemoglobin monoclonal antibody by flow cytometry. *Transfusion.* 1998;38:749-756.

Duguid JK. Antenatal serologic testing and preventing of hemolytic disease of the newborn. *J Clin Pathol.* 1997;50:193-196.

Eder AF. *Transfusion Medicine.* Chicago, IL:ASCP Press; 2003 Check Sample. *Transfusion Medicine* TM 03-5 (TM-265).

Eder AF. Update on HDFN: new information on long-standing controversies. *Immunohematology.* 2006;22(4):188-95. Review.

Finning K, Martin P, Summers J, Daniels G. Fetal genotyping for the K (Kell) and Rh C, c, and E blood groups on cell-free fetal DNA in maternal plasma. *Transfusion.* 2007 Nov;47(11):2126-33.

Hadley AG. In vitro assays to predict the severity of hemolytic disease of the newborn. *Transfus Med Rev.* 1995;9:302-313.

Hartwell EA. Use of Rh Immune Globulin–ASCP Practice Parameters. *Am J Clin Pathol.* 1998;110:281-292.

Hillyer CD, Shaz BH, Winkler AM, Reid M. Integrating molecular technologies for red blood cell typing and compatibility testing into blood centers and transfusion services. *Transfus Med Rev.* 2008 Apr;22(2):117-32.

Judd WJ for the Scientific Section Coordinating Committee of the AABB. Practice guidelines for prenatal and perinatal immunohematology, revisited. *Transfusion.* 2001;41:1445-1452.

Lo YMD, Hjelm NM, Path FRC et al. Prenatal diagnosis of fetal RhD status by molecular analysis of maternal plasma. *New Eng J Med.* 1998;339:1734-1738.

Moise KJ. Management of Rhesus alloimmunization in pregnancy. *Am Coll Obst Gyn.* 2002;100(3):600-611.

Moise KJ. Fetal anemia due to non-Rhesus-D red-cell alloimmunization. *Semin Fetal Neonatal Med.* 2008 Aug;13(4):207-14. Epub 2008 Apr 8. Review.

Moise KJ. Non-anti-D antibodies in red cell alloimmunization. *Eur J Obstet Gynecol Reprod Biol.* 2000;92:75-81.

Moise KJ. Changing trends in the management of red blood cell alloimmunization in pregnancy. *Arch Pathol Lab Med.* 1994;118:421-428.

Perinatal Issues in Transfusion Practice. *AABB Technical Manual*; 50th Anniversary ed., 14th ed. pp. 497-514.

Porter TF, Silver RM, Jackson GM et al. Intravenous immune globulin in the management of severe Rh D hemolytic disease. *Obstet Gynecol Surv.* 1997;52:193-197.

Queenan JT, Tomai TP, Ural SH, King JC. Deviation in amniotic fluid optical density at a wavelength of 450 nm in Rh-immunized pregnancies from 14 to 40 weeks' gestation: A proposal for clinical management. *Am J Obstet Gynecol.* 1993;168:1370-1376.

van Dijk BA, Dorren MC, Overbeeke MAM. Red cell antibodies in pregnancy: there is no 'critical titre.' *Transfus Med.* 1995;4:199-202.

Whitecar PW, Moise KJ. Sonographic methods to detect fetal anemia in red blood cell alloimmunization. *Obstet Gynecol Surv.* 2000;55:240-250.

Zupanska B. Assays to predict the clinical significance of blood group antibodies. *Curr Opin Hematol.* 1998;5:412-416.

Chapter 14

Drug-Related Extrinsic Hemolytic Anemia

Robert C. Blaylock, MD

Drug-related hemolysis is a rare event despite the prevalence of prescriptions and over-the-counter medications, and occurs at an approximate rate of one in a million people. Diagnosis can be difficult because patients with drug-related hemolysis are commonly on many medications, and interpretation of laboratory results is challenging because in-vitro testing does not always correlate with in vivo hemolysis. Additionally a few laboratories offer tests for diagnosis of drug-related hemolysis. Alternatives to a drug suspected of causing hemolysis may be limited and changes to medications may have an undesirable effect.

Drugs cause hemolysis by three main mechanisms: 1) drug-induced oxidation of hemoglobin, 2) drugs related to an antibody which destroys blood red cells, and 3) drugs associated with thrombotic microangiopathies (TMA) which result in mechanical destruction of red blood cells.

14.1 Pathophysiology

14.1.1 Drug-Induced Oxidation of Hemoglobin

Numerous drugs can oxidize hemoglobin. Normally, hemoglobin is readily returned to the reduced state; however, oxidation may lead to hemolysis in patients with an intrinsic deficiency in the pathways necessary to produce reduced glutathione or in patients with an unstable hemoglobin.

Glucose-6-phosphate dehydrogenase (G6PD) deficiency is the most common enzymatic deficiency associated with drug-induced hemolysis. The interaction of an oxidative drug with G6PD-deficient RBCs leads to depletion of glutathione and inadequate production of the reduced form of nicotinamide-adenine dinucleotide phosphate (NADPH). The depletion of GHS is followed by irreversible oxidation of hemoglobin. Hemoglobin degradation products polymerize to form Heinz bodies, with resultant membrane damage and reticuloendothelial phagocytosis by the spleen. Young RBCs have more NADPH and are less susceptible to oxidative damage, so as reticulocytosis increases, the effects of low doses of an oxidative drug tend to be self-limited. Drugs that induce hemolysis in patients with G6PD deficiency are listed in **t14.1**. Owing to variations in the deficiency phenotype, these drugs do not uniformly cause hemolysis in any person with G6PD deficiency.

Patients with unstable hemoglobins also may be more susceptible to oxidative damage to hemoglobin. An amino acid substitution in either the a or b chain near the attachment site of the heme group to hemoglobin renders the molecule more sensitive to oxidative injury and subsequent denaturation. This leads to the formation of Heinz bodies and hemolysis by reticuloendothelial cell activity.

t14.1 Drugs Commonly Associated With Hemolysis in G6PD

Drug Class	Specific Entities
Antimalarial agents	Primaquine Quinacrine
Sulfonamides	Sulfanilamide Salicylazosulfapyridine Sulfacetamide
Other antibacterial agents	Nitrofurantoin Nitrofurazone Para-aminosalicylic acid Nalidixic acid
Analgesics	Acetanilid
Sulfones	Diaminodiphenyl sulfone Thiazolsulfone
Miscellaneous	Dimercaprol Naphthalene (mothballs) Methylene blue Trinitrotoluene (TNT)

G6PD = glucose-6-phosphate dehydrogenase

14.1.2 Drug-Related Antibody Destruction of Red Blood Cells

Drug-related hemolysis involves many different mechanisms and proposed theories of pathogenesis. Some mechanisms discussed here will involve drugs which can cause an antibody to be produced that is indistinguishable from an antibody that causes warm autoimmune hemolytic anemia. Additionally, drugs can act as haptens and adsorb onto red blood cell membranes, or drugs can cause "immune complex" mediated hemolysis and passive administration of immunoglobulin with specificity to red blood cell alloantigens.

Drugs Associated with the Formation of Warm-Type Autoantibodies

Methyldopa is the prototypical drug that induces the formation of an IgG indistinguishable from a warm autoantibody. Fludarabine is a newer medication associated with the same mechanism of hemolysis. The antibody may arise within months of starting the drug, but can also arise after years of use. A direct antiglobulin test (DAT) will detect IgG antibody usually without complement. The red blood cells coated with antibody are removed by macrophages in the reticuloendothelial system. Occasionally complement can be detected on red blood cells and intravascular hemolysis is evident. The IgG antibody, eluted from the affected red blood cells, has broad and equal reactivity with all panel cells tested. The exact mechanism of the autoantibody formation is not understood, but these drugs may have a direct, aberrant effect on the immune system.

The antibody does not require the presence of the drug for reactivity. Discontinuation of the drug usually results in resolution of symptomatic hemolysis, however, the DAT may remain positive for as long as 24 months.

"Drug Adsorption" onto Red Blood Cell Surfaces

Drugs and drug metabolites are too small to initiate an immune response. Drugs act as haptens by closely binding to proteins either on the surface of red blood cells, or contained in plasma. In the 1970s penicillin was the prototype drug that "adsorbed," or bound, to proteins on the red blood cell surface. Antibodies in patient serum will react with red blood cells treated with the offending drug (autologous, drug coated red blood cells are not required). The hemolysis caused by this mechanism is usually mild to moderate and extravascular.

"Immune Complex" Mechanism

The "immune complex" mechanism of drug-related hemolysis involves complement activation and intravascular hemolysis. Patient plasma in the presence of an offending drug (drug not bound to patient red blood cells) causes immune complex intravascular hemolysis that can be severe and cause renal failure.

Drug-related immune hemolysis caused by hapten binding to red cells, or the immune complex mechanism are both considered drug dependent (drug must be on red cells or present in plasma). In the 1970s, drug dependent hemolysis was most commonly associated with penicillin use. Now, most drug dependent, drug-related, immune hemolysis is due to second and third generation cephalosporins. Not all cephalosporins cause hemolysis via one mechanism alone (immune complex versus hapten binding to red cells) but the most common is hapten binding to the red cell membrane. Cefotetan is the most immunogenic and problematic of the cephalosporins.

Passive Administration of Red Blood Cell Specific Antibodies

Intravenous immunoglobulin and intravenous administration of anti-D are used to treat autoimmune disorders such as idiopathic thrombocytopenic purpura. IVIG is thought to block the Fc receptors of macrophages in the reticuloendothelial system (RES), thus sparing the destruction of antibody-coated platelets. Anti-D is used in patients expressing the D antigen on red blood cells and is thought to be a better "blocker" (compared to IVIG) of the RES. Macrophages are preoccupied by antibody coated red blood cells instead of antibody alone. Anti-D basically causes a "controlled" transfusion reaction, unfortunately, hemolysis sometimes causes drastic drops in hemoglobin, and rarely, renal failure. IVIG is pooled from many different donors and sometimes contains alloantibodies, which can be clinically significant.

14.1.3 Drugs Associated with Thrombotic Microangiopathies

TMAs are disorders that result in thrombocytopenia and a microangiopathic hemolytic anemia. Platelet thrombi deposited in small arterioles cause turbulence and shear stress that mechanically fragment red blood cells. TMAs have many different etiologies. For example, hemolytic uremic syndrome is usually caused by bacteria like *E coli* 0157:H7 producing a "Shigella-like" exotoxin.

Thrombotic thrombocytopenic purpura can be caused by an autoantibody that neutralizes a plasma metalloprotease required to break down large molecular weight von Willebrand factor multimers. When these high molecular weight multimers accumulate, they activate platelets and thrombi develop.

Mitomycin, cyclosporine, and tacrolimus have been associated with thrombocytopenia and mechanical hemolysis. The exact mechanism is not understood, but may relate to drug toxicity to vascular endothelium.

14.2 Clinical Findings

Hemolysis related to G6PD deficiency is abrupt and occurs 1-3 days after initiation of the oxidative drug. Severe anemia ensues with hemoglobinemia, hemoglobinuria, and jaundice. Hemolysis may be somewhat self-limiting when there is an abundance of reticulocytes. Hemolysis will cease as the drug is metabolized and excreted.

Drug-related immune hemolysis is most commonly extravascular with mild to moderate anemia. However, severe intravascular hemolysis and anemia associated with renal failure can occur. Fatalities are uncommon.

Drugs can cause the entire classic pentad associated with TMAs (mental status changes, renal failure, fever, thrombocytopenia, and microangiopatic hemolytic anemia), or result in subtle thrombocytopenia and anemia.

14.3 Diagnostic Approach

Proper diagnostic evaluation requires a high index of suspicion in a patient who is currently receiving, or has recently received, hemolytic-inducing drugs with unexplained anemia. Evaluation proceeds with the following steps:

1. Hematologic findings show a normochromic anemia that may be actively hemolytic. Bone marrow aspiration is usually not needed.
2. Test results for Heinz bodies may be positive in patients with G6PD deficiency or unstable hemoglobins.
3. The direct antiglobulin test (DAT) result is positive in immunohemolytic processes, although to a variable degree depending on the mechanism of drug action.
4. Serum antibody screening tests with standard reagent RBCs looking for unexpected red cell alloantibodies are usually negative.
5. Special red cell testing using the drug suspected of causing hemolysis.

14.4 Hematologic Findings

The anemia may be severe or mild to moderate if well compensated by bone marrow activity. The degree of anemia may also vary, depending on the drug mechanism of action, dosage, and the type of antibody evoked. A reactive leukocytosis may appear. In G6PD deficiency and unstable hemoglobinopathies, hemolysis begins as Heinz bodies appear. As the hemolysis persists, Heinz bodies are removed in the spleen and tend to disappear.

14.4.1 Blood Cell Measurements

Hemoglobin can be markedly decreased to 3 g/dL (30 g/L) in severe hemolysis. Elevations in mean corpuscular volume (MCV) of 105-110 μm^3 (105-110 fL) reflect reticulocytosis. The WBC count is often elevated to 10-20 $\times 10^3/\mu L$ (10-20 $\times 10^9/L$), and a left shift to the myelocyte stage may be seen.

14.4.2 Peripheral Blood Smear Morphology

Nucleated RBCs and polychromasia are general findings. Spherocytes may be seen with a-methyldopa-type AIHAs. Schistocytes are seen with drugs associated with TMAs. Bite cells may be seen when Heinz bodies have been extracted by the spleen. Heinz bodies are not visualized on Wright-stained smears, but are seen with crystal violet stains.

14.4.3 Bone Marrow Examination

The bone marrow is often hypercellular with normoblastic erythroid hyperplasia and increased iron stores.

14.5 Other Laboratory Tests

Test 14.5.1 Direct Antiglobulin Test (DAT)

Purpose. The DAT determines if immunoglobulin, and/or complement, is coating the surface of the patient's red blood cells.

Principle. Patient red blood cells are incubated with poly-specific IgM reagent with specificity for human IgG and complement.

Specimen. Red blood cells are collected in EDTA.

Procedure. Washed patient red blood cells are incubated with poly-specific IgM reagent and observed for agglutination. Reagents specific for human IgG or complement component C3d are used if the initial poly-specific test is positive.

Interpretation. No matter what the mechanism of drug-related immune hemolysis, antibody and/or complement attached to the RBC will be detected. Drug-related immune hemolytic anemia is unlikely, but not completely ruled out with negative DAT results. The DAT result in G6PD-mediated drug hemolysis and drugs associated with TMAs is negative.

Often the result in drug-induced hemolytic anemia is weakly positive, and the use of eluates may be necessary. Eluates remove and harvest the antibody contained on the red blood cell. The harvested antibody can be used to determine specificity or to react with red blood cells coated with the drug in question. Findings for each category of drug-induced immune hemolysis are summarized in **t14.2**.

t14.2 Features of Drug-Mediated Immune Hemolysis

Parameter	Drug Absorption, Hapten Formation	Immune Complex	Warm-Type Autoantibodies	Passive Antibody Administration
Associated drugs	Penicillin	Quinine, quinidine, non-steroidal anti-inflammatory agents	α-methyldopa, procainamide, mefenamic acid, fludarabine	IVIG, Anti-D
Role of drug	Binds to RBC membrane	Forms antigen-antibody complex that binds to RBC	Unknown	Binds to RBC specific alloantigen
Antibody formed	To drug	Part drug, part RBC membrane	To RBC	Not formed, passively acquired
Antibody class	IgG	IgM or IgG	IgG	IgG
Proteins detected with direct antiglobulin test	IgG, rarely complement	Complement	IgG, rarely complement	IgG, rarely complement
Drug needed for hemolysis	Yes	Yes	No	Yes
Mechanism of RBC destruction	RES sequestration	Complement-mediated lysis	RES sequestration	RES sequestration

RBC = red blood cell; RES = reticuloendothelial system

Notes and Precautions. Warm autoimmune hemolytic anemia (WAIHA) is much more common than the warm autoantibodies induced by methyldopa or fludaribine. Any patient with a non-specific IgG antibody present in serum or eluted from red blood cells should be evaluated for an underlying disease associated with WAIHA such as lymphoma or lupus.

A positive DAT due to passive administration of antibody contained in IVIG or anti-D will demonstrate specificity when the eluate is tested.

Test 14.5.2 Serum Antibody Tests with Drug-Treated RBCs

Purpose. This test determines if the patient's serum reacts with cells coated with the drug in question.

Principle. Reagent red blood cells are incubated with the suspected drug, which acts as a hapten, and binds to the red cell surface.

Sample. Serum is used.

Procedure.

1. Group O reagent red blood cells are incubated with a known concentration of the drug in question for a specified period of time (usually 1-2 hours). Cells are washed after incubation with the drug and re-suspended.
2. Patient serum is incubated with drug-coated cells in the presence of polyspecific antiglobulin reagent and viewed for agglutination. Negative controls using cells not coated with drug must be used. A negative control serum must also be used and not agglutinate drug-coated cells.

Interpretation. Patient serum, which agglutinates drug-coated cells, is a positive test. Agglutination strength will vary.

Notes and Precautions. Antibodies to drug coated cells are common and in vitro testing does not always correlate with shortened red blood cell survival. Cross reactivity between drugs within a given class (eg, cephalosporins) or between classes of drugs (eg, penicillin and a cephalosporin) can occur.

Test 14.5.3 Immune Complex Antibody Detection Method

Purpose. Immune complex antibody detection determines if red blood cell destruction is due to drug-related immune complex deposition

Principle. Patient serum is incubated with the drug in the presence of reagent red blood cells. The mixture is assessed for agglutination, hemolysis, or complement on red cells.

Sample. Serum is used.

Procedure. Patient serum, a known concentration of drug, a source of complement, and reagent red blood cells are incubated together for a given period of time (usually 1 hour).

Interpretation. Hemolysis or agglutination indicates a positive test. The red blood cells are then tested using poly-specific antiglobulin reagent and viewed for agglutination (a DAT is performed). Reagent cells coated with IgG antibody and/or C3d is also considered a positive test.

Test 14.5.4 RBC Glucose-6-Phosphate Dehydrogenase Assay

Purpose. A deficiency of G6PD in a patient with acute hemolysis supports a diagnosis of drug-related hemolysis. Complete discussion of screening and quantitative assays are included in Chapter 9 and **Test 9.5.2**.

Test 14.5.5 Heinz Body Test

(See Test **9.5.3**)

14.6 Course and Treatment

Drug-induced hemolysis in G6PD deficiency is often self-limited as reticulocytes with greater concentrations of enzyme are produced. Drug-induced hemolysis may vary from mild to severe, depending on the subtype of disease and the oxidative stress (see Chapter 9).

When methyldopa or procainamide-type drugs incite a warm-type autoantibody, it may be difficult to determine whether the hemolysis is caused by an unrelated autoimmune disease or by the drug. Do not assume that a positive DAT is related to a drug-related immune response or an autoimmune disorder. Active hemolysis of the methyldopa type usually resolves spontaneously, but steroids may be necessary in severe or prolonged anemia. Steroids can then be tapered without relapse, although the positive DAT result may persist for up to 2 years. If clinical hemolysis is not present, steroid therapy is not indicated. In warm-type autoantibodies, such as those seen with methyldopa, antibody persists in the absence of the drug. If the DAT result is positive, but there is no detectable serum antibody, transfused RBCs survive normally. However, in the rare patient with severe warm-type autoantibody, transfused cells have a markedly decreased survival rate. Transfusions can be given if clinically indicated, but underlying alloantibodies, masked by the presence of the warm-type autoantibody, must be identified. Red blood cells lacking the corresponding alloantigen must be selected for transfusion.

Immune hemolysis due to drugs is usually mild to moderate, although rare cases of severe hemolysis and deaths have been reported. All suspicious drugs should be discontinued immediately until the cause of hemolysis is determined. If severe hemolysis has occurred, the patient can be supported with transfusion. In all cases, except for those where a true warm-type autoantibody has been generated, the antibody is dependent on the presence of the drug and transfusion is tolerated as soon as the drug is cleared from the circulation.

Drugs chemically similar to the inciting drug should be avoided due to possible cross reactivity. Re-exposure to a drug, documented as causing hemolysis, must be avoided. Cefotetan, a second-generation cephalosporin, is the most common cause of antibiotic-related immune hemolysis and 15 deaths have been reported with its use. Up to 8% of patients exposed develop antibodies 5-78 days after drug initiation. Studies demonstrate that cefotetan remains tightly bound to red blood cells for approximately a median of 9 weeks after exposure even though the half-life of the drug is 4 hours or less. Because hemolysis may occur after exposure, clinicians may not consider cefotetan the cause of the problem. A thorough and remote drug history must be obtained on any patient with unexplained hemolysis.

Drugs associated with TMAs must be discontinued for improvement to occur. This sometimes poses a clinical challenge since many of these drugs are immunosuppressants used in transplant settings and medication options are limited. Tough choices must be made because plasma exchange is not effective as a treatment for TMAs unless the etiology of the TMA is a deficiency of the metalloprotease responsible for breaking down large molecular weight von Willebrand multimers.

14.7 References

Ainsworth CD, Crowther MA, Treleaven D, Evanovitch D, Webert KE, Blajchman MA. Severe hemolytic anemia post-renal transplantation produced by donor anti-D passenger lymphocytes: case report and literature review. *Transfus Med Rev.* 2009 Apr;23(2):155-9. Review.

Arndt PA, Garratty G. The changing spectrum of drug-induced immune hemolytic anemia. *Semin Hematol.* 2005 Jul;42(3):137-44.

Arndt PA, Garratty G. Cross-reactivity of cefotetan and ceftriaxone antibodies associated with hemolytic anemia, with other cephalosporins and penicillin. *Am J Clin Pathol.* 2002;118:256-262.

Arndt P, Garratty G, Isaak E, Bolger M, Lu Q. Positive direct and indirect antiglobulin tests associated with oxaliplatin can be due to drug antibody and/or drug-induced nonimmunologic protein adsorption. *Transfusion.* 2009 Apr;49(4):711-8. Epub 2009 Dec 15.

Arndt PA, Leger RM, Garratty G. Serology of antibodies to second- and third-generation cephalosporins associated with immune hemolytic anemia and/or positive direct antiglobulin tests. *Transfusion.* 1999;39:1239-1246.

Beutler E. Glucose-6 phosphate dehydrogenze deficiency. In: Beutler E, Coller BS, Kipps TJ, et al, eds. *Williams Hematology. 5th ed.* New York, NY: McGraw-Hill;1995:564-580.

Christie DJ. Specificity of drug-induced immune cytopenias. *Transfus Med Rev.* 1993;7:230-241.

Chun NS, Savani B, Seder RH, Taplin ME. Acute renal failure after intravenous anti-D immune globulin in an adult with immune thrombocytopenic purpura. *Am J Hematol.* 2003 Dec;74(4):276-9.

Davenport RD, Judd J, Dake LR. Persistence of cefotetan on red blood cells. *Transfusion.* 2004;44:849-852.

Drug-Induced Immune Hemolytic Anemias. *AABB Technical Manual, 50th Anniversary Ed. 14th ed.* 439-450.

Gaines AR, Lee-Stroka H, Byrne K, Scott DE, Uhl L, Lazarus E, Stroncek DF. Investigation of whether the acute hemolysis associated with Rh(D) immune globulin intravenous (human) administration for treatment of immune thrombocytopenic purpura is consistent with the acute hemolytic transfusion reaction model. *Transfusion.* 2009;49:1050-8.

Gaines AR. Acute onset hemoglobinemia and/or hemoglobinuria and sequelae following Rh(o)(D) immune globulin intravenous administration in immune thrombocytopenic purpura patients. *Blood.* 2000 Apr 15;95(8):2523-9.

Gaines AR. Disseminated intravascular coagulation associated with acute hemoglobinemia or hemoglobinuria following Rh(O)(D) immune globulin intravenous administration for immune thrombocytopenic purpura. *Blood.* 2005 Sep 1;106(5):1532-7.

Garratty G. What is the mechanism for acute hemolysis occurring in some patients after intravenous anti-D therapy for immune thrombocytopenic purpura? *Transfusion.* 2009 June;49(6):1026-1031.

Garratty G. Drug-induced immune hemolytic anemia. In: Garratty G, ed. *Immunobiology of Tranfusion Medicine.* New York, NY: Dekker; 1994;523-551.

Garratty G. Guest editorial: drug-induced immune cytopenia. *Transfus Med Rev.* 1993;7:213-214.

Johnson ST, Fueger JT, Gottschall JL. One center's experience: the serology and drugs associated with drug-induced immune hemolytic anemia--a new paradigm. *Transfusion.* 2007 Apr;47(4):697-702.

Kees-Folts D, Abt AB, Domen RE, Freiberg AS. Renal failure after anti-D globulin treatment of idiopathic thrombocytopenic purpura. *Pediatr Nephrol.* 2002 Feb;17(2):91-6.

Leger RM, Arndt PA, Garratty G. Serological studies of piperacillin antibodies. *Transfusion.* 2008 Nov;48(11):2429-34. Epub 2008 Jul 22.

Martinengo M, Ardenghi DF, Tripodi G, Reali G. The first case of drug-induced immune hemolytic anemia due to hydrocortisone. *Transfusion.* 2008 Sep;48(9):1925-9. Epub 2008 Jun 29.

Garratty G. Immune cytopenia associated with antibiotics. *Transfus Med Rev.* 1993;7:255-267.

Moake JL. Thrombotic microangiopathies. *N Engl J Med.* 2002;347:589-600.

Packman CH, Leddy JP. Drug-related immune hemolytic anemia. In: Beutler E, Coller BS, Kipps TJ, et al, eds. *Williams Hematology.* 5th ed. New York, NY: McGraw-Hill; 1995:691-696.

Petz LD. Drug-induced autoimmune hemolytic anemia. *Transfus Med Rev.* 1993;7:242-254.

Rewald MD, Francischetti MM. After eight-year-tolerance minimal i.v. anti-D infusions unleash hemolysis in a patient with immune thrombocytopenic purpura (ITP). *Transfus Apher Sci.* 2004;30:105-10.

Shulman NR, Reid DM. Mechanisms of drug-induced immunologically mediated cytopenias. *Transfus Med Rev.* 1993;7:215-229.

Tarantino MD, Bussel JB, Cines DB, McCrae KR, Gernsheimer T, Liebman HA, Wong WY, Kulkarni R, Grabowski E, McMillan R. A closer look at intravascular hemolysis (IVH) following intravenous anti-D for immune thrombocytopenic purpura (ITP). *Blood.* 2007 Jun 15;109(12):5527; author reply 5528. No abstract available.

Tran MH, Fadeyi E, Scheinberg P, Klein HG. Apparent hemolysis following intravenous antithymocyte globulin treatment in a patient with marrow failure and a paroxysmal nocturnal hemoglobinuria clone. *Transfusion.* 2006 Jul;46(7):1244-7.

Chapter 15

Autoimmune Hemolytic Anemia

Robert C. Blaylock, MD

Autoimmune hemolytic anemia (AIHA) occurs when a patient produces antibodies directed at antigens on the patient's own red blood cells, resulting in decreased red blood cell survival. These autoantibodies are classified as warm or cold depending on the optimal thermal activity of the antibody. Patients with AIHA may have severe anemia necessitating emergent transfusions. All transfusions will involve incompatible units of blood and should only proceed if clinically necessary. Transfusion can be performed with relative safety, in patients with severe anemia, provided the presence of alloantibodies in patient plasma has been excluded. Unfortunately, autoantibodies can interfere with all routine blood bank tests used to screen, and identify, alloantibodies. Therefore, most morbidity associated with transfusion from AIHA is caused by unidentified alloantibodies. The most important information to obtain in a patient suspected of having AIHA is an accurate history of transfusion, pregnancy, and intravenous drug use. Alloantibodies are rarely found in patients without previous exposure to allogeneic red blood cells.

15.1 Pathophysiology

Warm AIHA occurs in both adult and pediatric patients. Warm autoantibodies react best at 37°C and are usually IgG. Hemolysis occurs via extravascular removal of antibody-coated red blood cells by macrophages in the reticuloendothelial system (RES) or intravascular hemolysis via activation of the complement system. Warm AIHA is rarely associated with renal failure and coagulopathy, unlike major hemolytic transfusion reactions. Autoantibodies in adults are commonly associated with underlying autoimmune disorders such as lupus, or associated with malignancies such as lymphomas. In pediatric patients, autoantibodies are more likely to be idiopathic or associated with a viral prodrome.

The most common warm autoantibodies react broadly to an epitope in the Rh system, but will not react with Rh null cells. Patients with severe anemia usually have antibody on red blood cells and in serum. Broadly reacting autoantibody in the serum makes alloantibody detection difficult.

Warm autoantibodies can have specificity for red blood cell alloantigens and appear as an alloantibody. When specificity exists, it is most commonly to one of the Rh antigens, in particular little e. Determining the presence of the corresponding antigen on a patient's native red blood cells can make the differentiation of alloantibody versus autoantibody.

Mimicking autoantibodies are another type of warm autoantibody. Mimicking autoantibodies initially appear to be broadly reacting, but during the course of a workup, the antibody will appear to have specificity and can be confused for an alloantibody. Mimicking antibodies will be described more in the discussion of autoantibody adsorptions.

Cold autoantibodies are usually IgM and are present in many healthy individuals when testing is performed at 4°C. These antibodies can have a thermal range that extends to room temperature. The antibodies can interfere with red blood cell alloantibody screening and compatibility testing because the IgM molecule is large and causes spontaneous red blood cell agglutination during testing. Most cold agglutinins are clinically insignificant and usually have specificity to I or IH antigens. Cold autoantibodies can become pathologic and cause hemolysis. The best method to differentiate a pathologic from non-pathologic cold agglutinin is to measure the thermal amplitude (thermal range) of the antibody. Cold autoantibodies capable of causing agglutination at 30°C or higher are very likely to cause in-vivo hemolysis. Antibodies, which react below 30°C, are unlikely to be pathologic.

Pathologic cold autoantibodies can be associated with lymphomas, but are more commonly associated with *Mycoplasma pnuemoniae* and Epstein-Barr infections. Many other viral infections can be associated with AIHA in both children and adults.

A Donath-Landsteiner antibody (also referred to as a biphasic antibody) is a unique autoantibody that classically requires a cold environment to bind to red blood cells and a warm temperature to activate complement and lyse cells. The hemolysis caused by this antibody is referred to as paroxysmal cold hemoglobinuria. These antibodies are IgG and have P blood group specificity. These biphasic antibodies were commonly found in patients with untreated syphilis, but are rare today.

Polyagglutination is another form of AIHA. Polyagglutination and hemolysis occur when red blood cell cryptantigens, which are normally hidden, become exposed. All patients have naturally occurring antibodies to these cryptantigens. Polyagglutination commonly occurs when organisms from a bacterial infection produce enzymes that cleave sugars and expose the cryptantigens. A prototype enzyme/organism combination is neuraminidase produced by *Clostridium perfringens* and exposure of the T antigen. Polyagglutination is also the cause of the acquired-B phenomenon where bacterial enzymes cleave a sugar from the blood group A antigen, causing the formation of a blood group B antigen. This type of polyagglutination can be discovered during the investigation of front and back-typing discrepancy. However, most forms of polyagglutination are not picked up during routine blood bank testing and lectin studies must be performed if polyagglutination is suspected.

Polyagglutination can also occur in association with myelodysplasia or leukemia and there are inherited forms that result in the incomplete biosynthesis of red blood cell antigens.

15.2 Clinical Findings

Patients with AIHA have anemia, malaise, easy fatigability, shortness of breath, pallor, and jaundice. Some patients may describe discolored urine secondary to either hemoglobin or bilirubin. Splenomegaly may be present. Anemia may be severe and any patient complaining of chest pain should be evaluated for myocardial ischemia. Patients with cold agglutinin disease (CAD) may present with Raynaud phenomenon, as the IgM autoantibody will agglutinate red blood cells and compromise circulation, primarily in the extremities. A comparison of the clinical characteristics of CAD versus warm AIHA is in **t15.1**.

t15.1 Clinical Characteristics of Autoimmune Hemolytic Anemias

Clinical Findings	Warm Type (70%)	Cold Type (30%)
Onset	Abrupt	Insidious
Jaundice	Usually present	Often absent
Splenomegaly	Yes	Absent
Age	All ages	All ages
Sex	Slightly more women	Women predominate
Origin of autoantibody		
Idiopathic	50%-60%	30%-40%
Drug-induced	25%-30%	1%-5%
Lymphoproliferative disorder	10%-15%	15%-20%
Viral or mycoplasma	0	25%-35%
Other (inflammatory diseases, other malignancies)	5%-10%	5%-10%

15.3 Diagnostic Approach

A thorough clinical history of the hemolytic episode with any recent infection and splenomegaly provide important diagnostic clues to the cause of AIHA and facilitate workup. Evaluation of the hemolysis proceeds with the following steps:

1. Hematologic analysis shows a normochromic, normocytic anemia, which may be hemolytic.
2. Results of direct antiglobulin test (DAT) or other methods of serum antibody detection should be positive and can identify the adsorbed globulins, allowing categorization of the process as a warm-type, cold-type, or mixed AIHA. If the DAT results are negative, immune hemolysis cannot be proven.
3. If a cold-type AIHA is suspected, further testing may include cold agglutinin titers, the Donath-Landsteiner test to exclude paroxysmal cold hemoglobinuria, antibody titers for viruses or mycoplasma, or search for an occult lymphoma or lymphoproliferative disorder in elderly patients to further characterize the type of hemolytic disease.
4. If a warm AIHA is suspected, further workup to identify an underlying cause, such as autoimmune disorders, malignancy, lymphoma, or other lymphoproliferative disorder, is required. Possible drug-induced causes should be considered.

15.4 Hematologic Findings

15.4.1 Blood Cell Measurements

Patients with warm AIHA have a normocytic, normochromic anemia, which can range from severe to moderate. Reticulocyte counts should be increased.

Automated red blood cell values in patients with CAD may be spurious due to the cold agglutinin, which clumps red blood cells in a cool in-vitro environment. This becomes evident when the hemoglobin approaches 40%-50% of the calculated hematocrit instead of the usual one third. The spontaneous clumps are due to the ability of the large IgM autoantibody to bridge the gap between red blood cells. The hemoglobin levels are usually accurate because clumped cells are lysed prior to the hemoglobin determination. The hematocrit is not accurate because it is calculated from the RBC count, which is falsely reduced because the clumped red blood cells are not part of the RBC count. The MCV, MCH, and MCHC are also inaccurate. Spun micro-hematocrits are usually valid. The peripheral smear in CAD will show red cell agglutination **t15.2**.

t15.2 Laboratory Characterization of Autoimmune Hemolytic Anemias

Laboratory Parameter	Warm Type	Cold Type
Usual immunoglobulin type	IgG	IgM
Direct antibody test	2+-4+	2+-4+
Monospecific sera		
Anti-IgG only	1+	0
Anti-IgG+ c3d	1+	0
Anti-c3d	Rare	1+
Complement activation	Little or none	Yes
Peripheral blood findings	Spherocytes, nucleated RBCs	RBC agglutination

15.4.2 Peripheral Blood Smear Morphology

The peripheral smear will demonstrate spherocytes due to red cell membranes being partially removed by macrophages in the RES. Polychromasia, poikilocytosis, anisocytosis, and nucleated red blood cells are also seen. CAD will show similar peripheral smear findings. One additional finding in CAD is the presence of red blood cell clumps i15.1.

15.4.3 Bone Marrow Examination

Bone marrow examination is usually not required. If performed, it demonstrates a hypercellular marrow with marked normoblastic erythroid hyperplasia. Usually marrow iron is markedly increased, reflecting the accelerated erythroid turnover. Prolonged severe hemolysis may result in relative deficiencies of folic acid or vitamin B12, causing superimposed megaloblastic maturation. Occasionally, bone marrow examination may reveal an underlying lymphoproliferative disorder associated with autoantibody production.

i15.1 Autoimmune hemolytic anemia

Red blood cell clumps. *(Wright stain)*

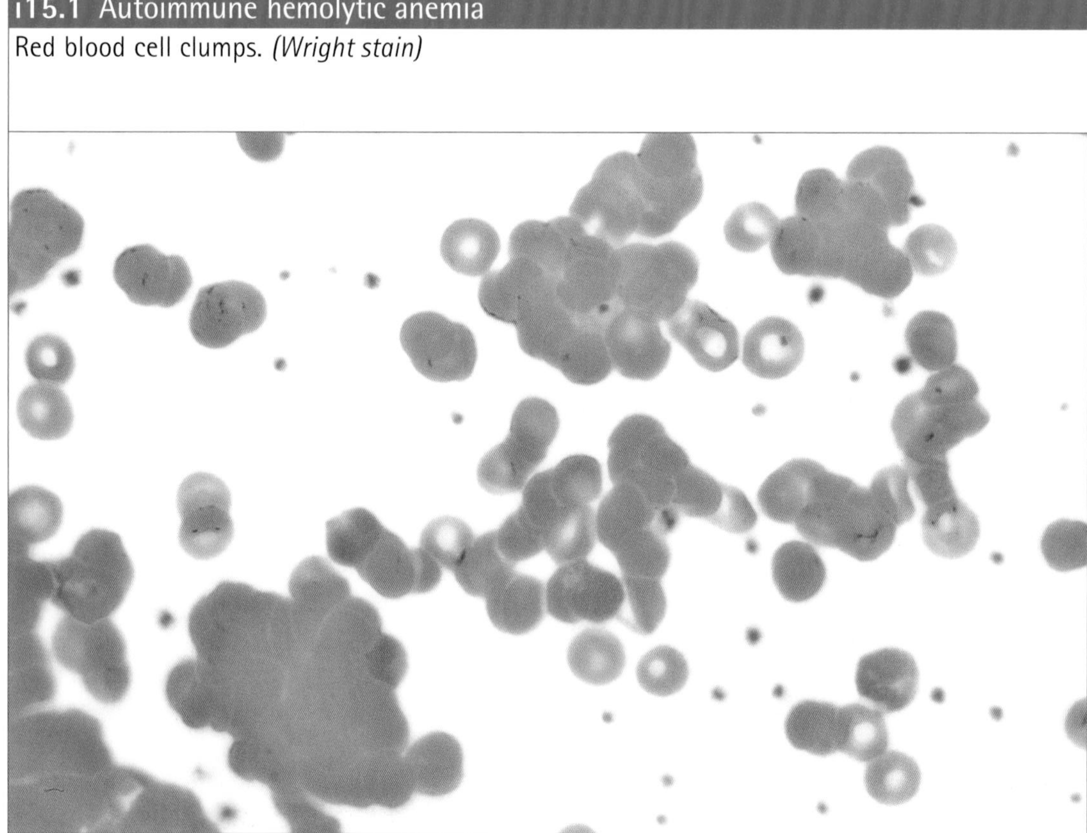

15.5 Other Laboratory Tests

Test 15.5.1 Blood Type

Purpose. Determine the ABO and D blood type of the patient.

Principle. Red blood cells contain major blood group antigens A, B, both, or neither, and is called the front type. Plasma contains the corresponding isohemagglutinin (back type). Failure to accurately identify blood type can lead to transfusion reactions.

Specimen. Serum or plasma sample with cells.

Procedure. To determine the front type, patient red blood cells are incubated with anti-A and anti-B reagents. Reagent IgM antibody will cause agglutination with patient cells expressing the corresponding antigen. The process for presence of the D antigen is the same. To determine the back type, patient plasma or serum is mixed with reagent red cells that contain A or B antigen. A large portion of isohemagglutinin is IgM, which will cause agglutination with reagent red cells.

Interpretation. The front and back type of the patient should match. For example, a patient with an A front type should contain anti-B in the back type. This patient would be typed as major blood group A.

Notes and Precautions. A typing discrepancy between the front and back type may exist in patients with CAD. The cold autoantibody can cause false-positive reactions with reagent cells used to determine the back type. Typing discrepancies can also exist in patients who have undergone bone marrow transplantation or have been massively transfused with blood other than their native type.

Test 15.5.2 Extended Phenotype

Purpose. To determine minor blood group antigens present on patient red blood cells. Antibodies directed at minor blood group antigens can cause hemolytic transfusion reactions and hemolytic disease of the newborn.

Principle. Extended phenotypes determine the presence of the Rh antigens C,c,D,E,e, and Kell, Kidd, Duffy, big S, and little s antigens.

Specimen. Red blood cells are collected in EDTA.

Procedure. Cells are washed and incubated with antisera of known specificity. Many reagents used to determine the presence or absence of a given antigen are IgM and cause spontaneous agglutination with the corresponding antigen. Some antiserum used to determine the presence of minor red cell antigens is IgG class and will require the addition of an IgM anti-IgG antibody to cause agglutination.

Interpretation. Agglutination determines the presence of a given antigen. Lack of agglutination means the antigen is absent.

Notes and Precautions. Recent transfusions make an extended phenotype difficult to determine since typing sera will not differentiate between autologous and allogeneic red blood cells. An extended phenotype can still be performed in patients with high reticulocyte counts by typing the reticulocytes after separation from non-reticulocytes using centrifugation. Incomplete removal of warm autoantibody prior to determining an extended phenotype can cause false-positive reactions with IgG typing reagents.

Test 15.5.3 Direct Antiglobulin Test (DAT)

Purpose. The DAT determines if immunoglobulin, and/or complement, is coating the surface of the patient's red blood cells.

Principle. Patient red blood cells are incubated with poly-specific IgM reagent with specificity for human IgG and complement.

Specimen. Red blood cells collected in EDTA.

Procedure. Washed patient red blood cells are incubated with poly-specific IgM reagent and observed for agglutination. Reagents specific for human IgG or complement component C3d are used if the initial poly-specific test is positive.

Interpretation. Red blood cells coated with either IgG or C3d will clump in the presence of the poly-specific reagent. In most cases of AIHA the poly-specific DAT will be positive. Further characterization of the DAT can be performed using mono-specific reagents, which are IgM anti-IgG or IgM anti-C3d. Red cells with warm AIHA typically demonstrate IgG on red blood cells and C3d may or may not be present. In CAD, C3d is usually found alone.

Notes and Precautions. It is important to determine if a mixed-field reaction is present. Mixed-field reactions are evident when some cells clump when incubated with poly-specific DAT reagent, while others are free floating. This can occur when two cell populations are present, one of which is coated with antibody or complement, and the other population is not. A mixed field reaction can be indicative of a delayed transfusion reaction instead of AIHA.

Test 15.5.4 Indirect Antiglobulin Test (IAT)

Purpose. The IAT detects autoantibodies, or unexpected alloantibodies in patient plasma or serum.

Principle. Commercially prepared screening red blood cells are collected from two to four individuals, depending on the vendor and methodology used in the test. The combination of cells is selected to ensure that all commonly encountered and problematic minor red blood cell antigens are present on at least one of the screening cells. Key antigens are homozygous so that alloantibodies are not missed due to reduced dosage of antigen.

Specimen. Serum or plasma is used.

Procedure. Patient plasma or serum is incubated with each individual screening cell. Most unexpected red cell alloantibodies are IgG class and will not clump red blood cells. IgM antiserum specific for human IgG and complement is added after the initial incubation. Agglutination with any of the screening cells determines a positive test.

Interpretation. Agglutination of one or all screening cells determines a positive test.

Notes and Precautions. Patients with AIHA often have autoantibody, which saturates red cells and spills into plasma. This autoantibody will cause the IAT to be positive and mask any underlying alloantibody.

Test 15.5.5 Elution

Purpose. An elution involves removing IgG from patient red blood cells. The antibody is harvested and used in an IAT.

Principle. Antibodies are removed from red blood cells using a variety of different methods.

Sample. Red blood cells are collected in EDTA.

Procedure. Patient red blood cells are placed in an environment which disassociates the IgG from the red cell membrane. Heat or acid environments are commonly used.

Interpretation. Once the antibody has been eluted, it is reacted with screening cells to see if the antibody has specificity. Patients with AIHA commonly have IgG lacking specificity (broadly reacting). Patients experiencing delayed hemolytic transfusion reactions will have IgG coating transfused cells, which demonstrate specificity for a blood group once eluted from the red cells.

Notes and Precautions. Patients with AIHA can have autoantibody with specificity for blood group alloantigens. This can lead to confusion regarding the etiology of the positive DAT. The extended phenotype of the patient can help differentiate alloantibody from autoantibody with specificity.

Test 15.5.6 Adsorptions

Purpose. This process removes autoantibodies from plasma or serum in order to facilitate detection of underlying alloantibodies.

Principle. Autoantibodies will adsorb onto all red blood cells. Autologous or allogeneic red blood cells with a known extended phenotype can be used to remove the autoantibody from plasma or serum.

Sample. Serum or plasma. Autologous red blood cells for autoadsorptions.

Procedure and Interpretation. This will be discussed independently for each type of adsorption.

Autologous Adsorption

Procedure. Autologous adsorptions are the preferred adsorption because of a reduced likelihood of missing an underlying alloantibody. To perform an auto-adsorption the antibody on the patient's cells must first be removed. This is commonly performed using enzymes. Once the autologous red blood cells are "free of antibody," they can be placed back into plasma where more of the autoantibody will attach to the red blood cell. If one adsorption does not remove all the autoantibody, the process can be repeated up to three times. Once the autoantibody is removed, the plasma can be screened against cells used for a routine IAT.

Interpretation. A negative IAT using adsorbed plasma will essentially rule out an underlying alloantibody.

Notes and Precautions. Autologous red blood cells will not adsorb blood alloantibodies, but weak alloantibodies may be diluted below detectable levels in the auto-adsorption process.

Unfortunately, auto-adsorptions are not always possible. Patients transfused within the prior four months may have transfused cells that could pull out an alloantibody, leading to a false-negative IAT. Transfusion histories are critical in the workup of an AIHA patient with extremely low hematocrits that make it impractical to collect enough cells to perform the auto-adsorption. In these situations allogeneic adsorptions must be used.

Single Cell Allogeneic Adsorption (SCAA)

Procedure. A SCAA can only be performed if the extended phenotype of the patient is known. The cells used to remove the autoantibody from the plasma are selected from a library of red blood cells, where the extended phenotypes have been previously determined. The cells used must duplicate the extended phenotype of the patient.

Once the duplicate cells are selected, testing proceeds as it would for autologous adsorptions, except the allogeneic cells are collected from donors that lack autoantibodies.

Interpretation. The allogeneic cells will adsorb the autoantibody, and leave any underlying alloantibodies behind in the plasma. A negative IAT after a single cell allogenic adsorption reduces the likelihood of an underlying alloantibody.

Notes and Precautions. The cell selected for the SCAA is only matched for commonly encountered and problematic minor blood group antigens. A chance exists, albeit small, that the allogeneic cell selected for the adsorption will express a minor antigen that the patient does not express. If the patient has formed an alloantibody to this minor antigen, the alloantibody will be removed by the allogeneic cell and lead to a false-negative IAT.

Three Cell Allogeneic Adsorption (TCAA)

Procedure. A TCAA is commonly used when patients with AIHA have a history of recent transfusion. The TCAA provides a method of removing autoantibody, and through a process of elimination, identifying any underlying alloantibodies. The key to a successful TCAA is the selection of cells used in the adsorption that are homozygous for the common blood group antigens involved in the formation of unexpected alloantibodies. The concept of a TCAA is illustrated **f15.1** and is simplified to demonstrate the identification of Rh antibodies only. However, the principle is the same

f15.1 Three Cell Allogeneic Absorption

a is a legend. We will pretend an alloantibody directed at the Rh antigen D is present along with the autoantibody.
b demonstrates the addition of allogeneic cells. Selection is based on homozygosity for antigens in the Rh system. They have been added to test tubes and patient plasma will be added to the test mix.
c demonstrates how the autoantibody will adsorb onto the allogeneic red cells. The alloantibody directed at the Rh antigen D will attach to the first two screening cells, but will not attach to the third screening cell, which facilitates identification.

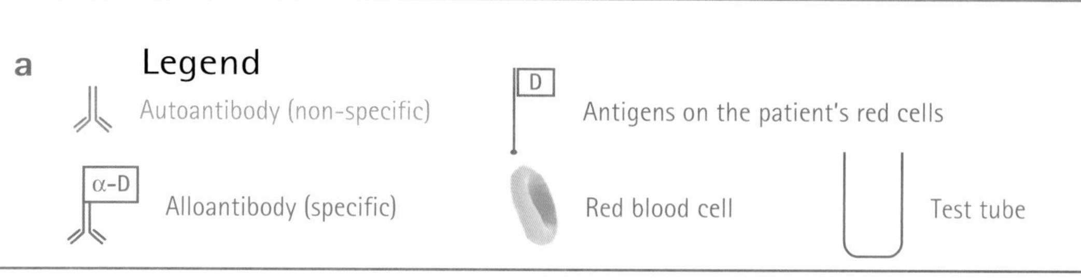

b Add the patient's serum...

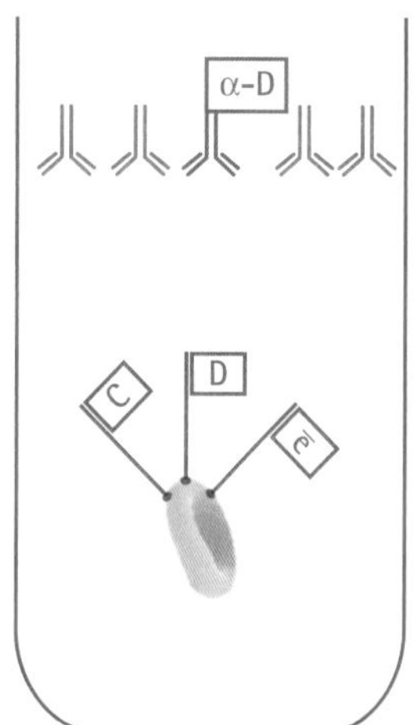

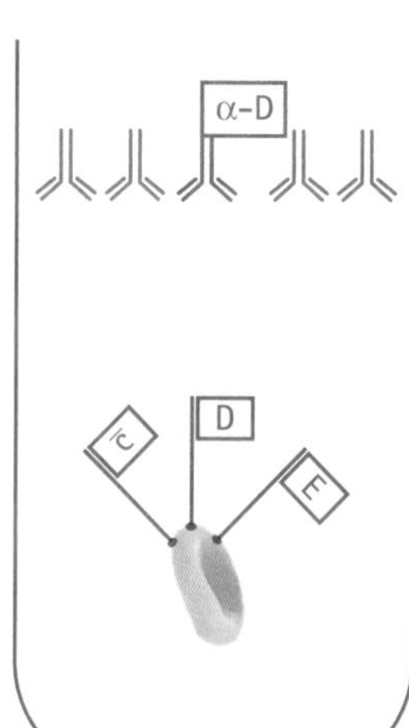

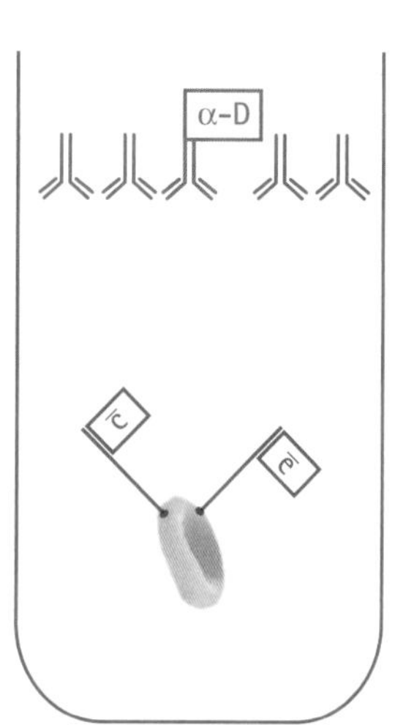

c Test the plasma...

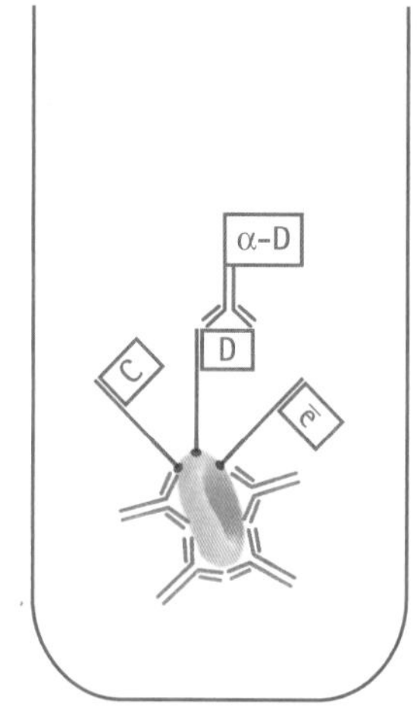

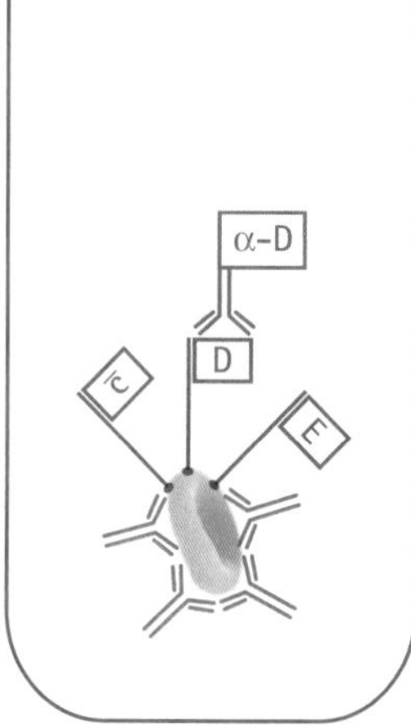

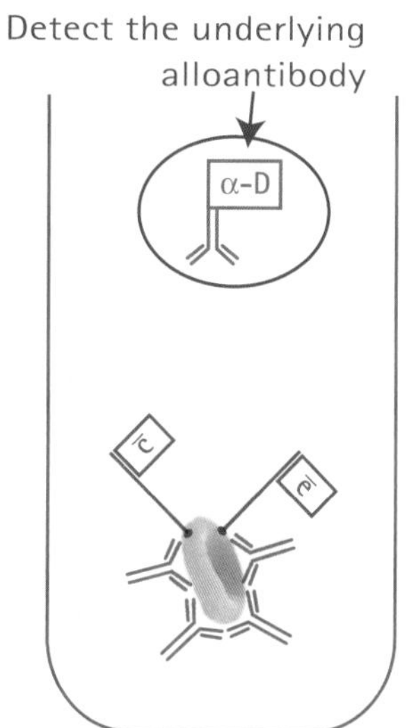

for other blood group systems. The process of identifying the five main Rh antibodies (anti-C,c,D,E,e) will follow.

The cells selected for identification of Rh alloantibodies must be homozygous. Cell number one should express a phenotype of CDe, cell number two should express cDE, and cell number three will be homozygous for ce. Each cell is placed into a separate test tube where they are incubated with patient plasma to adsorb the autoantibody. Once the autoantibody is adsorbed, the plasma is removed and an IAT is performed.

Interpretation. In this example we will pretend the patient has a warm autoantibody and an underlying anti-D alloantibody, and review how it is identified.

Cell number one is homozygous CDe/CDe. When this cell is placed in an environment containing a warm autoantibody and an anti-D, both antibodies will bind to the red blood cell. When the adsorbed serum is used to perform an IAT, a negative screen result is expected. While the anti-D is not identified, the negative screen does allow exclusion of anti-c and anti-E from the plasma, because these antibodies will not attach to red blood cells lacking the corresponding antigens. Therefore, this first adsorption has ruled out two of five Rh alloantibodies.

Cell number two is homozygous cDE/ cDE. Again the autoantibody and the anti-D will bind to the red blood cell. A negative IAT on the adsorbed plasma now allows exclusion of anti-C and anti-e since neither of these antibodies should bind to cell number two. Four of the five Rh antibodies have now been excluded.

Cell number three is homozygous ce/ce. When placed in patient plasma, the autoantibody will be removed, but the anti-D will not. The subsequent IAT will now be positive and further identification will identify the anti-D, which will not bind to a ce/ce positive cell. This process of elimination is complete, four of five Rh alloantibodies have been ruled out, and the anti-D identified.

Notes and Precautions. The cells selected for the TCAA will only be selected based on commonly encountered and problematic minor blood group antigens. A chance exists that the allogeneic cells selected for the TCAA will express a minor antigen that the patient does not express. If the patient has formed an alloantibody to this minor antigen, the alloantibody will be removed by the allogeneic cells and lead to a false-negative IAT.

Test 15.5.7 Thermal Amplitude

Purpose. Cold autoantibodies are commonly found in routine blood bank testing, but they are rarely clinically significant. The thermal amplitude characterizes the cold antibody to determine clinical significance.

Principle. The patient's plasma is reacted with reagent red blood cells at different temperatures.

Sample. Serum or plasma is used.

Procedure. Patient plasma is incubated with reagent red blood cells at temperatures of 37°C and 30°C as well as room temperature. All cells, reagents, and patient plasma must be at the desired test temperature before the test. The tubes are read for agglutination.

Interpretation. Autoantibodies causing agglutination at 30°C, or above, are considered clinically significant.

Notes and Precautions. False-positive reactions will occur if all components of the test are not allowed to equilibrate to the desired temperature prior to incubation.

Test 15.5.8 Donath-Landsteiner Test

Purpose. The Donath-Landsteiner test facilitates diagnosis of PCH, allowing it to be distinguished from cold-type AIHA. PCH is usually a self-limited disease that is treated conservatively by keeping the patient warm.

Principle. This test reproduces in vitro the biphasic reaction that characterizes PCH. The Donath-Landsteiner hemolysin is a complement-dependent IgG antibody that agglutinates cells at 4°C and lyses them at warmer temperatures (usually 37°C). Other hemolysins may react at a single temperature, 4°C or 37°C, but are not biphasic. The Donath-Landsteiner hemolysin does not lyse cells with reverse incubations of 37°C to 4°C.

Procedure. The patient's serum is incubated with test RBCs at 4°C for 30 minutes and then at 37°C for 30 minutes and observed for hemolysis, which is usually marked (3+ to 4+). If biphasic hemolysis is present, it is tested against panels of reagent RBCs to determine blood group specificity, which is often in the P or I system.

Interpretation. A biphasic hemolysin is diagnostic of PCH, which occasionally may clinically mimic cold-type AIHA. If intravascular hemolysis has recently occurred, the DAT results may be negative.

Notes and Precautions. PCH often occurs following a viral infection but can also be seen with syphilis, so follow-up serologic testing should be performed.

Test 15.5.9 Lectin Testing

Purpose. Polyagglutination involves the exposure of previously-hidden, red blood cell cryptantigens. Lectin testing determines if these antigens have been exposed.

Principle. Plant lectins will cause agglutination of red blood cells with exposed cryptantigens.

Sample. Red cells are collected in EDTA.

Procedure. Patient red blood cells are reacted with various plant lectins and the presence or absence of agglutination is determined. Examples of lectins used include Arachis hypogaea (peanut), Glycine max (soybean), or *Phaseolus lunatus* (lima bean).

Interpretation. The pattern of reactivity with these plant lectins can determine which cryptantigen is exposed. Examples of cryptantigens include T, Tk, Tn, and acquired B phenomenon.

Test 15.5.10 Serum Haptoglobin Quantitation

Purpose. Decreased or absent serum haptaglobin indicates hemolysis. Decreased haptoglobin also may be seen in liver failure or rarely as a genetic variant.

Principle. Haptoglobin is an a2-globulin produced in the liver that binds free hemoglobin on a molecule-for-molecule basis. The haptoglobin-hemoglobin complex is metabolized in the reticuloendothelial system, maintaining serum hemoglobin levels below renal thresholds. During intravascular hemolysis, haptoglobin binding is completely saturated. The excess hemoglobin is then bound by other serum proteins (hemopexin, transferrin, and albumin) before spilling into the urine. Absence of haptoglobin implies binding saturation and degradation. Decreased haptoglobin reflects active hemolysis or, alternatively, failure of production due to liver failure. Rare abnormal haptoglobins (such as Hp-) are genetic variants that do not bind hemoglobin but are of little clinical significance.

Specimen. Fresh serum is obtained atraumatically. To avoid extraneous hemolysis, serum should not be allowed to remain on RBCs. Testing specimens with macroscopic hemoglobinemia is superfluous.

Procedure. The haptoglobin molecule has separate sites for antibody and hemoglobin binding. Haptoglobin is quantitated with turbidimetric methods using a nephelometer. Antihaptoglobin is added to the patient's serum, forming immune complexes with serum haptoglobin (1:1). These immune complexes scatter light proportionate to their concentration.

Interpretation. The normal range for haptoglobin is 40-180 mg/dL (0.4-1.8 g/L). Less than 25 mg/dL (0.25 g/L) of haptoglobin is consistent with active hemolysis.

Notes and Precautions. Haptoglobin is an acute phase reactant, increasing three to four times in inflammation, infection, or tissue necrosis (eg, pneumonia or myocardial infarction). Such increases may mask changes in haptoglobin levels secondary to hemolysis. Haptoglobin levels greater than 200 mg/dL (2.0 g/L) are consistent with inflammation and not helpful in the diagnosis of hemolysis.

Molecular sites for hemoglobin binding are not the same as those for antibody binding by antihaptoglobin. With radial immunodiffusion testing, elevations of haptoglobin may be falsely interpreted due to measurement of saturated haptoglobin-hemoglobin complexes that have not been removed by the reticuloendothelial system.

Haptoglobin is decreased or absent in patients with liver failure, after a recent massive transfusion due to removal of senescent transfused RBCs, and in some abnormally functioning haptoglobin molecules (eg, Hp-).

15.6 Clinical Treatment

Patients with AIHA should first be assessed for severity of anemia. A patient with an extremely low hematocrit, chest pain, shortness of breath, and EKG changes consistent with myocardial ischemia will require an emergency transfusion. Hopefully, time will allow a front and back type in order to issue type specific blood. Patients in critical condition may require the release of type O negative red blood cells, however, every effort should be made to obtain samples for blood bank testing prior to transfusion.

If a patient does not exhibit signs and symptoms that are life threatening, obtain a thorough history of prior transfusions, pregnancy, and IV drug use. The history is extremely important and confidential interviews are especially critical in obtaining an accurate history of pregnancy or IV drug use.

Transfusions should be avoided if at all possible. However, transfusions can be performed if a patient starts to de-compensate, once underlying alloantibodies have been ruled out. This is hopefully accomplished using blood bank testing, but a complete blood bank workup will take a minimum of 6 hours and may be longer if reference testing is not performed in a given geographical area.

All red blood cell units selected for transfusion will be incompatible with autoantibodies in plasma. Blood should be started slowly when clinical circumstances permit. An infusion rate of 1 mL/minute for 30 minutes is a good starting point. If no adverse signs or symptoms are encountered, this can be increased to 2 mL/minute until the unit is infused. Patients with cold agglutinin disease must have blood infused through a blood warmer.

Some blood banks select red cells for transfusion that completely, or partially, match the extended phenotype of the patient. This is done to limit the potential of the patient to form unexpected alloantibodies. Limiting the potential for alloantibody formation can reduce the risk associated with emergent transfusions if they are required during a future admission. However, not all blood banks have the ability to provide this type of blood product, nor do some feel it is a cost-effective use of resources.

Medical evaluation for AIHA must include a search for an underlying disease. These usually involve malignancy (especially lymphoma) and autoimmune disorders such as systemic lupus erythematosus. CAD is commonly associated with infections such as *Mycoplasma pneumoniae* and other viral infections (Epstein-Barr). Pediatric patients with AIHA are more likely to have a viral prodrome, and less likely to have an autoimmune disease or lymphoma.

Warm AIHA, not associated with an underlying malignancy (lymphoma), usually responds to steroids and intravenous immune globulin. The use of IVIG should be communicated to the blood bank since it commonly contains red cell antibodies that can confound the blood bank workup. Splenectomy is reserved for patients unresponsive to initial therapy. Some success has been achieved with other forms of immunosuppression such as cytoxan or monoclonal anti-CD20. Plasmapheresis is of limited to no benefit, in the treatment of warm AIHA.

CAD is not responsive to steroid therapy or IVIG. Treating the underlying infection is of benefit. Some clinicians advocate the use of plasmapheresis for CAD. This can be technically challenging at times since blood will cool and agglutinate when placed in an extra-corporeal system.

The best approach to CAD involves keeping the patient warm. This should include instructions for wearing long sleeve clothes and gloves (even inside a home) and avoiding outside exposure. Cars should be pre-heated before the patient is transported. Bathing should be done quickly and in a bathroom with an elevated temperature. Cold food and drinks should be avoided as they will lower the temperature of gastrointestinal mucosa and increase the propensity of the temperature dependent autoantibody to cause hemolysis. Patients with chronic CAD may need to relocate to a geographical area with a warmer climate.

Patients with polyagglutination must have the underlying infection treated aggressively, since the infection is the source of the enzyme that modifies red cell antigens. The hemolysis that occurs will be somewhat self-limiting once the naturally occurring antibody is consumed. The transfusion of plasma containing blood products should be avoided since the plasma will be a fresh source of antibody and more hemolysis will ensue.

15.7 References

Arndt *PA*, Leger RM, Garratty G. Serologic findings in autoimmune hemolytic anemia associated with immunoglobulin M warm autoantibodies. *Transfusion.* 2009 Feb;49(2):235-42.

AABB Technical Manual, 50th Anniversary Edition 14th ed. 1953-2003.

Buetens OW, Ness PM. Red blood cell transfusion in autoimmune hemolytic anemia. *Curr Opin in Hematol.* 2003;10:429-433.

Garratty G. Autoimmune hemolytic anemia. In: Garratty G, ed. *Immunobiology of Transfusion Medicine.* New York, NY: Marcel Dekker, 1994;493-521.

Garratty G. Immune hemolytic anemia associated with negative routine serology. *Semin Hematol.* 2005 Jul;42(3):156-64. Review.

Garratty G. Immune hemolytic anemia-a primer. *Semin Hematol.* 2005 Jul;42(3):119-21.

Hashimoto C. Autoimmune hemolytic anemia. *Clin Rev Allergy Immunol.* 1998;16-285-295.

Issit PD, Combs MR, Bumgarner DJ, Allen J, Kirkland A, Melroy-Carawan H. Studies of antibodies in the sera of patients who have made red cell autoantibodies. *Transfusion.* 1996;36:481-486.

Judd WJ. Review: polyagglutination. *Immunohematology.* 1992;8:58-69.

King KE. Review: pharmacologic treatment of warm autoimmune hemolytic anemia. *Immunohematology.* 2007;23(3):120-9. Review. No abstract available.

Koppel A, Lim S, Osby M, Garratty G, Goldfinger D. Rituximab as successful therapy in a patient with refractory paroxysmal cold hemoglobinuria. *Transfusion.* 2007 Oct;47(10):1902-4.

Linz WJ, Tauscher C, Winters JL, Gastineau DA, Moore B. Cold agglutinin disease. *Transfusion Medicine Illustrated.* 2003;43:1185.

Petz LD. Bystander immune cytolysis. *Transfus Med Rev.* 2006 Apr;20(2):110-40. Review.

Petz LD. Cold antibody autoimmune hemolytic anemias. *Blood Rev.* 2008 Jan;22(1):1-15. Epub 2007 Sep 27. Review.

Petz LD. Diagnostic complexities in autoimmune hemolytic anemias. *Transfusion.* 2009 Feb;49(2):202-3. No abstract available.

Petz LD. Editorial: 'Least incompatible' units for transfusion in autoimmune hemolytic anemia: should we eliminate this meaningless term? A commentary for clinicians and transfusion medicine professionals. *Transfusion.* 2003;43:1503-1507.

Sokol RJ, Booker DJ, Stamps R. ACP Broadsheet No. 145. Investigation of patients with autoimmune haemolytic anemia and provision of blood for transfusion. *J Clin Pathol.* 1995;48:602-610.

Telen MJ, Rao N. Recent advances in immunohematology. *Curr Opin Hematol.* 1994;1:143-150.

Thomas AT. Autoimmune hemolytic anemias. In: Lee GR, Foerster J, Lukens JN, et al, eds. *Wintrobe's Clinical Hematology. 10th ed.* Baltimore, MD: Williams & Wilkins: 1999;1233-1263.

Part III

Reactive Disorders of Granulocytes and Monocytes

Chapter 16
Neutrophilia

Kathryn Foucar, MD

The normal range for absolute neutrophil count shows significant age variation **t16.1**. For example, a brisk neutrophilia, often exceeding 30 × 10^3/mm^3 (30 × 10^9/L) is typical at birth. Shortly after birth, the absolute neutrophil count plummets. The upper limit of normal for the absolute neutrophil count remains stable at approximately 7.0 × 10^3/mm^3 throughout infancy, childhood, and adulthood. Beyond the neonatal period, neutrophilia is generally defined as absolute neutrophil counts exceeding 8-10 × 10^3/mm^3.

Although the diagnostic approach to neutrophilia will be discussed later in this chapter, key concepts in the assessment of neutrophilia can guide the diagnostician **t16.2**. These concepts include a basic understanding of granulopoiesis, bone marrow reserves of readily available neutrophils, and basic strategies to recognize secondary neutrophilias and distinguish them from neoplastic disorders.

t16.1 Normal Absolute Neutrophil Count and Definition of Neutrophilia Based on Age

Age	ANC-Normal Range*	Neutrophilia (ANC)*
Birth	7.0 - 20.0 × 10^3/$mm^{3\dagger}$	> 28.0 × 10^3/mm^3
Infants	2.5 - 7.0 × 10^3/mm^3	> 10.0 × 10^3/mm^3
Children	1.5 - 7.0 × 10^3/mm^3	> 8.0 × 10^3/mm^3
Adults	1.5 - 6.0 × 10^3/mm^3	> 7.0 × 10^3/mm^3

**Only circulating pool of neutrophils measured in blood samples. ANC=absolute neutrophil count*
†Varies by altitude; higher absolute neutrophil counts detected in normal term babies born at high elevations

The causes of reactive neutrophilia include a broad spectrum of disorders, ranging from infections to metabolic defects **t16.3**. Bacterial infections are the predominant cause of neutrophilia in clinical practice. Other causes of reactive neutrophilia include therapeutic or endo¬genous drugs/hormones, acute stress, acute tissue necrosis, and other infectious/inflammatory processes **i16.1**, **i16.2**. More recently identified causes of secondary neutrophilia are Hantavirus pulmonary syndrome (HPS) and severe acute respiratory distress syndrome (SARS). In HPS, non-toxic neutrophilia with left shift, thrombocytopenia, hemoconcentration, and circulating immunoblasts are evident in patients with florid disease **i16.3**, **i16.4**. In patients with SARS, there was an association between neutrophilia and secondary bacterial infections. Constitutional neutrophilia is exceedingly rare and is generally linked to neutrophil migration defects (see Chapter 21).

Absolute neutrophilia is seen in various hematopoietic neoplasms, especially chronic myeloproliferative neoplasms. In affected patients the neutrophils are part of the neoplastic process. Because chronic myeloproliferative neoplasms represent clonal stem cell defects, the

t16.2 Neutrophilia—Key Concepts

- Bone marrow neutrophil production rates are astronomical.
- Exquisite regulation of granulopoiesis is required.
- A large reserve compartment of neutrophils, bands, and neutrophilic metamyelocytes is present in the bone marrow and can be readily released.
- Absolute neutrophil count shows age and race-related variations in normal ranges.
- Most notable is normal ANC at birth, which can exceed 20.0 x $10^3/mm^3$.
- Approximately equal numbers of neutrophils are circulating and marginated; only the circulating neutrophils are reflected in the WBC.
- Morphologic features of activation are present in most, but not all, reactive neutrophilias.
- In adults, left-shift is generally more limited in reactive neutrophilias compared to chronic myeloid neoplasms.
- A systematic evaluation of all hematopoietic lineages, clinical features, and other lab data is necessary to distinguish some secondary neutrophilias from chronic myeloid neoplasms.
- Genetic testing, although not confirmatory in all cases, is the optimal specialized test for neutrophilia-associated chronic myeloid neoplasms.

t16.3 Reactive Neutrophilias

Infections
- Primarily bacterial
- Less common in viral, mycobacterial, leptospiral, or toxoplasmal infections
- Hantavirus pulmonary syndrome (HPS)*
- Severe acute respiratory distress syndrome (SARS)†

Drugs, hormones
- Excess CSF (therapeutic, CSF-producing tumors)
- Epinephrine (therapeutic or endogenous production)
- Corticosteroids (therapeutic or endogenous production)
- Lithium
- Poisons/toxins/venoms

Tissue necrosis
- Burns
- Trauma
- Infarct
- Acute gout

Inflammatory disorders
- Collagen vascular disorders
- Other autoimmune disorders

Tumor-associated
- Carcinoma: CSF-producing
- Carcinoma: chemokine-producing
- Myeloma: interleukin-producing

Miscellaneous
- Stress/severe exercise/trauma
- Pregnancy
- Smoking
- Acute hemorrhage/hemolysis
- Postsplenectomy

Metabolic
- Ketoacidosis
- Uremia
- Eclampsia

Neonatal neutrophilia
- Infection
- Stressful labor
- Asphyxia, seizures
- Meconium aspiration
- Hemolytic disease
- Hypoglycemia
- Congenital anomalies
- Leukocyte adhesion deficiency

Constitutional (very rare)‡
- Hereditary neutrophilia
- Familial cold urticaria
- Leukocyte adhesion deficiency

**Neutrophilia in HPS secondary to acute, severe respiratory distress; neutrophils generally lack toxic changes*
†Neutrophilia in SARS often linked to secondary bacterial infections
‡These rare disorders are very rarely encountered in clinical practice
CSF = colony-stimulating factor

mature RBCs, WBCs, and platelets within the peripheral blood are all derived from the neoplastic clone. A variety of blood features and several specialized blood studies are useful in separating these clonal disorders from non-neoplastic neutrophilias.

i16.1 Toxic neutrophilia

Blood smear from a patient receiving pharmacologic doses of recombinant human granulocyte-colony-stimulating factor. A striking leukocytosis with pronounced toxic changes and left shift is evident. *(Wright stain)*

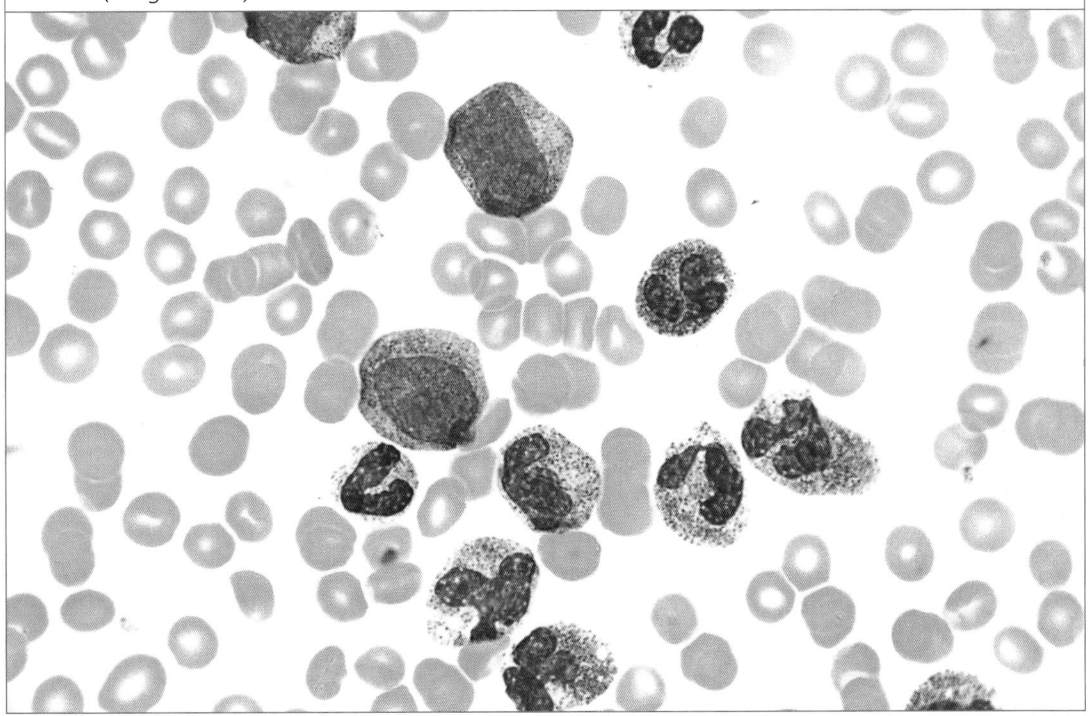

i16.2 Toxic neutrophilia with intracytoplasmic morulae

Blood smear from a patient with human granulocytic ehrlichiosis. Both toxic neutrophilia and intracytoplasmic morulae are present. *(Wright stain) (courtesy P Ward, MD)*

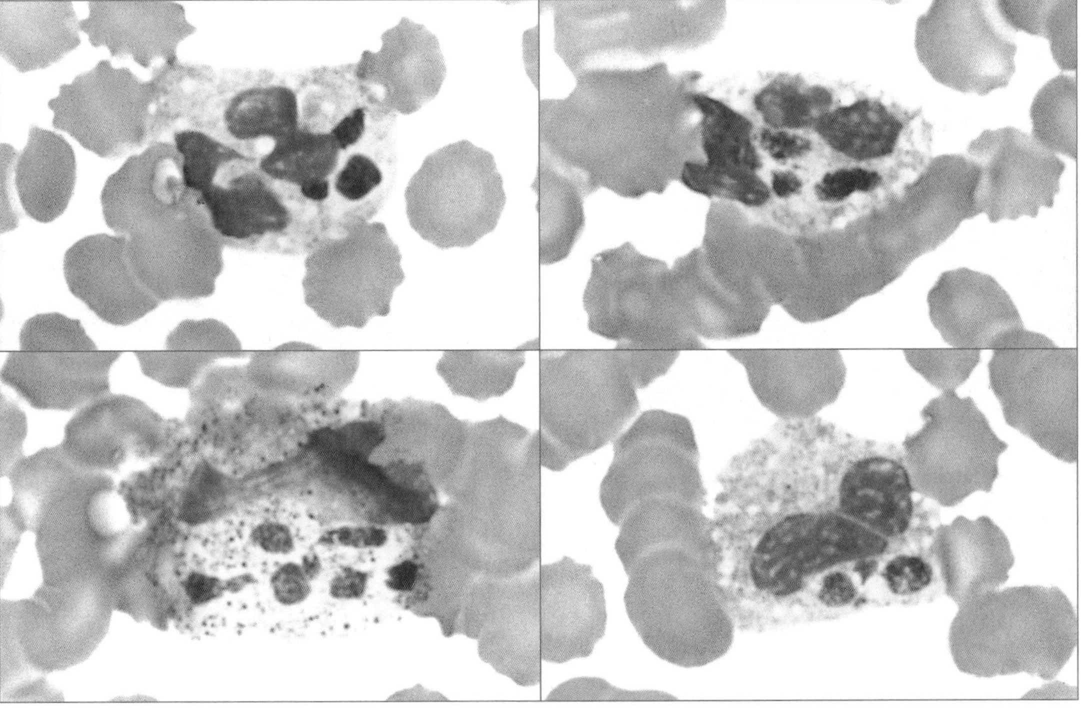

i16.3 Hantavirus cardiopulmonary syndrome

Features of Hantavirus cardiopulmonary syndrome in early capillary leak phase include gradually increasing absolute neutrophil count, circulating immunoblasts, and significant thrombocytopenia. *(Wright stain)*

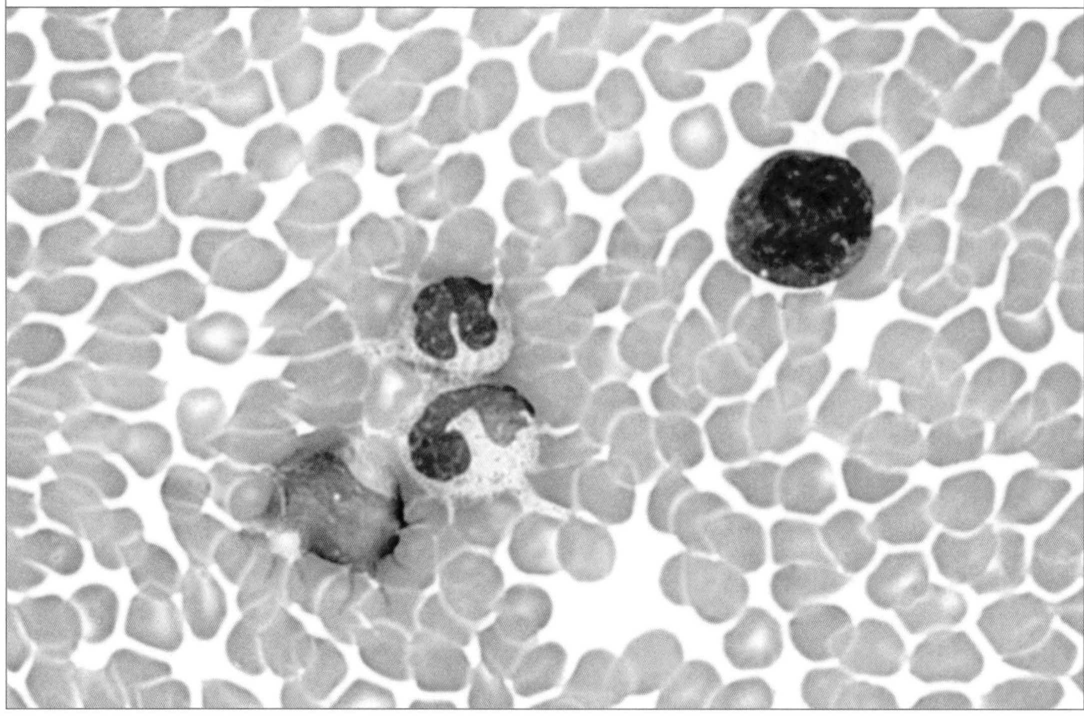

i16.4 Hantavirus cardiopulmonary syndrome

Progression to florid Hantavirus cardiopulmonary syndrome is characterized by progressive increase in hemoglobin/hematocrit, prominent neutrophilia with left shift without significant toxic changes, circulating immunoblasts, and marked thrombocytopenia. *(Wright stain)*

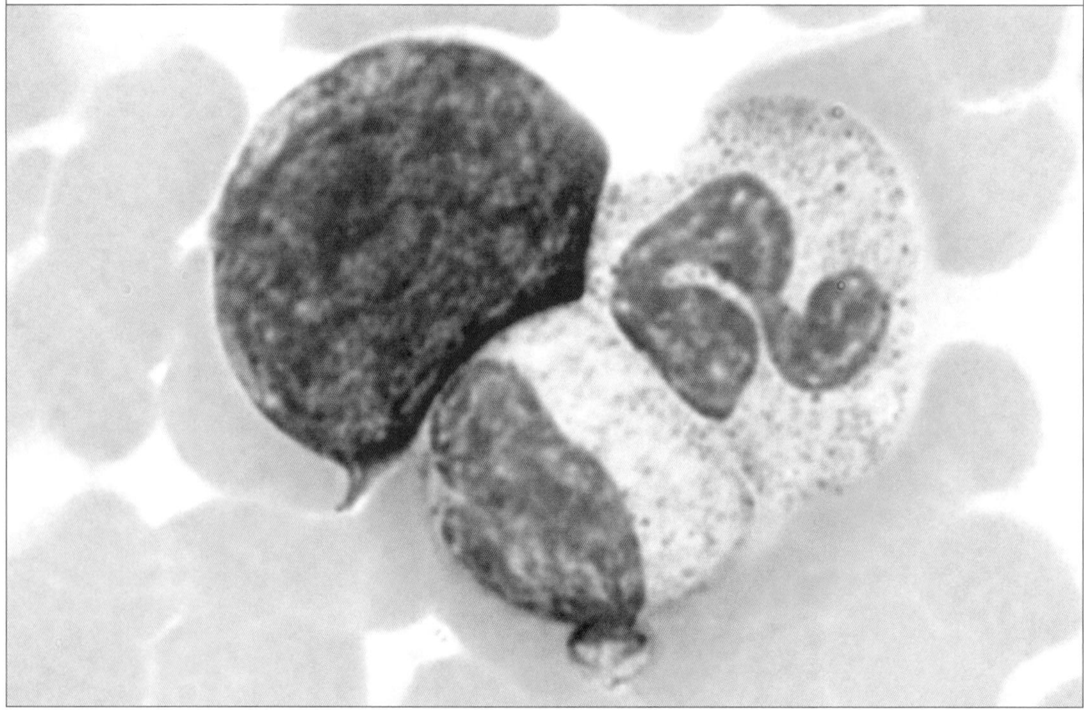

16.1 Pathophysiology

Granulopoiesis occurs when the bone marrow contains sufficient stem cells and progenitor cells, an adequate microenvironment for hematopoiesis, and sufficient regulatory factors. Granulopoiesis is a precisely regulated system of cell proliferation and maturation; regulation is largely achieved by factors produced within the bone marrow microenvironment. The most well-characterized of these regulatory factors is a family of glycoproteins called colony-stimulating factors (CSFs). By binding to an appropriate surface receptor on progenitor cells, these regulatory proteins stimulate production of granulocytes (granulocyte CSF [G-CSF]), monocytes (monocyte CSF [M-CSF]), or both (granulocyte-monocyte CSF [GM-CSF]). Colony-stimulating factors also induce a hyperfunctional state in mature neutrophils and monocytes, cells that also express CSF receptors. The hyperfunctional state of these mature cells is linked to morphologic changes such as toxic granulation, Döhle bodies, and prominent cytoplasmic vacuolization (see **i16.1**). CSFs are produced by various cells within the bone marrow including monocytes/macrophages and T lymphocytes; CSFs may also be aberrantly secreted by epithelial neoplasms.

Granulocyte maturation is characterized by both a progressive decrease in nuclear size with eventual segmentation and a progressive increase in cytoplasmic granularity. The arbitrarily defined stages of granulopoiesis consist of myeloblasts, promyelocytes, myelocytes, metamyelocytes, band neutrophils, and segmented neutrophils. Myeloblasts, promyelocytes, and myelocytes are capable of mitotic division, but metamyelocytes, band neutrophils, and segmented neutrophils have lost this capability. Primary granules are initially recognized in "late" myeloblasts and promyelocytes. These lysosomal granules contain numerous cytolytic enzymes, the most notable of which is myeloperoxidase. Secondary granules first appear at the myelocyte stage of maturation, and they eventually outnumber primary granules, giving the cytoplasm a homogeneous pink blush in Wright-stained slides. Like primary granules, secondary lysosomal granules contain numerous cytolytic enzymes. The most commonly evaluated secondary granule enzyme is leukocyte (neutrophil) alkaline phosphatase. A third type of granule subset, the gelatinase granule, has recently been identified in band and segmented neutrophils.

The time required for granulopoiesis varies from 1-3 weeks. Once neutrophils are released into the peripheral blood, they circulate for only a few hours before egressing to tissues. Homeostatic rates of neutrophil production exceed 1-2 × 10^9 neutrophils per kilogram per day.

Baseline granulopoiesis can be stimulated by infectious and inflammatory conditions **t16.4**. The primary mechanisms for neutrophilia include demargination of the marginated pool, release of the bone marrow maturation-storage compartment, and increased neutrophil production. Demargination of neutrophils is caused by epinephrine release and can occur within minutes. Because the circulating and marginating pools are approximately equal, this mechanism is predicted to approximately double the absolute neutrophil count. Greater increases in the absolute neutrophil count result from release of the bone marrow maturation-storage compartment, a phenomenon induced by corticosteroids, acute infections, and acute inflammation. In addition to a substantial absolute neutrophilia, a left shift with circulating band neutrophils, metamyelocytes, and even myelocytes is a predictable finding in patients in whom mobilization of the bone marrow reserve (maturation-storage) compartment has occurred.

For a neutrophilia to be sustained, increased bone marrow production must occur. This is the slowest mechanism of neutrophilia, but results in significant sustained neutrophilia. This process is mediated by CSFs; conditions linked to sustained increased CSF production include chronic infections, chronic inflammation, CSF-producing tumors, and therapy with recombinant human CSF.

t16.4 Mechanisms Causing Non-Neoplastic Neutrophilia

Mechanism	Time Course	Causes
Demargination*	Minutes	Epinephrine release, acute stress, exercise
Mobilization of maturation-storage compartment	Hours	Corticosteroids, infection, inflammation
Increased production	Days	Sustained infection, chronic inflammation, CSF-producing tumors, CSF therapy, lithium therapy

**Detachment of marginated neutrophils from endothelium into circulating pool*
CSF = colony stimulating factors

16.2 Clinical Findings

The clinical findings in patients with reactive neutrophilia are diverse, depending on the underlying disorder. Fever is a hallmark of acute infection, but various other signs and symptoms are linked to the specific site of infection. Patients in whom the neutrophilia is part of a bone marrow neoplasm (eg, patients with chronic myeloproliferative neoplasms) generally present with symptoms of fatigue and malaise. Fever is not present unless these patients have developed a secondary infection. Splenomegaly and variable hepatomegaly are common clinical findings in patients with chronic myeloid neoplasms (see Chapters 38-42).

16.3 Diagnostic Approach

The evaluation of a patient with an increased absolute neutrophil count must include both the distinction between a reactive and neoplastic process and the determination of the likely cause of a reactive neutrophilia. The distinction between a reactive neutrophilia and chronic myeloid neoplasms, notably chronic myelogenous leukemia (CML) and chronic neutrophilic leukemia (CNL), is based on the assimilation of clinical, hematologic, morphologic, and chemical parameters **t16.5-t16.7**. In general, pronounced toxic changes, a limited left shift, and normal absolute basophil count indicate a reactive neutrophilia, whereas CML is characterized by a strikingly elevated non-toxic leukocytosis with left shift, including blasts, abnormalities in other lineages, and prominent absolute basophilia.

t16.5 Morphologic Features of Reactive Neutrophilia

Blood	Comments
Leukocytosis	Usually <30 × $10^3/mm^3$ (<30 × $10^9/L$); higher WBC count in young children Rarely exceeds 50 × $10^3/mm^3$ (50 × $10^9/L$) except in patients receiving CSF therapy (or with CSF-producing tumor)
Left shift	Bands and metamyelocytes typical; may also see myelocytes In neonates with sepsis may see circulating myeloblasts along with other granulocytic elements
Döhle bodies	Retained portion of cytoplasm from more immature state of maturation
Toxic granulation	Etiology controversial; either retained primary granules or altered uptake of stain by secondary granules
Cytoplasmic vacuoles	Prominent neutrophil vacuoles correlates with sepsis
Other lineages	Thrombocytosis common; if DIC develops, thrombocytopenia is found Eosinophilia or monocytosis may accompany neutrophilia Basophilia not present

CSF = colony-stimulating factor; DIC = disseminated intravascular coagulation

t16.6 Morphologic Features of Blood in Patients Receiving Recombinant Growth Factor Therapy*

Leukocytosis with increase in neutrophils (increase in monocytes in patients receiving GM-CSF)
Prominent toxic changes in mature and immature granulocytes
Left shift with circulating blasts (usually low percent except during earliest recovery phase)
Transient increase in blasts prior to neutrophil recovery may mimic leukemia
Rare binucleate (tetraploid) neutrophils present (G-CSF)
Circulating myeloid cytoplasmic fragments

**Therapy may be recombinant human GM-CSF or recombinant human G-CSF*
GM-CSF = granulocyte-monocyte colony-stimulating factor; G-CSF = granulocyte colony-stimulating factor

t16.7 Comparison of Reactive Neutrophilia to Chronic Myeloid Neoplasms

Parameter	Reactive Neutrophilia	CML	CNL
WBC	Usually <30 × 10^3/mm^3 (<30 × 10^9/L)	Usually >50 × 10^3/mm^3 (>50 × 10^9/L)	Usually>25 × 10^3/mm (>25 × 10^9/L)
Toxic neutrophils	Present	Usually absent*	Often present
Left shift	Includes myelocytes	Includes blasts	Usually limited (<10%)
Basophilia	Absent	Present	Usually absent
Platelet count	Variable, decreased with sepsis	Increased	Normal
Platelet morphology	Unremarkable	Abnormal, variable micromegakaryocytes	Unremarkable
Nucleated erythroid cells in blood	Absent	Present	Absent
Splenomegaly	Absent	Present	Present
Fever	Usually present	Usually absent	Absent
Uric acid	Normal	Increased	Usually increased
LAP	Increased	Low*	Normal to increased
Karyotype	Normal	Philadelphia chromosome; t(9;22)(q34;q11)	Often normal (90%)
Molecular	Normal	*BCR-ABL1* gene rearrangement	Not available

**Except in patients with secondary infection*
LAP = leukocyte alkaline phosphatase; CML = chronic myelogenous leukemia (see Chapter 35); CNL = chronic neutrophilic leukemia (see Chapter 36)

The following approach to diagnosis should be considered:

1. Assess the complete blood count with differential.
2. Evaluate the morphology for toxic changes and for evidence of multilineage abnormalities.
3. Conduct appropriate microbacterial studies to evaluate for a possible infection.
4. Integrate the blood findings with clinical features and chemical analyses.
5. Examine bone marrow or perform cytogenetic/molecular evaluation in selected patients in whom a neoplastic disorder is the primary diagnostic consideration. (See Chapters 35-42)

16.4 Hematologic Findings

16.4.1 Blood Cell Measurements

In a reactive neutrophilia the WBC count rarely exceeds 30 × 10^3/mm^3 (30 × 10^9/L). In exceptional patients, including either young children with infection or patients receiving recombinant human CSF therapy, the WBC count may exceed 50 × 10^3/mm^3 (50 × 10^9/L). A neoplastic disorder should be strongly considered when the WBC count exceeds 100 × 10^3/mm^3 (100 × 10^9/L), except in the circumstance of pharmacologic doses of recombinant CSF (see **t16.6**).

Depending on the underlying disorder, the hemoglobin, hematocrit, and platelet values are highly variable in patients with reactive neutrophilia. For example, if an infectious or inflammatory condition is long-standing, an anemia of chronic disease may have developed (see Chapter 3). In patients with severe infections and secondary disseminated intravascular coagulation, RBC fragmentation and thrombocytopenia may be evident. Thrombocytosis, however, accompanies many cases of reactive neutrophilia that are secondary to acute stress.

16.4.2 Peripheral Blood Smear Morphology

The morphologic features of reactive neutrophilia are listed in **t16.5**. Although highly variable, the WBC count usually does not exceed 30 × 10^3/mm^3 (30 × 10^9/L); exceptions do occur, especially in patients receiving recombinant human CSF therapy **t16.6**. In addition to an increase in mature neutrophils, a left shift including bands and metamyelocytes is typical in patients with a marked reactive neutrophilia i16.5. In septic newborns, circulating blasts and promyelocytes also may be evident. However, circulating blasts are not a typical feature of reactive neutrophilia in adults, except in those receiving recombinant human CSF. Toxic

i16.5 Acute bacterial infection

Peripheral blood smear demonstrating marked absolute neutrophilia with left shift and toxic changes characteristic of acute bacterial infection. *(Wright stain)*

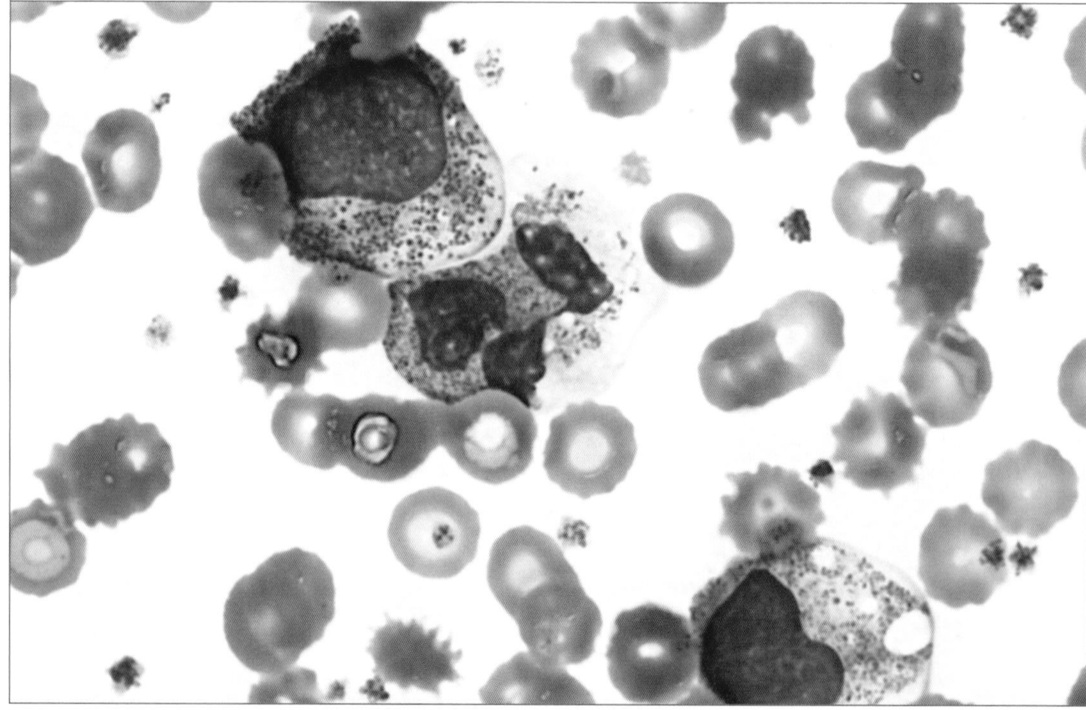

changes within the cytoplasm of reactive neutrophils include Döhle bodies, toxic granulation, and, when sepsis is present, prominent cytoplasmic vacuoles i16.6. In exceptional cases of sepsis, intra- and extracellular bacteria or fungi may be identified on the peripheral smear, usually a grave finding i16.6, i16.7. Some cases of reactive neutrophilia are characterized by nuclear hyposegmentation (pseudo–Pelger-Huët change). The absolute neutrophilia may be accompanied by eosinophilia or monocytosis in infectious and inflammatory processes. Notably, basophilia is not a feature of a reactive neutrophilia.

One area of particular controversy is the use of the band count in evaluating a patient for possible bacterial infection. Despite the reliance of clinicians, especially neonatologists and pediatricians, on the band count, both the accuracy of band counts and their sensitivity in predicting infection have been challenged. In several studies, the factors found most sensitive in predicting bacterial infection include WBC, absolute neutrophil count, and the presence of immature myeloid elements such as myelocytes and promyelocytes. One recent study suggests that the manual differential count contributes to the identification of infected patients who have normal or low absolute neutrophil counts.

In patients with chronic myeloid neoplasms, striking toxic changes are absent unless a concurrent acute infection is present, the left shift includes blasts, and basophilia is common, especially in CML. An exception is the rare chronic myeloid neoplasm, CNL, in which neutrophils often exhibit intense granulation. Numerical and morphologic abnormalities of

i16.6 Acute bacterial infection

a Prominent toxic granulation is evident in this neutrophil in a patient with acute bacterial infection. **b** Intracellular *diplococci* are evident in this circulating neutrophil in a patient with bacterial sepsis. *(Wright stain)*

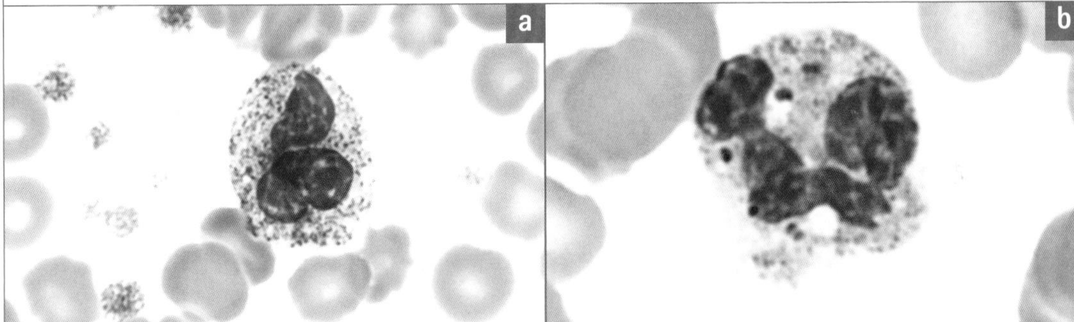

i16.7 Histoplasmosis

Fungal organisms confirmed to be histoplasmosis are evident in this circulating neutrophil in a patient with underlying immunodeficiency. *(Wright stain) (courtesy Dennis O'Malley, MD)*

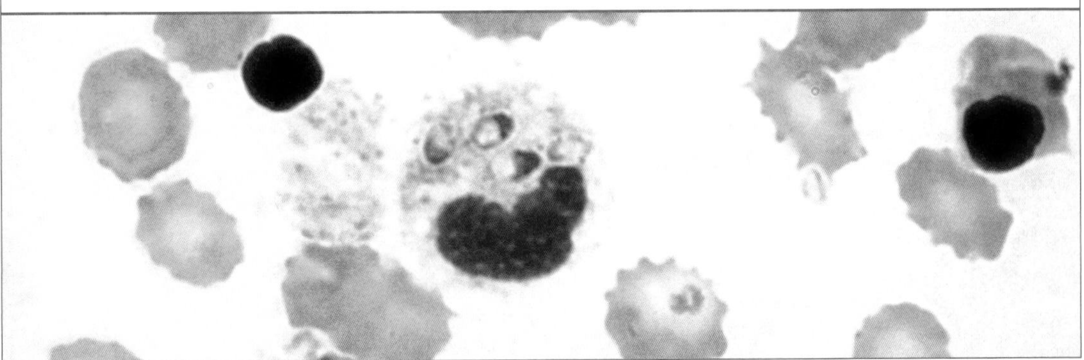

platelets and RBCs are common in CML, and both circulating erythroid and megakaryocytic precursors may be evident **t16.7** (see Chapters 35-42).

16.4.3 Bone Marrow Examination

In a straightforward reactive neutrophilia, bone marrow examination is generally unnecessary. In patients with a sustained reactive neutrophilia, the predicted bone marrow findings include a granulocytic hyperplasia. However, bone marrow examination may be warranted for culture or to exclude a possible neoplastic process.

16.5 Other Laboratory Tests

Test 16.5.1 Leukocyte (Neutrophil) Alkaline Phosphatase

Purpose. The leukocyte alkaline phosphatase (LAP) test provides evidence in differentiating CML from leukemoid reactions, although more precise diagnostic tests such as molecular/cytogenetic analyses have largely replaced the routine use of this test in clinical practice.

Principle. LAP is an enzyme present within the secondary (specific) granules of maturing neutrophils from the myelocyte stage onward. Stimulated neutrophils contain increased amounts of LAP. Therefore, the test helps distinguish reactive neutrophilia (increased LAP) from the abnormally maturing clonal granulocytes of CML (decreased LAP).

Procedure. LAP is usually determined semiquantitatively by specific cytochemical staining of peripheral blood smears. The LAP present in the neutrophils hydrolyzes a substrate that is then coupled to a dye, forming brown-to-black particles in the cytoplasm of these cells at the enzyme sites. The smears are then counterstained, examined microscopically, and 200 segmented or band neutrophils are counted and graded 0 to 4+ by evaluating the number of cytoplasmic particles. The LAP score is calculated by adding the products of the number of cells multiplied by the grades. The range of normal scores is 13 to 130, although there may be slight variation in each laboratory. Recently a quantitative flow cytometric technique to measure LAP has been developed, but this method is not commonly used in clinical practice.

Specimen. Freshly prepared patient and control blood smears are obtained from finger-stick capillary blood. Blood smears should be dried at least 1 hour before fixation. If not stained immediately, fixed slides may be stored overnight in a freezer without significant loss of enzyme activity.

Interpretation. The general LAP score is very low in CML, while increased scores are more characteristic of inflammatory disorders and other chronic myleoproliferative neoplasms. However, many exceptions exist. The LAP score may be increased in CML patients with secondary infections. A rising LAP score also characterizes some cases of CML in evolving blast phase.

Notes and Precautions. Improperly stored smears lose enzymatic activity and give falsely low LAP scores. Ethylenediaminetetraacetic acid (EDTA) anticoagulant inhibits this reaction. It is not recommended that LAP score replace more sensitive and specific molecular/genetic tests for CML and other chronic myeloid neoplasms.

16.6 Ancillary Tests

Other laboratory tests may be used to evaluate selected patients with neutrophilia. For example, serologic tests for collagen vascular disorders, uric acid levels, and gallium scans may be warranted for specific clinical indications. Either routine cytogenetic studies or molecular analyses for BCR/ABL gene rearrangements are essential in establishing the diagnosis of CML.

In addition, clonal cytogenetic abnormalities are identified in approximately 1/3 of patients with chronic myeloproliferative neoplasms; by gene mutation studies, a higher proportion of clonal abnormalities can be detected in patients with chronic myeloproliferative neoplasms (see Chapters 35-42).

16.7 Course and Treatment

The course and treatment of neutrophilia depend on the underlying disease process.

16.8 References

Bain BJ, Phillips D, Thomson K, et al. Investigation of the effect of marathon running on leucocyte counts of subjects of different ethnic origins: relevance to the aetiology of ethnic neutropenia. *Br J Haematol.* 2000;108:483-487.

Borregaard N, Sehested M, Nielsen BS, et al. Biosynthesis of granule proteins in normal human bone marrow cells: gelatinase is a marker of terminal neutrophil differentiation. *Blood.* 1995;85:812-817.

Buescher E. Neutrophil function and disorders of neutrophils in the newborn. In: de Alarcon P, Werner E, eds. *Neonatal Hematology.* Cambridge University Press; 2005:254-279.

Carballo C, Foucar K, Swanson P, et al. Effect of high altitude on neutrophil counts in newborn infants. *J Pediatr.* 1991;119:464-466.

Fernandes B, Hamaguchi Y. Automated enumeration of immature granulocytes. *Am J Clin Pathol.* 2007;128:454-463.

Foucar K. Neonatal hematopathology: special considerations. In: Collins R, Swerdlow S, eds. *Pediatric Hematopathology.* New York: Churchill Livingstone. 2001:173-184.

Foucar K. Normal anatomy and histology of bone marrow. In: King D, Gardner W, Sobin L, et al., eds. *Non-Neoplastic Disorders of Bone Marrow* (AFIP fascicle). Washington, DC: American Registry of Pathology; 2008:1-40.

Hamilton KS, Standaert SM, Kinney MC. Characteristic peripheral blood findings in human erlichiosis. *Mod Pathol.* 2004;17:512-517.

Helmus Y, Denecke J, Yakubenia S, et al. Leukocyte adhesion deficiency II patients with a dual defect of the GDP-fucose transporter. *Blood.* 2006;107:3959-3966.

Herring WB, Smith LG, Walker RI, et al. Hereditary neutrophilia. *Am J Med.* 1974;56:729-734.

Kimura N, Ogasawara T, Asonuma S, et al. Granulocyte-colony stimulating factor- and interleukin 6-producing diffuse deciduoid peritoneal mesothelioma. *Mod Pathol.* 2005;18:446-450.

Kinashi T, Aker M, Sokolovsky-Eisenberg M, et al. LAD-III, a leukocyte adhesion deficiency syndrome associated with defective Rap1 activation and impaired stabilization of integrin bonds. *Blood.* 2004;103:1033-1036.

Koster F, Foucar K, Hjelle B, et al. Rapid presumptive diagnosis of hantavirus cardiopulmonary syndrome by peripheral blood smear review. *Am J Clin Pathol.* 2001;116:665-672.

Meyerson HJ, Farhi DC, Rosenthal NS. Transient increase in blasts mimicking acute leukemia and progressing myelodysplasia in patients receiving growth factor. *Am J Clin Pathol.* 1998;109:675-681.

Moser B, Wolf M, Walz A, et al. Chemokines: multiple levels of leukocyte migration control. *Trends Immunol.* 2004;25:1471.

Tindall JP, Beeker SK, Rosse WF. Familial cold urticaria: a generalized reaction involving leukocytosis. *Arch Intern Med.* 1969;124:129-134.

Uzel G, Tng E, Rosenzweig SD, et al. Reversion mutations in patients with leukocyte adhesion deficiency type-1 (LAD-1). *Blood.* 2008;111:209-218.

Wickramasinghe S. Bone marrow. In: Mills S, ed. *Histology for Pathologists. 3rd ed.* Philadelphia: Lippincott Williams & Wilkins; 2007:799-836.

Wile MJ, Homer LD, Gaehler S, et al. Manual differential cell counts help predict bacterial infection: a multivariate analysis. *Am J Clin Pathol.* 2001;115:644-649.

Wilson C. Laboratory evaluation of blood and bone marrow in non-neoplastic disorders. In: King D, Gardner W, Sobin L, et al., eds. *Non-Neoplastic Disorders of Bone Marrow* (AFIP fascicle). Washington, DC: American Registry of Pathology; 2008:57-73.

Wilson C. Non-neoplastic granulocytic and monocytic disorders In: King D, Gardner W, Sobin L, et al., eds. *Non-Neoplastic Disorders of Bone Marrow* (AFIP fascicle). Washington, DC: American Registry of Pathology; 2008:125-175.

Wong RS, Wu A, To KF, et al. Haematological manifestations in patients with severe acute respiratory syndrome: retrospective analysis. *Br Med J.* 2003;326:1358-1362.

Chapter 17
Eosinophilia

Kathryn Foucar, MD

Eosinophils are normally present in the blood in low numbers, and there are no age-related variations in normal absolute eosinophil counts. Eosinophilia is defined as an absolute eosinophil count exceeding 0.6 × 10^3/mm^3 (0.6 × 10^9/L) i17.1. Cases of eosinophilia have been arbitrarily classified as mild (0.6-1.49 × 10^3/mm^3), moderate (1.5-5 × 10^3/mm^3), or severe (>5 × 10^3/mm^3) absolute eosinophilia. Sustained eosinophilia may be primary (the eosinophils are part of a clonal hematopoietic disorder) or secondary (eosinophils are non-neoplastic). Recent evidence suggests that production of cytokines (eg, interleukin [IL-1, IL-3, IL-5]) by activated T cells is responsible for many types of secondary eosinophilia. In an ambulatory setting eosinophilia is detected in fewer than 1% of adult and pediatric patients by screening complete blood counts (CBC), although a higher incidence would be expected in geographic

i17.1 Secondary eosinophilia

A moderate absolute eosinophilia in a patient with medication-associated secondary eosinophilia. *(Wright stain)*

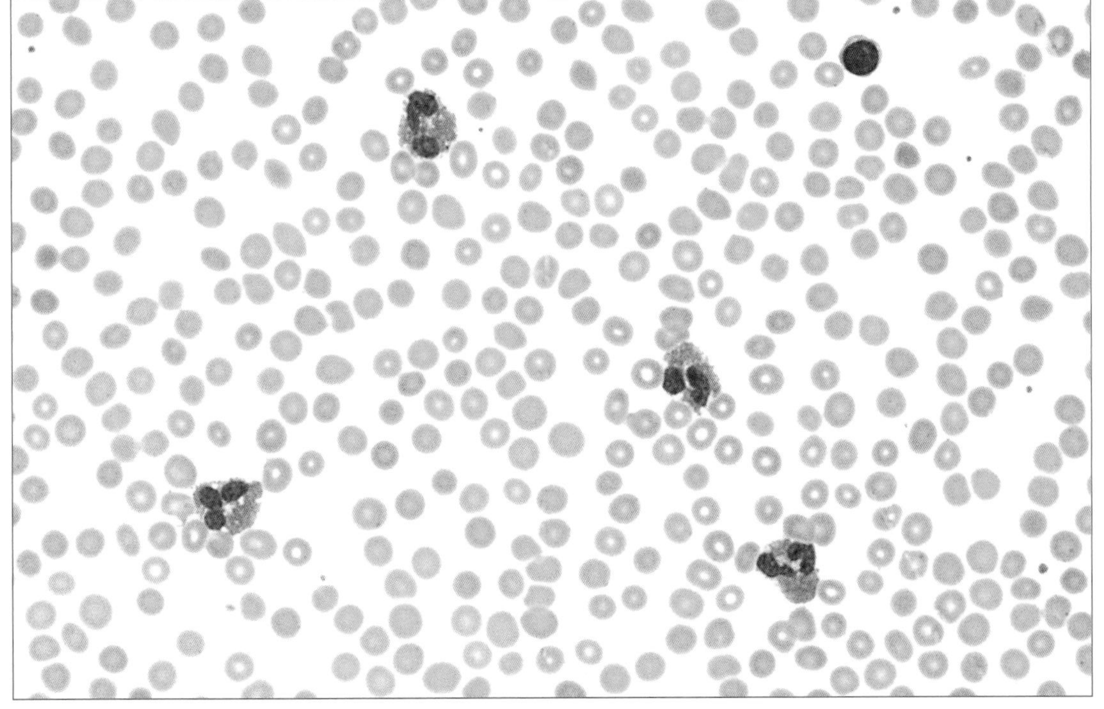

regions in which parasitic infections are common. Causes of reactive eosinophilia are summarized in **t17.1**; the most common causes are drug treatments, allergies, or parasitic infections. Parasites must invade tissues to produce eosinophilia. Worldwide, helminthic infections are the most common cause of eosinophilia, while allergic disorders are the most common cause in industrialized nations. More recently identified causes of reactive eosinophilia include therapy with pharmacologic doses of recombinant human interleukins, which are associated with a brisk, reactive eosinophilia. However, in most outpatients with a mild to moderate eosinophilia no inciting cause is identified.

t17.1 Causes of Reactive Eosinophilia*

Cause	Examples
Allergic/atopic disorders	Asthma, allergic rhinitis, atopic dermatitis, urticaria
Medications/vitamins/nutrient supplements	Many medications linked to secondary eosinophilia, recombinant interleukin, or other cytokine therapy, contaminant in L-tryptophan supplement (eosinophil-myalgia syndrome)
Parasitic infections	Helminthics (must invade tissue to produce eosinophilia)
Other infections	HIV-1, syphilis, rarely in other bacterial, protozoal, and fungal infections
Cutaneous disorders	Bullous pemphigoid, pemphigus, atopic dermatitis, eczema
Other inflammatory disorders	Celiac disease, vasculitides, inflammatory bowel disease, collagen vascular disease, sarcoidosis
Pulmonary disorders	Löffler syndrome, bronchiectasis, pneumonia, sarcoidosis, Churg-Strauss syndrome, cystic fibrosis
Neoplasms†	Occult clonal T-cell disorders, Hodgkin lymphoma, carcinomas, Langerhan cell histiocytosis, overt T-cell lymphomas/leukemias
Miscellaneous rarer causes of eosinophilia	Kimura disease, viral infections (HIV-1, HTLV-II), renal allograft rejections, dialysis

**In a substantial proportion of ambulatory patients the cause of the eosinophilia is not determined*
†Increased eosinophil production secondary to cytokines released by neoplastic cells; eosinophils are not neoplastic
HIV = human immunodeficiency virus; HTLV = human T-cell leukemia virus

Sustained eosinophilia is also linked to various hematolymphoid and non-hematolymphoid neoplasms. Increased blood eosinophils can be seen in various hematopoietic neoplasms, including myeloproliferative neoplasms and certain acute leukemias **t17.2**. In patients with these clonal myeloid conditions, the eosinophils are part of the neoplastic clone and often exhibit prominent morphologic abnormalities. In other patients, abnormal T-cell clones, sometimes clinically occult, may drive a secondary eosinophilia. In these cases molecular testing on blood and other tissues may be required to detect the clonal T cell population.

t17.2 Hematopoietic Neoplasms Demonstrating Clonal Mature Blood Eosinophilia

Myeloproliferative neoplasms

Chronic myelogenous leukemia
Chronic eosinophilic leukemia, NOS
Systemic mastocytosis*
Myeloid and lymphoid neoplasms with eosinophilia and abnormalities of *PDGFRA*, *PDGFRB*, or *FGFR1*

Acute leukemias

Acute myelomonocytic leukemia with eosinophilia (variable blood eosinophilia)
Other acute myeloid leukemias
B-lymphoblastic leukemia with eosinophilia and t(5;14)(q31;q32)*

**Evidence regarding whether the eosinophils are part of a neoplastic clone is controversial. Eosinophils may be reactive, non-clonal. PDGFRA = platelet-derived growth factor receptor alpha; PDGFRB = platelet-derived growth factor receptor beta; FGFR1 = fibroblast growth factor receptor 1.*
Reference: WHO Classification of Tumours of Haematopoietic and Lymphoid Tissues, 2008

17.1 Pathophysiology

Although eosinophils are derived from the same progenitor cells that give rise to other granulocytic elements within the bone marrow, eosinophil production is influenced by the synergistic action of IL-2, IL-3, IL-5, IL-9, and IL-13 produced in the bone marrow microenvironment. Like other regulatory factors, these interleukins (most notably, IL-5) not only stimulate production of eosinophils but also enhance functional activity of mature eosinophils. Although the distinctive granule used to identify the eosinophil is a secondary granule, the stages of eosinophil maturation are presumed to parallel other granulocytic cells and include myeloblasts, promyelocytes, eosinophilic myelocytes, eosinophilic metamyelocytes, and mature eosinophils. These mature eosinophils characteristically have bilobed nuclei and contain abundant large, refractile eosinophilic granules i17.2.

Eosinophils are present in low numbers in the peripheral blood, and normal eosinophil function is dependent on migration to solid tissue; eosinophil recruitment into tissue is mediated by chemokines such as eotaxin. Eosinophils demonstrate two main functions: (1) modulation of immediate hypersensitivity reactions and (2) destruction of parasites. Release of eosinophil secondary granules plays a key role in both of these functions. These secondary granules contain major basic protein, peroxidase, arylsulfatase, histamine oxidase, and eosinophil cationic protein. In addition, the surface membranes of eosinophils express Fc receptors for IgE, IgG, and certain complement components. Eosinophils also produce factors such as stem cell factor or c-kit ligand which influence mast cell activity.

i17.2 Secondary eosinophilia

Cytologically normal eosinophils with bilobed nuclei and prominent refractile granules are evident in this patient with medication-associated secondary eosinophilia. *(Wright stain)*

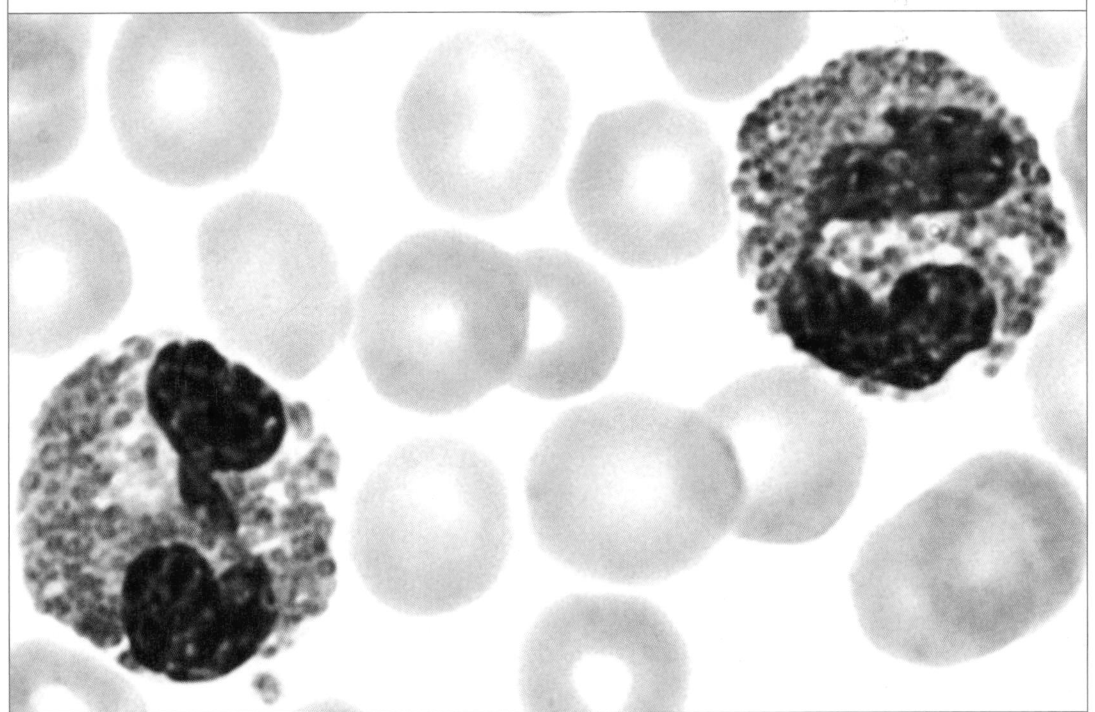

17.2 Clinical Findings

The cause of eosinophilia may be either clinically obvious or obscure. In outpatient settings the cause of isolated mild eosinophilia often is not determined. For patients with sustained eosinophilia, the clinical features of the diverse disorders that cause eosinophilia must be considered, along with the fact that the eosinophilia itself can produce distinctive clinical manifestations. A sustained peripheral blood eosinophilia can result in endothelial and endomyocardial damage from intravascular degranulation of these cells. The potent cytolytic enzymes contained within eosinophil secondary granules damage endothelial cells throughout the body. As a consequence, either thrombosis or endomyocardial fibrosis may result. Although both neoplastic and reactive eosinophils can be associated with this type of tissue damage, it is far more common in patients with neoplastic eosinophilic disorders such as chronic eosinophilic leukemia or other myeloproliferative neoplasms with a prominent eosinophilic component, including systemic mastocytosis. Patients with these myeloproliferative neoplasms may also exhibit organomegaly, pulmonary infiltrates, and central nervous system disease, in addition to the more common thrombotic and cardiac disorders.

Eosinophilia-myalgia syndrome causes peripheral blood eosinophilia, linked to L-tryptophan ingestion. Affected patients were usually women who presented with severe myalgia and arthralgia, fatigue, peripheral blood eosinophilia, and, less frequently, respiratory disorders, skin changes, and neuropathy. Following an isolated outbreak of cases, eosinophilia-myalgia syndrome was linked to L-tryptophan produced by a single Japanese manufacturer and was thought to have been caused by a toxic contaminant introduced in the manufacturing process.

Recent cloning studies have identified a unique fusion gene resulting from t(1;5)(q23;q33) involving platelet-derived growth factor receptor beta and a novel partner gene, myomegalin, in myeloproliferative neoplasms with eosinophilia. Similarly, other authors describe chronic eosinophilic myeloproliferative neoplasms resulting from fusion genes involving platelet-derived growth factor receptor alpha. The eosinophils in these cases are part of the neoplastic clone, and dramatic responses to imatinib therapy have been described.

17.3 Diagnostic Approach

In any patient with a sustained eosinophilia, it is important to distinguish a reactive (secondary) process from a hematopoietic neoplasm with an eosinophilic component. Once an eosinophilia is confirmed as reactive, an attempt should be made to determine the underlying cause, especially if the absolute eosinophilia is substantial and sustained.

The following approach to diagnosis should be considered:

1. Perform a clinical evaluation and assess the patient's history of drug treatments.
2. Evaluate for possible parasitic infection, including any history of travel to foreign countries.
3. Perform appropriate laboratory tests for possible parasitic infection if clinically warranted.
4. Perform a physical examination for evidence of organomegaly or pulmonary infiltrates.
5. A chest radiograph or lung biopsy may be warranted in patients with possible pulmonary infiltrates.
6. Evaluate the patient for neoplasms associated with secondary eosinophilia as a consequence of cytokine production by the tumor, including occult T-cell clones in blood or other tissues.
7. Assess for a possible myeloproliferative neoplasm, systemic mastocytosis, or other clonal disorder with primary eosinophilia.

17.4 Hematologic Findings

17.4.1 Blood Cell Measurements

Eosinophilia is present when the absolute eosinophil count exceeds $0.6 \times 10^3/mm^3$ ($0.6 \times 10^9/L$). Eosinophils have a diurnal variation, highest in the morning and decreasing in the afternoon.

17.4.2 Blood Morphology

In blood smears demonstrating a significant absolute eosinophilia, it is appropriate to assess all other lineages for evidence of morphologic abnormalities. In addition, it is important to scan the feather edge and the thick regions of the smear for possible parasites i17.3, i17.4. Circulating peosinophil morphology is of little help in distinguishing reactive from clonal eosinophil disorders, because eosinophil dysplasia such as hypogranularity and nuclear segmentation defects can be seen in both clonal and non-clonal populations. In particular, hypodense eosinophil morphology has been linked to sustained interleukin production, a mediator of secondary eosinophilia. In general, the combination of severe eosinophil dyspoiesis plus abnormalities or dysplasia in other lineages favors a neoplastic process that should be confirmed by cytogenetic/molecular studies i17.5, i17.6. Hypersegmented (trilobed), hypogranular, degranulated, or vacuolated eosinophils are especially prominent in myeloproliferative neoplasms formerly termed "idiopathic hypereosinophilic syndromes," a clinical designation that is no longer recommended if clonality of the disorder can be established.

17.4.3 Bone Marrow Examination

Bone marrow examination generally is not required in patients with straightforward reactive (secondary) eosinophilia unless indicated for other reasons such as tumor staging. However, both bone marrow examination and cytogenetic studies are valuable in patients with a possible myeloid neoplasm in which the eosinophils are likely to be part of a clonal process.

17.5 Ancillary Tests

1. In an ambulatory setting the detection of an isolated mild eosinophilia is generally not associated with a serious illness; consequently an extensive medical workup may not be necessary in otherwise healthy patients without distinctive clinical abnormalities or additional CBC abnormalities.
2. If a parasitic infection is suspected, both stool examination for ova and parasites and serologic tests for parasites may be warranted.
3. Molecular studies for T-cell receptor gene rearrangement may provide useful information in patients with possible occult T-cell neoplasms.
4. Fluorescence in situ hybridization (FISH), cytogenetic, or molecular analyses may be useful in both establishing the diagnosis of a clonal hematopoietic disorder.
5. Measurement of serum IL-5 levels may be useful in selected patients with presumed secondary eosinophilia.
6. Although non-specific, the determination of serum IgE levels may be useful in selected situations; elevated levels support allergy.

i17.3 Parasitic eosinophilia

A marked peripheral blood eosinophilia is evident in a patient who had recently emigrated from Africa. *(Wright stain)*

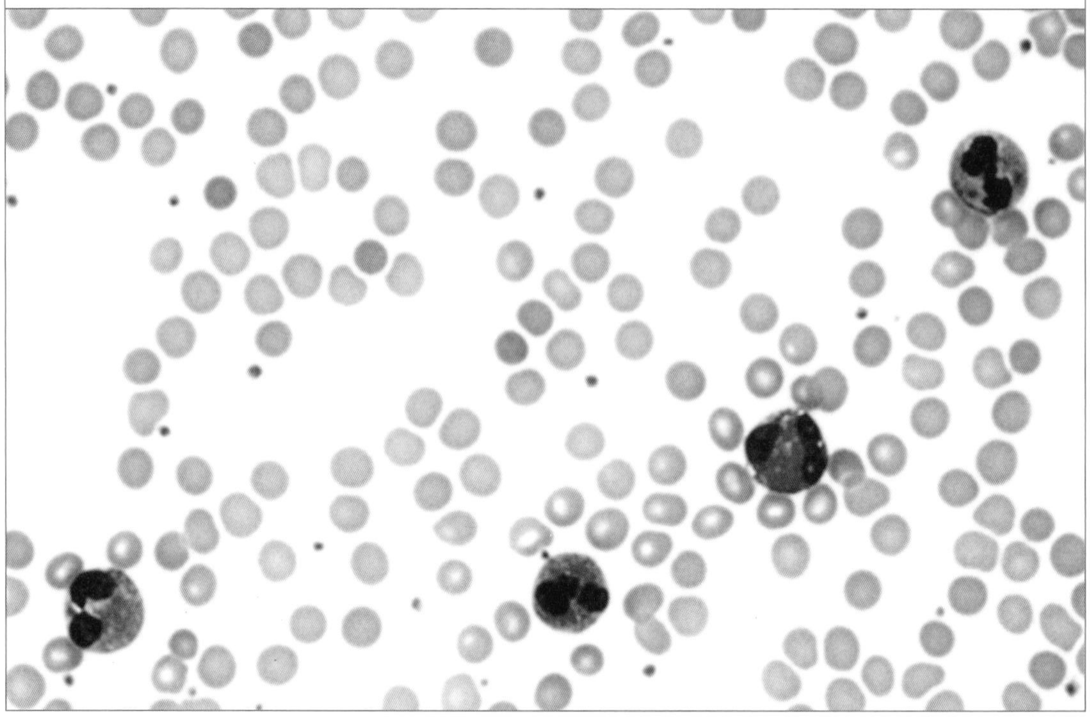

i17.4 Parasitic eosinophilia

Loa loa parasites were evident in the feather edge in this patient with marked eosinophilia (see i17.3). *(Wright stain)*

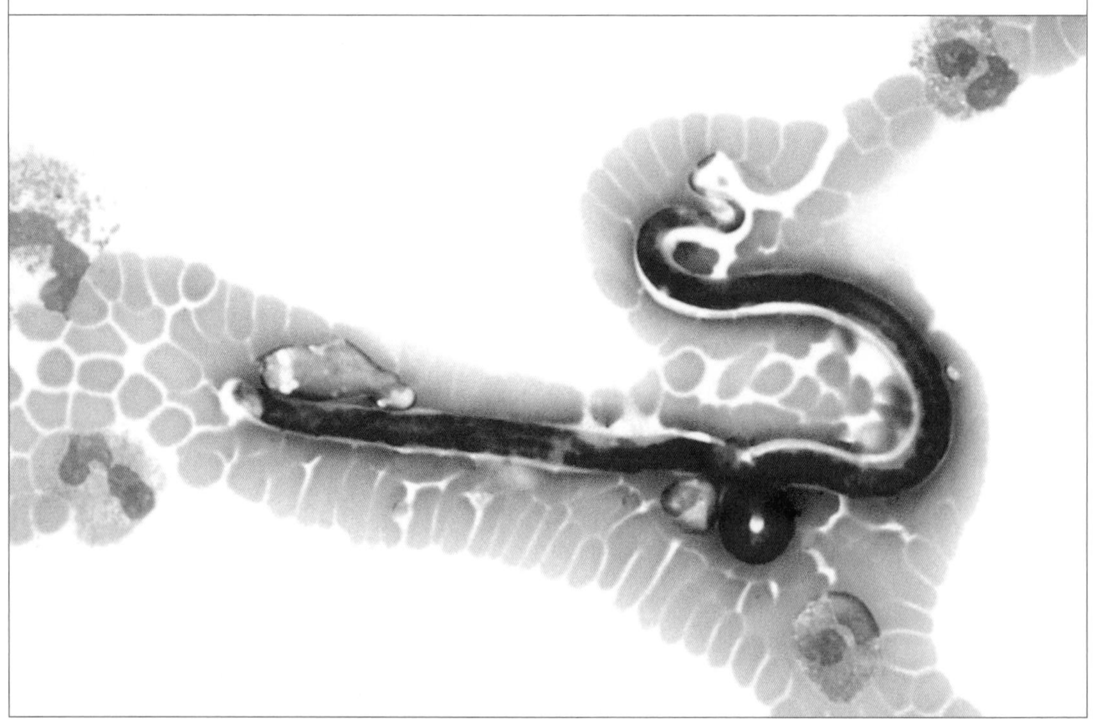

i17.5 Chronic eosinophilic leukemia

Peripheral blood smear from a patient with chronic eosinophilic leukemia. A striking eosinophilia with dysplastic changes is noted. *(Wright stain)*

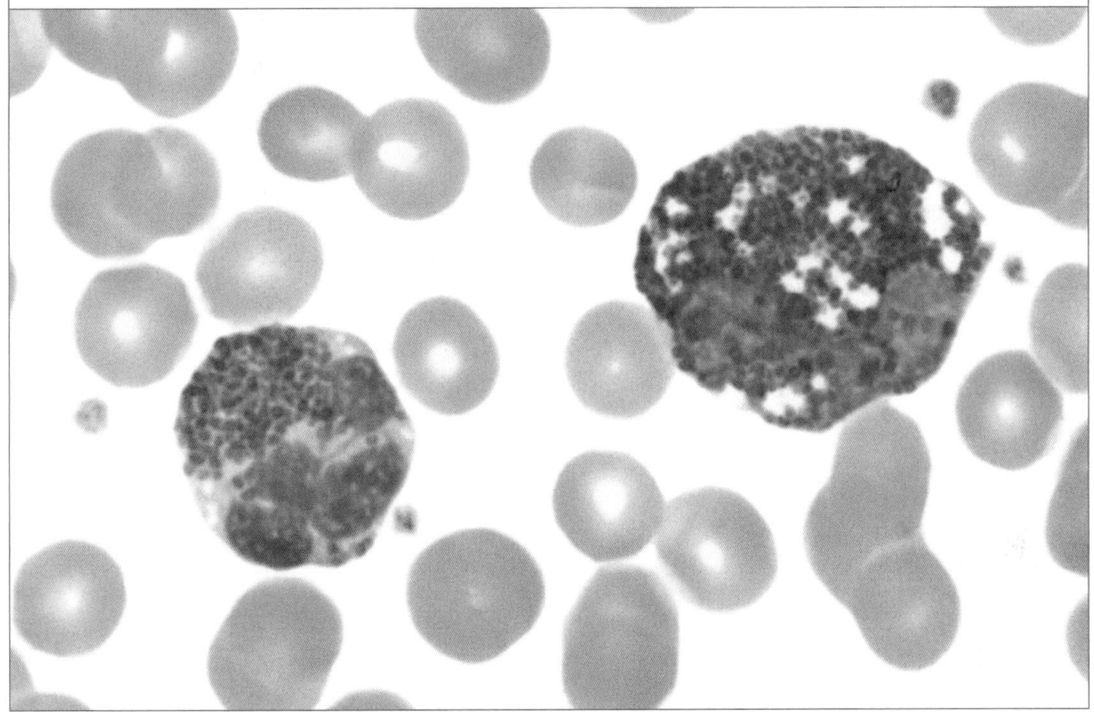

i17.6 B-lymphoblastic leukemia with t(5;14)

Markedly hypogranular eosinophils are evident in the peripheral blood of this patient with B-lymphoblastic leukemia and t(5;14) with associated eosinophilia. *(Wright stain)*

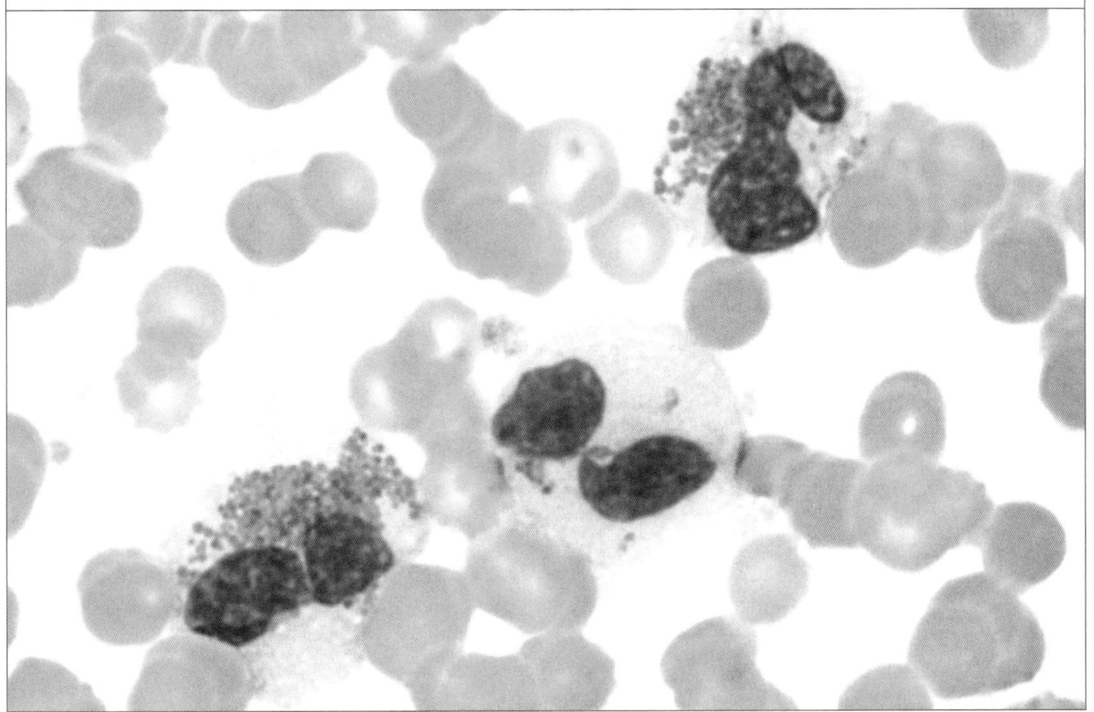

7. Nasal smears or sputum cytology for eosinophils may be useful in selected patients. Nasal eosinophilia is common in allergic rhinitis, and abundant eosinophils in sputum may be evident in patients with Löffler pneumonia. Charcot-Leyden crystals may be present.
8. A chest radiograph is useful to evaluate for either Löffler pneumonia or sarcoidosis.
9. Serologic tests for collagen vascular disorders may be helpful in selected patients.
10. Measurement of serum tryptase may be a sensitive marker of systemic mastocytosis-associated eosinophilia, some of which are imatinib responsive.

17.6 Course and Treatment

Treatment of reactive eosinophilia depends on the underlying cause. A primary eosinophilic disorder often requires therapy to arrest the progressive endothelial cell damage with associated subendocardial fibrosis that results from sustained intravascular eosinophil degranulation.

17.7 References

Bain B, Gilliland D, Horney H-P, Vardiman J. Myeloid and lymphoid neoplasms with eosinophilia and abnormalities of PDGFRA, PDGFRB, or FGFR1. In: Swerdlow S, Campo E, Harris N, et al., eds. *WHO Classification of Tumours of Haematopoietic and Lymphoid Tissues. 4th ed.* Lyon, France: IARC Press; 2008:68-73.

Bain B, Gilliland D, Vardiman J, Horney H-P. Chronic eosinophilic leukaemia, not otherwise specified. In: Swerdlow S, Campo E, Harris N, et al., eds. *WHO Classification of Tumours of Haematopoietic and Lymphoid Tissues. 4th ed.* Lyon, France: IARC Press; 2008:51-53.

Bain BJ. Hypereosinophilia. *Curr Opin Hematol.* 2000;7:21-25.

Brigden M, Graydon C. Eosinophilia detected by automated blood cell counting in ambulatory North American outpatients: incidence and clinical significance. *Arch Pathol Lab Med.* 1997;121:963-967.

Brito-Babapulle F. The eosinophilias, including the idiopathic hypereosinophilic syndrome. *Br J Haematol.* 2003;121:203-223.

Butterfield JH. Diverse clinical outcomes of eosinophilic patients with T-cell receptor gene rearrangements: the emerging diagnostic importance of molecular genetics testing. *Am J Hematol.* 2001;68:81-86.

Cilloni D, Messa F, Martinelli G, et al. WT1 transcript amount discriminates secondary or reactive eosinophilia from idiopathic hypereosinophilic syndrome or chronic eosinophilic leukemia. *Leukemia.* 2007;21:1442-1450.

Cools J, DeAngelo DJ, Gotlib J, et al. A tyrosine kinase created by fusion of the PDGFRA and FIP1L1 genes as a therapeutic target of imatinib in idiopathic hypereosinophilic syndrome. *N Engl J Med.* 2003;348:1201-1214.

Gounni AS, Gregory B, Nutku E, et al. Interleukin-9 enhances interleukin-5 receptor expression, differentiation, and survival of human eosinophils. *Blood.* 2000;96:2163-2171.

Hartman M, Piliponsky AM, Temkin V, et al. Human peripheral blood eosinophils express stem cell factor. *Blood.* 2001;97:1086-1091.

Kamb ML, Murphy JJ, Jones JL, et al. Eosinophilia-myalgia syndrome in L-tryptophan-exposed patients. *JAMA.* 1992;267:77-82.

Klion AD, Noel P, Akin C, et al. Elevated serum tryptase levels identify a subset of patients with a myeloproliferative variant of idiopathic hypereosinophilic syndrome associated with tissue fibrosis, poor prognosis, and imatinib responsiveness. *Blood.* 2003;101:4660-4666.

Klion AD, Law MA, Riemenschneider W, et al. Familial eosinophilia: a benign disorder? *Blood.* 2004;103:4050-4055.

Matsuyama W, Mitsuyama H, Ono M, et al. Discoidin domain receptor 1 contributes to eosinophil survival in an NF-kappaB-dependent manner in Churg-Strauss syndrome. *Blood.* 2007;109:22-30.

Moosbauer C, Morgenstern E, Cuvelier SL, et al. Eosinophils are a major intravascular location for tissue factor storage and exposure. *Blood.* 2007;109:995-1002.

Palframan RT, Collins PD, Williams TJ, et al. Eotaxin induces a rapid release of eosinophils and their progenitors from the bone marrow. *Blood.* 1998;91:2240-2248.

Pandit R, Scholnik A, Wulfekuhler L, Dimitrov N. Non-small-cell lung cancer associated with excessive eosinophilia and secretion of interleukin-5 as a paraneoplastic syndrome. *Am J Hematol.* 2007;82:234-237.

Pardanani A, Ketterling RP, Brockman SR, et al. CHIC2 deletion, a surrogate for FIP1L1-PDGFRA fusion, occurs in systemic mastocytosis associated with eosinophilia and predicts response to imatinib mesylate therapy. *Blood.* 2003;102:3093-3096.

Peters MS, Rodriguez M, Gleich GJ. Localization of human eosinophil granule major basic protein, eosinophil cationic protein, and eosinophil-derived neurotoxin by immunoelectron microscopy. *Lab Invest.* 1986;54:656-662.

Rothenberg ME, Owen WF Jr, Silberstein DS, et al. Human eosinophils have prolonged survival, enhanced functional properties, and become hypodense when exposed to human interleukin 3. *J Clin Invest.* 1988;81:1986-1992.

Roufosse F, Schandene L, Sibille C, et al. Clonal Th2 lymphocytes in patients with the idiopathic hypereosinophilic syndrome. *Br J Haematol.* 2000;109:540-548.

Ryan ET, Felsenstein D, Aquino SL, et al. Case records of the Massachusetts General Hospital. Case 39-2005. A 63-year-old woman with a positive serologic test for syphilis and persistent eosinophilia. *N Engl J Med.* 2005;353:2697-2705.

Sasano H, Virmani R, Patterson RH, et al. Eosinophilic products lead to myocardial damage. *Hum Pathol.* 1989;20:850-857.

Sidransky H. Eosinophilia-myalgia syndrome: a recent syndrome serving as an alert to new diseases ahead. *Mod Pathol.* 1994;7:806-810.

Simon HU, Plotz SG, Dummer R, et al. Abnormal clones of T cells producing interleukin-5 in idiopathic eosinophilia. *N Engl J Med.* 1999;341:1112-1120.

Tefferi A, Patnaik MM, Pardanani A. Eosinophilia: secondary, clonal and idiopathic. *Br J Haematol.* 2006;133:468-492.

Wilkinson K, Velloso ER, Lopes LF, et al. Cloning of the t(1;5)(q23;q33) in a myeloproliferative disorder associated with eosinophilia: involvement of PDGFRB and response to imatinib. *Blood.* 2003;102:4187-4190.

Wilson C. Non-neoplastic granulocytic and monocytic disorders In: King D, Gardner W, Sobin L, et al., eds. *Non-Neoplastic Disorders of Bone Marrow* (AFIP fascicle). Washington, DC: American Registry of Pathology; 2008:125-175.

Chapter 18
Basophilia

Kathryn Foucar, MD

Basophils are normally the least numerous granulated cells within the peripheral blood. These cells generally account for less than 1% of WBCs, and the absolute basophil count is characteristically less than $0.1 \times 10^3/mm^3$ ($0.1 \times 10^9/L$). There are no established age-related variations in absolute basophil count.

Basophilia is defined as an absolute basophil count that exceeds $0.2 \times 10^3/mm^3$ ($0.2 \times 10^9/L$). Reactive basophilia is an uncommon blood finding with an absolute basophil count that is only moderately increased. Conditions occasionally associated with reactive basophilia include allergic disorders and hypersensitivity reactions, inflammatory disorders such as ulcerative colitis and rheumatoid arthritis, chronic renal disease, and infections including influenza, chicken pox, and smallpox **t18.1**. The absolute basophil count also may be modestly increased following radiation exposure.

t18.1 Causes of Reactive Basophilia*

Cause	Example
Allergic/hypersensitivity reactions	Urticaria; allergies to food, medications (eg, estrogen, antithyroid agents), supplement allergies; erythroderma
Inflammatory disorders	Collagen vascular disease, rheumatoid arthritis, ulcerative colitis
Endocrinopathy	Diabetes; hypothyroidism estrogen administration
Renal disease	Chronic disorders
Infections	Influenza, chicken pox, smallpox, tuberculosis
Irradiation	Exposures
Carcinomas	Rare in lung carcinomas

**Degree of absolute basophilia typically modest*

In contrast, neoplastic disorders with a substantial mature basophilic component are encountered much more frequently in clinical practice than are reactive basophilias. The absolute basophil count is substantially higher in patients with these neoplastic conditions. Chronic myeloproliferative neoplasms, especially chronic myelogenous leukemia (CML), are the most common malignancies in which an absolute basophilia is present (see Chapters 35-42). Even though the percentage of basophils is generally less than 10% of the WBCs in patients with CML, because of the marked leukocytosis, the absolute basophil count is strikingly elevated. A rising absolute basophil count can precede overt blast phase in some CML patients. Basophilia is a consistent feature in the blood of patients with CML, whereas only about one third of patients with other myeloproliferative neoplasms demonstrate this characteristic. Various acute leukemias also can exhibit a basophilic component, but these cells are generally very immature, requiring special studies for their identification. Rarely, a more mature basophilia is noted in acute myeloid leukemias.

18.1 Pathophysiology

Although the mechanisms responsible for basophil production have not been completely delineated, regulatory factors currently thought to play a role in this process include interleukin (IL)-3, granulocyte-monocyte colony-stimulating factor (GM-CSF), and IL-5. Recent studies indicate that IL-3 is the main growth and differentiation factor for basophils. Even though the earliest stages of maturation are not distinguishable from other myeloid lineages, the proposed stages of basophil maturation include myeloblast, promyelocyte, basophilic myelocyte, basophilic metamyelocyte, and mature basophil. Basophils are recognized in the peripheral blood and bone marrow by their distinctive secondary granule, which is large, deeply basophilic, and often obscures the segmented nucleus. These secondary granules contain numerous proteins that are essential for basophil function, including heparin, histamine, eosinophil chemotactic factor, arylsulfatase A, and slow-reacting substance of anaphylaxis, as well as many other substances. By flow cytometric immunophenotyping, basophils express CD9, CD13, CD25 (dim), CD33, CD36, moderate CD45, and bright CD123.

Basophils may be closely related to tissue mast cells, although there are differences in maturation characteristics between these two cell types. However, despite the differences in immunophenotype and morphology between basophils and mast cells, the granule contents of these two cells are remarkably similar. Likewise, both basophils and mast cells function in immediate hypersensitivity reactions via granule release. Basophil degranulation occurs in response to the binding of IgE antibodies to Fc receptors on the cell membrane. Following allergen challenge, basophils are recruited rapidly from blood to tissue. Both the recruitment and the enhanced functional activity of these tissue basophils are mediated by IL-3, Il-5, and GM-CSF. In addition to basophil function by degranulation, other cytokine-mediated immune functions of basophils have been proposed, including IL-4 mediated induction of T helper 2 (Th 2) response.

18.2 Clinical Findings

The clinical findings in patients with reactive basophilia vary, reflecting the spectrum of disorders associated with this blood abnormality. Some patients with allergic and hypersensitivity reactions may have urticaria, whereas patients with collagen vascular disorders, endocrinopathy, or renal disease exhibit diverse symptomatology and clinical findings.

The clinical features of patients with neoplastic mature basophilia are more distinctive. As described earlier, a striking mature basophilia is typical of CML, and affected patients frequently have marked splenomegaly at presentation. These patients also may complain of malaise, fatigue, and left upper quadrant pain. Hepatomegaly is variable but present in a substantial number of CML patients (see Chapter 35).

18.3 Diagnostic Approach

Reactive basophilias must be distinguished from myeloproliferative neoplasms with a mature basophilic component. Various clinical and hematologic parameters are useful in making this distinction.

The following approach to diagnosis should be considered:

1. Perform a complete blood count with differential.
2. Determine the absolute basophil count and assess the morphology of basophils.
3. Be aware that basophils frequently degranulate on blood smears, making their identification challenging in manual differential cell counts.
4. Evaluate other lineages for evidence of a myeloproliferative neoplasm. For example, in patients with CML, a marked leukocytosis with left shift to myeloblasts is characteristic. In addition to an absolute basophilia, eosinophilia is also common. Likewise, most CML patients demonstrate a marked, atypical thrombocytosis.
5. Correlate findings with clinical features and assess for splenomegaly.
6. Evaluate the chemical indicators of increased cell turnover, such as uric acid.

18.4 Hematologic Findings

18.4.1 Blood Cell Measurements

Basophils are noteworthy when the absolute basophil count exceeds $0.2 \times 10^3/mm^3$ ($0.2 \times 10^9/L$). Most reactive basophilias are characterized by a modest increase in basophils, whereas in neoplastic disorders the absolute basophil count is often strikingly increased i18.1. Except for anemia (usually anemia of chronic disease), other peripheral blood abnormalities are not generally present in patients with reactive basophilia.

i18.1 Basophilia

Circulating basophils are the least numerous myeloid cell in blood. Note dark granules. *(Wright stain)*

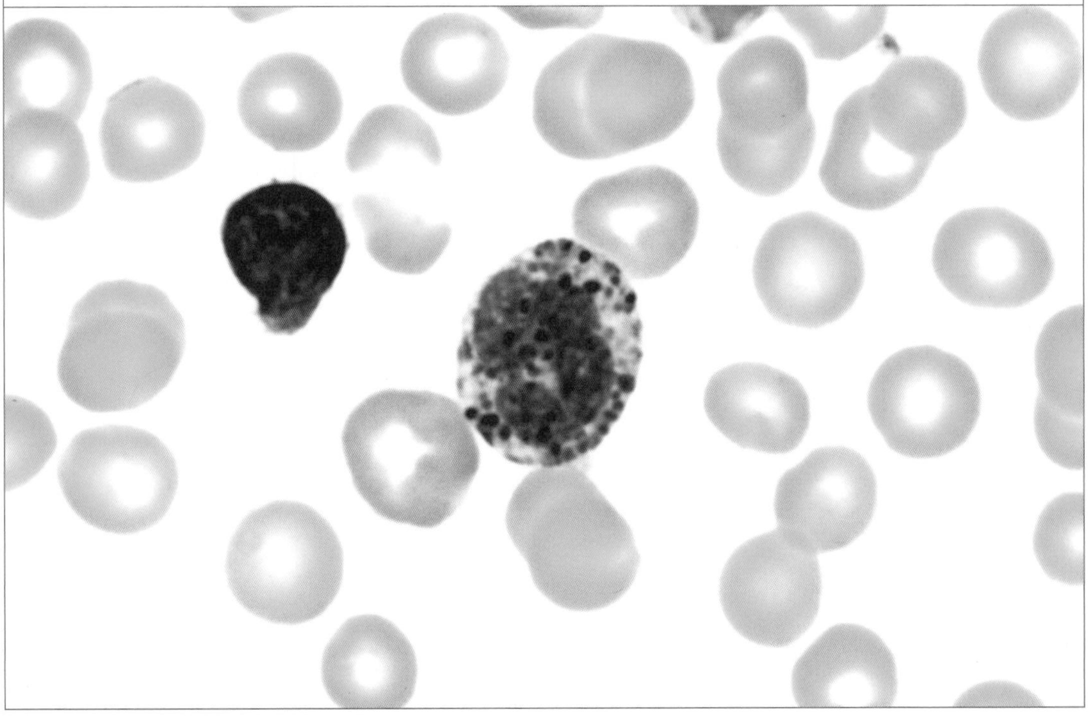

i18.2 Degranulated basophil

Basophil granules may be "washed out" during specimen transport and processing. *(Wright stain)*

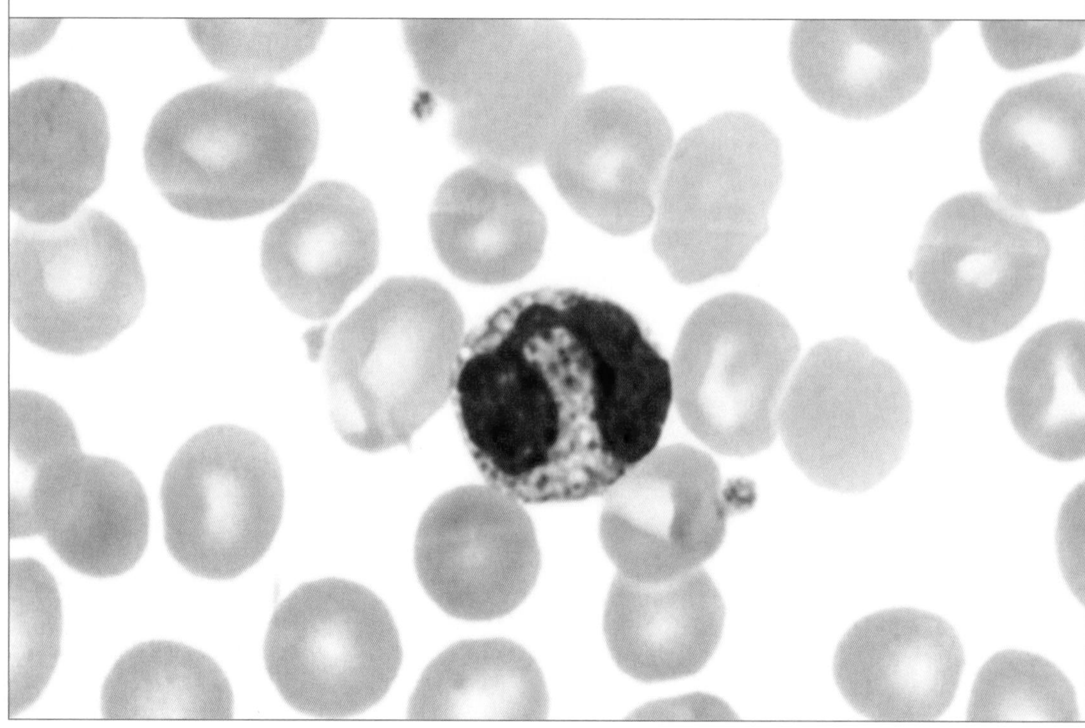

18.4.2 Blood Morphology

Basophils are morphologically unremarkable in reactive basophilia, although there may be some degranulation i18.2. In contrast, various morphologic abnormalities, including variable degranulation of basophils, may be present in the blood of patients with myeloproliferative neoplasms i18.3 (see Chapters 35-42). Although these basophils often appear normal by morphology, multiple aberrancies have been detected by flow cytometric immunophenotyping.

18.4.3 Bone Marrow Examination

Bone marrow examination generally is not required in the evaluation of patients with a reactive basophilia. In contrast, bone marrow examination with cytogenetic studies is often essential in establishing the diagnosis of various myeloproliferative neoplasms i18.3.

18.5 Course and Treatment

In patients with reactive (secondary) basophilia, both the clinical course and appropriate therapy are determined by the underlying disorder. In general, the increase in basophils within the peripheral blood is not associated with any specific disease manifestations. The treatment of myeloproliferative neoplasms such as CML is usually directed toward disease eradication (see Chapter 39).

i18.3 Chronic myelogenous leukemia

A marked absolute basophilia is evident in this blood smear from a patient with CML. Although these basophils are morphologically normal in appearance, they are part of the neoplastic clone. *(Wright stain)*

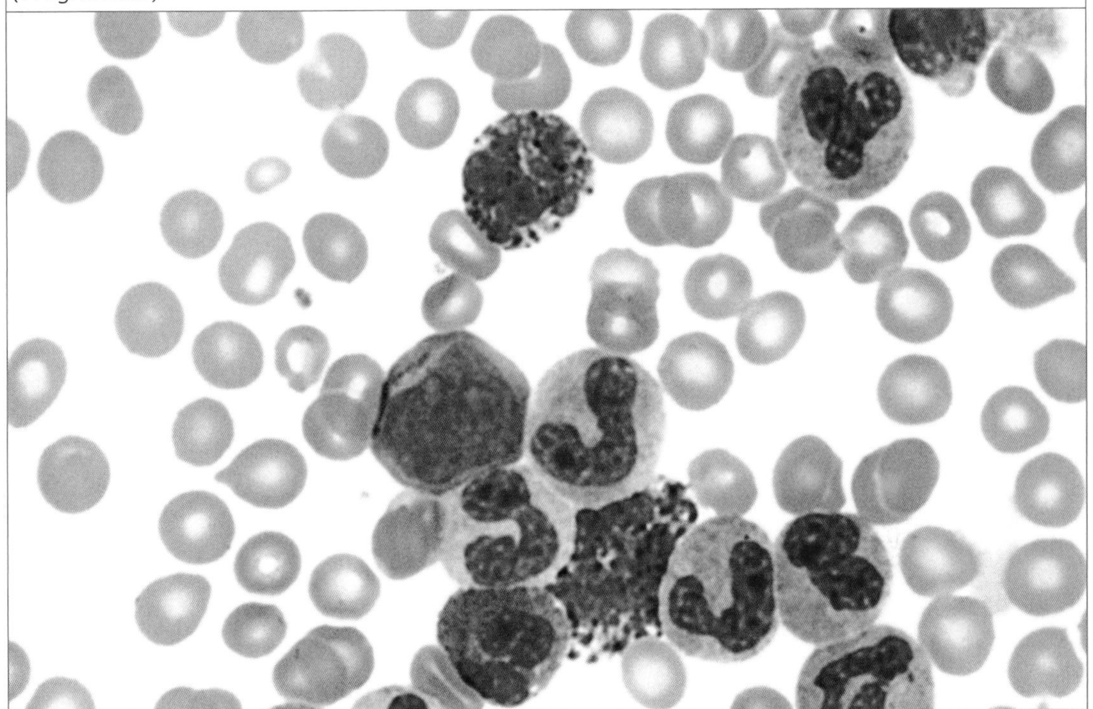

18.6 References

Arock M, Schneider E, Boissan M, et al. Differentiation of human basophils: an overview of recent advances and pending questions. *J Leukoc Biol.* 2002;71:557-564.

Costa JJ, Weller PF, Galli SJ. The cells of the allergic response: mast cells, basophils, and eosinophils. *JAMA.* 1997;278:1815-1822.

Grattan CE, Dawn G, Gibbs S, Francis DM. Blood basophil numbers in chronic ordinary urticaria and healthy controls: diurnal variation, influence of loratadine and prednisolone and relationship to disease activity. *Clin Exp Allergy* .2003;33:337-341.

Han X, Jorgensen JL, Brahmandam A, et al. Immunophenotypic study of basophils by multiparameter flow cytometry. *Arch Pathol Lab Med.* 2008;132:813-819.

Mitre E, Nutman TB. Basophils, basophilia and helminth infections. *Chem Immunol Allergy.* 2006;90:141-156.

Obata K, Mukai K, Tsujimura Y, et al. Basophils are essential initiators of a novel type of chronic allergic inflammation. *Blood.* 2007;110:913-920.

Takao K, Tanimoto Y, Fujii M, et al. In vitro expansion of human basophils by interleukin-3 from granulocyte colony-stimulating factor-mobilized peripheral blood stem cells. *Clin Exp Allergy.* 2003;33:1561-1567.

Uston PI, Lee CM. Characterization and function of the multifaceted peripheral blood basophil. *Cell Mol Biol.* (Noisy-le-grand) 2003;49:1125-1135.

Wilson C. Laboratory evaluation of blood and bone marrow in non-neoplastic disorders. In: King D, Gardner W, Sobin L, et al., eds. *Non-Neoplastic Disorders of Bone Marrow* (AFIP fascicle). Washington, DC: American Registry of Pathology; 2008:57-73.

Wilson C. Non-neoplastic granulocytic and monocytic disorders In: King D, Gardner W, Sobin L, et al., eds. *Non-Neoplastic Disorders of Bone Marrow* (AFIP fascicle). Washington, DC: American Registry of Pathology; 2008:125-175.

Chapter 19

Monocytosis

Kathryn Foucar, MD

Although generally present in low numbers, monocytes and related cell types are ubiquitous of all organ systems in the body. Monocytes generally comprise only 2%-9% of WBCs, with an absolute count of 0.1-0.9 × $10^3/mm^3$ (0.1-0.9 × $10^9/L$). Higher numbers of monocytes are identified within the blood of normal neonates and young infants. However, beyond infancy there are no striking age-related variations in normal absolute monocyte count.

Monocytosis is defined as an absolute monocyte count that exceeds 1.0 × $10^3/mm^3$ (1.0 × $10^9/L$) in adults and 1.2 × $10^3/mm^3$ (1.2 × $10^9/L$) in neonates. Both neoplastic and non-neoplastic disorders are associated with absolute monocytosis **t19.1**, **t19.2**. The most common cause of reactive monocytosis is a chronic infection secondary to many agents, including tuberculosis, *Listeria*, syphilis, subacute bacterial endocarditis, and certain protozoal and rickettsial infections. In general, a chronic infection is more likely than an acute infection to elicit monocytosis. In rare cases, either chronic Epstein-Barr or cytomegalovirus infection in children results in sustained monocytosis and neutrophilia. Other causes of reactive monocytosis include non-hematopoietic neoplasms such as Hodgkin lymphoma and occasional non-Hodgkin lymphomas. Often recovery from agranulocytosis is preceded by transient monocytosis; this is common in patients with cyclic neutropenia. Various immune-mediated disorders also are associated with mature reactive monocytosis, including collagen vascular diseases and gastrointestinal disorders such as ulcerative colitis and regional enteritis. Other less common causes of reactive monocytosis include hemolytic anemia, chronic neutropenia, and post-splenectomy states. Monocytes in post-traumatic conditions may exhibit aberrant phenotypic and cytochemical properties.

t19.1 Causes of Reactive Monocytosis

Cause	Examples
Infection	Chronic fungal, bacterial, protozoal, rickettsial, and viral infections
Other inflammatory conditions	Sarcoidosis, collagen vascular disorders, inflammatory bowel disease, sprue
Neoplasms	Hodgkin lymphoma, non-Hodgkin lymphomas, cytokine-producing carcinomas, multiple myeloma
Chronic neutropenia	Constitutional neutropenic disorders, during recovery phase from agranulocytosis (both acquired and cyclic neutropenia)
Miscellaneous	Post splenectomy, hemolytic anemia, immune thrombocytopenic purpura, acute stress, cytokine therapy

t19.2 Disorders With Circulating Neoplastic Monocytes

Myelodysplastic/myeloproliferative neoplasms, especially chronic myelomonocytic leukemia
Acute myelomonocytic leukemia
Acute monocytic leukemia
Chronic myelogenous leukemia
Other myeloproliferative neoplasms and myelodysplastic syndromes
Various pediatric myelodysplastic/myeloproliferative neoplasms that are linked to constitutional or acquired monosomy 7

Patients with primary hematopoietic neoplasms can also exhibit a peripheral blood monocytosis, but in these disorders the monocytes are part of the neoplastic clone (see **t19.2**). For example, monocytosis is a defining feature of myelodysplastic/myeloproliferative neoplasms such as chronic myelomonocytic leukemia. In addition, both acute myelomonocytic and acute monocytic leukemias demonstrate a dominant monocytic component. However, in these acute leukemias, the monocytes demonstrate marked immaturity, whereas more mature circulating monocytes are evident in chronic myelomonocytic leukemia and chronic myelogenous leukemia. Other myelodysplastic/ myeloproliferative neoplasms can sometimes demonstrate an increase in peripheral blood monocytes. In particular, monocytosis with immaturity can be striking in very young children with constitutional or acquired disorders frequently associated with monosomy 7 (see Chapters 35, 42).

19.1 Pathophysiology

Monocytes are derived from bone marrow myeloid progenitor cells, and regulatory factors linked to monocyte production include granulocyte-monocyte colony-stimulating factor (GM-CSF) and monocyte colony-stimulating factor (M-CSF). The proposed stages of monocyte differentiation within the bone marrow include monoblasts, promonocytes, and mature monocytes, although neither monoblasts nor promonocytes are typically identified in normal bone marrow specimens.

Monocytes circulate briefly in the peripheral blood and migrate to tissues where they mature into various cells of the monocyte/histiocyte/immune accessory cell system. Members of this diverse cell family exhibit various functions in both cellular and humoral immunity, in phagocytic and antimicrobial activities, and in tissue homeostasis and repair. Monocytes and other cells within this lineage secrete hundreds of proteins that modulate immune function, regulate hematopoiesis, stimulate inflammatory reactions, provide host defense against tumors, and remove either senescent blood cells or infectious organisms by phagocytosis. A partial list of proteins produced by cells within this complex lineage includes complement components, interferons, interleukins, prostaglandins, tumor necrosis factors, and colony-stimulating factors. Like neutrophils, monocytes contain granules within their cytoplasm that play a major role in the cell's antimicrobial function. These granules contain numerous enzymes, including lysozyme, acid phosphatase, collagenase, various esterases, and elastase. Monocytes express CD4, CD13, CD15, CD33, CD36, CD64, and HLA-DR.

19.2 Clinical Findings

The predicted clinical features in patients exhibiting reactive monocytosis are diverse because of the numerous disorders linked to this relatively non-specific peripheral blood finding. The most common cause of reactive monocytosis is chronic infection, and these patients are likely to be febrile with other symptoms related to the infection.

In patients in whom the monocytosis is a component of a hematopoietic neoplasm, additional blood abnormalities are expected. The clinical features in patients with primary hematopoietic neoplasms often include fatigue, fever, malaise, and signs of organ infiltration. Differentiation between reactive and neoplastic monocytosis is particularly challenging in young children because of the overlap between clinical and morphologic findings. Children with either viral infections (Epstein Barr virus–EBV, cytomegalovirus–CMV, parvovirus) or juvenile rheumatoid arthritis can have splenomegaly and prominent monocytosis with some immature forms. Likewise, young children may develop clonal myelodysplastic/myeloproliferative neoplasms characterized by hepatosplenomegaly, variable lymphadenopathy, and marked leukocytosis with monocytosis and neutrophilia (see Chapter 35).

19.3 Diagnostic Approach

Blood monocytosis occurs frequently in certain hematologic neoplasms; therefore, it is imperative that a distinction between reactive and neoplastic monocytosis be made. In patients with primary hematologic neoplasms such as chronic myelomonocytic leukemia, acute myelomonocytic and monocytic leukemias, and chronic myelogenous leukemia, the monocytes are an integral part of the neoplastic clone. The determination of the reactive or neoplastic nature of a blood monocytosis often requires the integration of a variety of hematologic, morphologic, and other laboratory and clinical parameters. A general approach to monocytosis includes:

1. A complete blood count with differential.
2. An evaluation of monocytes for evidence of nuclear immaturity or other atypical features.
3. An evaluation of other peripheral blood cells for quantitative and morphologic abnormalities including dysplasia and immaturity.
4. Correlation of clinical and hematologic findings.
5. Appropriate cultures to assess for possible chronic infection.
6. A bone marrow examination for culture or assessment for clonal cytogenetic abnormalities associated with specific hematopoietic neoplasms.
7. A cytogenetic/molecular evaluation for a possible hematopoietic neoplasm.
8. Flow cytometric immunophenotyping to assess for aberrant patterns of antigen expression on neoplastic monocytes.

19.4 Hematologic Findings

19.4.1 Blood Cell Measurements

In healthy children and adults, the absolute monocyte count is characteristically less than $1.0 \times 10^3/mm^3$ ($1.0 \times 10^9/L$) i19.1. Depending on the cause of the monocytosis, many other peripheral blood abnormalities may be evident i19.2. For example, reactive monocytosis secondary to infection may be accompanied by a neutrophilia i19.3-i19.5. In infected patients, the platelet count is highly variable, and a mild to moderate anemia (most likely anemia of chronic disease) also may be evident. The WBC count also is highly variable in patients with a neoplastic monocytosis, but it is typically elevated, with increased monocytes and a variable proportion of immature myeloid and monocytic elements. In patients with hematopoietic neoplasms, the hemoglobin, hematocrit, and platelet count may be markedly reduced.

i19.1 Normal monocyte

Monocyte compared to lymphocyte; note voluminous, minimal vacuolated cytoplasm and folded mature nucleus of monocyte. *(Wright stain)*

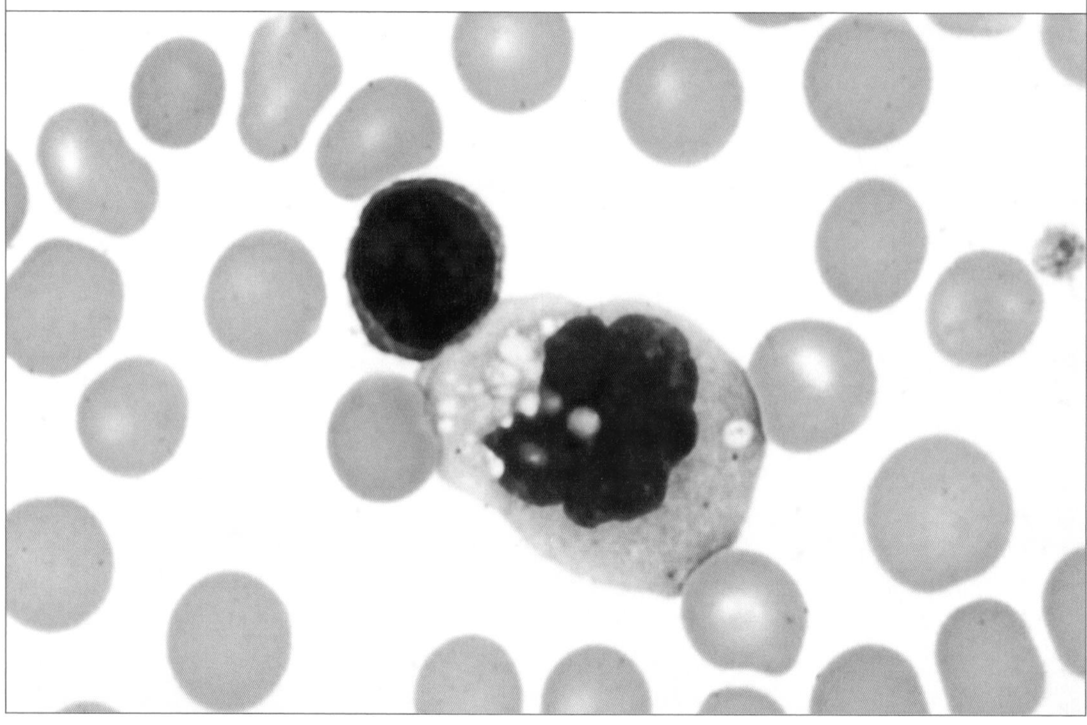

i19.2 Kostmann syndrome

Peripheral blood monocytes in child with severe absolute neutropenia secondary to Kostmann syndrome (severe congenital neutropenia). *(Wright stain) (courtesy Parvin Izadi, MD)*

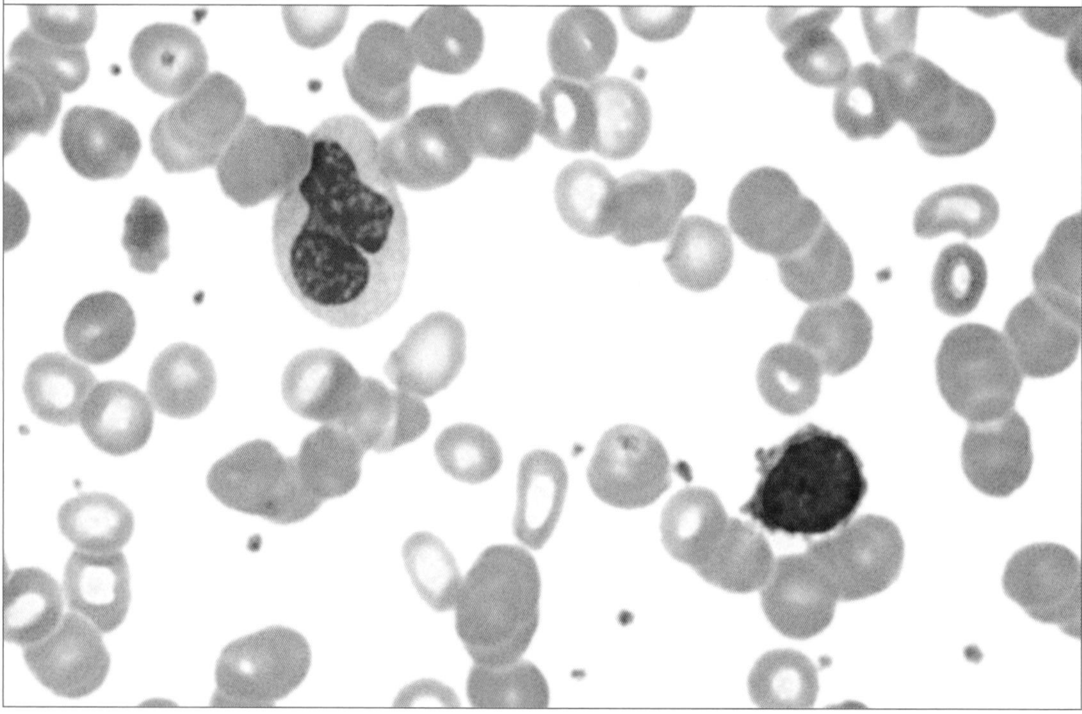

i19.3 Sepsis

Peripheral blood smear from a septic infant. Prominent cytoplasmic vacuolization of both neutrophils and monocytes is evident. *(Wright stain)*

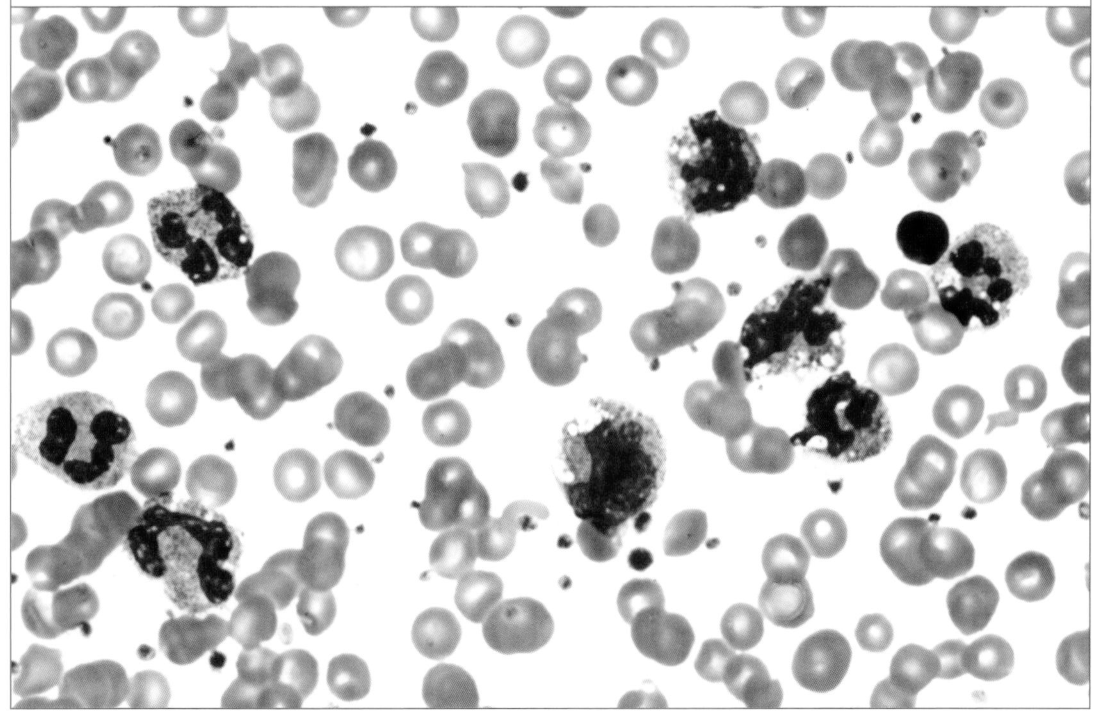

i19.4 Histoplasmosis

Ingestion of fungal elements by both monocytes and neutrophils is evident in this immunosuppressed patient with disseminated histoplasmosis. (*Wright stain) (courtesy Dennis O'Malley, MD)*

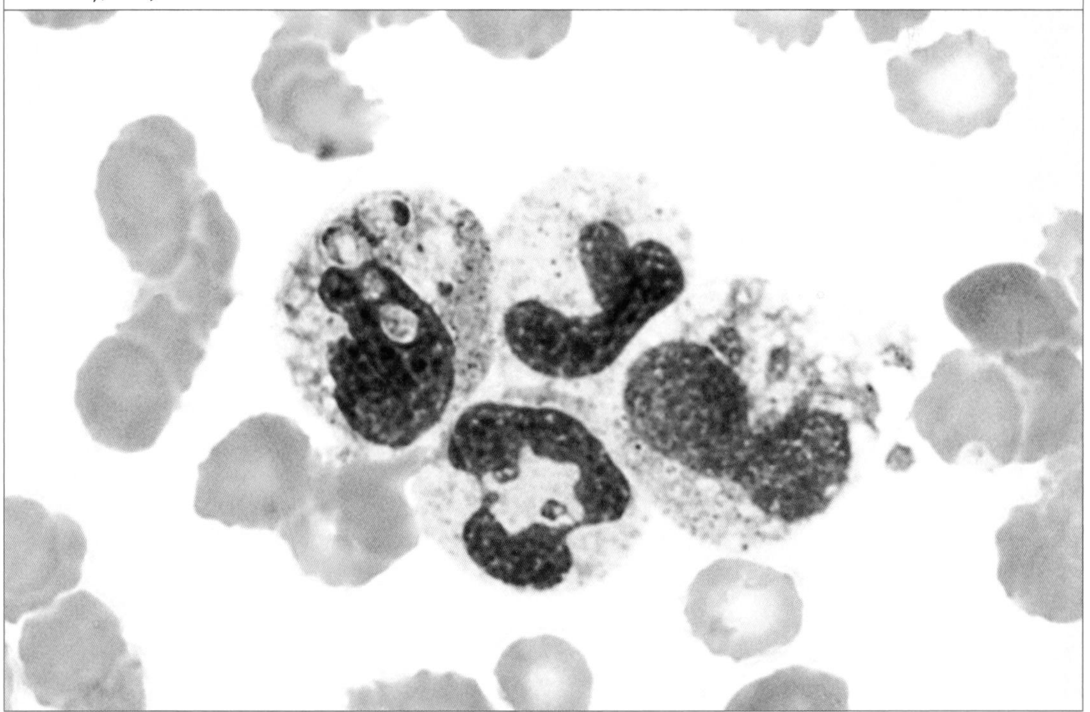

i19.5 Reactive monocytosis

Both a toxic neutrophilia and reactive monocytosis are evident on this blood smear in an infected newborn. *(Wright stain)*

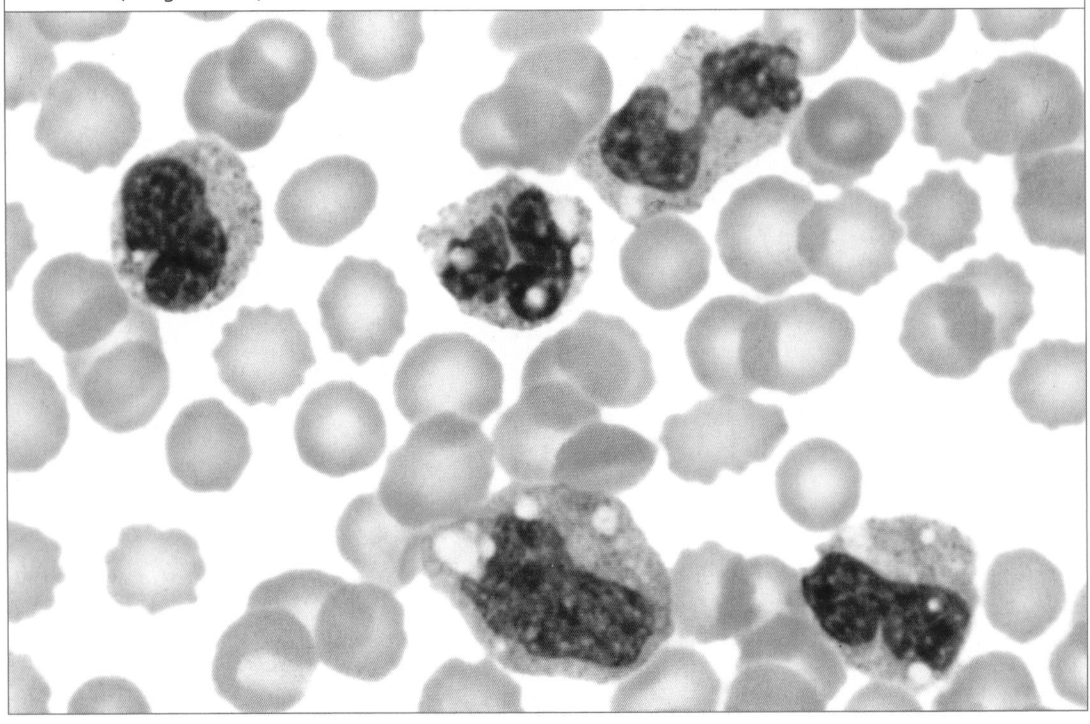

i19.6 Congenital leukemia

a Both a mature neutrophilia and monocytosis are evident in the peripheral blood of this 5-month-old baby with congenital leukemia. *(Wright stain)* **b** Dysplastic neutrophil and circulating blasts are evident in this peripheral blood smear from a 5-month-old baby with congenital leukemia. Note striking mature and immature monocytic elements. *(Wright stain)* **c** Circulating immature monocytic element with nucleolus in conjunction with dysplastic neutrophil is evident in the peripheral blood in this 5-month-old baby with congenital leukemia. *(Wright stain)*

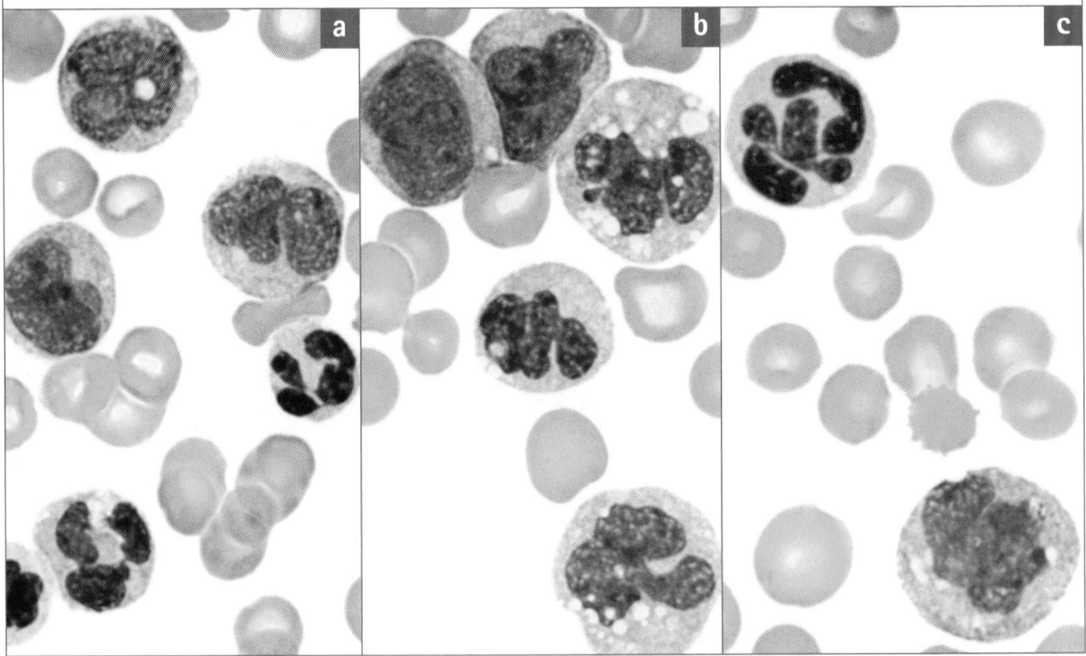

19.4.2 Peripheral Blood Smear Morphology

Reactive monocytes characteristically exhibit indented or folded nuclei, relatively mature nuclear chromatin, and cytoplasm that is frequently vacuolated (see i19.3). Cytoplasmic granulation also may be prominent. Organisms may be evident in blood smears from immunosuppressed patients i19.4. Evidence of monocyte immaturity, such as finely dispersed nuclear chromatin, nucleoli, and variable abnormal nuclear configurations, suggests a neoplastic process i19.6. Circulating monoblasts also suggest a neoplastic process. In addition to evaluating monocyte morphology, an evaluation of the morphology of other cell types can help in distinguishing benign from neoplastic monocytosis. If there is either prominent dysplasia of any lineage or substantial left shift, the patient probably has a neoplastic hematologic disorder with involvement of many cell lines, including the monocyte lineage (see i19.6). This multilineage dysplasia with atypical monocytes is especially prominent in either myelodysplastic syndromes or hybrid myelodysplastic/myeloproliferative neoplasms.

19.4.3 Bone Marrow Examination

Bone marrow examination may be warranted in selected patients with blood monocytosis. Indications for bone marrow examination in this patient population include culture or evaluation for a possible hematopoietic neoplasm.

19.5 Ancillary Tests

1. Blood or bone marrow culture.
2. Serologic studies for infectious agents.
3. Cytogenetic/molecular studies in patients with possible hematopoietic neoplasm.
4. Special stains for monocytic differentiation on bone marrow aspirate smears if monocytic leukemia is suspected (ie, a-naphthol butyrate esterase).
5. Flow cytometric immunophenotyping, especially in disorders with marked immaturity.

19.6 Course and Treatment

The clinical course varies with the underlying disorder, as does the treatment of patients with monocytosis. In general, patients with a neoplastic monocytosis follow an aggressive disease course requiring antileukemic therapy.

19.7 References

Cline MJ. Laboratory evaluation of benign quantitative granulocyte and monocyte disorders. In: Bick RL, ed. *Hematology Clinical and Laboratory Practice.* Vol 2. St. Louis: Mosby. 1993:1155-1160.

Dale DC, Boxer L, Liles WC. The phagocytes: neutrophils and monocytes. *Blood.* 2008;112:935-945.

Devaraj S, Jialal I. Validation of the circulating monocyte being representative of the cholesterol-loaded macrophage: biomediator activity. *Arch Pathol Lab Med.* 2008;132:1432-1435.

Dunphy CH, Orton SO, Mantell J. Relative contributions of enzyme cytochemistry and flow cytometric immunophenotyping to the evaluation of acute myeloid leukemias with a monocytic component and of flow cytometric immunophenotyping to the evaluation of absolute monocytoses. *Am J Clin Pathol.* 2004;122:865-874.

Foucar K. Constitutional and reactive myeloid disorders. In: *Bone Marrow Pathology. 2nd ed.* Chicago: ASCP Press. 2001:146-172.

Kampalath B, Cleveland RP, Chang CC, et al. Monocytes with altered phenotypes in posttrauma patients. *Arch Pathol Lab Med.* 2003;127:1580-1585.

Liu CZ, Persad R, Inghirami G, et al. Transient atypical monocytosis mimic acute myelomonocytic leukemia in post-chemotherapy patients receiving G-CSF: report of two cases. *Clin Lab Haematol.* 2004;26:359-362.

Perkins S. Disorders of hematopoiesis. In: Collins R, Swerdlow S, eds. *Pediatric Hematopathology.* New York: Churchill Livingstone. 2001:105-140.

Wilson C. Non-neoplastic granulocytic and monocytic disorders In: King D, Gardner W, Sobin L, et al., eds. *Non-Neoplastic Disorders of Bone Marrow* (AFIP fascicle). Washington, DC: American Registry of Pathology; 2008:125-175.

Xu Y, McKenna RW, Karandikar NJ, et al. Flow cytometric analysis of monocytes as a tool for distinguishing chronic myelomonocytic leukemia from reactive monocytosis. *Am J Clin Pathol.* 2005;124:799-806.

Yetgin S, Cetin M, Yenicesu I, et al. Acute parvovirus B19 infection mimicking juvenile myelomonocytic leukemia. *Eur J Haematol.* 2000;65:276-278.

Chapter 20

Neutropenia

Kathryn Foucar, MD

In normal adults, the range for an absolute neutrophil count is 1.5-7.0 × $10^3/mm^3$ (1.5-7.0 × $10^9/L$). Both patient age and race have an impact on the established lower limit of the normal range. For example, in neonates and infants, the lower limit is approximately 2.5 × $10^3/mm^3$ (2.5 × $10^9/L$), whereas the lower limit of normal for children and adults is 1.5 × $10^3/mm^3$ (1.5 × $10^9/L$). Approximately 1/4 of healthy black children and adults demonstrate an absolute neutrophil count that ranges from 1.0-1.5 × $10^3/mm^3$ (1.0-1.5 × $10^9/L$). Because these patients demonstrate no evidence of clinically significant neutropenia, this value is presumed to represent a normal race variation.

Consequently, the definition of neutropenia varies by patient age and race. An absolute neutrophil count less than 2.5 × $10^3/mm^3$ (2.5 × $10^9/L$) constitutes neutropenia in infants; an absolute neutrophil count less than 1.5 × $10^3/mm^3$ (1.5 × $10^9/L$) is generally used to define neutropenia in all other patient age groups. Neutropenias are subclassified into mild, moderate, and severe based on the absolute neutrophil count. A mild neutropenia generally ranges from 1.0-1.5 × $10^3/mm^3$ (1.0-1.5 × $10^9/L$), while moderate neutropenias range from 0.5-0.999 × $10^3/mm^3$ (0.5-1.0 × $10^9/L$). Patients with severe neutropenia (<0.5 × $10^3/mm^3$ [<0.5 × $10^9/L$]) are at the greatest risk for serious bacterial infection, usually of endogenous origin.

In evaluating a patient for a neutropenia, it is important to distinguish neoplastic disorders in which neutrophils are a component of the malignant clone from non-neoplastic neutropenias. Abnormalities in other lineages are often clues to neoplastic processes, while most cases of isolated absolute neutropenia are linked to either constitutional or acquired non-neoplastic disorders. This chapter will focus on non-neoplastic neutropenias.

Although the diagnostic approach to neutropenia will be delineated in a later section of this chapter, a review of key concepts is provided to guide the diagnostician and provide a conceptual framework for consideration before specific neutropenic disorders are discussed **t20.1**.

t20.1 Key Neutropenia Concepts

- Granulopoiesis requires adequate progenitor cells, an intact bone marrow microenvironment, and essential regulatory factors such as G-CSF.
- Because neutrophil lifespan in blood is only a few hours, the absolute neutrophil count is a reflection of current and ongoing bone marrow granulopoiesis.
- Neutrophils within blood are about equally divided between the circulating and the marginated pools; only the circulating pool is reflected in the absolute neutrophil count.
- There are significant age and race-related variations in normal range for absolute neutrophil count.
- Age at onset and duration of neutropenia are critical factors in diagnostic decision-making.
- Similarly, differential diagnoses vary substantially for an isolated neutropenia vs. multilineage abnormalities.
- Morphologic abnormalities of neutrophils can be seen in both constitutional and acquired non-neoplastic neutropenias.

t20.2 Age-Related Causes of Neutropenia

Patient Age	Causes of Neutropenia
Neonate	Infection
	Maternal hypertension and/or drug treatment
	Maternal antibody production
	Constitutional disorders such as cyclic neutropenia, Kostmann syndrome, and Chédiak-Higashi syndrome
Infant/child	Infection
	Autoimmune neutropenia
	Neoplasms replacing bone marrow
	Idiosyncratic drug reactions
	Secondary autoimmune neutropenia in collagen vascular disorders
	Immunodeficiency disorders
	Myeloablative therapies
	Constitutional neutropenic disorders (rare)
	Megaloblastic anemia (rare)
	Copper deficiency (rare)
Adult	Idiosyncratic drug reactions
	Infections
	Neoplasms replacing bone marrow
	Myeloablative therapies
	Secondary autoimmune neutropenia in collagen vascular disorders
	Autoimmune disorders including white cell aplasia
	T-cell large granular lymphocytic leukemia
	Aplastic anemia
	Immunodeficiency disorders
	Hypersplenism
	Megaloblastic anemia
	Copper deficiency (may be zinc-induced)

The primary causes of neutropenia, based on patient age, are listed in **t20.2**. Infection is by far the most common cause of neutropenia in neonates. However, neonates also may develop neutropenia from maternal factors such as hypertension, drug treatments given to the mother during late gestation, and maternal antibodies that cross the placenta and attack fetal granulocytes. Although rare, various distinct constitutional neutropenic disorders also may manifest during the neonatal period **t20.3**. Because of their rarity in clinical practice, constitutional neutropenias will not be discussed in detail. However, the diagnostician should be aware of the general features of molecular classification, patterns of inheritance, and prototypic blood and bone marrow findings **t20.3**. Of these hereditary disorders, the more prevalent are cyclic neutropenia, severe congenital neutropenia (including Kostmann syndrome), and Chédiak-Higashi syndrome (see Chapter 22). Severe sustained neutropenia characterizes Kostmann syndrome and Chédiak-Higashi syndrome, whereas patients with cyclic neutropenia exhibit episodic loss of neutrophils followed by a rebound recovery. In addition to the hematologic features listed on **t20.3**, many of these constitutional disorders are associated with multiple phenotypic and functional abnormalities of other organ systems.

As with neonates, infection is a common cause of neutropenia in older children. Other causes of neutropenia in infants and children include autoimmune disorders, bone marrow replacement by neoplasms, myeloablative therapy, and idiosyncratic drug reactions. In adults, idiosyncratic drug reactions are the most common cause of neutropenia in ambulatory patients. Numerous drug treatments are linked to acquired neutropenia, and patients should always be queried regarding both medications and homeopathic remedies/supplements. Other common causes of neutropenia in adults include infections, bone marrow replacement disorders, myeloablative therapy, megaloblastic anemia, and various autoimmune/immune disorders including acquired white cell aplasia. Although rare, an increased number of cases of zinc-induced copper deficiency with associated anemia and neutropenia have been noted due to excess homeopathic supplemental zinc ingestion.

t20.3 Hematologic and Genetic Features of Constitutional Disorders Associated with Neutropenia

Disorder	Age of Onset	Blood Findings	Bone Marrow Features	Molecular Defect	Usual Inheritance
Cyclic neutropenia	Early infancy	Periodicity in ANC (usual 21 day cycle with rebound neutrophilia)	Cyclical myeloid aplasia followed by rebound*	Primary granule formation	Autosomal dominant
Severe congenital neutropenia (Kostmann)	Birth/early infancy	Isolated, profound neutropenia	Sustained myeloid aplasia with only scattered myeloblasts and promyelocytes	Primary granule formation	Autosomal dominant/ recessive
Shwachman-Diamond syndrome	Birth/early infancy	Initial neutropenia; may develop other cytopenias	Variable picture with myeloid aplasia/ hypoplasia in a substantial proportion	Ribosome biogenesis	Autosomal recessive
Chédiak-Higashi syndrome	Early infancy	Neutropenia; abnormal granulation of neutrophils, monocytes, and lymphocytes	Hypercellular bone marrow with abnormal granule formation in many lineages	Lysosomal trafficking regulation	Autosomal recessive
Myelokathexis	Early infancy	Neutropenia; pronounced thin nuclear stands between lobes, hypersegmentation	Granulocytic hyperplasia; thin nuclear stands between lobes, hypersegmentation	Chemokine receptor	Autosomal dominant
Fanconi anemia	Infancy/ childhood/ rare adult presenta-tion	Variable cytopenias over time	Variable picture initially, but eventual development of aplastic picture	DNA repair pathway	Recessive
Dyskeratosis congenita	Infancy	Variable cytopenias over time	Gradual development of aplastic picture	Telomere maintenance	Variable

**Impaired survival of progenitor cells ANC=absolute neutrophil count*

Neutropenia secondary to splenic pooling of neutrophils can be present in patients with hypersplenism (see **t20.2**).

20.1 Pathophysiology

Normal numbers of circulating neutrophils are maintained by adequate bone marrow proliferation, unimpeded bone marrow maturation and release into blood, and normal survival time in blood. Defects both within and outside the bone marrow may be responsible for neutropenia, and these mechanisms can be broadly classified as proliferation, maturation, survival, and distribution defects **t20.4**. Often, more than one of these mechanisms is operational in the production of neutropenia. For example, a patient with an infection may develop neutropenia because of bone marrow suppression by the infectious agent, decreased neutrophil survival, and increased egress of neutrophils from the blood to infection sites. Likewise, the mechanisms that are operative in patients who develop neutropenia secondary to idiosyncratic drug reactions also are overlapping and variable. In some of these patients, the drug causes abrupt loss of the granulocyte lineage (ie, agranulocytosis, proliferation defect), while drug-induced immune-mediated neutrophil destruction is operative in other patients (ie, a survival defect). Recent studies document increased apoptosis of bone marrow myeloid progenitor cells as the cause of chronic idiopathic neutropenia; overproduction of inflammatory cytokines by the bone marrow microenvironment is linked to apoptosis. Finally, in constitutional neutropenic disorders genetic aberrations may be identified. For example, a truncation mutation of the cytoplasmic region of the G-CSF receptor has been detected in patients with Kostmann syndrome.

t20.4 Mechanisms Causing Neutropenia

Mechanism	Comments
Proliferation defect	Failure of granulocytic lineage Often only scattered myeloblasts and promyelocytes present Occurs in many constitutional neutropenias, many idiosyncratic drug reactions, bone marrow replacement disorders, aplastic anemia, and following myeloablative therapy In addition, bone marrow effacement by fibrosis or a neoplasm is also a type of proliferation defect. The neutropenia is not the consequence of failed or suppressed granulopoiesis, but rather due to marrow effacement; all hematopoietic lineages are affected.
Maturation defect	Granulocytic lineage abundant but maturation does not proceed normally and many cells die within the bone marrow Occurs in neutropenias associated with megaloblastic anemia and rare constitutional disorders such as myelokathexis
Survival defect	Bone marrow production and release of neutrophils is increased, but cells are rapidly removed from blood Occurs in many infections and immune disorders characterized by accelerated destruction/removal of neutrophils
Distribution abnormality	Total body granulocyte pool is normal, but number of circulating neutrophils is reduced Occurs in patients with hypersplenism and patients with defective release of bone marrow neutrophils (rare) Seldom the primary mechanism responsible for neutropenia

20.2 Clinical Findings

Because of the various underlying causes, patients with neutropenia have diverse clinical manifestations. However, all neutropenic patients must be assessed for possible underlying infections that may be either the cause or the consequence of the neutropenia. Secondary infections in neutropenic patients are often derived from endogenous organisms, and commonly involved sites include skin, oral pharynx, gingiva, gastrointestinal tract, and the anal region. The detection of infection may be challenging in neutropenic patients, because many of the clinical "clues" to a specific site of infection are the consequence of the migration of huge numbers of neutrophils to that site. Consequently, in severely neutropenic patients, findings such as swelling, induration, erythema, and even infiltrates on chest radiograph are less conspicuous.

20.3 Diagnostic Approach

The evaluation of a patient with neutropenia requires the integration of multiple clinical and laboratory parameters. The severity and duration of the neutropenia will guide the extent of

i20.1 Chédiak-Higashi syndrome

Abnormal cytoplasmic granules in both eosinophil and neutrophil in child with Chédiak-Higashi syndrome-associated neutropenia. *(Wright stain) (courtesy Parvin Izadi, MD)*

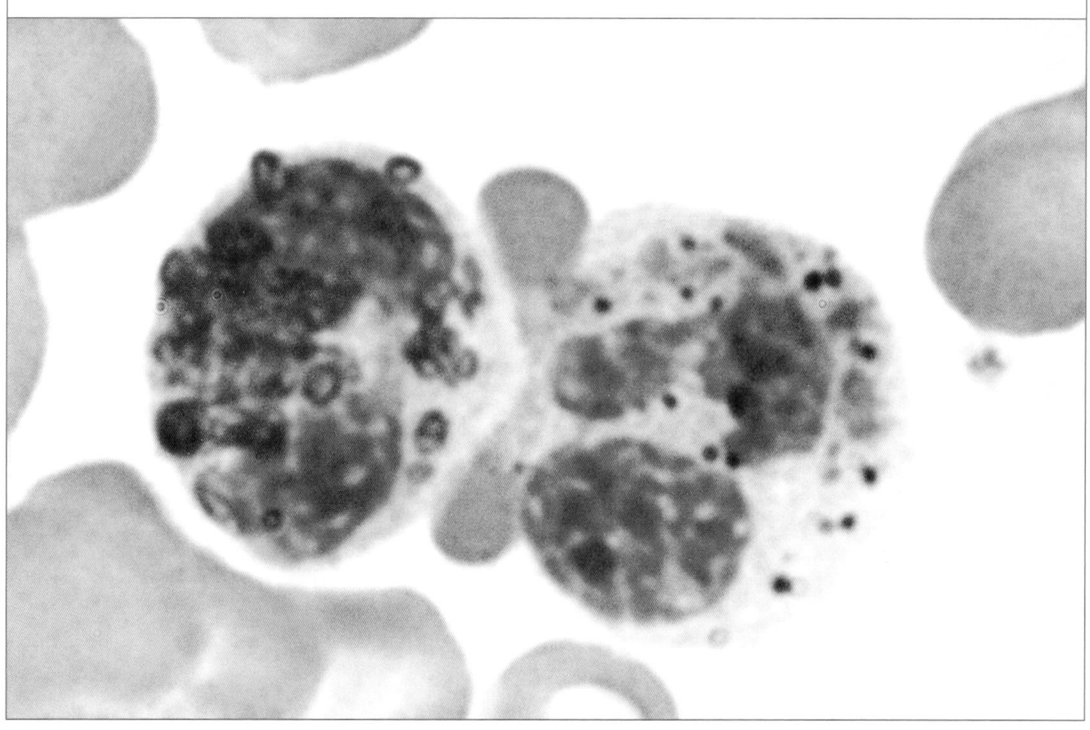

i20.2 Cyclic neutropenia

Severe absolute neutropenia in a 1-year-old boy. *(Wright stain)*

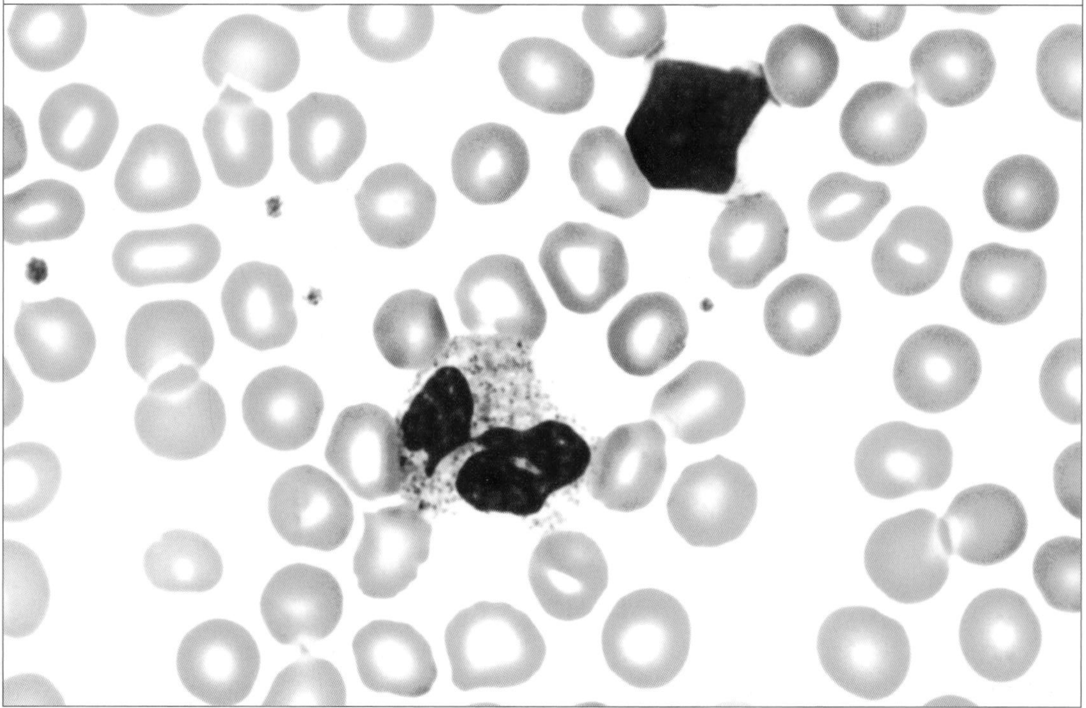

i20.3 Toxic changes

Metamyelocyte demonstrating toxic changes including Döhle body in the peripheral blood of a patient with an infection. *(Wright stain)*

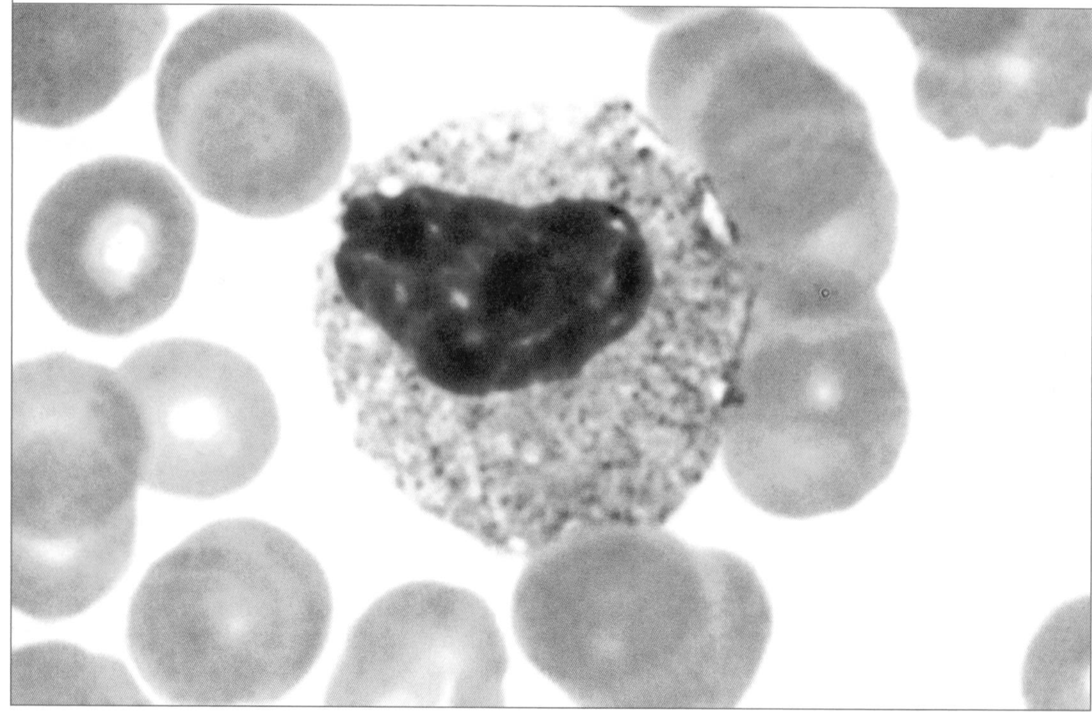

workup. Although the appropriate workup varies with patient age, in general, the evaluation of a neutropenia should include the following steps:

1. A detailed history for evidence of a current or recurrent infection, findings suggestive of a constitutional disorder, and symptoms of an underlying immunologic disorder or occult neoplasm.
2. An investigation for drug therapy, homeopathic remedies/supplements, toxin, or alcohol exposure.
3. A physical examination for possible splenomegaly, evidence of occult infection or evidence of neoplasm, or phenotypic abnormalities linked to constitutional neutropenic disorders.
4. A complete blood count with differential. Serial complete blood counts document either a cyclic pattern or neutrophil recovery in patients with transient neutropenia.
5. A morphologic review of blood smear for evidence of hematopoietic neoplasms, infection-related changes, megaloblastic features, and features of constitutional disorders such as Chédiak-Higashi syndrome.
6. An evaluation of other hematopoietic lineages for morphologic or numeric abnormalities.
7. A laboratory workup for possible infection, if clinically suspected.
8. In selected patients, a laboratory assessment of immune status, tests for collagen vascular disorders, or serologic studies for viral infections.
9. Various radiographic studies in selected patients, including those with suspected constitutional neutropenic disorders, to assess for constitutional bony defects, evidence of neoplasm, or evidence of infection.
10. A bone marrow examination. This is generally required in adult patients with new-onset neutropenia. Likewise, bone marrow evaluation is necessary in children with suspected

t20.5 Bone Marrow Findings in Non-Neoplastic Neutropenic Disorders

Disorder	Comments
Aplastic anemia (proliferation defect)	All lineages absent or reduced
Radiation/chemotherapy (proliferation defect)	All lineages suppressed or absent
Myelophthisis (proliferation effect)	Bone marrow replaced by infiltrative disorder
Drug-induced neutropenia (proliferation or survival defect)	Variable; most cases exhibit almost complete granulocytic aplasia with occasional blasts and promyelocytes Other cases characterized by granulocytic hyperplasia with a decrease in mature forms (eg, drug-induced immune destruction)
Immune-mediated neutropenia (survival or proliferation defect)	Generally find granulocytic hyperplasia with decreased mature neutrophils, although immune mechanisms also responsible for suppressing granulocyte and other lineages Prominent ingestion of neutrophils by macrophages possible Immune aberrations may be primary or secondary to neoplastic or non-neoplastic disorders
Vitamin B_{12} or folate deficiency (maturation defect)	Markedly hypercellular bone marrow with pronounced megaloblastic changes; intramedullary cell death
Infection-associated neutropenia (proliferation or survival defect)	Variable bone marrow morphology; some infections (especially viral) suppress progenitor cells, inducing hypoplasia Other infections cause decreased neutrophil survival and bone marrow shows granulocytic hyperplasia

i20.4 Severe bacterial infection

Scattered immature myeloid elements are evident in this bone marrow aspirate smear from a patient with severe bacterial infection-associated neutropenia. Note toxic changes with prominent paranuclear hof. *(Wright stain)*

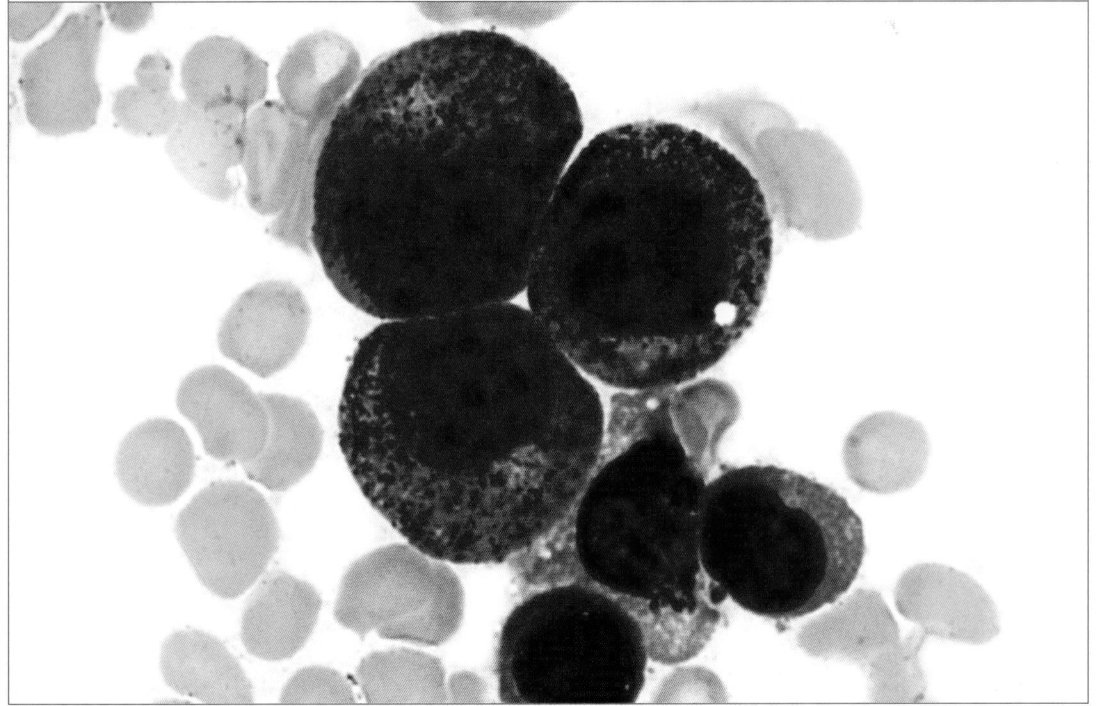

i20.5 Agranulocytosis in infant

Bone marrow aspirate shows rare left-shifted granulocytic precursors without maturation. *(Wright stain)*

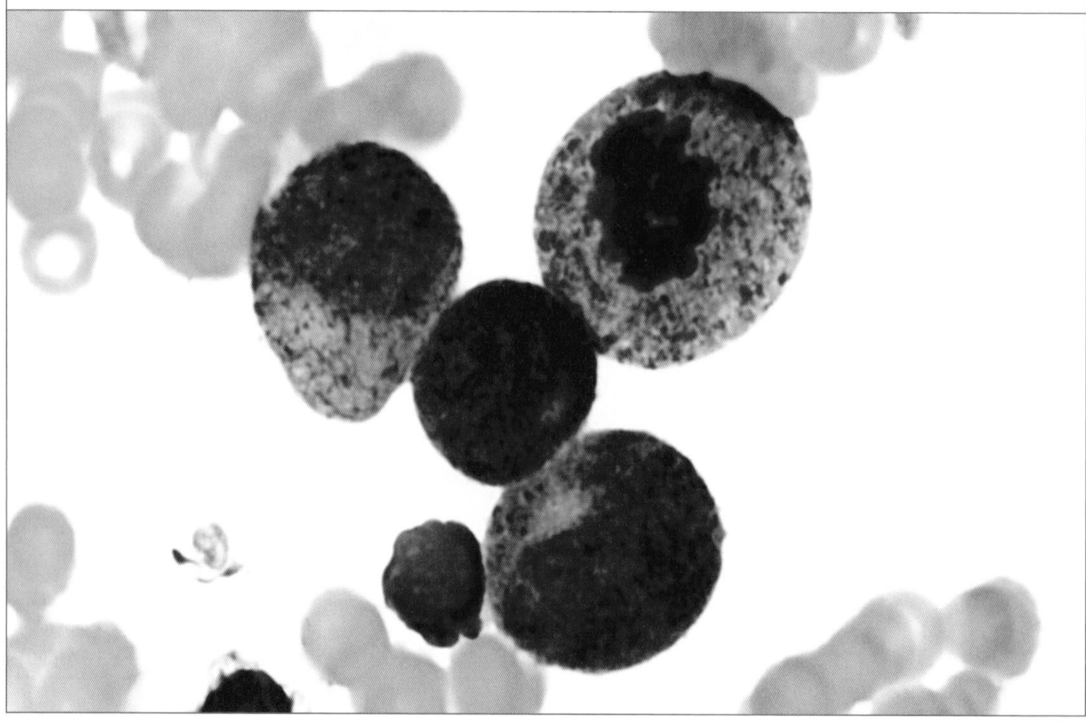

i20.6 Agranulocytosis without maturation

Bone marrow core biopsy shows immature paratrabecular granulocytic cells; note absence of central maturation storage compartment. *(H& E)*

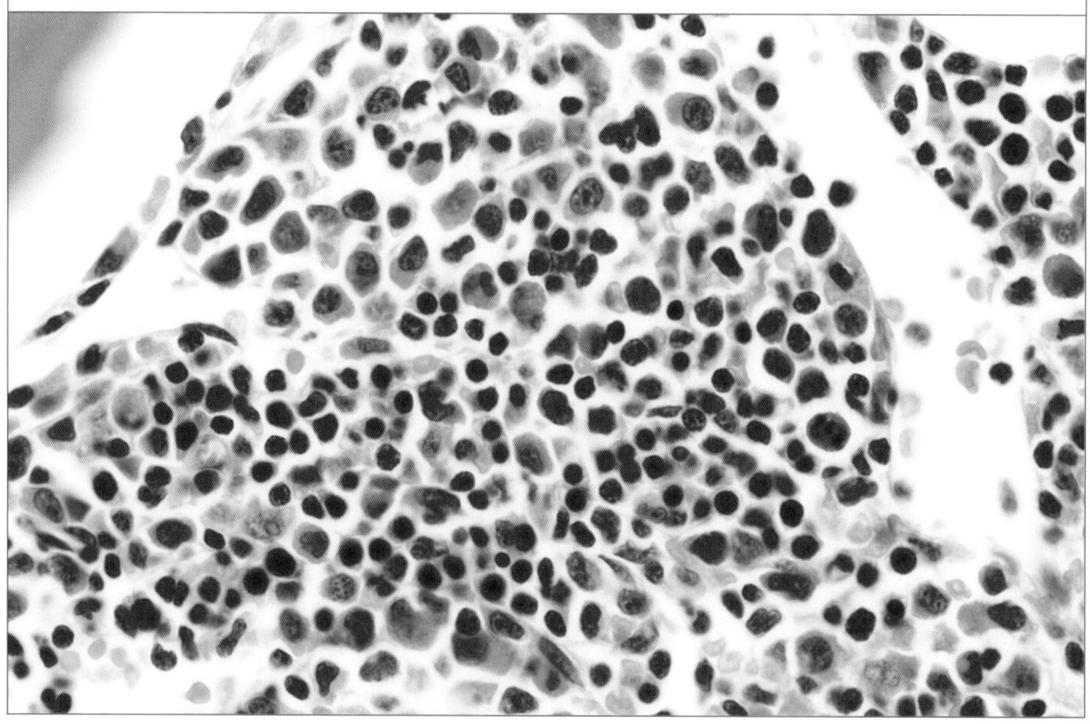

i20.7 Felty syndrome

Peripheral blood smear from patient with Felty syndrome and profound neutropenia. *(Wright stain)*

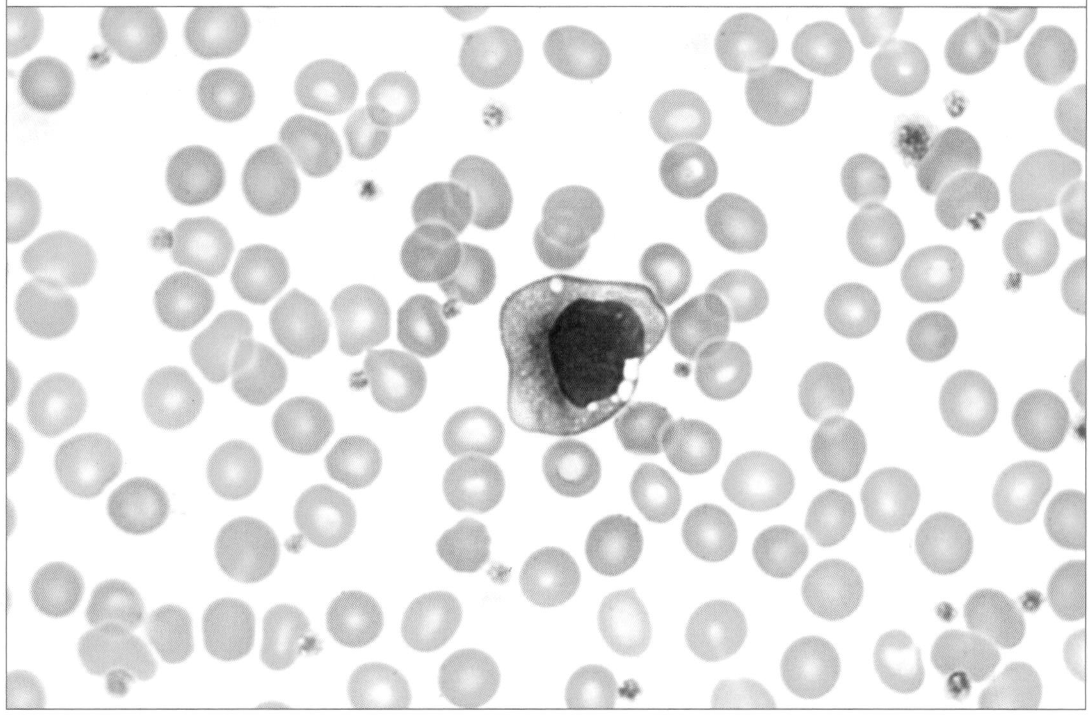

i20.8 Felty syndrome

Brisk granulocytic hyperplasia in this bone marrow aspirate smear in a patient with Felty syndrome (see **i20.7**). *(Wright stain)*

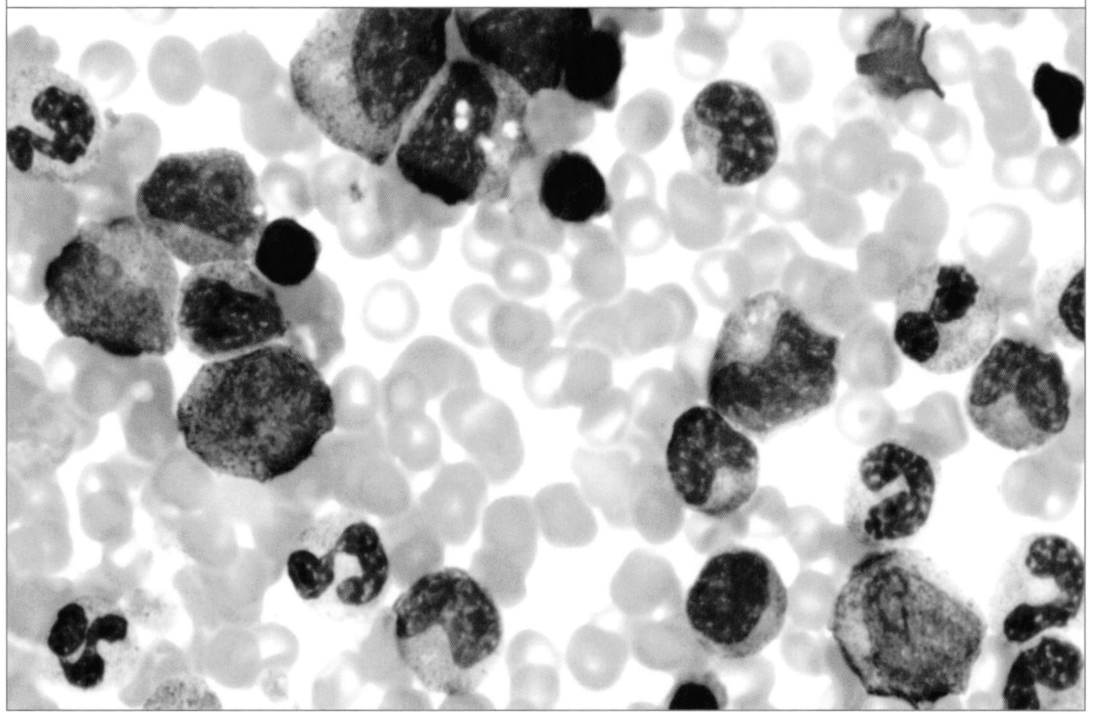

neoplasms, aplasia, bone marrow infiltration in storage disorders/other disorders, and selected infections. However, many children develop transient neutropenia following presumed viral infections. In these children, who are otherwise healthy and have only isolated neutropenia, a "watch and wait" approach is often taken. A bone marrow examination is unlikely to be considered in these children unless spontaneous neutrophil recovery fails to occur within 1-2 months.

20.4 Hematologic Findings

20.4.1 Blood Cell Measurements

The neutrophil count is less than $1.5 \times 10^3/mm^3$ ($1.5 \times 10^9/L$). Depending on the cause of the neutropenia, the other hemogram parameters are highly variable.

20.4.2 Peripheral Blood Smear Morphology

Although the total number is decreased, the morphology of granulocytes is generally normal, except in rare constitutional disorders such as Chédiak-Higashi syndrome **i20.1**, and myelokathexis. In other constitutional neutropneias granulocyte morphology is normal **i20.2**. Toxic changes and left shift may be evident in infected patients **i20.3**. A compensatory monocytosis may be present especially prior to the recovery of neutrophils in patients with cyclic neutropenia.

20.4.3 Bone Marrow Examination

Bone marrow findings vary with the mechanism responsible for the neutropenia **t20.3-t20.5**. In patients with proliferation defects, the granulocytic lineage is largely absent **i20.4**. This may be the consequence of some hematopoietic regulatory defect, or the bone marrow may be effaced by a neoplasm or fibrosis. In patients with constitutional neutropenias such as severe congenital neutropenia (Kostmann syndrome), the myeloid lineage is virtually absent except for rare myeloblasts and promyelocytes, which often are enlarged and binucleate. In infants with sustained severe neutropenia, the bone marrow aspirate and biopsy may show markedly reduced and left-shifted granulocytic cells without a maturation storage compartment **i20.5, i20.6**. In patients with maturation defects, the granulocytic lineage is hyperplastic, and morphologic abnormalities are generally prominent. The defective myeloid elements generally die within the medullary cavity, often by apoptosis. In patients with survival defects, the granulocytic lineage also is hyperplastic **i20.7, i20.8**. However, as a consequence of the rapid release of mature forms into the blood, the granulocyte maturation pyramid may exhibit left shift in patients with survival defects. If the survival defect is immune-mediated, bone marrow macrophages may contain ingested neutrophils **i20.9**.

20.5 Ancillary Tests

Numerous ancillary tests may be warranted in selected neutropenic patients, including tests for folate and vitamin B_{12} levels, collagen vascular disease, immune status, granulocyte antibody studies, cytogenetics, serologic tests for infectious agents, neutrophil survival studies, and copper levels.

Screening and confirmatory testing is available for some constitutional disorders including chromosome breakage analysis for Fanconi's anemia and telomere length assessment for dyskeratosis congenita. Although genetic testing for specific mutations can be performed for some constitutional neutropenis, they generally identify only a subset of cases.

i20.9 Autoimmune neutropenia

Imprint smear of bone marrow cone biopsy from child with autoimmune neutropenia. Macrophages contains ingested neutrophils *(Wright stain)*

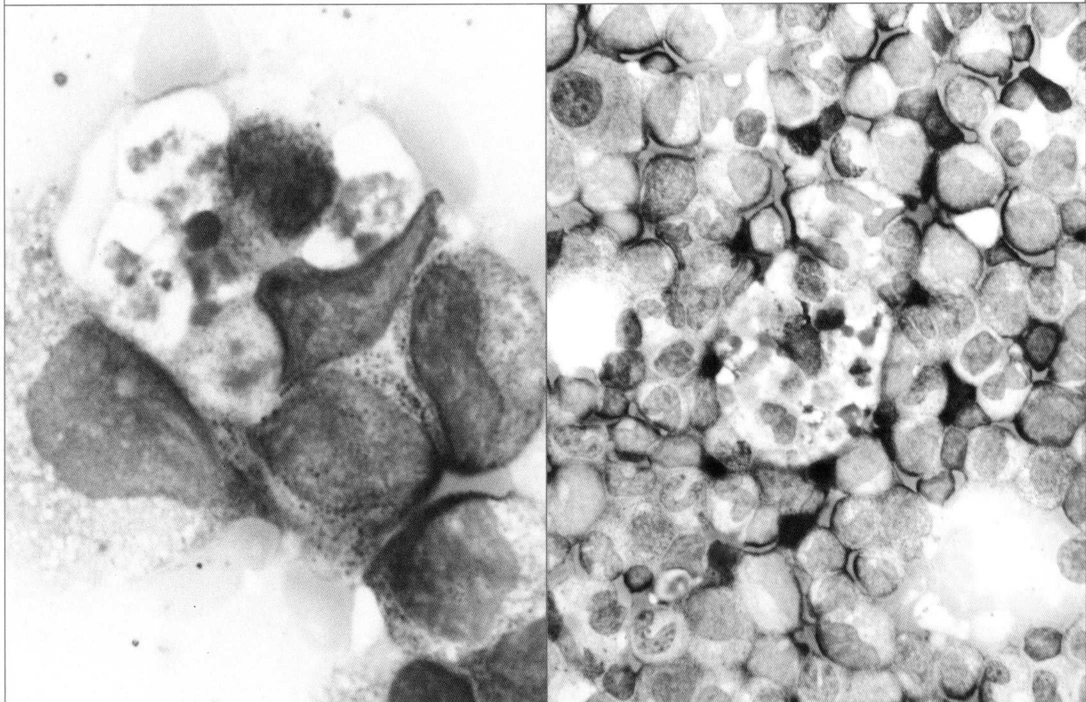

20.6 Course and Treatment

The management of a patient with neutropenia includes the following components:

1. Prompt antibiotic therapy for patients with bacterial infections.
2. The determination and management of the underlying cause of neutropenia.
3. Possible recombinant human colony-stimulating factor therapy to stimulate neutrophil production.

The development of recombinant human colony-stimulating factor has been a major breakthrough in the treatment of neutropenias of diverse etiology, including both constitutional and acquired neutropenic disorders. The most consistent increases in absolute neutrophil count are achieved with granulocyte colony-stimulating factor therapy. In these patients, brisk neutrophilia with prominent toxic changes results from pharmacologic doses of granulocyte colony-stimulating factor (see Chapter 16). However, there is a substantial risk of progression to myelodysplasia and acute myeloid leukemia in patients with severe congenital neutropenia who receive sustained recombinant G-CSF therapy.

20.7 References

Bain BJ, Phillips D, Thomson K, et al. Investigation of the effect of marathon running on leukcocyte counts of subjects of different ethnic origins: relevance to the aetiology of ethnic neutropenia. *Br J Haematol.* 2000;108:483-487.

Balabanian K, Lagane B, Pablos JL, et al. WHIM syndromes with different genetic anomalies are accounted for by impaired CXCR4 desensitization to CXCL12. *Blood.* 2005;105:2449-2457.

Berliner N. Lessons from congenital neutropenia: 50 years of progress in understanding myelopoiesis. *Blood.* 2008;111:5427-5432.

Boxer L, Dale DC. Neutropenia: causes and consequences. *Semin Hematol.* 2002;39:75-81.

Bux J, Behrens G, Jaeger G, et al. Diagnosis and clinical course of autoimmune neutropenia in infancy: analysis of 240 cases. *Blood.* 1998;91:181-186.

Cham B, Bonilla MA, Winkelstein J. Neutropenia associated with primary immunodeficiency syndromes. *Semin Hematol.* 2002;39:107-112.

Dale DC, Bolyard AA, Aprikyan A. Cyclic neutropenia. *Semin Hematol.* 2002;39:89-94.

Dale DC, Cottle TE, Fier CJ, et al. Severe chronic neutropenia: treatment and follow-up of patients in the Severe Chronic Neutropenia International Registry. *Am J Hematol.* 2003;72:82-93.

Dale DC, Boxer L, Liles WC. The phagocytes: neutrophils and monocytes. *Blood.* 2008;112:935-945.

Dokal I, Vulliamy T. Inherited aplastic anaemias/bone marrow failure syndromes. *Blood Rev.* 2008;22:141-153.

Dror Y, Sung L. Update on childhood neutropenia: molecular and clinical advances. *Hematol Oncol Clin N Am.* 2004;18:1439-1458.

Foucar K. Constitutional and reactive myeloid disorders. In: *Bone Marrow Pathology. 2nd ed.* Chicago: ASCP Press. 2001:146-172.

Grenda DS, Murakami M, Ghatak J, et al. Mutations of the ELA2 gene found in patients with severe congenital neutropenia induce the unfolded protein response and cellular apoptosis. *Blood.* 2007;110:4179-4187.

Harless W, Crowell E, Abraham J. Anemia and neutropenia associated with copper deficiency of unclear etiology. *Am J Hematol.* 2006;81:546-549.

Horwitz MS, Duan Z, Korkmaz B, et al. Neutrophil elastase in cyclic and severe congenital neutropenia. *Blood.* 2007;109:1817-1824.

Kameoka J, Funato T, Miura T, et al. Autoimmune neutropenia in pregnant women causing neonatal neutropenia. *Br J Haematol.* 2001;114:198-200.

Kaufman DW, Kelly JP, Issaragrisil S, et al. Relative incidence of agranulocytosis and aplastic anemia. *Am J Hematol.* 2006;81:65-67.

Kobayashi M, Sato T, Kawaguchi H, et al. Efficacy of prophylactic use of trimethoprim-sulfamethoxazole in autoimmune neutropenia in infancy. *J Pediatr Hematol Oncol.* 2003;25:553-557.

Neth OW, Bajaj-Elliott M, Turner MW, Klein NJ. Susceptibility to infection in patients with neutropenia: the role of the innate immune system. *Br J Haematol.* 2005;129:713-722.

Pagliuca A, Carrington PA, Pettengell R, et al. Guidelines on the use of colony-stimulating factors in haematological malignancies. *Br J Haematol.* 2003;123:22-33.

Palmblad JE, von dem Borne AE. Idiopathic, immune, infectious, and idiosyncratic neutropenias. *Semin Hematol.* 2002;39:113-120.

Papadaki HA, Eliopoulos AG, Kosteas T, et al. Impaired granulocytopoiesis in patients with chronic idiopathic neutropenia is associated with increased apoptosis of bone marrow myeloid progenitor cells. *Blood.* 2003;101:2591-2600.

Rosenberg PS, Alter BP, Bolyard AA, et al. The incidence of leukemia and mortality from sepsis in patients with severe congenital neutropenia receiving long-term G-CSF therapy. *Blood.* 2006;107:4628-4635.

Rosenberg PS, Alter BP, Link DC, et al. Neutrophil elastase mutations and risk of leukaemia in severe congenital neutropenia. *Br J Haematol.* 2008;140:210-213.

Shimamura A. Shwachman-Diamond syndrome. *Semin Hematol.* 2006;43:178-188.

Shimizu H, Sawada K, Katano N, et al. Intramedullary neutrophil phagocytosis by histiocytes in autoimmune neutropenia of infancy. *Acta Haematol.* 1990;84:201-203.

Starkebaum G. Chronic neutropenia associated with autoimmune disease. *Semin Hematol.* 2002;39:121-127.

Sternberg A, Eagleton H, Pillai N, et al. Neutropenia and anaemia associated with T-cell large granular lymphocyte leukaemia responds to fludarabine with minimal toxicity. *Br J Haematol.* 2003;120:699-701.

Vulliamy T, Dokal I. Dyskeratosis congenita. *Semin Hematol.* 2006;43:157-166.

Vulliamy TJ, Marrone A, Knight SW, et al. Mutations in dyskeratosis congenita: their impact on telomere length and the diversity of clinical presentation. *Blood.* 2006;107:2680-2685.

Welte K, Zeidler C, Dale DC. Severe congenital neutropenia. *Semin Hematol.* 2006;43:189-195.

Wilson C. Laboratory evaluation of blood and bone marrow in non-neoplastic disorders. In: King D, Gardner W, Sobin L, et al., eds. *Non-Neoplastic Disorders of Bone Marrow.* (AFIP fascicle). Washington, DC: American Registry of Pathology; 2008:57-73.

Wilson C. Non-neoplastic granulocytic and monocytic disorders In: King D, Gardner W, Sobin L, et al., eds. *Non-Neoplastic Disorders of Bone Marrow* (AFIP fascicle). Washington, DC: American Registry of Pathology; 2008:125-175.

CHAPTER 21

Functional Defects of Granulocytes

Kathryn Foucar, MD

Adequate neutrophil function is essential for protection from invading bacteria and fungi. Patients with significant neutrophil function defects, especially from constitutional disorders, are susceptible to recurrent bacterial and fungal infections. All genetic disorders of neutrophil function are extremely rare and infrequently encountered in clinical practice. In contrast, acquired neutrophil function defects are much more common but generally are not severe. In fact, many acquired neutrophil function defects, although apparent by various in vitro tests using normal donor neutrophils as controls, may lack clinical significance.

21.1 Pathophysiology

Neutrophil function is a complex and highly regulated process requiring normal levels and functional activity of various cytoplasmic components and membrane proteins, as well as an external environment that contains adequate chemotactic factors, complement levels, cytokines, and normal endothelial cell function. A series of interrelated activities are required to accomplish neutrophil destruction of invading bacteria and fungi. Neutrophils must be produced in adequate numbers by the bone marrow and appropriately released into the peripheral blood (see Chapters 16 and 20). Circulating neutrophils must be able to sense chemotactic factors released in the vicinity of bacterial or fungal invasion. Appropriate ligands on the surface of the neutrophil are necessary to bind these chemotactic factors, which include immunoglobulins, complement components, bacterial metabolites, and denatured neutrophil proteins. These neutrophils must then attach to endothelial cells, egress through the blood vessel wall, and migrate to the specific site of invasion. Adhesion of neutrophils to endothelial cells is accomplished by the binding of neutrophil adhesion molecules (integrins such as CD11a,b/CD18, the selectin CD62L, or selectin ligand CD162) to the surface of the endothelial cells. The complex role of endothelial cell/neutrophil interactions is an area of active investigation. Newly identified roles for CD157 and CD177 in response to acute infection and in enhanced neutrophil diapedisis have been recognized.

Neutrophil migration involves a repetitive sequential series of receptor binding, signal transduction, and remodeling of the neutrophil cytoskeleton. Neutrophils must subsequently recognize, bind, and surround tightly with cell membrane, phagocytose, and finally destroy these invading bacteria or fungi. This destruction is achieved by degranulation (fusion of a granule with phagolysosome) and activation of nicotinamide adenine dinucleotide phosphate (NADPH)-dependent oxidase. Neutrophil granules contain microbicidal enzymes, which are of high concentration when released into the small phagolysosomes.

Both chemotaxis and microbial phagocytosis/destruction require the integrated activity of cytoplasmic cytoskeletal proteins, cytoplasmic granules, and surface membrane constituents of neutrophils. In addition, many factors external to granulocytes are essential for normal function. For example, the complement system, various immunoglobulins, and several inflammatory cytokine mediators are all required for many of these neutrophil activities. Cytokines such as the colony-stimulating factors also enhance functional activities of mature neutrophils by binding to specific cell membrane receptors. Once microorganisms have been engulfed by neutrophils, an oxidative reaction called "respiratory burst" is often required for their destruction. Neutrophil constitutive death is also critical for modulating neutrophil number and function as well as maintaining homeostasis.

Any abnormality in this complex series of neutrophil functions can result in increased susceptibility to bacterial or fungal infections, including infections with low-virulence organisms. These neutrophil function abnormalities can be either constitutional (genetic) or acquired, and are generally classified as defects in adhesion, motility, granule formation, and phagocytic/killing activity **t21.1**. In some disorders, especially in acquired conditions, more than 1 type of defect is evident. Because sophisticated methods to investigate neutrophil function are relatively new, many neutrophil function defects have been only recently categorized. In addition to intrinsic neutrophil abnormalities, disorders in the complement cascade and immunoglobulins also cause neutrophil dysfunction.

All constitutional neutrophil function defects are exceedingly rare; these hereditary disorders are typically manifested during infancy and early childhood. Hereditary neutrophil function disorders are often severe; consequently, patients develop numerous recurrent and progressive bacterial and fungal infections, often associated with poor wound healing.

Chédiak-Higashi syndrome was the first recognized constitutional neutrophil function disorder. This autosomal recessive, multisystem disease is the consequence of defects in granule structure and function that affect many cells throughout the body. Because of abnormalities in melanosome structure, affected patients often have oculocutaneous albinism; platelet granule defects are linked to bleeding disorders. Abnormal granules are apparent within all granulated hematopoietic cells and even within lymphocytes (see Chapter 22). Because of this defective cytoplasmic granulation, many cells die within the bone marrow, resulting in neutropenia and thrombocytopenia. Although neutrophil defects are primarily responsible for the increased susceptibility to infection in patients with Chédiak-Higashi syndrome, functional defects of eosinophils, basophils, and monocytes also are present. The abnormal cytoplasmic granulation in Chédiak-Higashi syndrome results in both impaired motility (ie, defective chemotaxis) and defective degranulation.

Chronic granulomatous disease is another rare type of constitutional neutrophil function disorder that results from mutations in the genes encoding subunits of NADPH oxidase. Most cases of this disease are X-linked recessive disorders, although autosomal recessive subtypes of chronic granulomatous disease also have been described. The onset of disease is characteristically within the first year of life, although milder forms may not manifest until adulthood. Patients with this disease frequently have lymphadenopathy, hepatosplenomegaly, and anemia of chronic disease. Dominant sites of recurrent infection include lung, skin, gastrointestinal tract, and lymph node; widespread multiorgan granuloma formation is a hallmark of this disease. Older patients often demonstrate restrictive lung disease; severe gastrointestinal disease is seen less frequently. Patients with chronic granulomatous disease demonstrate multiple types of defects related to the generation of NADPH oxidase that result in failed oxidative reactions (respiratory burst). Consequently, ingested organisms are not killed.

Three types of leukocyte adhesion deficiency (LAD types I, II, and III) have been described. These rare genetic disorders of neutrophil adhesion/chemotaxis are characterized by severe, recurrent bacterial infections. Children affected by LAD type II may manifest dysmorphic features. In LAD type I the adhesion molecule CD11/CD18 is defective, whereas defects in selectin-dependent leukocyte rolling adherence characterize the more uncommon LAD type II. Multiple mutations

t21.1 Classification of Constitutional and Acquired Functional Defects of Neutrophils

General Type of Defect	Constitutional Disorders	Acquired Disorders/Conditions*
Adhesion defects	Leukocyte adhesion deficiency (Types I, II, III)	Aging Alcohol-induced Drug effects (corticosteroids, epinephrine, aspirin) Diabetes Renal disorders Chronic infections Paraproteinemias Sickle cell anemia
Defects in granule structure/function	Chédiak-Higashi syndrome Specific (secondary) granule deficiency Myeloperoxidase deficiency	Myeloproliferative neoplasms, AML, myelodysplasia (hematologic neoplasms) Severe thermal injury Trauma/surgery Pregnancy
Motility/chemotaxis defects	Chédiak-Higashi syndrome Complement disorders Leukocyte adhesion deficiency Neutrophil actin deficiency Other actin and microtubular defects Specific granule deficiency Hyperimmunoglobulin E syndrome with associated chemotactic defects of neutrophils and monocytes Storage disease, eg, Gaucher Rac 2 deficiency	Autoimmune disorders (collagen vascular disorders) Diabetes, cirrhosis Renal failure Numerous medications interfere with neutrophil migration (eg, colchicine, numerous anti-inflammatory agents) Chronic infections including HIV-1 Malnutrition Hematologic neoplasms Thermal injury Bone marrow transplant Paroxysmal nocturnal hemoglobinuria Graft-versus-host disease Recombinant interleukin-2 therapy
Phagocytic/killing defects	Chronic granulomatous disease (several types) Complement disorders Myeloperoxidase deficiency Specific granule deficiency Immunodeficiency disorders with decreased immunoglobulins	Autoimmune disorders (collagen vascular disorders) Thermal injury Hematologic neoplasms Diabetes, cirrhosis Trauma/surgery/splenectomy Bone marrow transplant Graft-versus-host disease Malnutrition Chronic infections including HIV-1 Sickle cell anemia

**Many acquired disorders/conditions are associated with multiple types of neutrophil function defects as determined by in vitro studies; clinical significance variable*
HIV-1 = human immunodeficiency virus-1; AML = acute myeloid leukemia

have been identified primarily in the gene encoding the b2 subunit of CD18; CD18 is a component of 4 major adhesion molecules (the integrins CD11a, CD11b, CD11c, and CD11d). Reduced expression of these integrins in patients with LAD type I results in 2 key functional defects: (1) neutrophils fail to adhere to and migrate through the endothelium and (2) neutrophils cannot bind CD3bi opsonized microorganisms. Mutations in golgi GDP-fucose transporter have been identified in patients with LAD type II. A third type of LAD with severe defects in integrin activation by chemokine signals has also been described.

Acquired neutrophil function disorders are usually less severe than constitutional defects. Either in patients with a wide variety of diseases/conditions or in patients receiving numerous types of therapeutic agents, neutrophils may demonstrate many functional aberrations by in vitro techniques when compared with control neutrophils obtained from normal volunteers **t21.1**. Whether these in vitro aberrations represent true functional defects or a physiologic response to the underlying disorder is unknown, especially in patients with non-neoplastic conditions. In contrast, in patients with hematologic neoplasms such as acute myeloid leukemia (AML) or myelodysplasia (MDS), neutrophil function abnormalities are a reflection of a defective myeloid clone and are linked to increased susceptibility to bacterial infections. However, in both AML and MDS, the concurrent decrease in absolute neutrophil count is a key factor in the increased risk of bacterial infections. Neutrophil function defects also are readily identifiable in patients with chronic myeloproliferative disorders, especially chronic myelogenous leukemia, although generally these defects are not clinically significant.

In the non-neoplastic acquired disorders/conditions/drug treatments listed in **t21.1**, the significance of the detection of in vitro neutrophil defects is less clear-cut. Although some patients, such as those with either chronic renal failure or poorly controlled diabetes mellitus, are clearly at increased risk for bacterial infections, the cause of this increased susceptibility is complex, involving many environmental factors that interfere with neutrophil function. The significance of drug-mediated neutrophil function defects is similarly unclear, because drug interference with neutrophil function has typically been documented using in vitro techniques with very high drug concentrations. Consequently, these neutrophil function defects may not be clinically relevant, except in patients receiving exceptionally high doses of the specific medication.

Finally, there are physiologic age variations in neutrophil function. Neonates, especially those born prematurely, frequently demonstrate impaired functional activities of neutrophils and monocytes, including defects in bone marrow release, cellular activation, and chemotaxis. This, in part, explains the increased susceptibility of newborns to serious bacterial infections. Likewise, elderly patients may develop aberrations in neutrophil adhesion, resulting in mild functional impairment.

21.2 Clinical Findings

Most constitutional neutrophil function defects are manifested in infancy or early childhood, whereas acquired defects are substantially more prevalent in adults. The clinical findings vary, depending on the severity of the defect. However, patients with profound neutrophil function defects characteristically present with severe recurrent bacterial and (less often) fungal infections that involve skin, oral cavity, sinuses and lung, lymph nodes, and gastrointestinal tract. Gingivitis is particularly prevalent in these patients. Progressive organ damage can result from recurrent infections. Recurrent pneumonias may lead to bronchiectasis, and recurrent infections along the gastrointestinal tract may cause fistulas and abscesses.

In patients with either adhesion or motility defects, inadequate numbers of neutrophils reach infection sites. The lack of pus is a unique feature in such patients, and there may be few localizing clinical signs and symptoms of infection.

21.3 Diagnostic Approach

Although a neutrophil function defect should be considered in children and adults with severe recurrent bacterial and fungal infections, in actual practice most patients with recurrent infections do not exhibit a demonstrable neutrophil function defect. However, in the subgroup of patients with a likely defect, the approach should include both the distinction between a constitutional and acquired defect and an attempt to categorize the nature of the abnormality. In general, the evaluation of these patients should comprise the following elements:

1. A complete blood count with differential.
2. A quantitative and morphologic evaluation of neutrophils and other lineages.
3. A detailed history regarding the frequency, severity, sites, and types of recurrent infections; age of onset; and family history.
4. A physical examination to assess for scars, abscesses, and pulmonary infiltrates; a careful evaluation of skin, oral cavity, respiratory tract, and anal region.
5. An evaluation for other features of constitutional neutrophil function defects, such as oculocutaneous albinism in Chédiak-Higashi syndrome.
6. An evaluation for evidence of underlying disorders and drug treatments linked to acquired neutrophil function defects in adults.
7. An assessment of immune status, complement component levels, immunoglobulin levels, and CH50.
8. Testing for HIV-1 in appropriate situations.

Specialized tests for neutrophil function also should be considered. Because these tests are ordered infrequently in clinical practice, most are performed only in specialized referral laboratories. The appropriateness and sequence of specialized neutrophil function testing should be determined on an individual basis. These specialized tests include:

Nitroblue tetrazolium test (indirect measurement of respiratory burst activity)
Flow cytometric assessment for oxidative burst
Myeloperoxidase stain of neutrophils
Flow cytometric evaluation of neutrophil surface membrane for expression of CD11/CD18 (adhesion molecules), CD15s (selectin ligand), CD157, CD177, and other molecules
Assessment of neutrophil motility, chemotaxis, and adhesion properties
Superoxidase generation (other tests of oxidation)
Electron microscopy to evaluate neutrophil granules, especially in patients with possible specific (secondary) granule deficiency

21.4 Hematologic Findings

21.4.1 Blood Cell Measurements

Depending on both the nature of the neutrophil function defect and whether the patient is actively infected, the blood cell measurements are variable. Patients with ongoing infection often demonstrate an absolute neutrophilia with toxic changes. Extremely high elevations of the absolute neutrophil count are characteristic of constitutional leukocyte adhesion disorders because of the inability of these cells to bind to endothelium and consequently migrate to tissues. In affected patients, the absolute neutrophil count may exceed $100 \times 10^3/mm^3$ ($100 \times 10^3/L$). In contrast, neutropenia is a frequent finding in Chédiak-Higashi syndrome secondary to ineffective granulopoiesis from intramedullary cell death. Patients with recurrent infections also may develop anemia of chronic disease.

21.4.2 Peripheral Blood Smear Morphology

Except for the massively enlarged granules that characterize Chédiak-Higashi syndrome, morphologic findings in patients with neutrophil function defects generally are not distinctive, although both bilobed nuclei with abnormal nuclear membranes and absent secondary granules have been noted in cases of neutrophil-specific granule deficiency (see i22.1, 22.4). Other morphologic aberrations, such as Pelger-Huët and May-Hegglin anomalies, are described in Chapter 22.

21.4.3 Bone Marrow Examination

Granulocytic hyperplasia is an anticipated finding in patients with neutrophil function defects who suffer from recurrent infections. In addition, granulomas may be evident, especially in patients with recurrent fungal infections. Indications for bone marrow examination in patients with neutrophil function abnormalities include assessment for infection, unexplained blood cytopenia, and evaluation for possible secondary hemophagocytic syndrome or secondary lymphoproliferative disorder (notably in patients with Chédiak-Higashi syndrome).

21.5 Other Laboratory Tests

Test 21.5.1 Nitroblue Tetrazolium Dye Test

Purpose. The nitroblue tetrazolium (NBT) test is used to indirectly detect the production of superoxide by neutrophils, such as during a respiratory burst.

Principle. NBT is a soluble yellow dye that is converted to an insoluble blue-black compound when neutrophils are capable of undergoing oxidative metabolism. This insoluble material precipitates within neutrophil cytoplasm and can be seen by light microscopy. Neutrophils that fail to reduce NBT lack this oxidative capability.

Specimen. Heparinized blood can be used for activated NBT tests.

Procedure. Stimulated neutrophils are incubated with NBT. The dye is reduced by oxidative enzymes within granules in neutrophils and monocytes. Following incubation, blood smears are prepared and stained with Wright stain. A differential cell count is performed by separating neutrophils into those containing or lacking the blue-black precipitate. Appropriate controls are used.

Interpretation. Indirect evidence of production of superoxide is present when neutrophils contain the blue-black precipitate. Neutrophils that fail to reduce NBT are evident in chronic granulomatous disease, as well as in other neutrophil enzyme deficiency disorders, some complement deficiency conditions, and agammaglobulinemias. Abnormal test results also can be useful in identifying female carriers. Normal ranges should be determined within individual laboratories.

Notes and Precautions. The NBT test cannot be performed on ethylenediaminetetraacetic acid (EDTA)–anticoagulated specimens. Likewise, heparin forms complexes with NBT that are ingested by neutrophils, making heparin an undesirable anticoagulant for examining spontaneous NBT-reducing activity. However, the incubated NBT-reducing activity using stimulated neutrophils is not affected by heparin anticoagulation. Although the NBT test is still used to assess superoxide production, it has largely been replaced by flow cytometric techniques that employ fluorescence detection methods to measure oxidant production.

Test 21.5.2 Myeloperoxidase Stain

Purpose. This cytochemical stain is used to evaluate the presence of myeloperoxidase within neutrophil granules.

Principle. The myeloperoxidase enzyme of granulocyte primary granules reduces substrate dyes in a colorimetric reaction, producing an insoluble compound that precipitates within the cytoplasm of neutrophils.

Specimen. Freshly prepared air-dried blood smears are used for this test.

Procedure. A colorless substrate (usually benzidine dihydrochloride) and hydrogen peroxide are layered on the peripheral blood smear. During the incubation, the myeloperoxidase present within neutrophil primary granules converts hydrogen peroxide into water and oxygen, which oxidizes the substrate and produces a blue-black precipitate. After counterstaining, cells are viewed under a light microscope, and the proportion of positive neutrophils is determined.

Interpretation. Normal neutrophils demonstrate strong positive granular reactivity throughout the cytoplasm. In patients with myeloperoxidase deficiency, no staining or weak staining may be identified; Sudan black B staining is typically negative in these patients.

Notes and Precautions. Optimal pH is essential for this enzymatic reaction. Myeloperoxidase is degraded by exposure to light, and the test should generally be performed within a few hours of obtaining the specimen. Although deficiency of myeloperoxidase is the most common inherited disorder of neutrophil function, most patients do not suffer from infectious complications. However, myeloperoxidase deficiency may be a cofactor in infectious complications in patients with systemic illnesses, notably diabetes. Detection of this generally clinically insignificant condition has increased with the use of automated hematology instruments that identify and quantitate neutrophils based on myeloperoxidase activity.

Test 21.5.3 Flow Cytometry

Flow cytometric immunophenotype or surface antigenic profile of neutrophils as well as flow cytometry utilizing dihydrorhodamine to assess oxidative burst. (See 63.1–63.5 for specimens, procedure, principle, and interpretation of flow cytometry).

21.6 Ancillary Tests

Many tests have been developed to assess different types of neutrophil function activities (see "21.3 Diagnostic Approach" above). The decision to perform these sophisticated tests should be determined on a case-by-case basis. Likewise, the sequence of testing strategies in patients with a presumed neutrophil function abnormality should be determined individually. Additional specialized tests of neutrophil function include:

1. Adherence of neutrophils to nylon wool fiber or to plastic tissue culture plates.
2. Measurements of various granule constituents, such as lactoferrin, as well as degranulation.
3. Assessment of bacterial killing ability, in addition to respiratory burst.
4. Flow cytometric methods to assess neutrophil oxidant production.

21.7 Course and Treatment

In patients with severe neutrophil function defects (typically constitutional defects), significant morbidity and mortality is associated with recurrent bacterial or fungal infections; prompt antibiotic therapy for established or suspected infections is essential. In addition, antibiotic prophylaxis is commonly prescribed. Patients should avoid cats, plants that have thorns, and other sources of skin infection, since these infections typically spread rapidly. Despite aggressive management, affected patients may develop severe organ failure, most commonly pulmonary failure as a result of tissue destruction from repeated infections. Response to immune-modulating agents such as recombinant human interferon-g has been achieved in patients with chronic granulomatous disease, presumably through stimulation of the macrophage oxidative pathway, although this mechanism was not documented in a recent clinical trial. Bone marrow transplantation has been attempted, with suboptimal results, in small numbers of patients with constitutional neutrophil function defects. Because the specific gene mutations in many of the constitutional disorders of granulocyte function are known, the potential for gene therapy to correct these genetic abnormalities is being actively investigated. Genetic tests also can be used for prenatal diagnosis using chorionic villus biopsy samples.

21.8 References

Bogomolski-Yahalom V, Matzner Y. Disorders of neutrophil function. *Blood Rev.* 1995;9:183-190.

Boxer LA, Blackwood RA. Leukocyte disorders: quantitative and qualitative disorders of the neutrophil, part 2. *Pediatr Rev.* 1996;17:47-50.

Brown J, Thrasher A. Disorders of phagocyte function. In: Wickramasinghe S, McCullough J, eds. *Blood and Bone Marrow Pathology.* Edinburgh: Churchill Livingstone. 2003:321-329.

Cacciapuoti C, Terrazzano G, Barone L, et al. Glycosyl-phosphatidyl-inositol-defective granulocytes from paroxysmal nocturnal haemoglobinuria patients show increased bacterial ingestion but reduced respiratory burst induction. *Am J Hematol.* 2007;82:98-107.

Dale DC, Boxer L, Liles WC. The phagocytes: neutrophils and monocytes. Blood 2008;112:935-945.

Fletcher J, Haynes AP, Crouch SM. Acquired abnormalities of polymorphonuclear neutrophil function. *Blood Rev.* 1990;4:103-110.

Gohring K, Wolff J, Doppl W, et al. Neutrophil CD177 (NB1 gp, HNA-2a) expression is increased in severe bacterial infections and polycythaemia vera. *Br J Haematol.* 2004;126:252-254.

Gombart AF, Shiohara M, Kwok SH, et al. Neutrophil-specific granule deficiency: homozygous recessive inheritance of a frameshift mutation in the gene encoding transcription factor CCAAT/enhancer binding protein--epsilon. *Blood.* 2001;97:2561-2567.

Helmus Y, Denecke J, Yakubenia S, et al. Leukocyte adhesion deficiency II patients with a dual defect of the GDP-fucose transporter. *Blood.* 2006;107:3959-3966.

Kinashi T, Aker M, Sokolovsky-Eisenberg M, et al. LAD-III, a leukocyte adhesion deficiency syndrome associated with defective Rap1 activation and impaired stabilization of integrin bonds. *Blood.* 2004;103:1033-1036.

Larson RS. Immunodeficiency disorders. In: Collins RD, Swerdlow S, eds. *Pediatric Hematopathology.* New York, NY: Churchill Livingstone. 2001:21-40.

Latger-Cannard V, Besson I, Doco-Lecompte T, Lecompte T. A standardized procedure for quantitation of CD11b on polymorphonuclear neutrophil by flow cytometry: potential application in infectious diseases. *Clin Lab Haematol.* 2004;26:177-186.

Luo HR, Loison F. Constitutive neutrophil apoptosis: mechanisms and regulation. *Am J Hematol* 2008;83:288-295.

Matzner Y. Acquired neutrophil dysfunction and diseases with an inflammatory component. *Semin Hematol.* 1997;34:291-302.

Newburger PE. Disorders of neutrophil number and function. *Hematology Am Soc Hematol Educ Program.* 2006:104-110.

Ortolan E, Tibaldi EV, Ferranti B, et al. CD157 plays a pivotal role in neutrophil transendothelial migration. *Blood.* 2006;108:4214-4222.

Rae J, Noack D, Heyworth PG, et al. Molecular analysis of 9 new families with chronic granulomatous disease caused by mutations in CYBA, the gene encoding p22(phox). *Blood.* 2000;96:1106-1112.

Romano M, Dri P, Dadalt L, et al. Biochemical and molecular characterization of hereditary myeloperoxidase deficiency. *Blood.* 1997;90:4126-4134.

Szczur K, Xu H, Atkinson S, et al. Rho GTPase CDC42 regulates directionality and random movement via distinct MAPK pathways in neutrophils. *Blood.* 2006;108:4205-4213.

Uzel G, Tng E, Rosenzweig SD, et al. Reversion mutations in patients with leukocyte adhesion deficiency type-1 (LAD-1). *Blood.* 2008;111:209-218.

Wagner C, Iking-Konert C, Denefleh B, et al. Granzyme B and perforin: constitutive expression in human polymorphonuclear neutrophils. *Blood.* 2004;103:1099-1104.

Walrand S, Valeix S, Rodriguez C, et al. Flow cytometry study of polymorphonuclear neutrophil oxidative burst: a comparison of three fluorescent probes. *Clin Chim Acta.* 2003;331:103-110.

Chapter 22

Granulocytic Disorders With Abnormal Morphology

Kathryn Foucar, MD

Both hereditary and acquired disorders are associated with morphologic abnormalities of neutrophils. These abnormalities include both nuclear and cytoplasmic aberrations. NucleaBoth hereditary and acquired disorders are associated with morphologic abnormalities of neutrophils. These abnormalities include both nuclear and cytoplasmic aberrations. Nuclear defects include hyposegmentation and hypersegmentation; cytoplasmic abnormalities include various types of inclusions, hypergranular cytoplasm, and hypogranular cytoplasm.

Although all hereditary disorders with abnormal neutrophils are rare, the more prevalent of these genetic disorders include Pelger-Huët anomaly, May-Hegglin anomaly, Chédiak-Higashi syndrome, and Alder-Reilly anomaly **t22.1**. Pelger-Huët anomaly is characterized by either bilobed or non-segmented neutrophil nuclei. The nuclear chromatin of these cells tends to be uniformly dense, their cytoplasm is unremarkable, and they demonstrate no significant functional abnormalities. Mutations in lamin B-receptor have been identified recently in kindreds with constitutional Pelger-Huët anomaly.

The neutrophils in May-Hegglin anomaly contain large blue cytoplasmic inclusions that resemble Döhle bodies. Similar inclusions also are evident in other granulated cells. Multiple mutations in MYH9 gene have been noted in patients with a spectrum of MYH9-related disorders. Additional hematologic abnormalities include thrombocytopenia, enlarged platelets, and variable neutropenia. Many of these patients are asymptomatic.

In contrast, patients with Chédiak-Higashi syndrome suffer from recurrent severe pyogenic infections and often die in childhood. Chédiak-Higashi syndrome is characterized by giant cytoplasmic granules that are present within all granulated cells (even in natural killer cells/lymphocytes) within the blood, bone marrow, and solid tissues. These giant granules represent fused lysosomes and are linked to many functional defects. Other abnormalities include neutropenia and thrombocytopenia, which are likely secondary to ineffective hematopoiesis. As a consequence of immunosuppression from decreased natural killer cell function, patients with Chédiak-Higashi syndrome may develop secondary viral infections (especially Epstein-Barr virus) that induce either florid hemophagocytic syndromes or lymphoproliferative disorders.

Intense azurophilic granulation of neutrophil cytoplasm characterizes the Alder-Reilly anomaly, which is associated with several types of genetic mucopolysaccharide disorders. Abnormalities of eosinophils, basophils, and lymphocytes also are evident in patients with these mucosaccharidoses.

Acquired morphologic neutrophilic abnormalities are substantially more common than their hereditary counterparts and are associated with both neoplastic and non-neoplastic hematologic disorders, as well as with other conditions **t22.2**. Morphologic abnormalities of both neutrophil nuclei and cytoplasm are common in patients with hematologic neoplasms such as myelodysplasia, acute myeloid leukemias, and chronic myelogenous leukemias, especially in transformation, reflecting the clonal nature of even mature blood elements in these neoplasms. For example, patients with these hematologic malignancies may demonstrate neutrophil pseudo–Pelger-Huët nuclei in conjunction with hypogranular cytoplasm. Less commonly, nuclear hypersegmentation may be evident in neutrophils from affected patients with clonal hematopoietic neoplasms. These morphologic aberrations are associated with functional defects.

t22.1 Hereditary Granulocyte Disorders With Abnormal Morphology

Disorder	Granulocyte Feature	Other Blood, Bone Marrow Abnormalities	Inheritance	Other Findings
Pelger-Huët anomaly **i22.1**	Bilobed or non-segmented neutrophil nuclei; cytoplasm normal	No other lineage abnormalities No functional abnormalities	Autosomal dominant	Mutations in lamin β-receptor identified in several kindreds
May-Hegglin anomaly **i22.1**	Large blue cytoplasmic inclusions resembling giant Döhle bodies	Thrombocytopenia Enlarged platelets Variable neutropenia Inclusions also in eosinophils, basophils, and monocytes	Autosomal dominant	Many patients are asymptomatic Multiple mutations in MYH9 gene described
Chédiak-Higashi syndrome **i22.1, i22.7**	Giant cytoplasmic granules	Neutropenia, thrombocytopenia All granulated cells and even lymphocytes/natural killer cells affected Represent fused lysosomes Functional defects of neutrophils Some patients develop infection, usually Epstein-Barr virus-associated hemophagocytic syndrome (accelerated phase) or Epstein-Barr virus–induced lymphoproliferative disorders	Autosomal recessive	Partial oculocutaneous albinism Frequent pyogenic infections Both neutrophil function defects and immunodeficiency from decreased natural killer cell function Mild bleeding tendency Progressive peripheral neuropathy
Alder-Reilly anomaly	Intense azurophilic granulation of neutrophil cytoplasm	Eosinophils and basophils contain large basophilic granules Vacuolated/abnormally granulated lymphocytes in some cases	Autosomal recessive	Associated with several different types of genetic mucopoly-saccharide disorders
Specific granule deficiency	Absence of secondary granules in cytoplasm imparts a pale appearance; nuclear hypo-segmentation also present	Abnormal granules (subset) in platelets and eosinophils	Autosomal recessive	Severe recurrent infections Mutations in C/EBP_{ε} gene Multiple functional defects of neutrophils
Myelokathexis **i22.8**	Shape abnormalities, pyknotic nuclei, hypersegmentation	Striking bone marrow abnormalities affecting all stages of granulopoiesis Neutropenia; intramedullary death of granulocytes Functional defects of neutrophils and monocytes	Autosomal dominant	Growth retardation Skeletal abnormalities Chemokine reception gene mutations
Hereditary hyperseg-mentation of neutrophils	Increased mean nuclear lobe index	No other abnormalities	Autosomal dominant	No associated findings
Hereditary giant neutrophils	Enlarged overall neutrophil size with hypersegmentation	Only a subset of neutrophils affected Other lineages unremarkable	Autosomal dominant	No associated findings

t22.2 Acquired Neutrophil Disorders With Abnormal Morphology †

Morphologic Abnormality	Other Hematologic Findings	Comments/Causes
Pseudo-Pelger-Huët change **i22.2, i22.3, i22.4**	Dependent on underlying cause	Found in patients with hematologic neoplasms (myelodysplasia, AML, CML) Small neutrophils with pseudo-Pelger-Huët nuclei and vacuolated cytoplasm described in myelodysplasia and AML associated with del(17p) Result of drug exposure (colchicine, sulfonamides, valproic acid, mycophenolate mofetil, tacrolimus) Linked to mycoplasma, HIV-1, influenza infections Rare finding after bone marrow transplantation
Hypersegmentation of neutrophils **i22.5, i22.9**	Varies depending on cause: pancytopenia, macrocytosis in patients with folate or vitamin B_{12} deficiency	Vitamin B_{12}or folate deficiency (occasional iron deficiency) Myelodysplasia, acute myeloid leukemia, other myeloid neoplasms Corticosteroid therapy, certain chemotherapeutic agents Hyperthermia, cocaine abuse
Hypogranular cytoplasm **i22.3**	Cytoplasmic hypogranulation and other lineage dyspoiesis common in myelodysplasia or myeloid leukemias Often found in association with nuclear segmentation abnormalities Dysplasia of other lineages common	Myelodysplasia Acute myeloid leukemias Chronic myeloid neoplasms, often in transformation
Cytoplasmic vacuoles	Variable; cytopenias common in copper deficiency	Distinct cytoplasmic vacuoles in granulocytic and erythroid precursors characteristic features of copper deficiency which may be secondary to excess zinc ingestion from homeopathic remedies Vacuoles in circulating neutrophils seen in sepsis and in ethanol toxicity
Cytoplasmic inclusions **i22.6**	Neutrophils and monocytes	Cryoglobulinemia Nuclear fragments (pseudo Howell-Jolly bodies) noted in HIV-1 infection and in other settings with immunosuppression
Giant neutrophils **i22.9**	Other hematologic abnormalities common in AIDS patients especially cytopenias	Advanced HIV-1 infection Pharmacologic G-CSF therapy
Striking karyorrhexis, other dyspoietic features	Striking dyserythropoiesis and karyorrhexis; megaloblastic changes; abnormal megakaryocytes	Arsenic poisoning; toxicity may also occur in APL patients treated with arsenic

†Mild dysplastic features common in bone marrow samples from normal elderly subjects.
AML = acute myeloid leukemia; CML = chronic myelogenous leukemia; G-CSF = granulocyte colony-stimulating factor; APL = acute promyelocytic leukemia

Other causes of acquired neutrophil hypersegmentation include vitamin B_{12} or folate deficiency, occasional drug treatments, iron deficiency, and renal insufficiency (see **t22.2**). Acquired Pelger-Huët change also is associated with certain drug exposures, notably colchicine, sulfonamide, and valproic acid therapy. This nuclear segmentation defect can be found in patients with mycoplasma infection, HIV-1 infection, and (rarely) in bone marrow transplant recipients. Likewise, several morphologic abnormalities of neutrophils, including pseudo–Pelger-Huët nuclear hyposegmentation, giant neutrophils, and neutrophils with Howell-Jolly–like cytoplasmic inclusions, have been described in patients with AIDS. Similar nuclear remnants (pseudo Howell-Jolly bodies) have been described within the cytoplasm of iatrogenically immunosuppressed patients. Prominent cytoplasmic inclusions are seen in neutrophils and monocytes in patients with cryoglobulinemia. Copper deficiency is associated with distinct cytoplasmic vacuoles in granulocytic and erythroid precursors, as well as in some maturing forms. Finally, mild dysplastic features have been noted in bone marrow specimens from healthy adults, especially elderly patients.

22.1 Pathophysiology

The pathophysiology of hereditary granulocytic disorders is linked to the underlying genetic defect. The cause of acquired neutrophil abnormalities is not always clear-cut. In patients with vitamin B_{12} or folate deficiency, the basic defect is an inability to undergo cell division (see Chapter 5), whereas the various nuclear and cytoplasmic abnormalities identified in patients with hematologic neoplasms are the consequence of an acquired clonal genetic defect. The cause of medication- or infection-associated morphologic abnormalities of neutrophils is generally unknown, but these changes should regress following successful treatment of the infection or cessation of the drug treatment.

22.2 Clinical Findings

Associated clinical findings in patients with hereditary neutrophil disorders are listed in **t22.1**. The clinical findings in patients with acquired neutrophil disorders are associated with the specific underlying disorder. Patients with hematologic neoplasms often experience fatigue, malaise, and fever if secondary infection has occurred. Likewise, splenomegaly and hepatomegaly may be evident in some of these patients.

22.3 Diagnostic Approach

When a morphologic neutrophilic abnormality is encountered, it is essential to determine whether it is a hereditary or an acquired defect. The cause of acquired defects, either neoplastic or non-neoplastic, also must be determined. The integration of clinical findings, other hematologic parameters, medical history, and the physical examination generally allow for these distinctions. The evaluation of a patient with neutrophil morphologic abnormalities generally includes the following steps:

1. A complete blood count (CBC) with differential.
2. A morphologic review of neutrophils and other lineages.
3. A family history and possible evaluation of other family members.
4. An evaluation for evidence of underlying infection.
5. An evaluation for evidence of bleeding.
6. An evaluation for evidence of a hematologic neoplasm.

7. An assessment for drug treatments and other conditions linked to specific morphologic abnormalities of neutrophils.
8. An evaluation for phenotypic abnormalities that occur in constitutional neutrophil disorders.
9. An evaluation for possible secondary lymphoproliferative disorders or infection-associated hemophagocytic syndrome in selected patients with genetic disorders, especially Chédiak-Higashi syndrome.

22.4 Hematologic Findings

22.4.1 Blood Cell Measurements

Several of the hereditary and acquired granulocytic disorders with abnormal morphology are associated with cytopenias, most notably neutropenia and/or thrombocytopenia. Anemia also may be evident in patients with recurrent chronic infections and in patients with underlying hematologic malignancies.

22.4.2 Peripheral Blood Smear Morphology

The various morphologic abnormalities of neutrophil nuclei and cytoplasm in patients with either hereditary or acquired granulocytic disorders are delineated in **t22.1** and **t22.2** (i22.1–i22.6). In addition, enlarged platelets characterize May-Hegglin anomaly; cytoplasmic abnormalities of other granulated cells or lymphocytes/natural killer cells may be encountered in patients with May-Hegglin anomaly, Chédiak-Higashi syndrome, and Alder-Reilly anomaly (see **t22.1**). In patients with acquired neutrophil abnormalities, other blood findings suggestive of myeloid neoplasms may be evident; multilineage abnormalities also are evident in megaloblastic anemia i22.2, i22.3, i22.5.

i22.1 Morphologic abnormalities

Blood smears illustrating morphologic abnormalities in **a** Pelger-Huët anomaly, **b** May-Hegglin anomaly, and **c** Chédiak-Higashi syndrome. *(Wright stain) (image* **c** *courtesy P Ward, MD)*

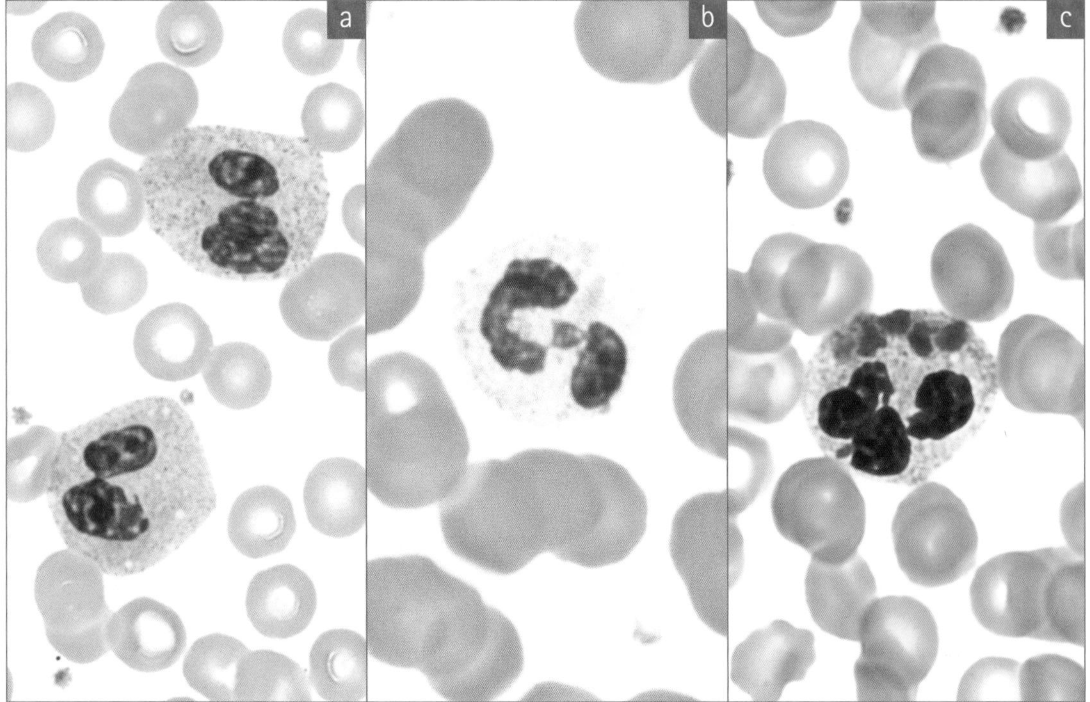

i22.2 Pseudo–Pelger-Huët anomaly

Peripheral blood showing circulating myeloblasts along with mononuclear pseudo–Pelger-Huët neutrophil in patient with acute myeloid leukemia. *(Wright stain)*

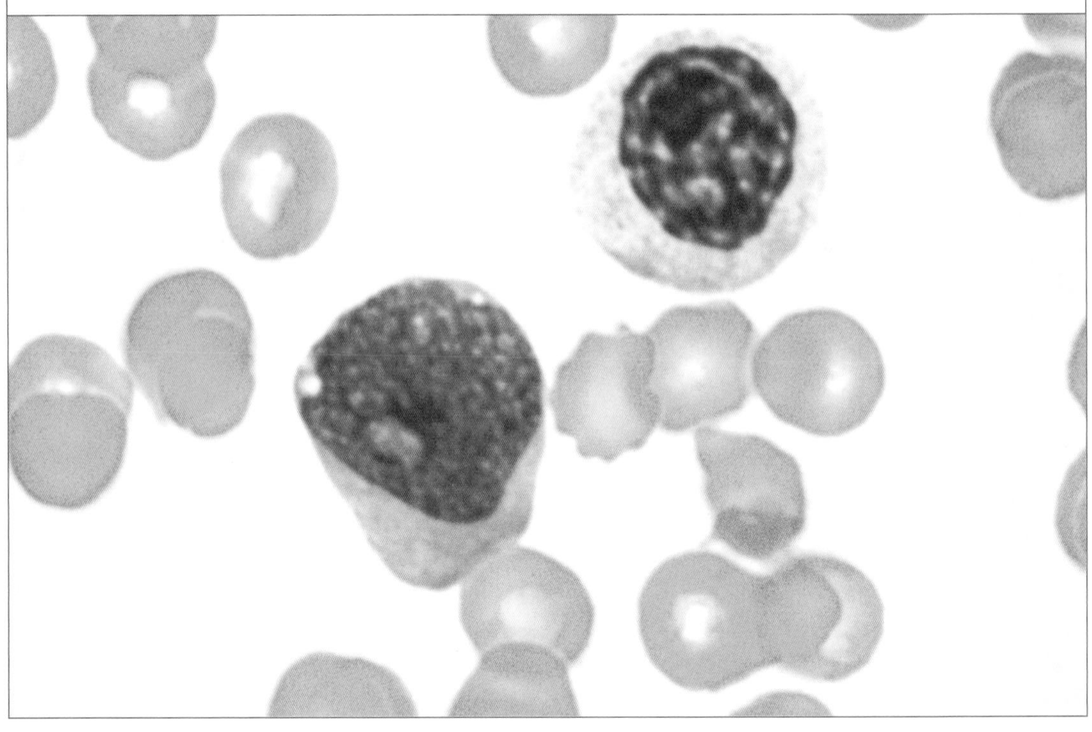

i22.3 Pseudo–Pelger-Huët anomaly

a Typical bilobed pseudo–Pelger-Huët neutrophil in patient with acute myeloid leukemia. Note hypogranular cytoplasm. **b** Pseudo–Pelger-Huët neutrophil with normally granulated cytoplasm evident in peripheral blood of patient receiving valproic acid. (**b** *courtesy M T Elghetany, MD*)

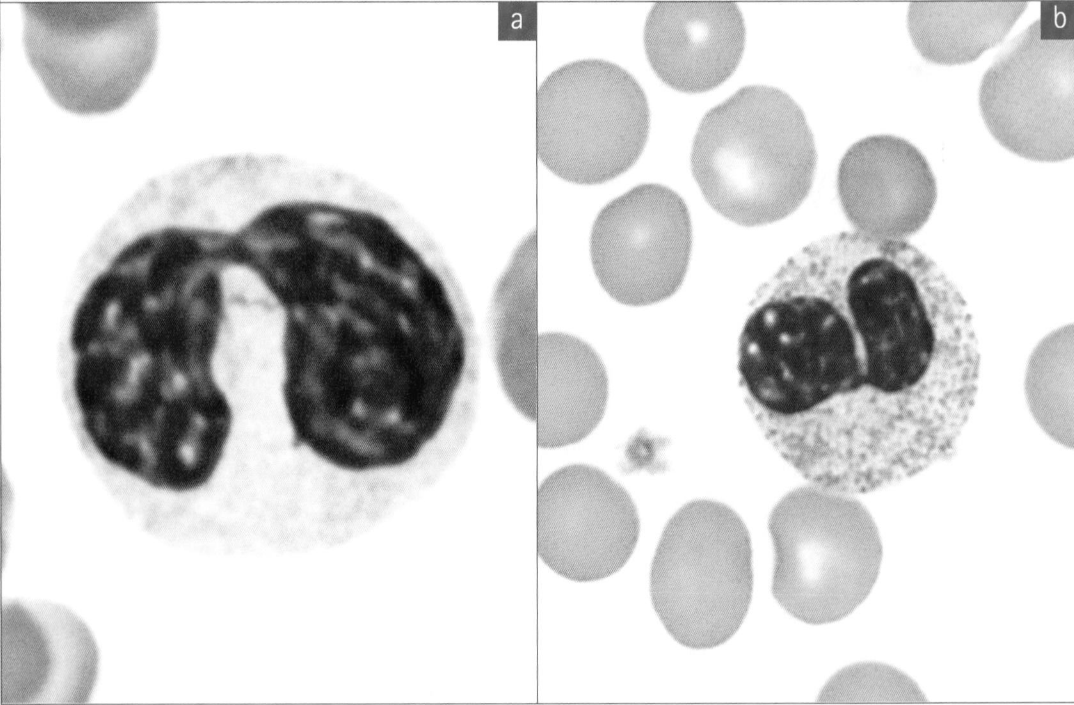

i22.4 Pseudo Pelger-Huët anomaly

Mononuclear pseudo Pelger-Huët cell in blood following chemotherapy. *(Wright stain)*

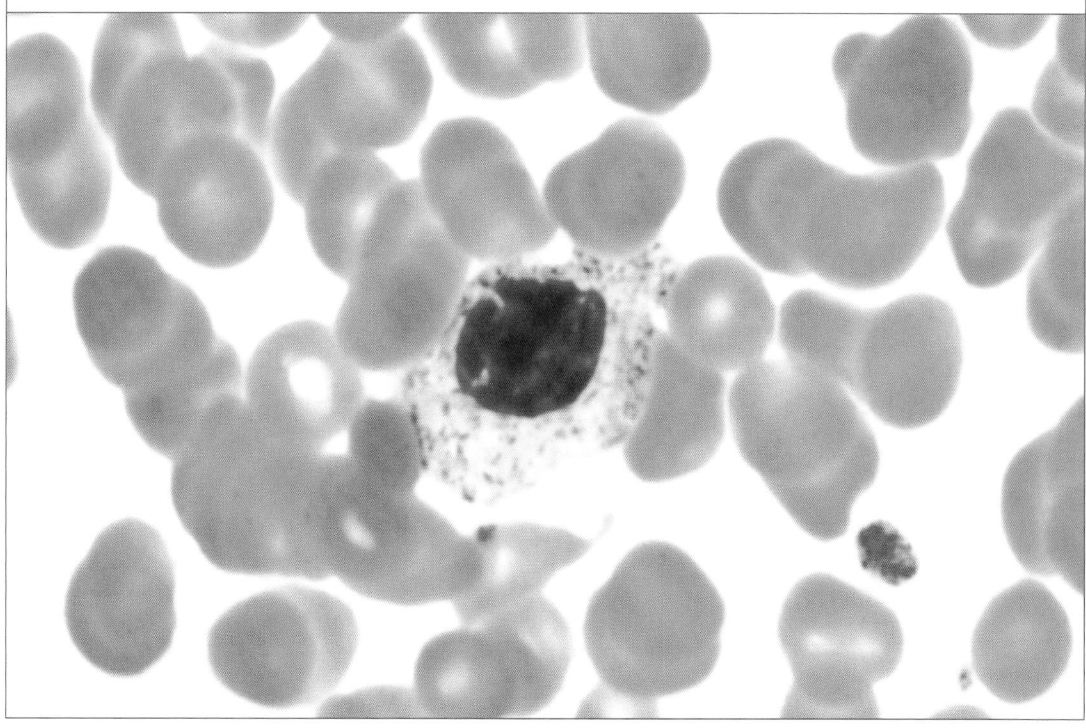

i22.5 Neutrophil hypersegmentation

a Blood composite illustrating neutrophil hypersegmentation in iron deficiency. **b** AML; note myeloblast. *(Wright stain)*

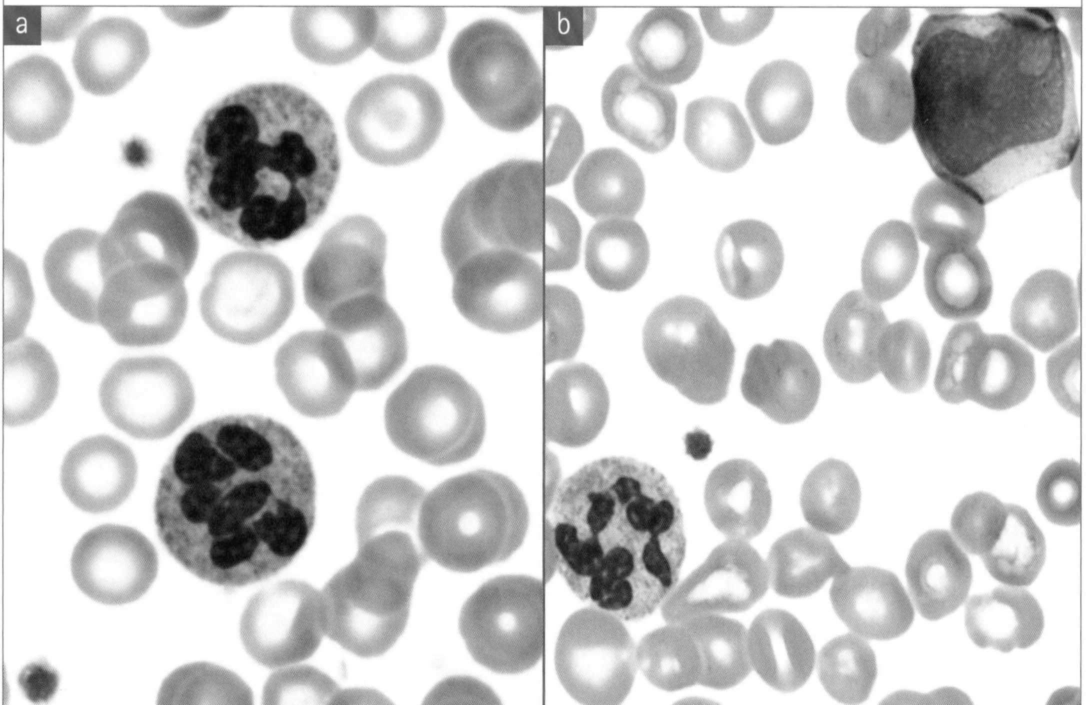

i22.6 Pseudo Howell-Jolly body

Pseudo Howell-Jolly body in neutrophil cytoplasm in child with Costelle syndrome. *(Wright stain)*

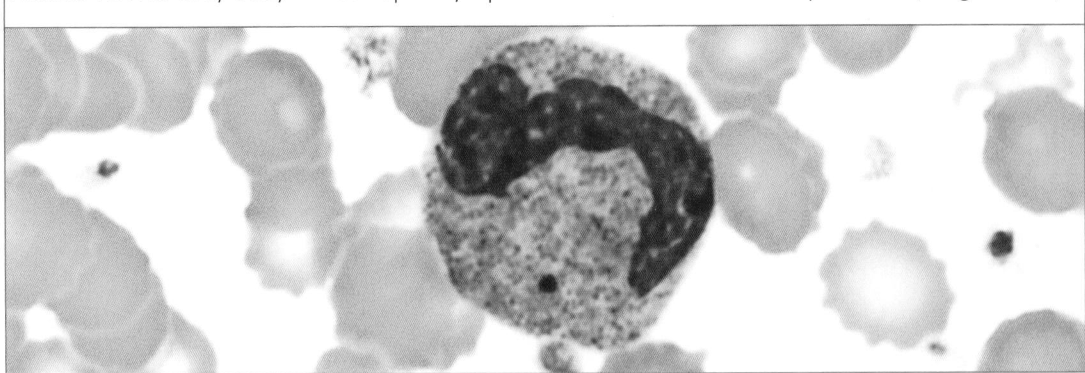

i22.7 Chédiak-Higashi syndrome

Bone marrow aspirate smear from patient with Chédiak-Higashi syndrome illustrating myeloid hyperplasia with dysmorphic granules in granulocytic and eosinophilic lineages. *(Wright stain) (courtesy Russell Brynes, MD)*

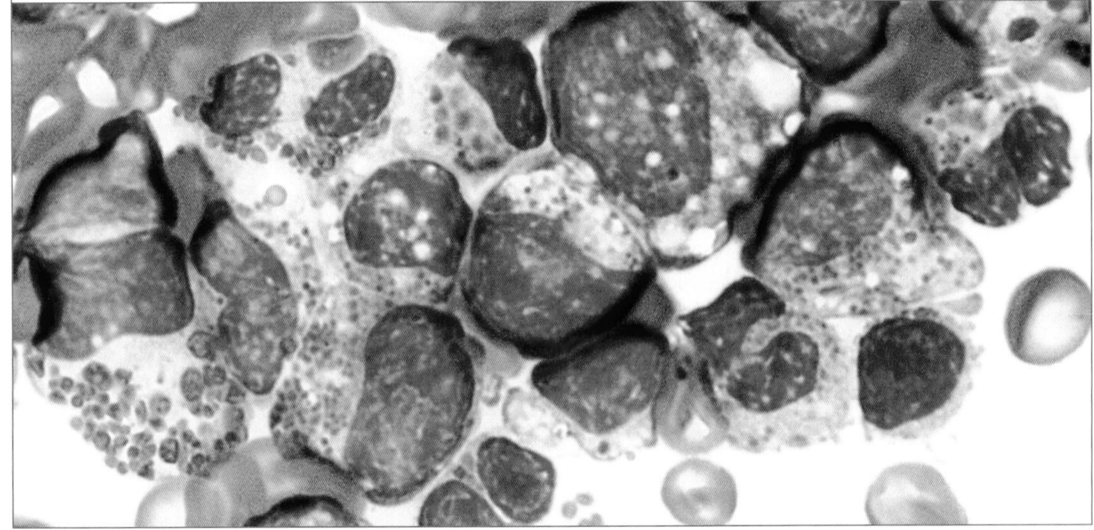

22.4.3 *Bone Marrow Examination*

Bone marrow examination generally is not required in patients with hereditary granulocytic disorders, unless warranted for cultures, assessment for a secondary neoplasm, or a possible infection-associated hemophagocytic disorder i22.7, i22.8. In contrast, bone marrow examination may be necessary to determine whether an acquired neutrophil disorder is the consequence of a hematologic neoplasm.

22.5 Ancillary Tests

Neutrophil function tests may be warranted in selected patients with morphologic neutrophil abnormalities. In addition, assessment of vitamin B_{12} or folate levels is appropriate in patients demonstrating nuclear hypersegmentation. Cytogenetic studies are warranted for patients with likely hematologic neoplasms.

i22.8 Myelokathexis

Bone marrow aspirate in patient with myelokathexis illustrating marked myeloid hyperplasia with nuclear segmentation abnormalities of maturing granulocytic elements. *(Wright stain) (courtesy Steve Kroft, MD)*

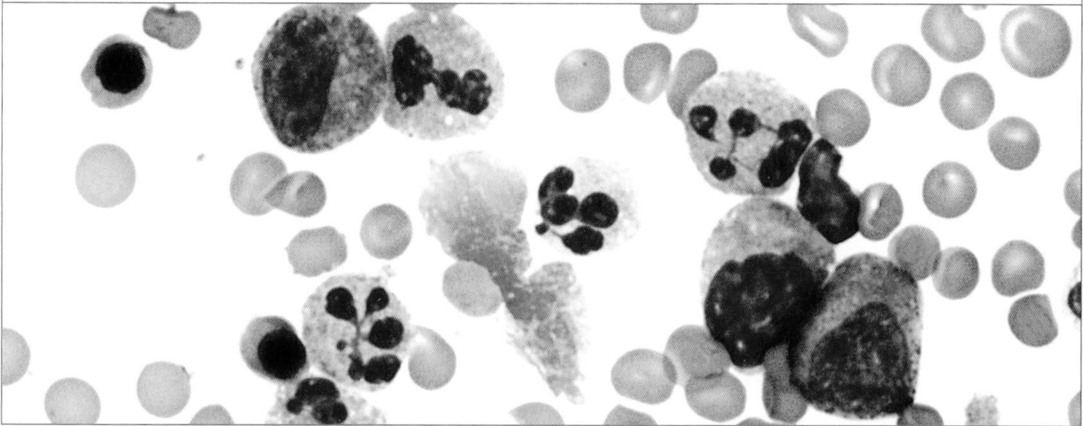

i22.9 Chemotherapy effect

Bone marrow aspirate smear from patient receiving induction chemotherapy demonstrating markedly enlarged and hypersegmented mature neutrophil secondary to chemotherapy effect. *(Wright stain)*

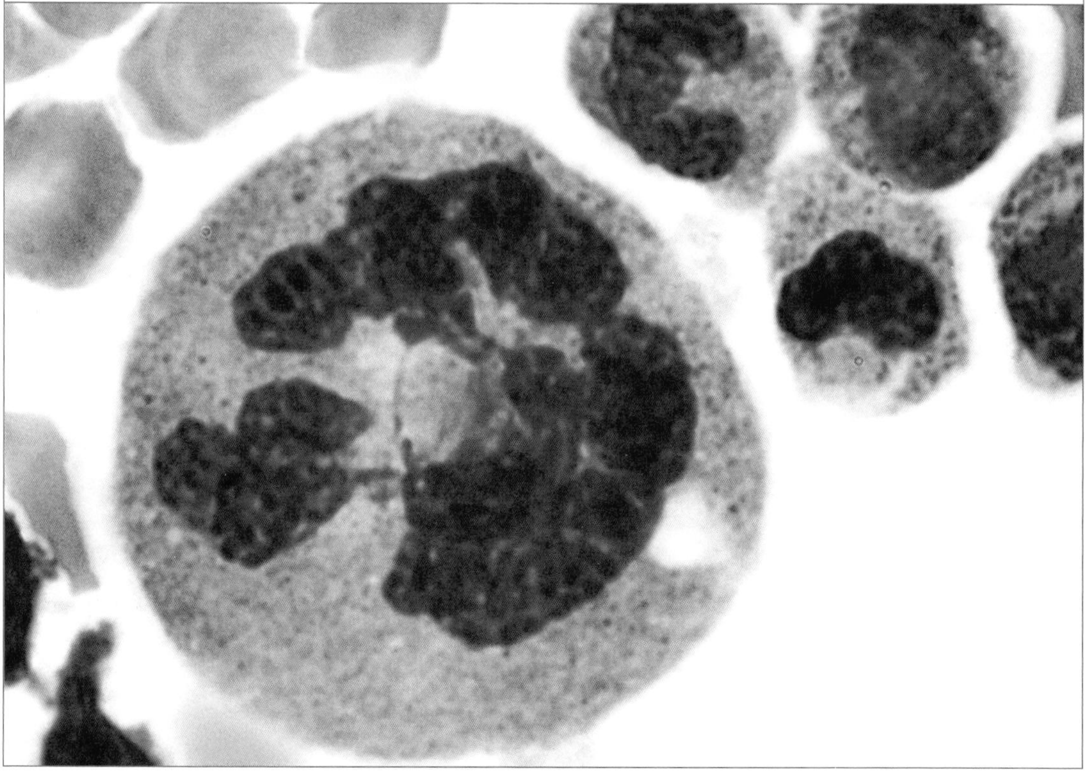

22.6 Course and Treatment

The clinical course is highly variable in patients with hereditary and acquired morphologic neutrophil disorders. For example, patients with Pelger-Huët anomaly, hereditary hypersegmentation of neutrophils, and hereditary giant neutrophils, and most patients with May-Hegglin anomaly are asymptomatic. In contrast, those with Chédiak-Higashi syndrome experience severe recurrent infections, infection-associated hemophagocytic syndrome, and secondary neoplasms.

Allogeneic bone marrow transplantation has been successful in some patients with this syndrome. Likewise, patients with hematologic neoplasms demonstrate a variable disease course, typically requiring aggressive multiagent chemotherapy or possible bone marrow transplantation (see Chapters 26, 27, and 32).

22.7 References

Aprikyan AA, Liles WC, Park JR, et al. Myelokathexis, a congenital disorder of severe neutropenia characterized by accelerated apoptosis and defective expression of bcl-x in neutrophil precursors. *Blood.* 2000;95:320-327.

Asmis LM, Hadaya K, Majno P, et al. Acquired and reversible Pelger-Huët anomaly of polymorphonuclear neutrophils in 3 transplant patients receiving mycophenolate mofetil therapy. *Am J Hematol.* 2003;73:244-248.

Balabanian K, Lagane B, Pablos JL, et al. WHIM syndromes with different genetic anomalies are accounted for by impaired CXCR4 desensitization to CXCL12. *Blood.* 2005;105:2449-2457.

Best S, Salvati F, Kallo J, et al. Lamin B-receptor mutations in Pelger-Huët anomaly. *Br J Haematol.* 2003;123:542-544.

Brunning RD. Morphologic alterations in nucleated blood and marrow cells in genetic disorders. *Hum Pathol.* 1970;1:99-124.

Chen Z, Naveiras O, Balduini A, et al. The May-Hegglin anomaly gene MYH9 is a negative regulator of platelet biogenesis modulated by the Rho-ROCK pathway. *Blood.* 2007;110:171-179.

Chetty-Raju N, Cook R, Erber WN. Vacuolated neutrophils in ethanol toxicity. *Br J Haematol.* 2004;127:478.

d'Onofrio G, Mancini S, Tamburrini E, et al. Giant neutrophils with increased peroxidase activity: another evidence of dysgranulopoiesis in AIDS. *Am J Clin Pathol.* 1987;87:584-591.

Eapen M, DeLaat CA, Baker KS, et al. Hematopoietic cell transplantation for Chediak-Higashi syndrome. *Bone Marrow Transplant.* 2007;39:411-415.

Etzell JE, Wang E. Acquired Pelger-Huet anomaly in association with concomitant tacrolimus and mycophenolate mofetil in a liver transplant patient: a case report and review of the literature. *Arch Pathol Lab Med.* 2006;130:93-96.

Girodon F, Favre B, Carli PM, et al. Minor dysplastic changes are frequently observed in the bone marrow aspirate in elderly patients without haematological disease. *Clin Lab Haematol.* 2001;23:297-300.

Harless W, Crowell E, Abraham J. Anemia and neutropenia associated with copper deficiency of unclear etiology. *Am J Hematol.* 2006;81:546-549.

Huang SY, Chang CS, Tang JL, et al. Acute and chronic arsenic poisoning associated with treatment of acute promyelocytic leukaemia. *Br J Haematol.* 1998;103:1092-1095.

Huff JD, Keung YK, Thakuri M, et al. Copper deficiency causes reversible myelodysplasia. *Am J Hematol.* 2007;82:625-630.

Kahwash E, Gewirtz AS. Howell-Jolly body-like inclusions in neutrophils. *Arch Pathol Lab Med.* 2003;127:1389-1390.

Khanna-Gupta A, Sun H, Zibello T, et al. Growth factor independence-1 (Gfi-1) plays a role in mediating specific granule deficiency (SGD) in a patientlacking a gene-inactivating mutation in the C/EBPepsilon gene. *Blood.* 2007;109:4181-4190.

Kunishima S, Hamaguchi M, Saito H. Differential expression of wild-type and mutant NMMHC-IIA polypeptides in blood cells suggests cell-specific regulation mechanisms in MYH9 disorders. *Blood.* 2008;111:3015-3023.

Lai J-L, Preudhomme C, Zandecki M, et al. Myelodysplastic syndromes and acute myeloid leukemia with 17p deletion: an entity characterized by specific dysgranulopoiesis and a high incidence of P53 mutations. *Leukemia.* 1995;9:370-381.

Maitra A, Ward PC, Kroft SH, et al. Cytoplasmic inclusions in leukocytes: an unusual manifestation of cryoglobulinemia. *Am J Clin Pathol.* 2000;113:107-112.

Masat T, Feliu E, Tassies D, et al. Pseudo–Pelger-Huët anomaly after bone marrow transplantation. *Hematol Pathol.* 1991;5:89-91.

Ramos F, Fernandez-Ferrero S, Suarez D, et al. Myelodysplastic syndrome: a search for minimal diagnostic criteria. *Leuk Res.* 1999;23:283-290.

Rezuke WN, Anderson C, Pastuszak WT, et al. Arsenic intoxication presenting as a myelodysplastic syndrome: a case report. *Am J Hematol.* 1991;36:291-293.

Slagel DD, Lager DJ, Dick FR. Howell-Jolly body-like inclusions in the neutrophils of patients with acquired immunodeficiency syndrome. *Am J Clin Pathol.* 1994;101:429-431.

So CC, Wong KF. Valproate-associated dysmyelopoiesis in elderly patients. *Am J Clin Pathol.* 2002;118:225-228.

van Hook L, Spivack C, Duncanson FP. Acquired Pelger-Huët anomaly associated with Mycoplasma pneumoniae pneumonia. *Am J Clin Pathol.* 1985;84:248-251.

Summerfield AL, Steinberg FU, Gonzalez JG. Morphologic findings in bone marrow precursor cells in zinc-induced copper deficiency anemia. *Am J Clin Pathol.* 1992;97:665-668.

Ward PC, McKenna RW, Kroft SH. White blood cell changes in hyperthermia. *Br J Haematol.* 2007;138:130.

Westerman DA, Evans D, Metz J. Neutrophil hypersegmentation in iron deficiency anaemia: a case-control study. *Br J Haematol.* 1999;107:512-515.

Part IV

Reactive Disorders of Lymphocytes

Chapter 23

Infectious Mononucleosis and Other Reactive Disorders of Lymphocytes

LoAnn Peterson, MD

The hallmark of a benign lymphocytosis is a transient increase in circulating lymphocytes. Most benign lymphocytoses are characterized by morphologically reactive or atypical lymphocytes. Several conditions are associated with a reactive lymphocytosis **t23.1**, but the most common is infectious mononucleosis (IM) caused by Epstein-Barr virus (EBV). Infections with several other agents, primarily viruses, also can elicit a reactive lymphocytosis. In some of these disorders, such as cytomegalovirus (CMV) infection, the clinical and peripheral blood picture may be indistinguishable from EBV-IM. These disorders are referred to as "IM-like syndromes." Other less frequent causes of reactive lymphocytosis include viral hepatitis, childhood viral infections, and drug reactions. Some benign lymphocytoses are typified by lymphocytes with mature or non-reactive morphology **t23.1**; these disorders include whooping cough, infectious lymphocytosis, transient stress lymphocytosis, and persistent polyclonal B-cell lymphocytosis. This chapter focuses on IM, but also addresses other causes of benign lymphocytosis.

t23.1 Causes of Benign Lymphocytosis

Reactive morphology
Infectious mononucleosis (EBV)
Infectious mononucleosis-like syndromes
  Cytomegalovirus
  Toxoplasmosis
  Adenovirus
  Acute HIV infection
  Human herpesvirus-6
Other viral infections
  Viral hepatitis
  Rubella
  Roseola
  Mumps
  Chickenpox
Drug reactions
Mature or non-reactive morphology
  Whooping cough
  Infectious lymphocytosis
  Transient stress lymphocytosis
  Persistent polyclonal B-cell lymphocytosis

EBV = Epstein-Barr virus; HIV = human immunodeficiency virus

23.1 Pathophysiology

Infectious mononucleosis is caused by an acute primary infection with EBV, a member of the herpesvirus family. The route of transmission of EBV is by intimate contact of a susceptible person with oral secretions from a previously infected individual who is shedding EBV. EBV infects B lymphocytes in the oropharynx, which then disseminate the virus throughout the reticuloendothelial system, provoking an intense immunologic response. The cellular response is complex and responsible for control of the acute infection. Most of the reactive lymphocytes in the blood during this time are cytotoxic T lymphocytes; NK cells are also increased. A humoral response also is elicited and is characterized by the production of heterophil antibody and EBV-specific antibodies directed against viral capsid antigen (VCA), early antigen (EA), and Epstein-Barr nuclear antigen (EBNA). After convalescence, EBV is present in the peripheral blood within latently infected B cells. These cells occasionally undergo lytic replication, shedding the virus, but are kept in check by cytotoxic T cells.

23.2 Clinical Aspects

Infectious mononucleosis typically occurs in persons between the ages of 10 and 25 years. Classic IM is characterized by sore throat, fever, headache, malaise, nausea, and anorexia. Lymphadenopathy, usually cervical, is almost always present. More than 50% of patients have splenomegaly, and mild hepatitis may be present. Acute EBV infections are also common in early childhood but these children often are asymptomatic or exhibit clinical symptoms not recognized as IM. Infectious mononucleosis is rare in persons older than 40 years, since most patients are immune to the virus by that time. When it does occur, the presenting features may be atypical, including prolonged fever, often without pharyngitis and lymphadenopathy.

23.3 Approach to Diagnosis

In a patient suspected of having IM, the initial laboratory workup should include the following:

1. CBC with leukocyte differential.
2. Morphologic examination of the peripheral blood smear.
3. Testing for IM heterophil antibody.
4. EBV-specific serologic studies (if indicated).

The appearance of increased numbers of reactive lymphocytes in the blood is one of the earliest laboratory signs of IM and is essential for the diagnosis. The diagnosis of IM is confirmed by detection of the heterophil antibody. EBV-specific serologic studies may be indicated to document IM in some cases.

23.4 Hematologic Findings

23.4.1 Blood Cell Measurements

Hemoglobin and hematocrit measurements usually are normal in IM. Mild hemolysis occasionally is present in persons with IM, but clinically significant anemia is uncommon, occurring only in about 1%-3% of patients. When anemia is present, it is usually an autoimmune hemolytic anemia caused by RBC autoantibodies. RBC autoantibodies with anti-i, anti-N, and anti-I specificities have been described in IM. An absolute lymphocytosis greater than $4.0 \times 10^3/mm^3$ ($4.0 \times 10^9/L$) usually is present. The total leukocyte count is increased and ranges from $10.0\text{-}30.0 \times 10^3/mm^3$ ($10.0\text{-}30.0 \times 10^9/L$); counts exceeding this range are rare. The leukocytosis begins about 1 week after the onset of symptoms, peaks during the second or third week, and persists for 2-8 weeks. A mild to moderate neutropenia often is present and is most prominent during the third or fourth week of the illness. Rarely, agranulocytosis may complicate IM. Mild thrombocytopenia ($100\text{-}140 \times 10^3/mm^3$ [$100\text{-}140 \times 10^9/L$]) is present in about 1/3 of patients with IM; severe thrombocytopenia is rare. The neutropenia and thrombocytopenia apparently are secondary to an immune mechanism.

23.4.2 Peripheral Blood Smear Morphologic Findings

The most striking morphologic finding in the peripheral blood smear from a patient with IM is the presence of an increased number of reactive lymphocytes. Reactive lymphocytes are benign activated cells with a characteristic morphologic appearance. Various terms are used to describe these cells, including "atypical," "variant," "transformed," and "Downey cells." Reactive lymphocytes are found in the blood of healthy individuals but usually account for less than 5-10% of the total lymphocyte population.

Reactive lymphocytes in the blood of patients with IM have a heterogeneous appearance. However, they usually are large with abundant cytoplasm i23.1. The most commonly encountered cells are large lymphocytes with abundant pale blue cytoplasm and coarse but dispersed chromatin. Nucleoli are absent or indistinct. Peripheral or radiating basophilia of the cytoplasm often is present, and scattered azurophilic granules may be noted. Immunoblasts also are observed frequently in IM. They are typically seen early in the disease, usually comprising only

i23.1 Infectious mononucleosis

Reactive lymphocytes from a patient with infectious mononucleosis. These cells exhibit abundant cytoplasm with radiating basophilia. Lymphocytes with this morphology have been referred to as Downey type II cells.

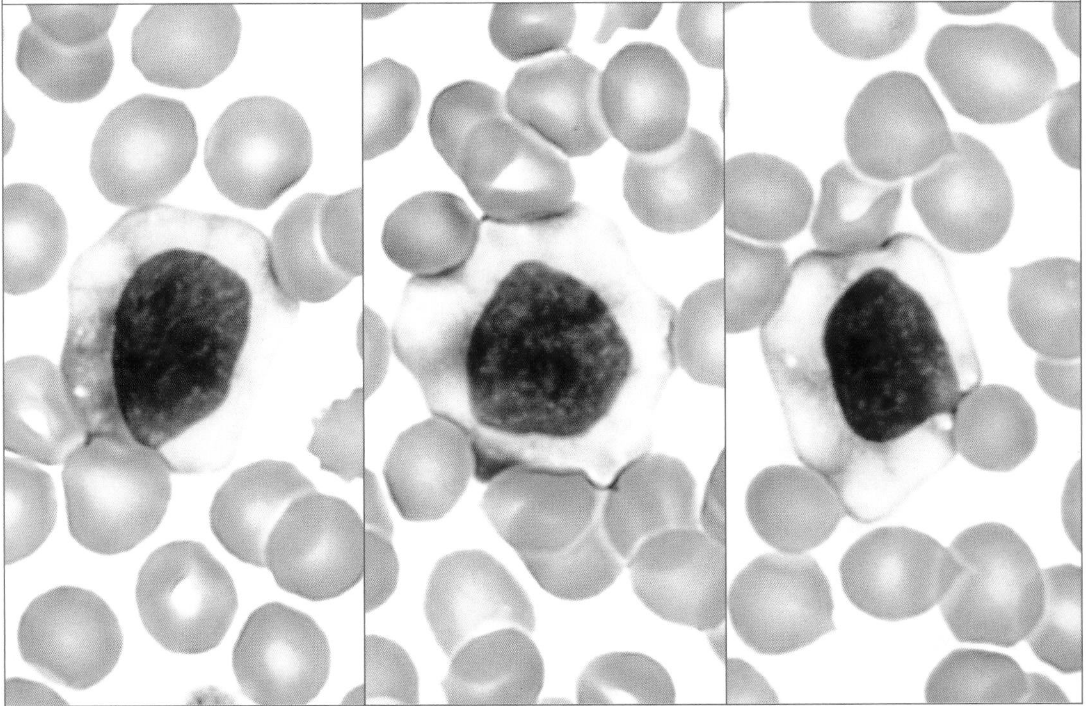

1% or 2% of the total lymphocyte population. Immunoblasts are medium to large lymphocytes with moderate amounts of basophilic cytoplasm, round to oval nuclei with a coarsely reticular chromatin pattern, and visible nucleoli i23.2. Large granular lymphocytes also are increased frequently in IM and contribute to the morphologic heterogeneity of the lymphocytes in this disorder. In addition, circulating plasma cells often are present in small numbers in IM.

The minimal morphologic criteria t23.2 for the diagnosis of IM include the following: (1) at least 50% mononuclear cells in the blood smear, (2) at least 10 reactive lymphocytes per 100 leukocytes, and (3) marked lymphocyte heterogeneity.

t23.2 Minimal Morphologic Criteria for Diagnosis of Infectious Mononucleosis
≥50% mononuclear cells (lymphocytes and monocytes) in blood smear
At least 10 reactive lymphocytes per 100 leukocytes
Marked lymphocyte heterogeneity

The erythrocytes in blood smears from patients with IM usually are normochromic and normocytic, but spherocytes and increased polychromasia may be apparent if an autoimmune hemolytic anemia is present. The platelets have normal morphologic features, but the number may be slightly decreased.

23.4.3 Bone Marrow Examination

A bone marrow biopsy is not indicated to diagnose IM.

i23.2 Infectious mononucleosis

Blood smear from a patient with infectious mononucleosis. The lymphocyte on the left has an increased amount of pale blue cytoplasm, a common finding in reactive lymphocytes. The lymphocyte on the right is large with a moderate amount of basophilic cytoplasm, loosely condensed chromatin, and a visible nucleolus. These are morphologic features of an immunoblast.

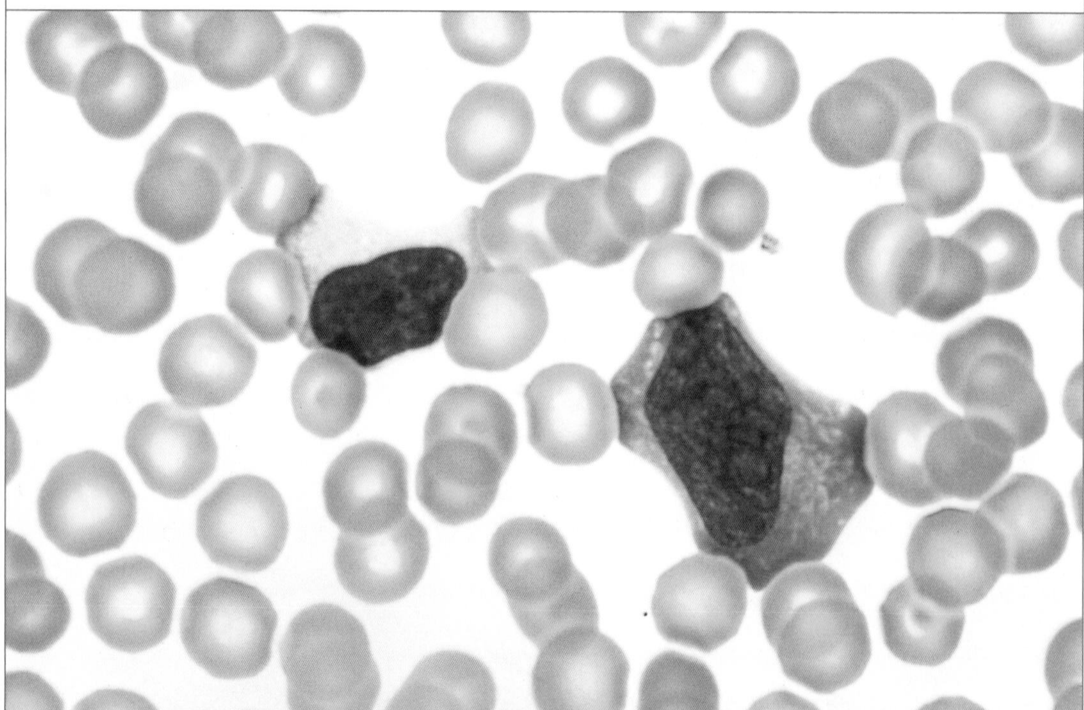

23.4.4 Flow Cytometric Immunophenotyping

Flow cytommetric immunophenotyping is not necessary to diagnose IM but may be performed if the differential diagnosis includes a neoplastic lymphoproliferative disorder. IM is characterized by an activated (HLA-DR+, CD38+) CD8+ cytotoxic T cell population. It is important to recognize that downregulation of CD7 and occasionally CD5 can be seen in IM.

23.5 Other Laboratory Tests

23.5.1 Tests for Detection of Heterophil Antibody

Purpose. Heterophil antibodies are produced in EBV-IM; they appear within the first 2 weeks of illness and usually are undetectable 3-6 months after the acute illness. The diagnosis of IM is confirmed by the detection of heterophil antibodies.

Principle. The IM heterophil antibody is of the IgM class and reacts with beef, sheep, and horse erythrocytes; it does not react with guinea pig kidney tissue. This characteristic separates the IM heterophil antibody from cross-reacting Forssman-type antibodies.

Specimen. Serum or plasma is used.

Procedure. Most clinical laboratories use one of the several commercially available rapid tests or "monospot tests" to detect heterophil antibodies. These tests are usually latex agglutination assays or ELISA (enzyme-linked immunoabsorbent assays).

Interpretation. The presence of heterophil antibodies in conjunction with the characteristic appearance of the peripheral blood smear is highly specific for the diagnosis of IM. When serial studies are done, heterophil antibody test results are positive in more than 96% of the teenagers and young adults with EBV-IM. False-positive results occur but are uncommon. Heterophil antibodies are not present in other conditions associated with a reactive lymphocytosis, such as the CMV mononucleosis-like syndrome.

A small percentage of teenagers and young adults with EBV-IM do not produce heterophil antibodies. These cases represent heterophil-negative IM. The incidence of heterophil negativity is much higher in infants and young children. About 75% of children with IM from ages 2-4 years and fewer than 25% of children with IM younger than 2 years produce heterophil antibodies. When the heterophil antibody cannot be detected, EBV-specific serologic tests can be used to confirm the diagnosis of EBV-IM. These tests are based on the detection of antibodies produced against specific antigens encoded by the EBV, such as VCA, EA, and EBNA (see Test 23.5.2).

23.5.2 EBV-Specific Serologic Tests

Purpose. EBV-specific serologic tests can establish the diagnosis of EBV-IM. These tests are especially useful in patients with suspected IM and a negative heterophil test.

Principle. EBV-specific serologic tests are based on the detection of antibodies produced against specific antigens encoded by the virus. During the EBV infection, there is sequential appearance and disappearance of different antibodies t23.3. Almost all patients develop IgG and IgM antibodies to VCA early in the course of the disease. The IgM anti-VCA titers diminish rapidly during convalescence and usually are undetectable at 12 weeks, while the IgG anti-VCA titers persist for life. Antibodies to EA (anti-EA) appear during the acute phase of the disease and then decline, however, antibodies to EA are not consistently present in IM. Antibodies to EBNA do not appear until symptoms have resolved and then persist indefinitely.

Procedure. Assays for EBV-specific antibodies are usually done with indirect immunofluorescence microscopy. Enzyme-linked immunosorbent assays, Western blot analysis, and other immunoassays are also available.

Interpretation. An acute primary infection is indicated by the following: (1) the presence of IgM anti-VCA, (2) high titers of IgG anti-VCA, and (3) the absence of anti-EBNA. The presence of IgG anti-VCA and anti-EBNA with absence of IgM anti-VCA indicates a remote infection.

t23.3 Serologic Profile in Infectious Mononucleosis (EBV)

Antibody	Acute (0-3 mo)	Recent (3-12 mo)	Past (>12 mo)
Heterophil	Positive*	Negative†	Negative
EBV-specific			
VCA-IgM	Positive	Negative	Negative
VCA-IgG	Positive	Positive	Positive
EA	Positive/Negative	Positive/Negative	Negative
EBNA	Negative	Positive	Positive

EBV = Epstein-Barr virus; VCA = viral capsid antigen; EA = early antigen; EBNA = Epstein-Barr early antigen;
**Occasionally negative in teenagers and young adults; frequently negative in children <4 years of age.*
†Heterophile antibody occasionally may persist for about 3-12 months

23.6 Practical Approach to the Diagnosis of Infectious Mononucleosis

A practical diagnostic approach for IM that is useful in most clinical settings is shown in **t23.4**. This approach uses the blood smear morphologic findings and a commercially available rapid test for heterophil antibody as the initial diagnostic workup in patients suspected of having EBV-IM. Although automated differential counters may flag a specimen as possibly containing reactive lymphocytes, a stained smear should be examined for blasts and other abnormal cells that are not reliably distinguished from reactive lymphocytes. Four diagnostic possibilities exist:

1. If the peripheral blood smear does not exhibit the morphologic features of IM and the results of the rapid test are negative for heterophil antibody, the diagnosis of IM usually is excluded. No further testing for IM is indicated. Other causes for the patient's symptoms should be considered.
2. If the morphologic features of IM are present in the blood smear and the results of the rapid test for heterophil antibody are positive, the diagnosis of IM is confirmed. No further testing is required. Determination of the heterophil titer is unnecessary since it does not correlate with clinical course.
3. When the results of the rapid test are positive for the heterophil antibody but the blood smear lacks the morphologic characteristics of IM, the diagnosis of IM is not confirmed.

t23.4 Workup of Patients with Clinically Suspected Infectious Mononucleosis*

Reactive Lymphocytosis†	Rapid Test for Heterophile Antibody	Diagnosis of Infectious Mononucleosis	Further DiagnosticTests
Absent	Negative	Not confirmed	Not indicated
Present	Positive	Confirmed	Not indicated
Absent	Positive	Inconclusive	EBV serologic tests
Present	Negative	Suspicious for IM or IM-like illness	Repeat rapid heterophile test in 1-2 weeks or perform EBV serologic tests; consider CMV serology, etc

EBV = Epstein-Barr virus; CMV = cytomegalovirus
**Modified from Horwitz CA. Practical approach to diagnosis of infectious mononucleosis.* Postgrad Med. *1979;65:179-184.*
†Blood smear meets minimal morphologic criteria for infectious mononucleosis (see **t23.2***)*

Another blood smear could be evaluated in a few days, because occasionally the appearance of reactive lymphocytes lags behind positive serologic findings. Since heterophil antibodies in some persons may persist for more than a year after acute IM, it also may be useful to ask the patient about past symptoms of IM. Another approach in this situation is to perform EBV-specific serologic tests to determine whether the rapid slide test result was a false-positive or whether there is additional evidence for IM.

4. If the blood smear meets the minimal morphologic criteria for IM and the results of the rapid test for heterophil antibody are negative, the diagnosis of IM still should be suspected. The serologic findings frequently lag behind the appearance of reactive lymphocytes, and retesting may yield a positive result in 1-2 weeks. If a negative rapid test result persists, the patient may still have IM but may not produce the heterophil antibody. In this instance, EBV-specific serologic tests may be necessary to establish the diagnosis. Other disorders that may result in an IM-like syndrome unrelated to EBV, such as acute CMV infection, also should be considered.

23.7 Treatment

IM is a self-limited disease. In patients with normal immunity, the syndrome resolves within days or weeks. Primary EBV infection rarely requires therapy. Steroid therapy is controversial but occasionally is used for the treatment of severe complications related to IM, including severe pharyngitis with obstructing tonsils, autoimmune hemolytic anemia, and other severe cytopenias. Rare complications include splenic rupture, neurologic complications, myocarditis, and pericarditis.

23.8 Other Causes of Reactive Lymphocytosis

Although IM is the most common cause of reactive lymphocytosis, other benign conditions also are associated with an increase in circulating reactive lymphocytes. Selected tests that are useful in the diagnosis of several of these conditions are listed in **t23.5**.

23.8.1 Infectious Mononucleosis-like Syndromes

Approximately 10% of patients with a clinical and morphologic syndrome similar to EBV-IM have a condition not caused by EBV **t23.1**. These disorders are referred to as "IM-like syndromes." The most common of these is caused by acute CMV infection. CMV-induced IM-like syndromes usually occur in adults between the ages of 20 and 30 years. The clinical syndrome may be indistinguishable from EBV-IM, but pharyngitis and lymphadenopathy typically are less severe than in EBV-IM. Hepatitis is almost always present. The peripheral blood morphologic features are the same as those of EBV-IM. The pathogenesis of CMV infection is less well understood than that of EBV-IM, but the peripheral lymphocytosis, like that of EBV-IM, is a T-cell response consisting primarily of cytotoxic-suppressor T-cells. The diagnosis can be made by documenting IgM antibodies to CMV.

Patients undergoing seroconversion to HIV also occasionally have an IM-like syndrome. Predominant symptoms include fatigue, malaise, fever and lymphadenopathy. The symptoms of the acute viral syndrome usually subside within a few weeks. The peripheral blood picture may be similar to EBV-IM but the incidence of a lymphocytosis is lower and the number of reactive cells is typically fewer than in EBV-IM.

Other rare causes of an IM-like syndrome include infection with human herpesvirus 6 (also the causative agent of roseola), adenovirus, and the parasite *Toxoplasma gondii*.

t23.5 Selected Tests in the Differential Diagnosis of Benign Lymphocytosis

Disease	Test	Interpretation
Infectious mononucleosis (EBV)	Heterophile test	Positive results in association with characteristic blood smear morphology indicate EBV-IM
	EBV-specific serologic tests	IgM and IgG antibodies to viral capsid antigens indicate acute infection
CMV	Serologic tests for antibodies to CMV	Positive result for IgM or increase in IgG titers in paired specimens indicates acute infection
Toxoplasmosis	Serologic tests for *Toxoplasma*-specific antibodies	Elevated *Toxoplasma*-specific IgM and IgG antibodies are suggestive of acute infection
Adenovirus	Culture or detection of virus or viral antigens	Positive results in acute infection
Acute HIV infection	Test for HIV-specific antibody with confirmation (eg, Western blot) of positives	Positive results indicate infection with HIV
Human herpesvirus (HHV)-6	Serologic tests for HHV-6 IgG or IgM antibodies	Seroconversion indicates acute infection
Hepatitis A, B, C	Serologic or molecular tests	Hepatitis A-specific IgM is positive in acute infection
		Presence of hepatitis B surface antigen (HBsAg) or high titer IgM-specific anti-HBcAg (HB core Ag) indicates acute infection
		Antibody to hepatitis C virus (HCV) and detection of HCV RNA indicate acute infection
Rubella	Serologic test for virus specific IgM antibody	Presence of rubella virus-specific IgM indicates acute infection
Bordetella pertussis	Direct fluorescent-antibody procedure for clinical specimens or cultures	Identification of bacteria indicates acute infection

EBV = Epstein-Barr virus; IM = infectious mononucleosis; CMV = cytomegalovirus; EIA = enzyme immunoassay; HIV = human immunodeficiency virus

23.8.2 Other Viral Infections

Occasionally, patients with viral hepatitis exhibit a reactive lymphocytosis. Patients with rubella, roseola, mumps, and chickenpox also may have a reactive lymphocytosis. The morphologic features of the lymphocytes in these disorders are similar to those of IM, but the lymphocytosis often is less intense and not as long lasting. In addition, circulating plasma cells frequently are prominent (i23.3).

23.8.3 Drug Reactions

Lymphocytosis also may be observed in patients with drug reactions, particularly anticonvulsants such as phenytoin. The leukocyte count is variable in these patients, and eosinophilia and neutrophilia may accompany the lymphocytosis. These patients also frequently exhibit circulating plasma cells.

i23.3 Viral hepatitis

Blood smear from a patient with viral hepatitis showing a reactive lymphocytosis and circulating plasma cells.

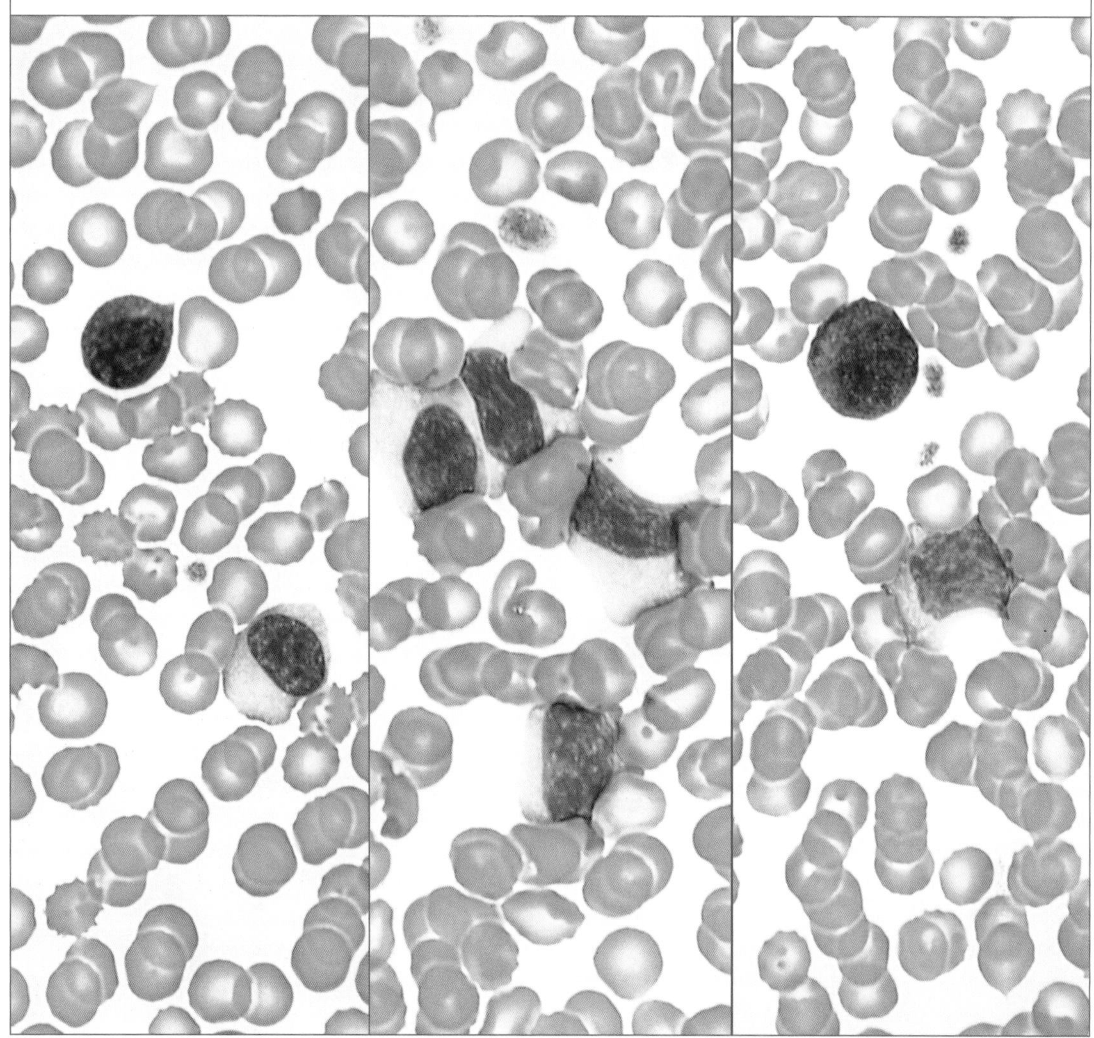

23.9 Lymphocytosis with Non-Reactive Morphology

23.9.1 Whooping Cough

Acute bacterial infections rarely cause lymphocytosis. An exception is whooping cough, in which a striking lymphocytosis may be seen. Whooping cough (pertussis) usually occurs in infants and young children who have not been immunized and is characterized clinically by severe paroxysmal coughing and prominent lymphocytosis. The causative organism, *Bordetella pertussis*, produces a toxin that seems to have a role in the accumulation of lymphocytes in the blood by preventing them from homing normally back to lymphoid tissue. In whooping cough, the peak lymphocyte counts average about $10.0 \times 10^3/mm^3$ ($10.0 \times 10^9/L$); however, counts higher than $30.0 \times 10^3/mm^3$ ($30.0 \times 10^9/L$) are not unusual. Neutrophilia also may be present. Unlike the previous disorders, the lymphocytes in whooping cough appear mature with condensed chromatin patterns and scant cytoplasm; they frequently exhibit cleaved or convoluted nuclei i23.4. Surface marker studies show that these cells are predominantly of the T-helper (CD4+) phenotype. Adults with pertussis do not exhibit a peripheral lymphocytosis.

23.9.2 Infectious Lymphocytosis

Infectious lymphocytosis is a benign illness of young children that is presumably of viral origin. The patients often are asymptomatic, but fever, abdominal pain, or diarrhea may be present. Organomegaly does not occur. The symptoms resolve within a few days. Leukocyte counts in infectious lymphocytosis range from 35.0-100.0 × $10^3/mm^3$ (35.0-100.0 × $10^9/L$). The predominant lymphocyte has been reported to be a T cell or natural killer cell, but increased numbers of B lymphocytes also have been observed. The lymphocytes appear morphologically mature, and eosinophilia may be present in the later stages of the disease. The lymphocytosis may persist for several weeks.

23.9.3 Transient Stress Lymphocytosis

Transient stress lymphocytosis occasionally is observed in patients with trauma, myocardial infarction, status epilepticus, and other acute medical conditions. In transient stress lymphocytosis, the lymphocytosis is mild to moderate, averaging about 6.0-8.0 × $10^3/mm^3$ (6.0-8.0 × $10^9/L$). The lymphocytes in transient stress lymphocytosis consist of mature-appearing lymphocytes. Large granular lymphocytes occasionally are prominent. The lymphocytosis resolves quickly, often within a few hours, followed by a neutrophilia. The lymphocytosis in this situation represents an expansion of the normal lymphocyte population and is similar to responses seen following epinephrine injection.

i23.4 ***Bordatella pertussis***

Blood smear from a child with whooping cough shows lymphocytes with scant cytoplasm, condensed chromatin, and occasional cleaved nuclei.

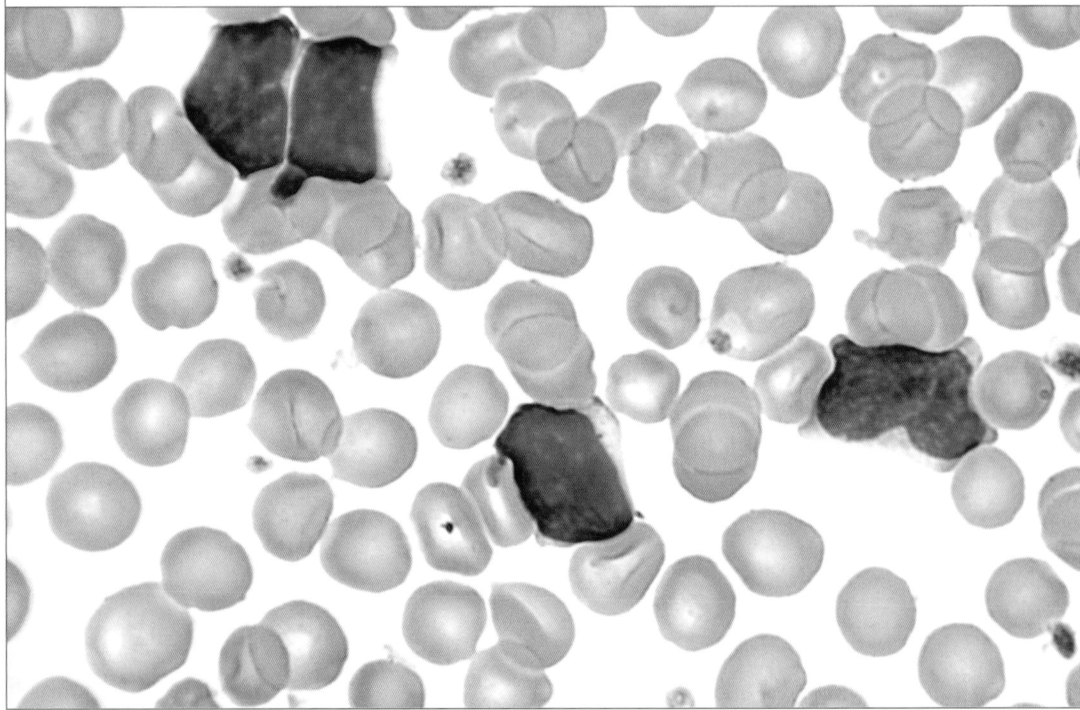

23.9.4 Persistent Polyclonal B-Cell Lymphocytosis

Persistent polyclonal B-cell lymphocytosis is a stable, presumably benign lymphocytosis diagnosed almost exclusively in women. The cause of the lymphocytosis is unknown, but there is a strong association with cigarette smoking. The patients usually are asymptomatic. The lymphocytosis has been documented over decades in some patients. The absolute lymphocyte counts in this disorder are typically mildly elevated but may exceed $10.0 \times 10^3/mm^3$ ($10.0 \times 10^9/L$) with total leukocyte counts greater than $15.0 \times 10^3/mm^3$ ($15.0 \times 10^9/L$). Flow cytometry shows a B-cell population (CD19+) with a normal κ/λ ratio. The hemoglobin level, platelet count, and neutrophil count are normal. A polyclonal increase in IgM often is present, and an association with HLA-DR7 has been reported. Morphologically, the lymphocytes appear mature; binucleate forms or bilobed nuclei are present in a variable proportion of the cells. Despite the long, indolent course, isochromosome (3q+) and multiple bcl-2/Ig gene rearrangements have been identified in several of these patients. Nevertheless, no increase in hematologic malignancies has been documented.

23.9.5 Increases of Large Granular Lymphocytes

Increased numbers of large granular lymphocytes can be transiently increased in various conditions including acute viral infections such as IM in which they are intermixed with reactive lymphocytes. In some cases, blood smears demonstrate an increase consisting predominantly of large granular lymphocytes. Clinical settings in which this occurs include post bone marrow transplantation, autoimmune disorders, and post-splenectomy. These expansions may be clonal or non-clonal. If other clinical and laboratory findings suggest a clonal process, a workup for a T-cell or NK-cell leukemia should be considered (see Chapter 58). However, it should be noted that the finding of clonality does not always indicate an overt neoplastic process.

23.10 Differential Diagnosis

The differential diagnosis of a patient with a benign lymphocytosis occasionally includes a malignant lymphoproliferative disorder, most notably acute lymphoblastic leukemia (ALL) and chronic lymphocytic leukemia (CLL). Confusion of a reactive lymphocytosis with ALL is most likely to occur when the leukocyte count is unusually high (ie, $>30 \times 10^3/mm^3$ [$>30 \times 10^9/L$]). This problem is compounded when the serologic test results are negative. Familiarity with the morphologic appearance of reactive lymphocytes, however, will aid in this differential diagnostic dilemma. In addition, anemia and thrombocytopenia are almost always present in acute leukemia but usually absent or mild in benign reactive conditions such as IM. Moreover, the diagnosis of ALL should be confirmed with a bone marrow aspirate and biopsy and other ancillary studies, including immunophenotypic analysis (see Chapter 48).

Benign lymphocytoses occasionally can be difficult to distinguish from chronic lymphoproliferative disorders such as CLL. This is more of a problem in patients older than 40 years because of the relative frequency of CLL in comparison with reactive disorders such as IM in this age group. In addition, when IM occurs in an older patient, the clinical findings may be atypical for IM. The morphologic characteristics of the lymphocytes in CLL (see **i55.1**) may help in this differential diagnosis since, in general, they appear mature and more monotonous than the lymphocytes in a reactive process. However, immunophenotypic studies are required to confirm a diagnosis of CLL or other chronic lymphoproliferative disorders (see Chapter 55).

23.11 References

Cohen JI, Corey RC. Cytomegalovirus infection in the normal host. *Medicine.* 1985;64:100-114.

Cohen JI. Epstein-Barr virus infection. *N Engl J Med.* 2000;343:481-492.

Garcia-Suarez J, Prieto A, Reyes E, et al. Persistent lymphocytosis of natural killer cells in autoimmune thrombocytopenic purpura (ATP) patients after splenectomy. *Br J Haematol.* 1995;653-655.

Groom DA, Kunkel LA, Brynes RK, et al. Transient stress lymphocytosis during crisis of sickle cell anemia and emergency trauma and medical conditions. *Arch Pathol Lab Med.* 1990;114:570-576.

Hickey SM, Strasburger VC. What every pediatrician should know about infectious mononucleosis in adolescents. *Pediatr Clin North Am.* 1997;44:1541-1556.

Horwitz CA. Practical approach to diagnosis of infectious mononucleosis. *Postgrad Med.* 1979;65:179-184.

Horwitz CA, Henle W, Henle G, et al. Clinical and laboratory evaluation of infants and children with Epstein-Barr virus–induced infectious mononucleosis: report of 32 patients (aged 10–48 months). *Blood.* 1981;57:933-938.

Horwitz CA, Henle W, Henle G, et al. Heterophil-negative infectious mononucleosis and mononucleosis-like illnesses: laboratory confirmation of 43 cases. *Am J Med.* 1977;63:947-957.

Horwitz CA, Henle W, Henle G, et al. Infectious mononucleosis in patients aged 40-72 years: report of 27 cases, including 3 without heterophil-antibody responses. *Medicine.* 1983;62:256-262.

Juneja, S, Januszewicz E, Wolf M, et al. Post-splenectomy lymphocytosis. *Clin Lab Haematol.* 1995;17:335-337.

Karandikar NJ, Hotchkiss EC, McKenna RW, et al. Transient stress lymphocytosis: an immunophenotypic characterization of the most common cause of newly identified adult lymphocytosis in a tertiary hospital. *Am J Clin Pathol.* 2002;117:819-825.

Kubic VL, Kubic PT, Brunning RD. The morphologic and immunophenotypic assessment of the lymphocytosis accompanying *Bordetella pertussis* infection. *Am J Clin Pathol.* 1990;95:809-815.

Mazzulli T, Drew LW, Yen-Lieberman B, et al. Multicenter comparison of the digene hybrid capture CMV DNA assay (version 2.0), the pp65 antigenemia assay, and cell culture for detection of cytomegalovirus viremia. *J Clin Microbiol.* 1999;37;958-963.

Mossafa H, Malaure M, Maynadie M, et al. Persistent polyclonal lymphocytosis with binucleated lymphocytes: a study of 25 cases. *Br J Haematol.* 1999;104:486-493.

Peterson L, Hrisinko MA. Benign lymphocytosis and reactive neutrophilia: laboratory features provide diagnostic clues. *Clin Lab Med.* 1993;13:863-877.

Shuart MC, Gretch DR. Hepatitis C and G viruses in Murray PR, Baron EJ, Jorgenson JH, et al, eds. *Manual of Clinical Microbiology. 8th ed.* ASM Press, Washington D. C. 2003: 1480-1494.

Steeper TA, Horwitz CA, Ablashi DV. The spectrum of clinical and laboratory findings resulting from human herpesvirus-6 (HHV-6) in patients with mononucleosis-like illnesses not resulting from Epstein-Barr virus or cytomegalovirus. *Am J Clin Patho*l. 1990;93:776-783.

Steeper TA, Horwitz CA, Hanson M, et al. Heterophil-negative mononucleosis-like illnesses with atypical lymphocytosis in patients undergoing seroconversions to the human immunodeficiency virus. *Am J Clin Pathol.* 1988;89:169-174.

Teggatz JR, Parkin J, Peterson L. Transient atypical lymphocytosis in patients with emergency medical conditions. *Arch Pathol Lab Med.* 1987;111:712-714.

Weisberger J, Cornfield D, Wojciech G, Liu Z. Down-regulation of pan-T-cell antigens, particularly CD7, in acute infectious mononucleosis. *Am J Clin Pathol.* 2003;120:49-55.

CHAPTER 24

Lymphocytopenia

LoAnn Peterson, MD

Lymphocytopenia in adults usually is defined as a total lymphocyte count in the blood of less than $1.0 \times 10^3/mm^3$ ($1.0 \times 10^9/L$). In children younger than 16 years, absolute lymphocyte counts are higher; the lower reference value is about $2.0 \times 10^3/mm^3$ ($2.0 \times 10^9/L$). Since approximately 80% of circulating lymphocytes in the blood are CD3+ T lymphocytes and about 2/3 of the T lymphocytes are CD4+ (helper) T lymphocytes, most patients with lymphocytopenia have a decrease in the absolute number of T lymphocytes and CD4+ T lymphocytes in particular.

24.1 Pathophysiology

t24.1 lists the major conditions associated with lymphocytopenia. The pathogenesis of the lymphocytopenia in many of these disorders is unknown.

24.1.1 Congenital Immunodeficiency Disorders

Patients with congenital immunodeficiency disorders may exhibit an associated lymphocytopenia. In many of these disorders, the lymphocytopenia is secondary to decreased lymphocyte production. For example, severe combined immunodeficiency disease (SCID), a syndrome characterized by profound defects in cellular and humoral immunity, almost always is associated with prominent lymphocytopenia. Severe combined immunodeficiency disease is caused by a heterogeneous group of genetic abnormalities; the most common form is X-linked SCID. X-linked SCID is characterized by a defect in the common γ chain (γc), an essential component of the interleukin cytokine receptor complex that is essential for normal B-, T-, and NK-cell development. The early lymphoid progenitor cells lack intact interleukin receptors and fail to be stimulated by the growth factors essential to the normal development and differentiation of T cells and the late phase of B-cell development. T cells are absent or decreased and NK cells are absent. B cells are present but are of naïve B-cell phenotype and do not function normally. Adenosine deaminase deficiency accounts for about 20%-50% of cases of SCID. The lack of this enzyme results in accumulation of toxic metabolites that inhibit DNA synthesis.

Infants with congenital thymic aplasia (DiGeorge syndrome) usually exhibit profound lymphocytopenia. Aplasia of the thymus and the parathyroid gland probably results from a defect in embryogenesis of the third and fourth pharyngeal pouches. The T-cell areas of all tissues, including lymph nodes and spleen, are depleted. Most patients with DiGeorge syndrome have microdeletions of chromosome 22q11.2 although other chromosomal abnormalities have also been reported, such as deletion of 10p.

t24.1 Major Conditions Associated With Lymphocytopenia

Congenital immunodeficiency disorders
Severe combined immunodeficiency disease
Congenital thymic aplasia (DiGeorge syndrome)
Wiskott-Aldrich syndrome

Nutritional deficiencies
Protein-calorie malnutrition
Zinc deficiency

Infectious diseases
Acquired immunodeficiency syndrome (AIDS)
Severe acute respiratory syndrome (SARS)
Influenza
Hepatitis
Tuberculosis
Typhoid fever
Babesiosis
Pneumonia
Sepsis
Other

Autoimmune disorders
Rheumatoid arthritis
Systemic lupus erythematosus
Myasthenia gravis

Systemic diseases
Burns
Protein-losing enteropathy
Sarcoidosis
Renal insufficiency
Hodgkin lymphoma
Carcinoma

Iatrogenic
Radiation therapy
Anti-neoplastic chemotherapy
Immunosuppressive agents
Glucocorticoid therapy
Anesthesia and surgery
Thoracic duct drainage or rupture

Idiopathic
Idiopathic CD4+ T-lymphocytopenia

Modified from Kipps 2006:1090.

Wiskott-Aldrich syndrome, an X-linked recessive disease characterized by eczematoid dermatitis, thrombocytopenia, and recurrent opportunistic infections, also is associated with lymphocytopenia. This disorder is caused by a defect in the WAS protein (WASP) gene on the X chromosome. Lymphocytes are normal early in the disease, but with increasing age, B and T lymphocytes decrease.

24.1.2 Nutritional Deficiencies

Nutritional deficiencies are associated with lymphocytopenia. Protein-calorie malnutrition is a common cause of lymphocytopenia worldwide and probably is due to decreased production of lymphocytes. Deficiency of zinc, an element required in protein synthesis, is also associated with lymphocytopenia and is characterized by decreased numbers of circulating CD4+ T-cells and increased CD8+ T-cells.

24.1.3 Infectious Diseases

Lymphocytopenia is prominent in AIDS and is due to selective loss of the CD4+ T lymphocytes. The lymphocytopenia in AIDS is, in part, secondary to a direct cytopathic effect of the HIV. It also could be related to exaggerated expression of inhibitors of T-lymphocyte production such as transforming growth factor-β (TGF-β). The host immune response also may contribute to the progressive loss of CD4+ T lymphocytes.

Some patients with other viral or bacterial infections also exhibit lymphocytopenia (see **t24.1**). The pathogenesis of the decrease in circulating lymphocytes for most infectious diseases is unclear. In viral infections, the lymphocytes may be destroyed by the virus, travel to the respiratory tract, or be trapped in spleen and lymph nodes.

24.1.4 Autoimmune Disorders

The lymphocytopenia seen in autoimmune disorders such as systemic lupus erythematosus is likely mediated by autoantibodies.

24.1.5 Systemic Diseases

Lymphocytopenia is associated with severe burns and is possibly related to redistribution of the T lymphocytes to the tissues. Lymphocytes are lost through the intestinal lymphatics in association with severe congestive heart failure, protein-losing enteropathies, or other primary diseases of the gut or intestinal lymphatics. The lymphocytopenia of renal insufficiency and sarcoidosis may be secondary to defective T-lymphocyte proliferative responses.

24.1.6 Iatrogenic

Radiotherapy induces lymphocytopenia through lymphocyte death by direct exposure. T-helper lymphocytes are more sensitive than are T-suppressor cells; the helper/suppressor ratio can be decreased for months after exposure to radiation. Chemotherapeutic agents, such as alkylating agents or purine analogs, can cause profound lymphocytopenia that may persist for years. The administration of antilymphocyte globulin leads to lymphocytopenia by destruction of lymphocytes. The mechanism by which glucocorticoids cause lymphocytopenia is not completely clear but may be due to redistribution of lymphocytes away from the peripheral blood component and to cell destruction. Lymphocytopenia often is associated with anesthesia and surgical stress and is secondary to redistribution, perhaps related to endogenous steroid release. In thoracic duct drainage, lymphocytes are lost from the body.

24.1.7 Idiopathic

A syndrome of isolated CD4+ T-cell depletion in the absence of evidence for a retroviral infection has been identified. The cause of this condition is unknown.

24.2 Clinical Aspects

The signs and symptoms of patients with lymphocytopenia are those characteristic of the underlying disease process associated with the lymphocytopenia. Whether the patient exhibits clinical signs of immunodeficiency depends on the pathophysiology of the disease, the duration of the disorder, the lymphocyte subsets affected, and the degree of functional disturbance of cellular or humoral immunity. In general, patients with cellular immunodeficiency disorders have recurrent infections with low-grade or opportunistic infectious agents. In congenital disorders, growth retardation, wasting, and a short life span often are observed. A high incidence of malignant neoplasms, especially lymphomas, also is observed in some patient groups.

Severe combined immunodeficiency disease is the most severe congenital immune deficiency state involving both cellular and humoral immunity. Affected patients suffer from recurrent bacterial, fungal, viral, or protozoan infections starting as early as 3 months of age. Transfusion with non-irradiated blood products may lead to severe graft-vs-host reactions. Persistent pulmonary infection, diarrhea, and wasting dominate the clinical picture. Infants with congenital thymic aplasia have severely impaired cellular immunity. They also have hypocalcemia and other congenital anomalies, including cardiac defects. Those who survive the neonatal period are susceptible to overwhelming viral, fungal, and bacterial infections. Wiskott-Aldrich syndrome also appears in early childhood with a triad of eczematoid dermatitis, thrombocytopenia with bleeding, and recurrent opportunistic infections. Patients are at high risk for developing malignant neoplasms, most commonly lymphomas and leukemias.

Patients with AIDS can have life-threatening infections. Opportunistic infections are prominent and include *Pneumocystis carinii* pneumonia, *Mycobacterium avium-intracellulare* complex pneumonia or disseminated disease, cryptosporidiosis diarrhea, oral candidiasis, hepatitis B, and cytomegalovirus and herpesvirus infections. Malignant neoplasms (Kaposi sarcoma, lymphoma), autoimmune diseases (thrombocytopenia), and neurologic disorders also occur in patients with AIDS.

24.3 Approach to Diagnosis

A clinical history—including the age and sex of the patient, family history, history of medication use, social and medical history, and physical examination—is needed to determine the subsequent workup. Unless the cause of the lymphocytopenia is clinically apparent or the lymphocytopenia is transient, the approach to the diagnosis should involve a comprehensive assessment of the integrity of the immune system. A thorough workup of patients with immunodeficiency diseases such as the congenital disorders can be complex and should be performed at referral medical centers that have expertise and experience in the diagnosis and treatment of these disorders.

In many cases, the workup of patients with lymphocytopenia includes the following:

1. CBC count with differential and platelet count. A bone marrow aspirate and biopsy may be indicated if the reason for the lymphocytopenia is unclear or to confirm a suspected diagnosis.
2. Quantitative immunoglobulin determination.
3. Immunophenotypic analysis of peripheral blood lymphocytes by flow cytometry.
4. Ancillary tests such as skin tests to evaluate cellular immunity.
5. Other tests dependent on the clinical setting to determine the underlying cause. These include tests for HIV, antinuclear antibodies (systemic lupus erythematosus), and lymph node biopsy (sarcoidosis).
6. Cultures for patients suspected of having infection.

24.4 Hematologic Findings

24.4.1 Blood Cell Measurements

In adults, the lymphocyte count is less than $1.0 \times 10^3/mm^3$ ($1.0 \times 10^9/L$) in lymphocytopenia. In children, it is less than $2.0 \times 10^3/mm^3$ ($2.0 \times 10^9/L$). Granulocytopenia also may be present. The presence or absence of thrombocytopenia depends on the underlying condition. Thrombocytopenia with small platelets is characteristic of the Wiskott-Aldrich syndrome. Normochromic, normocytic anemia is present in many of the diseases associated with lymphocytopenia.

24.4.2 Bone Marrow Examination

Findings depend on the underlying disorder and recent therapeutic approaches. In some congenital immunodeficiency states, lymphocytes are decreased.

The bone marrow in patients with HIV is usually hypercellular, even in the setting of peripheral cytopenias. Dysplasia may be present in all cell lines. Plasma cells frequently are increased, especially late in the course of the disease. Lymphohistiocytic aggregates may be present in bone marrow core biopsy specimens and may be large and atypical. These must be distinguished from lymphomas, since the occurrence of lymphomas is increased in AIDS and may involve the bone marrow. Disseminated infections, especially *M avium-intracellulare* complex and histoplasmosis, often involve the bone marrow. The marrow granulomas in association with these agents may be loosely formed or absent.

24.5 Other Laboratory Tests

Test 24.5.1 Quantitation of Immunoglobulins

Purpose. Immunodeficiency states associated with lymphocytopenia often are combined with deficient production of immunoglobulins. Quantitation of serum immunoglobulins aids in evaluating the presence and severity of any immunoglobulin abnormality.

Immunoglobulin production is altered when there is a defect in the B-cell population alone or when a combined defect involving B and T lymphocytes exists. Defects in antibody production also can result from severe defects in T-lymphocyte function, since in humans, all antigens seem to be T-lymphocyte dependent.

Principle, Specimen, Procedure. See Test 56.9.4.

Interpretation. The level of serum immunoglobulins depends on the cause of the lymphocytopenia. In SCID and congenital thymic aplasia, serum immunoglobulin concentrations are normal. In Wiskott-Aldrich syndrome, serum IgG concentrations are low, but the concentrations of IgA and IgE are elevated. In AIDS, polyclonal hypergammaglobulinemia is often present.

Test 24.5.2 Immunophenotypic Analysis of Peripheral Blood Lymphocytes

Purpose. Lymphocyte markers are used to identify and enumerate lymphocyte subsets, which aid in diagnosing and classifying disorders associated with lymphocytopenia.

Principle, Specimen, Procedure. See Chapter 63.

Interpretation. About 60%-80% of circulating lymphocytes are T-cells, 10%-20% B-cells, and 5%-10% natural killer (NK) cells. The T-cell population consists of T-helper (CD4+) and T-suppressor (CD8+) cells; the T-helper cells outnumber the T-suppressor cells 2:1.

In X-linked SCID, T lymphocytes are absent or decreased. NK-cells are absent. The number of B lymphocytes is normal or elevated, but they are of a naïve B-cell phenotype, expressing surface IgM. In adenosine deaminase deficiency, T and B lymphocytes are markedly decreased. NK-cells are usually decreased. Congenital thymic aplasia is associated with a markedly decreased number of T lymphocytes. In Wiskott-Aldrich syndrome, the number of lymphocytes may be normal at first but with increasing age both B- and T-cells decrease. Identification of affected individuals can be performed by evaluating for expression of WASP on lymphocytes and monocytes by flow cytometry.

In AIDS, CD4+ cells are depleted and an inverted CD4/CD8 ratio is found. In patients with HIV, there is a strong association between CD4+ lymphocyte levels and development of opportunistic infections, progression to AIDS, and eventual death. Measurement of the CD4 subset is useful not only for assessing prognosis but also for making management decisions and for evaluating response to therapy.

24.6 Treatment

The clinical course and treatment of lymphocytopenia depends on the underlying cause. The prognosis for patients with SCID is dismal without therapy. This disorder can be rapidly fatal if affected infants are not rendered immunocompetent by bone marrow transplantation. Transplants of fetal thymic tissue reverse the T-cell defects in children with congenital thymic aplasia. In the past, patients with Wiskott-Aldrich syndrome usually died within the first year of life, but improved management with splenectomy, intravenous immune globulin therapy, and other measures, including bone marrow transplantation, has improved their life expectancy.

Patients with HIV are being treated with antiretroviral agents. Most patients with AIDS eventually die of infection or malignant neoplasms associated with AIDS, although survival continues to increase with treatment advances.

24.7 References

Bagby GC. Leukopenia and leukocytosis. In: Goldman L, Bennett JC, eds. *Cecil Textbook of Medicine. 21st ed.* Philadelphia: WB Saunders; 2000:919–933.

Bonilla FA, Geha RS. Primary immunodeficiency diseases. In: Nathan DG, Orkin SH, Ginsburg D, Look AT, eds. *Nathan and Oski's Hematology of Infancy and Childhood.* Philadelphia: Saunders; 2003:1043–1078.

Buckley RH. Primary immunodeficiency diseases due to defects in lymphocytes. *N Engl J Med.* 2000;343:1313-1324.

Castelino DJ, McNair P, Kay TWH. Lymphocytopenia in a hospital population–what does it signify? *Aust N Z J Med.* 1997;27:170–174.

Hoxie JA. Hematologic manifestations of HIV infection. In: Hoffman R, Benz, Jr EJ, Shattel SJ, et al, eds. *Hematology: Basic Principles and Practice. 3rd ed.* New York: Churchill-Livingstone; 2000:2430–2457.

Illoh OC. Current applications of flow cytometry in the diagnosis of primary immunodeficiency diseases. *Arch Pathol Lab Med.* 2004;128:23-32.

Kim N, Rosenbaum GS, Cunha BA. Relative bradycardia and lymphopenia in patients with babesiosis. *Clin Infect Dis.* 1998;26:1218–1219.

Kipps TJ. Lymphocytosis and lymphocytopenia. In: Lichtman MA, Beutler E, Kipps TJ, et al, eds. Williams *Hematology. 7th ed.* New York: McGraw-Hill; 2006:1087–1097.

Laurence J. T-cell subsets in health, infectious disease, and idiopathic CD4+ T lymphocytopenia. *Ann Intern Med.* 1993;119:55–62.

Schoentag RA, Cangiarella J. The nuances of lymphocytopenia. *Clin Lab Med.* 1993;13:923–936.

Toft P, Svendsen P, Tonnesen E, et al. Redistribution of lymphocytes after major surgical stress. *Acta Anaesthesiol Scand.* 1993;37:245–249.

Part V

Reactive Disorders of Lymph Nodes

Chapter 25

Reactive Disorders of Lymph Nodes

Carl Kjeldsberg, MD

The immediate and most important problem for the clinician or surgeon when a patient presents with lymphadenopathy is to determine whether the patient has (1) a benign, reactive hyperplasia caused by infectious or non-infectious agents, or (2) a malignant disease. The term "lymphadenopathy" refers to an enlarged lymph node or group of nodes. It is a common physical finding that requires an explanation as to its cause. Lymphadenopathy is often a transient response to localized infection and, in infected patients, the pathologic condition should be sought in the area drained by the node. In other patients, the lymphadenopathy may be due to a response to a systemic disease or a metastatic malignancy. Lymphadenopathies caused by a neoplastic proliferation of lymphoid cells are known as malignant lymphomas and are discussed in Chapters 53 and 61.

25.1 Pathophysiology

Enlargement of the lymph nodes is caused by a proliferation of lymphoid cells and the associated cells of the mononuclear phagocytic system. In addition, there is frequently a variable degree of vascular proliferation. The intensity and pattern of reaction depends on the nature and duration of the antigenic stimulus and on the age and immune status of the patient. As noted in **t25.1**, a wide variety of disorders are associated with lymphadenopathy. These disorders may be divided into 5 categories: infections, autoimmune, iatrogenic, malignant, and others. In approximately 40%-60% of patients who undergo lymph node biopsy, no specific diagnosis can be reached. Of the specific benign lymphadenopathies, the most common causes encountered are infectious, including mononucleosis (Epstein-Barr virus), cytomegalovirus (CMV), toxoplasmosis, and human immunodeficiency virus (HIV) among others.

25.2 Clinical Findings

The cause of the lymphadenopathy frequently is not apparent from microscopic changes observed in a lymph node biopsy specimen alone. The patient's clinical history, physical examination, and the results of other tests are usually essential for an accurate diagnosis. Certain benign lymphadenopathies, such as Kikuchi-Fujimoto lymphadenitis, are much more common in women than in men (4:1), whereas malignant lymphadenopathies are more common in men. Infectious mononucleosis is rarely seen in patients older than 35 years. Sexual behavior, drugs, previous surgery/biopsy, vaccination, occupation, exposure to pets, and duration of lymphadenopathy are other important aspects of the clinical history **t25.2**.

t25.1 Causes of Lymphadenopathy

Infections

Viral
- Infectious mononucleosis*
- Cytomegalovirus*
- HIV†
- Postvaccinial lymphadenitis‡

Bacterial
- *Staphylococcus**
- *Streptococcus**
- *Mycobacterium tuberculosis**
- Cat-scratch disease‡
- Syphilis*
- Chancroid‡

Protozoal
- Toxoplasmosis*

Fungal
- Cryptococcus*

Histoplasmosis*
Coccidioplasmosis*
Chlamydial*
Lymphogranuloma venereum‡

Autoimmune

Sjögren syndrome‡
Rheumatoid arthritis*

Iatrogenic

Drug hypersensitivity (phenytoin, phenylbutazone, methyldopa, meprobamate, hydralazine)*
Serum sickness*
Silicone‡

Malignant

Hodgkin lymphoma*
Non-Hodgkin lymphoma*
Acute and chronic leukemias*
Metastatic cancer*

Other disorders

Castleman disease*
Kikuchi-Fujimoto lymphadenitis‡
Sarcoidosis*
Dermatopathic lymphadenopathy‡
Histiocytosis X*
Sinus histiocytosis with massive lymphadenopathy*
Abnormal immune response*

**Localized or generalized lymphadenopathy*
†Generalized lymphadenopathy
‡Localized lymphadenopathy

t25.2 Useful Clinical Information in the Evaluation of Lymphadenopathy

Clinical Parameter	Description
History	Sex, age, duration of lymphadenopathy, symptoms, sexual behavior, drug history, pets, occupation
Physical examination	Location of lymphadenopathy; size, tenderness, and texture of lymph node; presence or absence of splenomegaly; ear-nose-throat examination or genital-pelvic examination (depending on site of lymphadenopathy)

Lymphadenopathy with a duration of several months and progressive increase in the size of the lymph node strongly suggests a malignant condition. Fever and weight loss are common symptoms in many benign and malignant lymphoproliferative disorders. A sore throat is frequently present in infectious mononucleosis. The presence of toothache, earache, or lesions in the region drained by the enlarged lymph nodes may explain the cause of lymphadenopathy in some patients.

Once a significant lymph node enlargement has been detected, a careful physical examination must be done to seek other sites of lymphadenopathy, and the presence or absence of splenomegaly should be noted. The location of the enlarged lymph node is important because certain lymph nodes are more frequently affected by certain disease processes than others **t25.3**. In inflammatory disorders, the lymph nodes are frequently tender, whereas in malignant lymphomas they are usually firm, rubbery, and painless. A hard, fixed, rock-like lymph node usually indicates metastatic tumor. The lymph node size is of little help in establishing the diagnosis. With inguinal lymphadenopathy, a genital and perineal examination is imperative. A careful ear, nose, oral, and throat examination is indicated in patients with cervical lymphadenopathy to identify a possible source of infection or a primary tumor.

t25.3 Correlations Between Lymph Node Locations and Disease Origin

Lymph Node Groups	Associated Causes
Occipital	Scalp infections, insect bites, ringworm infection
Posterior auricular	Rubella
Anterior auricular	Eye or conjunctival infections
Posterior cervical	Toxoplasmosis, scalp infections, cat-scratch disease
Submental/submandibular	Dental infections, metastatic disease (oral cavity)
Anterior cervical	Infections of pharynx and oral cavity, tuberculosis, Epstein-Barr virus, nasopharyngeal carcinoma
Supraclavicular	Lymphomas, metastatic disease (lung, gastrointestinal tract)
Mediastinal	Lymphoma, sarcoidosis, histoplasmosis, coccidioidomycosis, tuberculosis, metastatic disease
Axillary	Lymphoma, cat-scratch disease, pyogenic infections of upper arms, brucellosis, dermatopathic lymphadenopathy, metastatic disease (breast)
Epitrochlear	Viral diseases, sarcoidosis, tularemia, infections of hands, lymphoma
Abdominal/retroperitoneal	Lymphoma, metastatic disease, tuberculosis
Inguinal	Herpes, lymphogranuloma venereum, syphilis, gonococcal infection, HIV, lymphoma, metastatic disease

Lymphadenopathy in the supraclavicular area is always a pathologic significance, usually due to lymphoma or metastatic malignancy, especially in the lung or gastrointestinal tract.

25.3 Diagnostic Approach

Following a clinical history and physical examination, the workup for a patient with lymphadenopathy should include the following elements as clinically indicated:

1. Complete blood cell count, including evaluation of the peripheral blood smear.
2. Erythrocyte sedimentation rate (ESR).
3. Throat culture and culture for gonorrhea (if clinically indicated).
4. Chest radiograph and computed tomography (CT) when needed.
5. Serologic tests for infectious disorders and autoimmune disorders.
6. Blood chemistry tests, including transaminase levels, serum calcium, and angiotensin-converting enzyme levels (test for sarcoidosis).

7. Tuberculin skin test or in vitro gamma interferon tests for TB infection.
8. Lymph node fine-needle aspiration (FNA).
9. Lymph node biopsy for histologic examination and culture.
10. Bone marrow aspirate (culture when indicated) and biopsy examination.

25.4 Hematologic Findings

The hematologic findings in reactive lymphadenopathies vary greatly depending on the cause of the disease. Examination of the peripheral blood smear may be particularly helpful.

25.4.1 Blood Cell Measurements

When anemia is present, it is usually mild, normochromic, and normocytic. The leukocyte count is usually elevated. The platelet count may be normal, decreased, or increased, depending on the cause of the lymphadenopathy.

25.4.2 Peripheral Blood Smear Morphology

The RBCs are usually normochromic and normocytic, or they may sometimes be macrocytic as often seen in patients with AIDS. Neutrophilic leukocytosis is often present in pyogenic infections or in the early stages of viral infections such as infectious mononucleosis. The presence of many reactive (atypical) or transformed lymphocytes, together with the characteristic clinical setting, suggest infectious mononucleosis. Such lymphocytosis is also frequently found in CMV infections and toxoplasmosis.

25.4.3 Bone Marrow Examination

Examination of the bone marrow aspirate is rarely helpful in diagnosing benign lymphadenopathies. The bone marrow specimen may show granulomas in patients with tuberculosis, sarcoidosis, or disseminated fungal disease. Special stains for organisms and cultures may occasionally be helpful in the diagnosis.

25.5 Other Laboratory Tests

Test 25.5.1 Serologic Tests for Infectious Agents

Purpose. A variety of infectious diseases and autoimmune disorders associated with lymphadenopathy may be detected with immunoassays.

Principle. Specific and non-specific antibodies and antigens produced by infection with various organisms are detected by methods such as complement fixation and enzyme-linked immunosorbent assay (ELISA) methods.

Specimen. Serum is used as a specimen. (Urine and cerebrospinal fluid are rarely used.) Specimens from the acute and convalescent phases are needed to detect rises in titer in complement fixation tests.

Procedure. A variety of methods can be used. The indirect immunofluorescent technique is performed by incubating serum dilutions with organisms fixed to glass slides. Specific antibody adheres to the organism. In complement fixation tests, specific antibody attaches to antigen (organism) with complement binding.

ELISA methods are extremely sensitive and are used for detecting antibodies to a variety of bacteria, viruses, and parasites. In this technique, an enzyme, such as alkaline phosphatase, is conjugated to an antigen specific immunoglobulin such as antihuman IgG or IgM. An antigen specific to the infectious agent is used to coat a polystyrene well. Dilutions of the patient's serum are added and allowed to react. Excess serum is removed by washing. To detect the antibody specific to the infectious agent, the enzyme-linked antihuman immunoglobulin is then added and allowed to bind. Unbound immunoglobulin is removed by washing. The appropriate substrate for the enzyme is added to measure the enzyme activity, correlating to the amount of bound antihuman immunoglobulin.

The indirect immunofluorescent technique (IFA) is still used in the diagnosis of many emergent infectious diseases where ELISA testing has not yet been developed such as for cat-scratch disease (*Bartonella henselae*) or ehrlichial diseases.

Other tests include Western blot (for HIV infection) and polymerase chain reaction (PCR) technology. The PCR assays for infectious disease associated lymphadenopathy include HIV, CMV, Epstein-Barr virus (EBV), tuberculosis, and cat-scratch disease. Molecular tests for other less frequently encountered infectious agents have also been described.

Interpretation. Serologic tests are available for infectious mononucleosis; CMV lymphadenitis; HIV lymphadenitis; toxoplasmosis; histoplasmosis; lymphogranuloma venereum; cat-scratch disease; syphilis; and autoimmune disorders such as rheumatoid arthritis, systemic lupus erythematosus (SLE), and Sjögren syndrome. A variety of techniques are used, including immunofluorescence, complement fixation, latex fixation, and ELISA. Even when the same basic procedure is used, the results from different laboratories may vary; reference values change frequently due to modifications in techniques and reagents. It is therefore important to be familiar with the particular method used and the reference values given by the laboratory.

In children and young adults with lymphadenopathy, the detection of heterophile antibodies (MonoSpot test) may be very helpful in the diagnosis of infectious mononucleosis. However, this test may be negative in approximately 50% of patients in the first 2 weeks of illness and is less sensitive in children less than 5 years of age. Tests for EBV and/or CMV also may be useful. Other serologic tests that may be helpful include ELISA for HIV, toxoplasmosis, and cat-scratch disease.

Test 25.5.2 Fine-Needle Aspiration (FNA)

Purpose. FNA is done either to render a diagnosis or to decide whether a (surgical) lymph node biopsy should be performed.

Principle. This simple technique is less risky, associated with less patient discomfort, and less costly than a surgical biopsy. It is particularly useful in the diagnosis of metastatic malignancy.

Specimen. Cells are aspirated from the lymph node and can be submitted for cytologic analysis, flow cytometry, microbial culture, or molecular diagnostics.

Procedure. A 23- or 25-gauge needle attached to a disposable syringe is inserted into the lymph node and tissue is aspirated. Small amounts of the aspirated material are smeared across glass slides and stained with Diff-Quik®, May-Grünwald, Giemsa, and/or Papanicolaou methods. Accuracy of the FNA may be improved by performing flow cytometry on the same specimen. A portion of the aspirated material is submitted to the flow cytometry laboratory in heparin (green-top tube) or citrate (yellow-top tube) anticoagulant. When indicated, a sterile specimen is submitted for culture.

Interpretation. FNA can provide a rapid diagnosis in metastatic malignancy, reactive hyperplasia, and some lymphomas when interpreted by an experienced cytopathologist. In select cases, immunohistochemistry and/or flow cytometry done on the aspirated material can provide additional information, such as the demonstration of light chain restriction and/or aberrant phenotypic expression.

Notes and Precautions. FNA does not replace a lymph node biopsy but is a complementary diagnostic technique. The main purpose of FNA is to decide whether a lymph node biopsy is indicated. A diagnosis of metastatic malignancy often obviates the need for a surgical biopsy. Cytologic suspicion of lymphoma is an indication for lymph node biopsy.

Test 25.5.3 Lymph Node Biopsy

Purpose. Lymph node biopsy is the final step in the workup for a patient with lymphadenopathy. It provides a histopathologic diagnosis and, if indicated, sterile tissue should be submitted for culture. Frequently, a specific diagnosis cannot be made. It is then the responsibility of the pathologist to provide the physician with a differential diagnosis.

Principle. Biopsy should be performed when a significantly enlarged lymph node persists and/or increases in size and other tests have failed to provide a diagnosis. A lymph node biopsy should not be performed if a viral infection such as infectious mononucleosis is suspected, because the histopathologic features often resemble malignant lymphoma.

Specimen. If several enlarged lymph nodes are present, an attempt should be made to remove the largest node. The lymph node should be submitted to the laboratory, intact and unfixed, as soon as possible.

Procedure. Histologic interpretation of lymph node biopsy specimens is often difficult, and special care is required in specimen handling. The accuracy of diagnosis is proportional to the quality of the histologic sections. The major reason for difficulty in interpretation is technical and results from improper handling of the biopsy specimen. It is extremely important that the complete lymph node be submitted intact and fresh to the pathology laboratory, where a portion of fresh tissue should be frozen for possible molecular studies, and another portion submitted for flow cytometry, when indicated. If clinically indicated, sterile culture should be performed. A portion of the tissue should then be fixed in formalin and another portion should be fixed in B5 or a similar fixative. (For a more detailed discussion of the handling of lymph node specimens, see Chapter 53).

Interpretation. Optimal interpretation of a lymph node biopsy specimen often requires the collaboration of an experienced surgeon, a hematopathologist, and a hematologist/oncologist. Benign lymphoproliferative disorders may be difficult to differentiate from malignant disorders, in both lymph nodes and extranodal sites. Detailed clinical information, excellent histologic sections, and marker studies are important to attain a correct diagnosis.

A helpful approach to the histologic diagnosis is the pattern approach, or the low-magnification appearance of the lymph node. **t25.4** lists the most common patterns of cellular infiltrate and the disorders associated with each. Once the general pattern is determined at low power, a higher-power examination determines the cellular components present. **t25.5** outlines features that may be useful in differentiating benign hyperplasia from malignant lymphoma.

Notes and Precautions. As previously noted, a number of benign disorders may clinically and histopathologically resemble a malignant lymphoproliferative disorder. Therefore, a hematopathologist should be consulted if the primary pathologist reviewing the tissue does not have experience in examining lymph nodes. Immunoperoxidase studies, flow cytometry, in situ hybridization studies, gene rearrangement studies, and other molecular studies can be extremely helpful in the final diagnosis in difficult cases. These studies are described in more detail in Chapter 53.

In 40%-60% of patients only a diagnosis of reactive, non-specific hyperplasia can be made. However, even a non-specific diagnosis is helpful to the clinician and reassuring to the patient, because the main aim of the lymph node biopsy is to exclude a malignant disease or a treatable disorder.

The term "atypical hyperplasia" refers to a condition where the pathologist cannot distinguish with certainty between a benign and a malignant process. Patients with such conditions must have a careful follow-up and a repeat biopsy if there is persistent lymphadenopathy or if new lymphadenopathy develops. In 18%-25% of affected patients (adults and children), a specific diagnosis is made on repeat biopsy. In adults (particularly in older patients), approximately 50% of patients whose lymph nodes are interpreted as atypical hyperplasia are subsequently diagnosed with malignant lymphoma.

t25.4 Patterns Observed in Reactive Lymphadenopathies

Pattern	Cause of Lymphadenopathy
Follicular pattern	Non-specific hyperplasia (most common) Rheumatoid arthritis HIV Castleman disease Toxoplasmosis Syphilis
Macronodular pattern	Progressive transformation of germinal centers
Interfollicular pattern	Viral lymphadenitis (infectious mononucleosis, cytomegalovirus)
Mixed pattern (follicular and interfollicular)	Viral lymphadenitis (infectious mononucleosis, cytomegalovirus) Toxoplasmosis Kimura disease Lymphogranuloma venereum
Sinusoidal pattern	Non-specific histiocytosis Sinus histiocytosis with massive lymphadenopathy Langerhans cell histiocytosis (histiocytosis X) Whipple disease Monocytoid B-cell hyperplasia Early metastatic disease Lymphangiogram effect
Diffuse pattern	Infectious mononucleosis Abnormal immune response Drug reactions Metastatic disease
Necrotizing pattern	Cat-scratch disease Kikuchi-Fujimoto lymphadenitis Infarction Toxoplasmosis
Granulomatous pattern	Sarcoidosis Tuberculosis Fungal disease Leprosy Drug exposure

t25.5 General Features Differentiating Benign Hyperplasia From Malignant Lymphoma in Lymph Nodes

Feature	Benign Hyperplasia	Malignant Lymphoma
Architecture	Distorted	Often effaced
Sinuses	Open or focally compressed	Often obliterated
Normal cell components	Hyperplastic	Often obliterated
Cell type	Mixture, often transformed cells	Atypical, often monomorphic cells
Immunophenotype	Polyclonal	Usually monoclonal

25.6 Examples of Reactive Lymphadenopathies

25.6.1 Follicular Hyperplasia

Follicular hyperplasia is a common finding in reactive lymph nodes i25.1a. When many follicles are seen in the cortical and medullary regions, it may be difficult to differentiate follicular hyperplasia from follicular lymphoma. The most useful histopathologic feature in the differential diagnosis is the low power appearance. In reactive conditions, compared to follicular lymphoma, the follicles are less numerous, less evenly distributed, and more irregular in shape. In follicular lymphoma, the follicles characteristically have a back-to-back appearance.

In difficult cases, an immunoperoxidase study for BCL-2 protein is useful i25.1b,c.

25.6.2 Infectious Mononucleosis

This disease is caused by EBV and usually affects teenagers and young adults. Typically, the patients have fever, pharyngitis, and cervical or generalized lymphadenopathy. Occasionally splenomegaly and hepatomegaly may be present.

Interpretation of lymph node biopsies from patients with infectious mononucleosis may be very difficult because of the frequent florid proliferation of immunoblasts i25.2a-h. It may be mistaken for non-Hodgkin lymphoma or Hodgkin lymphoma. Immunoperoxidase studies may also be difficult to interpret because many of the large, atypical cells express CD30, suggesting a diagnosis of anaplastic large cell lymphoma or Hodgkin lymphoma i25.2i-k.

The Epstein-Barr virus can be demonstrated within the large transformed cells (immunoblasts) with in situ hybridization studies i25.2l.

To minimize the danger of mistaking infectious mononucleosis from malignant lymphoma it is useful to remember that immunoblastic proliferations, together with lymphoid cells at varying stages of transformation, in teenagers and young adults, is usually a benign, reactive process. A serologic test (MonoSpot test) should always be done, and repeated if necessary, in such situations.

25.6.3 Cytomegalovirus (CMV) Lymphadenopathy

CMV infection may be seen in immunocompromised adults, but more often CMV infection affects immunosuppressed patients. Lymph nodes are usually involved, and the morphologic features resemble infectious mononucleosis. Follicular hyperplasia, clusters of monocytoid cells, and sheets of immunoblasts are often seen i25.3a-c. Viral inclusions may be seen within immunoblasts i25.3c.

In contrast to infectious mononucleosis, CD15 positivity may be seen within the large, atypical cells, suggesting a diagnosis of Hodgkin lymphoma. CMV can be detected within affected cells using an immunoperoxidase method or in situ hybridization.

25.6.4 Cat-Scratch Disease

This necrotizing granulomatous lymphadenitis is caused by *Bartonella henselae*. It is usually unilateral and involves axillary, epitrochlear, cervical, or inguinal lymph nodes. The disease is usually a benign, self-limited disorder, most common in children having had contact with a cat.

Early changes consist predominantly of follicular hyperplasia. Later microabscesses are seen, which finally develop into stellate necrotizing granulomas i25.4.

For a more specific diagnosis, serologic tests are available. Also PCR tests are available to identify the *Bartonella* organism.

i25.1 Follicular hyperplasia

a Multiple reactive follicles are seen in this lymph node section. **b** Immunoperoxidase study demonstrates expression of BCL-2 protein within the mantle zone, but not within the germinal center. **c** Follicular lymphoma. In contrast to follicular hyperplasia, the expression of BCL-2 protein is within the germinal center.

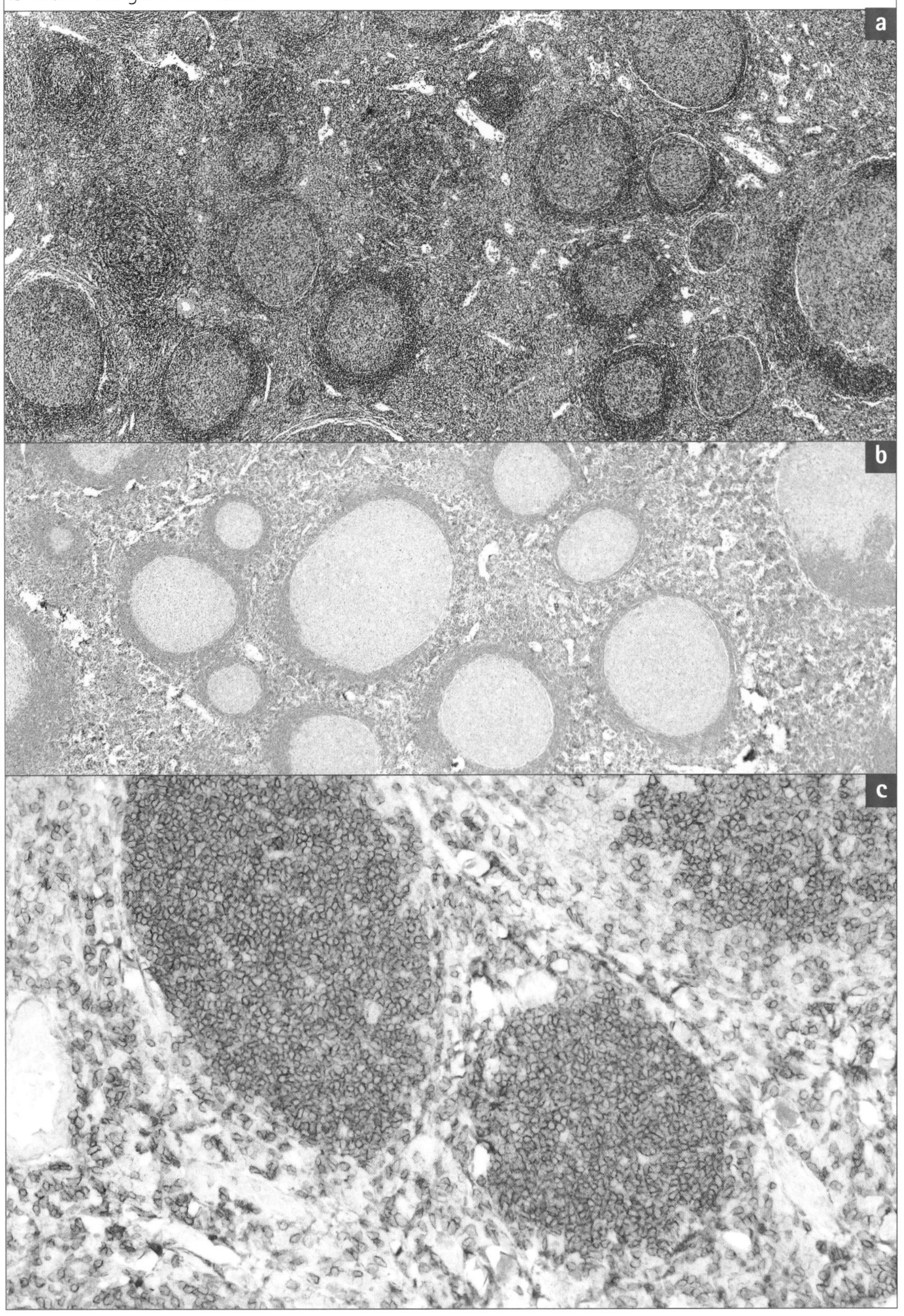

i25.2a–f Infectious mononucleosis

a Section of lymph node biopsy shows a prominent interfollicular infiltrate. **b** Interfollicular infiltrate is composed of lymphoid cells at various stages of transformation. **c** A "starry sky" pattern is created by the presence of many tingible-body macrophages together with sheets of transformed lymphoid cells. **d** The interfollicular infiltrate seen in **i25.2a** consists of immunoblasts, plasmacytoid lymphocytes, and plasma cells. **e** A Reed-Sternberg-like cell (arrow) surrounded by many large transformed lymphocytes and scattered plasma cells. **f** A low-power view of lymph node shows a prominent interfollicular infiltrate and an area of necrosis (arrow).

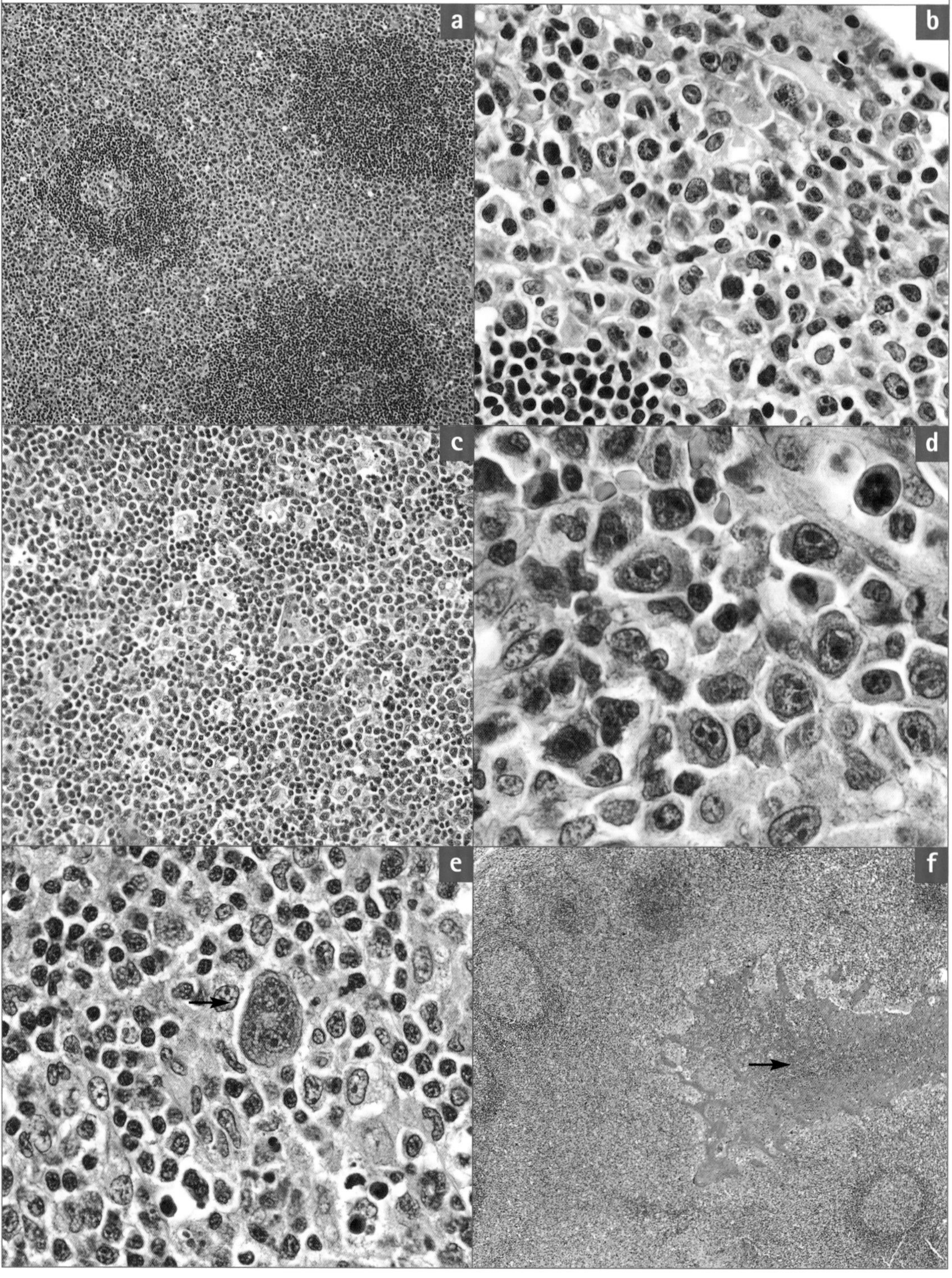

i25.2g–l Infectious mononucleosis

g A high-power view of the interfollicular infiltrate in **i25.2a** shows lymphoid cells at various stages of transformation with a predominance of large cells. Also present are several mitotic figures. **h** Interfollicular infiltrate contains many large cells resembling Reed-Sternberg cells or anaplastic large cell lymphoma cells. **i** CD30 is expressed in many of the large atypical cells present in **i25.2h**. **j** CD20 is expressed in a majority of the large cell interfollicular infiltrate. **k** CD3 is expressed predominantly in the small lymphocytes and not in the large transformed cells. At a later stage of the disease, many of the larger cells express T-cell markers. **l** Numerous large lymphoid cells are positive for the Epstein-Barr virus RNA antigen EBER.

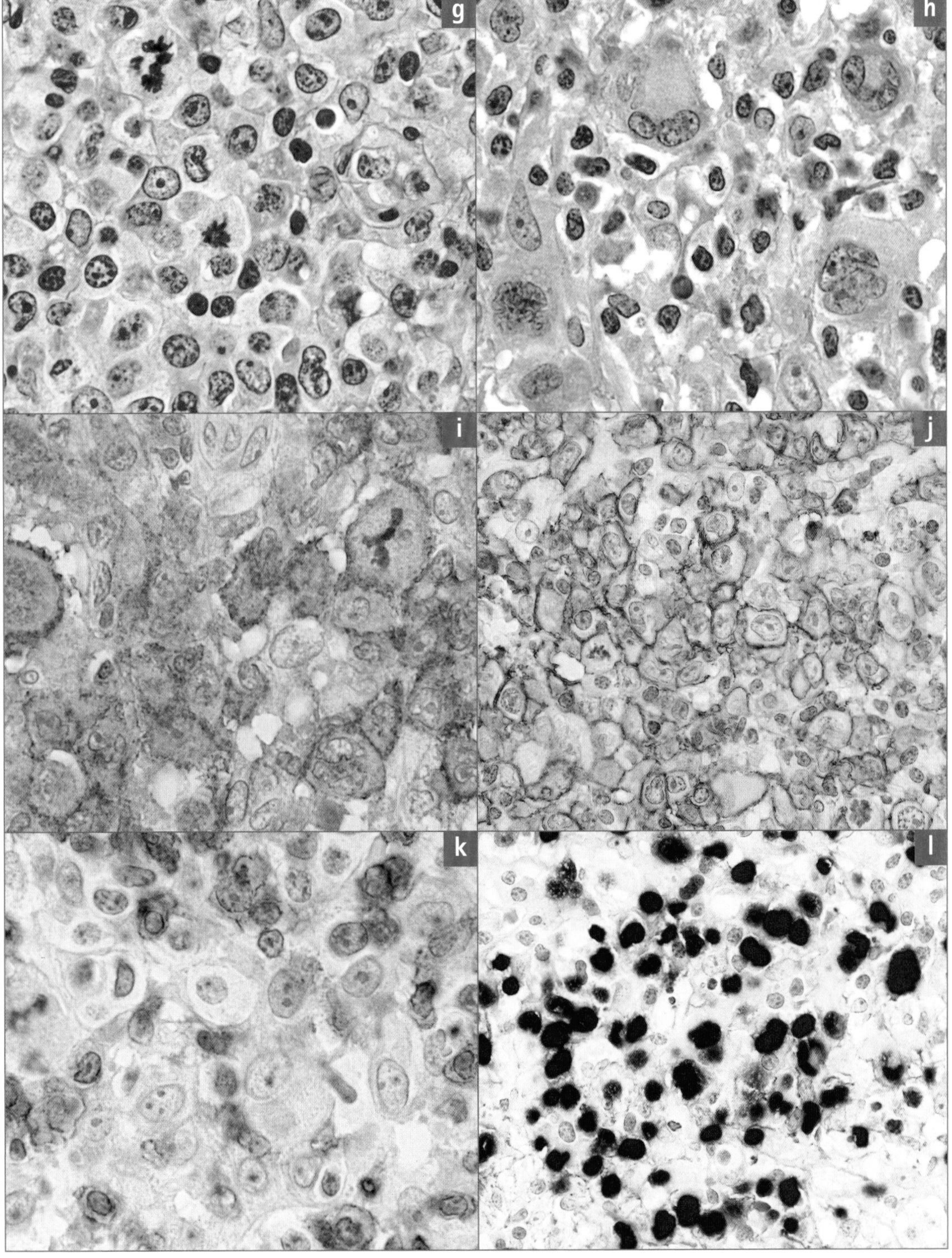

i25.3 Cytomegalovirus lymphadenopathy

a Lymph node biopsy shows follicular hyperplasia and sheets of monocytoid cells (arrow). **b** Numerous transformed lymphocytes and scattered plasma cells are present within interfollicular areas. **c** Intranuclear viral inclusion in a large lymphoid cell (arrow).

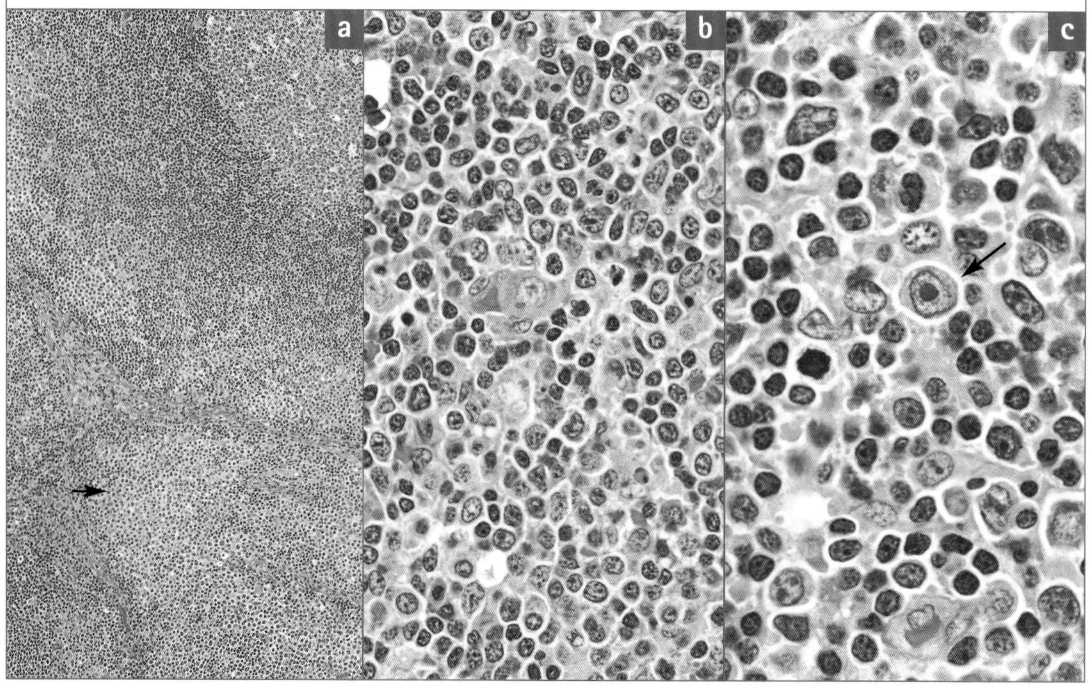

i25.4 Cat-scratch disease

a A hard, immobile, tender mass in the neck is shown. **b** Pus is aspirated from the mass . **c** Polymerase chain reaction assay was done on the pus with primers specific for the *Bartonella henselae* citrate synthase gene. The DNA band pattern is shown . Lanes 2 and 3 show pus specimen from the patient; lanes 1,5,7, and 8 show pus specimens from patients without cat-scratch disease. Lane 4 shows *B henselae* DNA; lane 6 shows pus specimen from another patient with cat-scratch disease; lane 9 shows the molecular size marker. **d** Histopathologic features typical of lymph node biopsy specimens from patients with cat-scratch disease are shown. *(courtesy of Michael Giladi, MD, with permission from* N Engl J Med. *1999;24:108)*

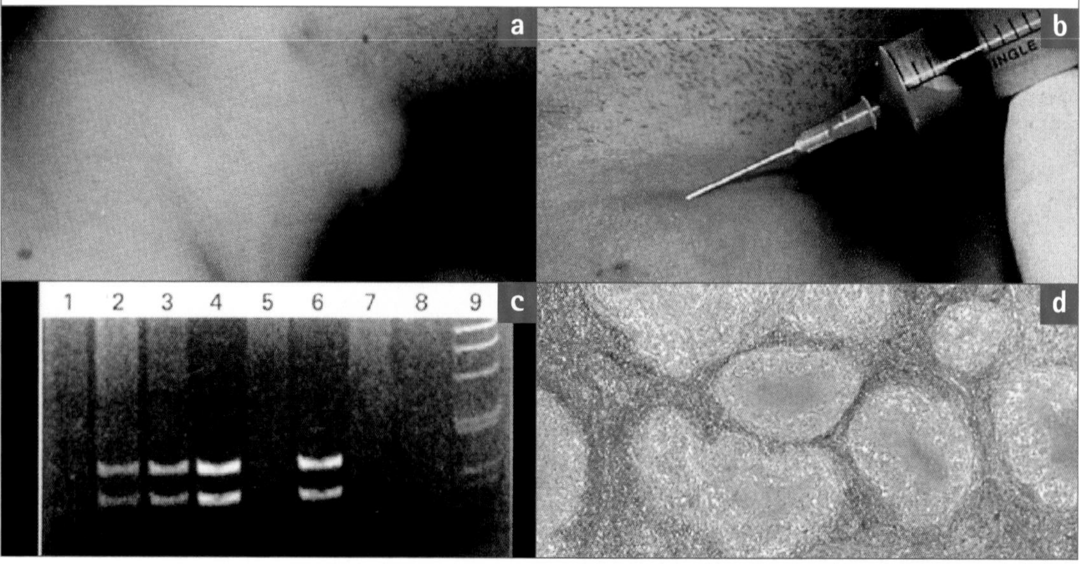

25.6.5 Toxoplasmosis

This is a common parasitic disease worldwide. Approximately 50% of Americans have antibodies to toxoplasma, indicative of chronic asymptomatic infection. In normal adults, localized, asymptomatic lymphadenopathy is the most common presentation. In immunocompromised patients, the infection becomes acutely disseminated.

The classic histopathologic features in the lymph nodes are follicular hyperplasia, large germinal centers surrounded by and/or containing epithelioid histiocytes, and aggregates of monocytoid B-cells within nodal sinuses i25.5a,b.

Serologic tests are available to confirm the histologic diagnosis. A PCR test for toxoplasma is also available.

25.6.6 Dermatopathic Lymphadenopathy

This lymphadenopathy is usually, but not always, associated with a chronic dermatologic lesion. The lymph node shows hyperplastic follicles and expansion of the paracortical T zone caused by many histiocytes, interdigitating reticulum cells, Langerhans cells, and pigment (melanin, lipids, or hemosiderin) i25.6a,b.

25.6.7 Kikuchi Lymphadenopathy

This subacute necrotizing lymphadenopathy is relatively frequent in Asia, but is also not uncommon in Western countries. It usually involves cervical lymph nodes and is most commonly seen in young women (20-30 years old). The etiology of the lesion is unknown.

The histopathologic features are characterized by patchy areas of necrosis in a lymph node where the normal architecture is partially maintained. The areas of necrosis show extensive

i25.5 Toxoplasmosis

a Section of lymph node biopsy shows a large germinal center containing many epithelioid histiocytes (arrows). **b** Monocytoid B-cells (arrow) with abundant cytoplasm surround a lymphoid follicle.

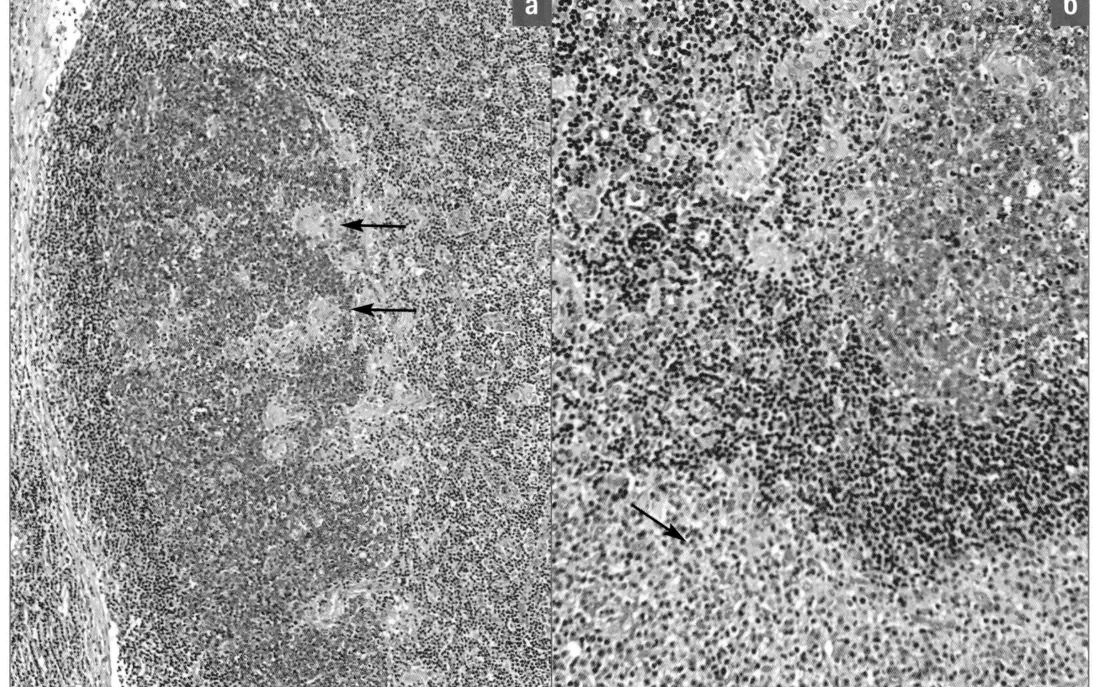

i25.6 Dermatopathic lymphadenopathy

a The paracortex shows pale staining areas of histiocytic aggregates (arrows). b The paracortex contains various types of histiocytes, including Langerhans cells and interdigitating dendritic cells. The brown pigment (arrow) represents melanin, lipid or hemosiderin.

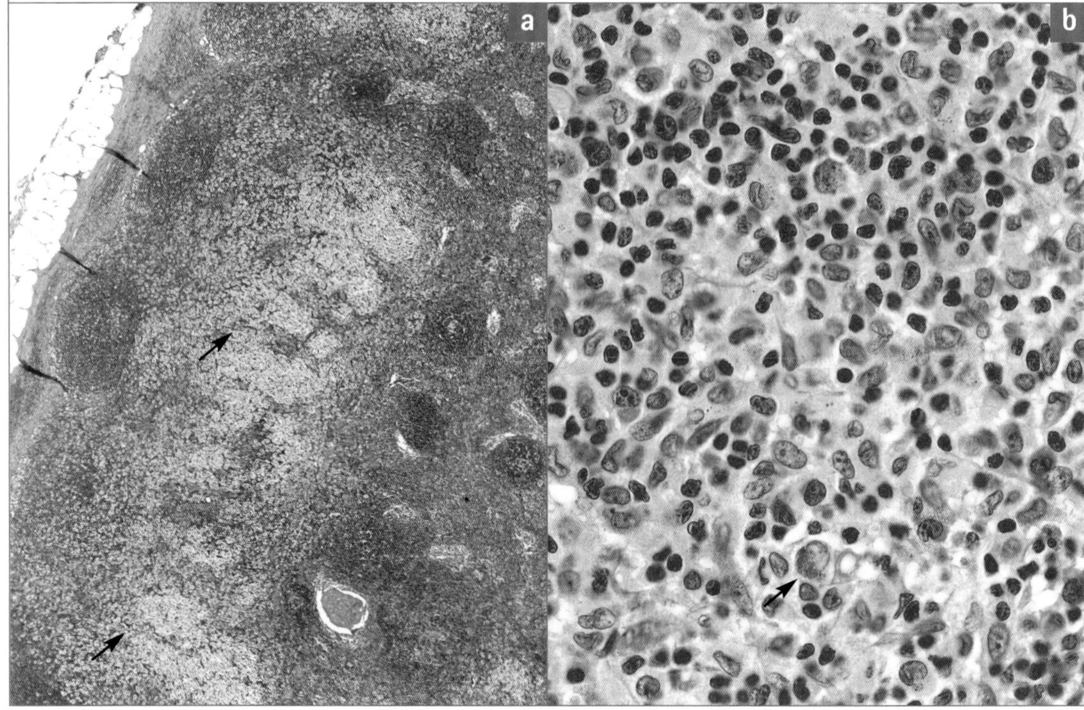

apoptosis with nuclear debris surrounded by large sheets of proliferating histiocytes, plasmacytoid monocytes, and immunoblasts i25.7a–e.

A characteristic feature is the absence of neutrophils and eosinophils, and the crescent shaped nuclei of the mononuclear phagocytes. Immunoperoxidase studies show the histiocytes to express CD68, and myeloperoxidase is expressed in many cells i25.7d,e. In addition, there are variable numbers of T lymphocytes.

Occasionally the sheets of histiocytes and plasmacytoid monocytes partially replacing the normal architecture are misdiagnosed as non-Hodgkin large cell lymphoma.

25.6.8 Castleman Lymphadenopathy

There are 3 main types of Castleman disease: the hyaline vascular type, the plasma cell type, and the multicentric type. Recently an aggressive plasmablastic variant, associated with HHV8+, has been described.

The hyaline vascular type lesions are usually localized, often in the mediastinum and usually asymptomatic. It is characterized by reactive follicles with involuted and hyalinized germinal centers and prominent interfollicular vascular proliferation i25.8a–c. These findings are non-specific and may also be seen in a variety of other disorders, including autoimmune disorders and Hodgkin lymphoma.

The plasma cell type is also non-specific and is seen in such disorders as rheumatoid arthritis and syphilis. It is not restricted to the mediastinum and is more often associated with systemic symptoms such as fever, myalgia, hypergammaglobulinemia and leukocytosis.

The histologic features are follicular hyperplasia with an interfollicular expansion of plasma cells i25.9a,b.

i25.7 Kikuchi lymphadenopathy

a There are localized areas (arrows) of eosinophilic zones of necrosis. b Areas of necrosis with karyorrhectic debris and eosinophilic debris. c Areas distant from the necrosis reveal an infiltrate consisting of histiocytes, transformed lymphocytes, and plasmacytoid monocytes. These areas could be mistaken for a non-Hodgkin large cell lymphoma. d Many of the large cells seen in i25.7c express CD68. e Many cells express myeloperoxidase.

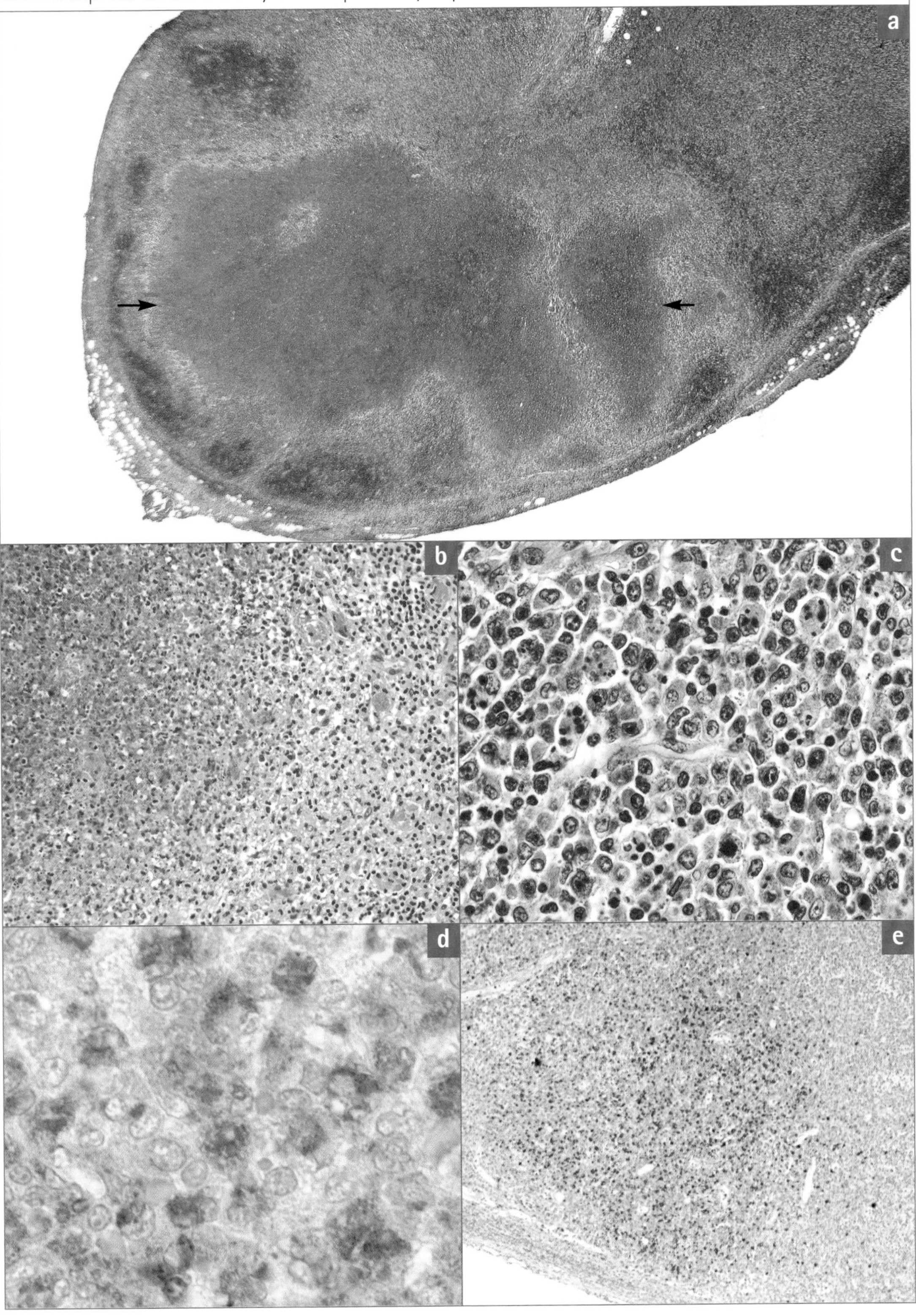

i25.8 Castleman disease, hyaline vascular variant

a There is proliferation of lymphoid follicles of varying size and shape containing several germinal centers. **b** Mantle zone cells are arranged in concentric rings ("onion skin" pattern) around atrophic hyalinized germinal center. **c** Atrophic hyalinized germinal centers are penetrated by blood vessels.

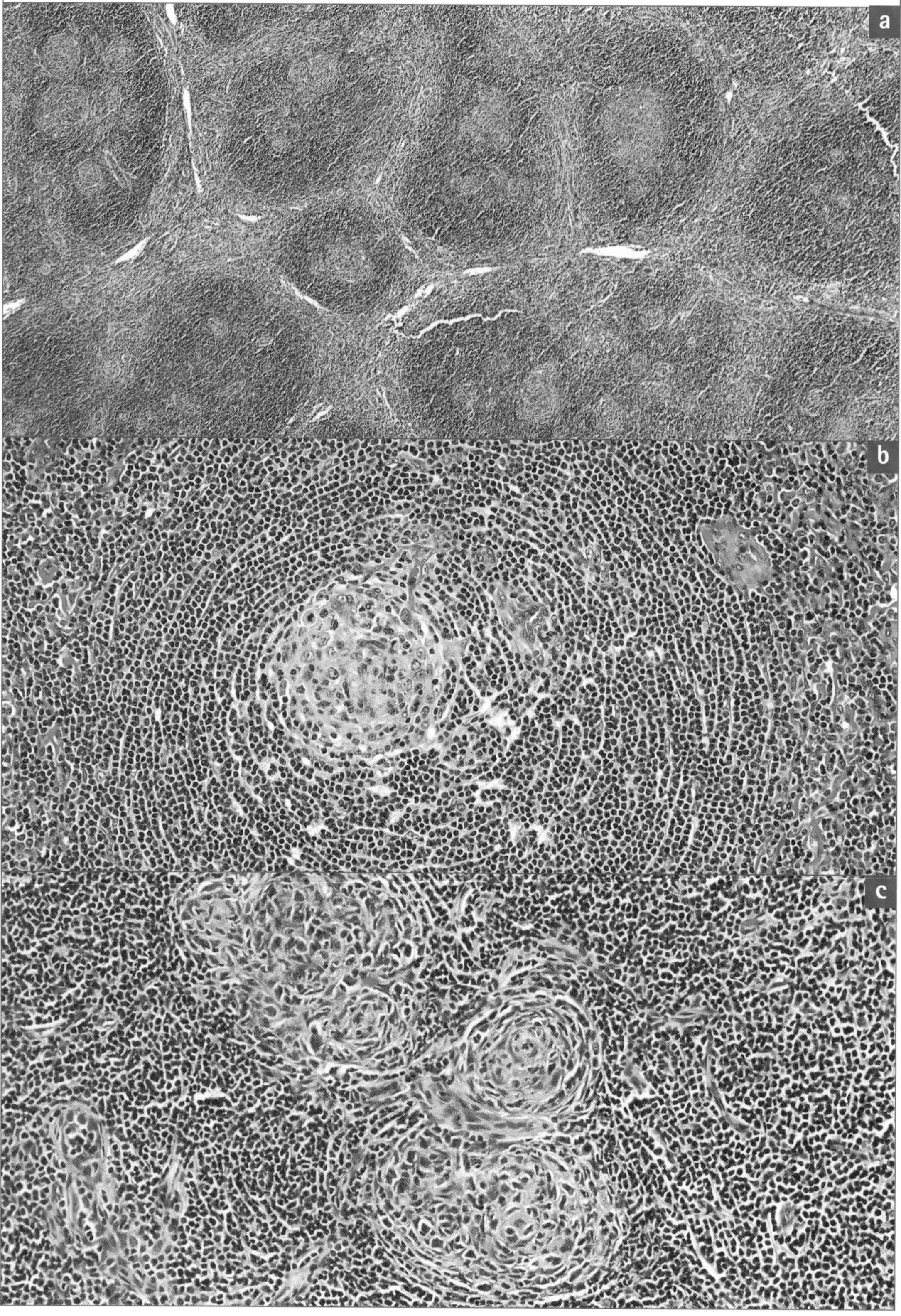

i25.9 Castleman disease, plasma cell variant

a Lymph node sections shows follicular hyperplasia and an interfollicular expansion of plasma cells.
b High power view shows sheets of plasma cells.

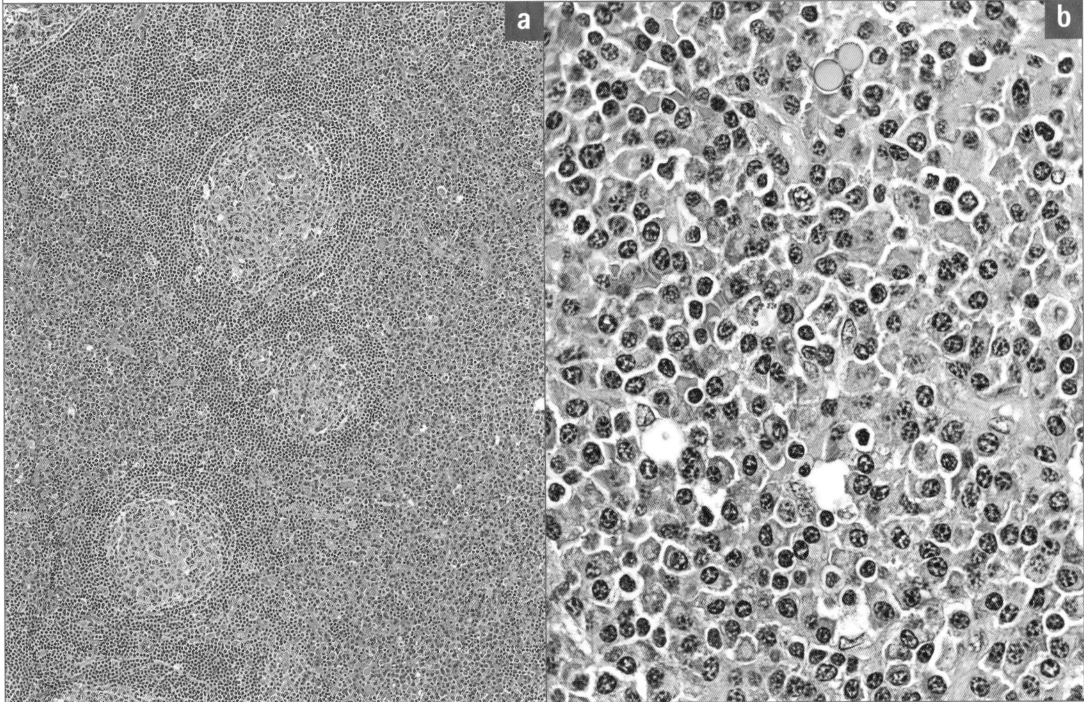

The multicentric Castleman disease has a median age of 50 and appears to be associated with immunoregulatory deficit. The disease may wax and wane, but is sometimes aggressive. The histopathologic features are similar to those seen in the plasma cell type.

The prognosis for the localized forms of Castleman disease is good and can usually be cured with surgery. The multicentric forms of hyaline vascular and plasma cell types may need treatment with steroids or chemotherapy.

25.6.9 Sinus Histiocytosis with Massive Lymphadenopathy (Rosai-Dorfman Disease)

The most common presentation is prominent, bilateral lymphadenopathy in the neck, associated with fever, leukocytosis, and hypergammaglobulinemia. The majority of cases occur during the first 2 decades of life, but any age group may be affected. In addition to affecting the lymph nodes, multiple other body sites may be involved.

Sinuses are dilated and filled with histiocytes i25.10a. Many of the histiocytes contain intact lymphocytes (emperipolesis) i25.10b. The lymph node capsule is usually thickened and the intersinusoidal tissue often contains many plasma cells. The histiocytes express S-100 but not CD1a.

25.6.10 Progressive Transformation of Germinal Centers

Progressive transformation of germinal centers usually presents in young men as a solitary lymph node enlargement. In rare cases there has been an association with Hodgkin lymphoma, usually nodular lymphocyte predominant type, but in the great majority of cases there is no connection with Hodgkin lymphoma. The etiology is unknown. It can be seen with a wide variety of other reactive lymphadenopathies.

i25.10 Sinus histiocytosis with massive lymphadenopathy (Rosai-Dorfman disease)

a Lymph node sections show a thick capsule and multiple pale histiocytes within distended sinuses (arrows). b Many histiocytes contain intact-appearing lymphocytes (emperipolesis) (arrows).

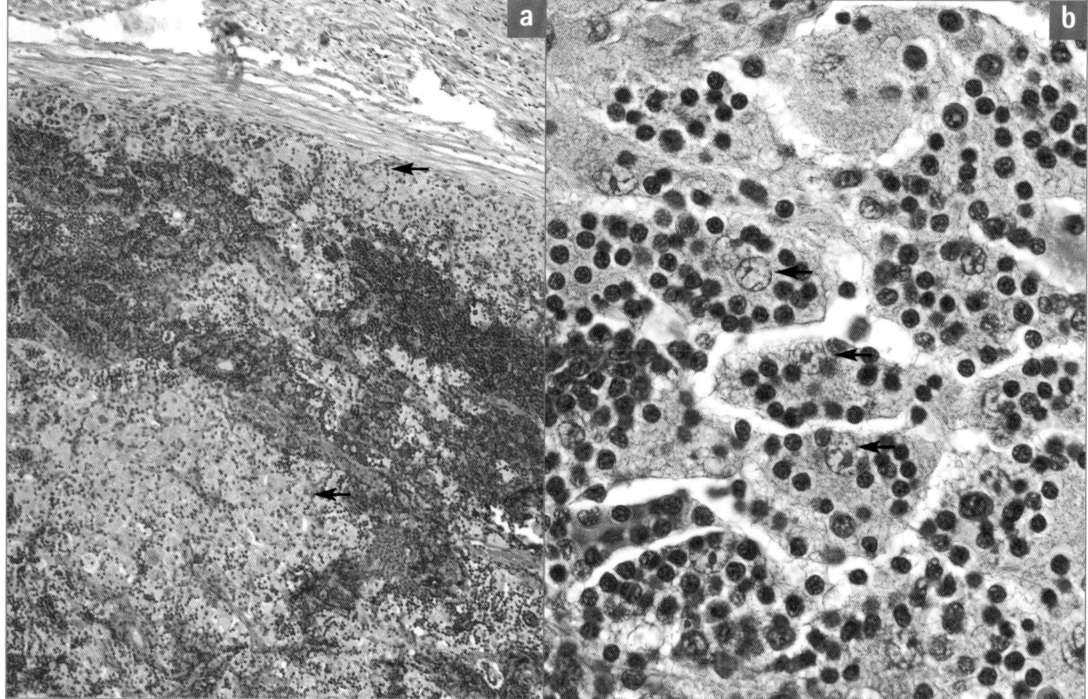

The lesion is characterized by small lymphocytes infiltrating and expanding the germinal centers and forming large nodules i25.11. The small lymphocytes are phenotypically equivalent to polyclonal mantle zone B-cells.

The disorder is benign, but may recur particularly in children.

25.6.11 Metastatic Nasopharyngeal Carcinoma

Nasopharyngeal carcinoma is uncommon in the United States, but in southern China and Malaysia it represents 18% of all malignant tumors. It occurs in children and adults and metastasizes early on to the cervical lymph nodes. Misdiagnosis of the lymph node is common due to absence of obvious primary malignancy and because of the poor differentiation of this tumor i25.12a. It may be mistaken for non-Hodgkin or Hodgkin lymphoma. Immunoperoxidase study will show that the tumor cells express cytokeratin i25.12b.

A more detailed description of reactive lymphadenopathies is available in the references listed.

25.7 Ancillary Tests

25.7.1 Chest Radiograph

A chest radiograph, although normal in most cases, is often indicated. It may show enlarged mediastinal lymph nodes, which may indicate malignant lymphoma, tuberculosis, sarcoidosis, histoplasmosis, or metastatic malignancy. In addition, primary lung parenchymal lesions may be detected.

i25.11 Progressive transformation of germinal centers in a lymph node biopsy

There is follicular hyperplasia surrounding a large nodule containing predominantly small lymphocytes.

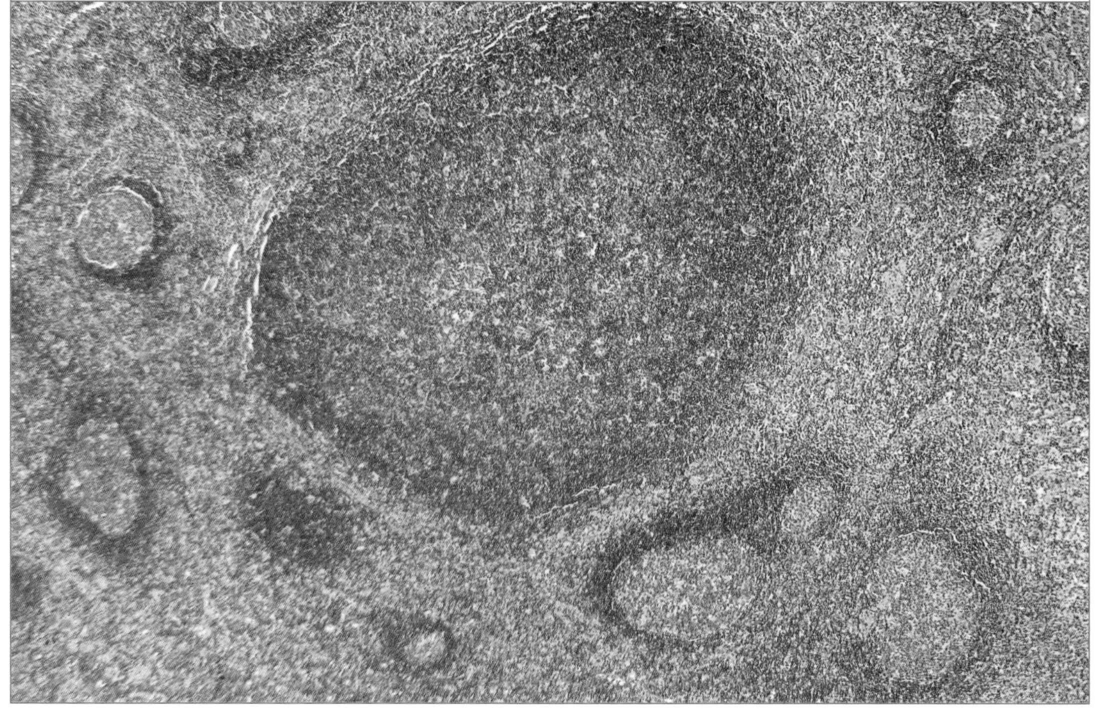

i25.12 Metastatic nasopharyngeal carcinoma

a A large cell interfollicular infiltrate is seen in a lymph node biopsy.
b An antibody to cytokeratin demonstrates that the large cell infiltrate is a carcinoma.

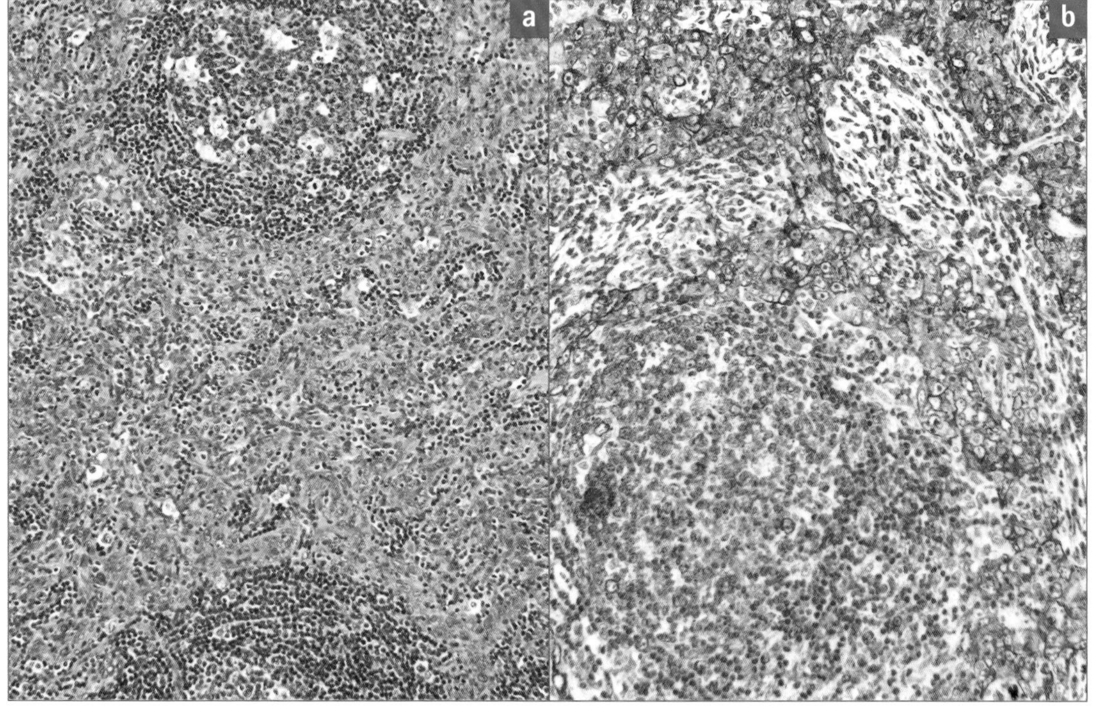

25.7.2 Serum Chemistry

Elevated serum calcium levels and antiotensin-converting enzyme may suggest sarcoidosis. Elevated transaminase levels are frequently seen in infectious mononucleosis.

25.7.3 Tuberculin Skin Test

A positive tuberculin skin test may be helpful in differentiating tuberculosis from sarcoidosis. Alternatively, serum quantity FERON®–TBGOLD testing can confirm latent M-tuberculosis infection.

25.7.4 Course and Treatment

As expected, the clinical course and treatment of lymphadenopathy depends on the cause of the disease.

25.8 References

Dispenzieri A, Gertz MA. Treatment of Castleman's disease. *Curr Treat Options Oncol.* 2005;6:255-266.

Dorfman RF, Berry GJ. Kikuchi's histiocytic necrotizing lymphadenitis: an emphasis on differential diagnosis. *Semin Diagn Pathol.* 1988;5:329-345.

Ferry JA, Harris NL. *Atlas of Lymphoid Hyperplasia and Lymphoma.* Philadelphia: Saunders; 1997.

Ioachim HL, Ratech H. *Ioachim's Lymph Node Pathology. 4th ed.* Philadelphia: Lippincott Williams and Wilkins, 2009.

Jaffe ES. *Surgical Pathology of Lymph Nodes and Related Organs.* Philadelphia: Saunders; 1995.

Lennet K, Diebold T. Reactive and Inflammatory Lymphadenopathies. Atlas Series on Pathology. Springer Verlag, 2001.

Pangalis GA, Boussiotis VA, Fessas PH, et al. Clinical approach to patients with lymphadenopathy. In: Pangalis GA, Pollack A, eds. *Benign and Malignant Lymphadenopathies: Clinical and Laboratory Diagnosis.* London, England: Hardword Academic Publishers; 1993:19-30.

Ramsay AD. Reactive lymph nodes in pediatric practice. *Am J Clin Pathol.* 2004;122(Suppl 1):587-597.

Rosai J. *Rosai and Ackerman Surgical Pathology. 9th ed.* Volume 2 Chapter 21 Lymph Nodes Mosby, 2004:1877-2018.

Segal G, Perkins S, Kjeldsberg CR. CD30 antigen expression on florid immunoblastic proliferations: a clinicopathologic study of 14 cases. *Am J Pathol.* 1994;102:292-298.

Waterston A, Bower M. Fifty years of multicentric Castleman's disease. *Acta Oncol.* 2004;43:698-704.

Weiss LM. *Pathology of Lymph Nodes.* New York: Churchill Livingstone; 1996.

Zardarvi IM, Jain S, Bennet S. Flow cytometric algorithm on fine needle aspiration for the clinical workup of patients with lymphadenopathy. *Diagn Cytopathol.* 1998;19:274-278.

Part VI

Bleeding Disorders

CHAPTER 26

Diagnosis of Bleeding Disorders

George Rodgers, MD, PhD

26.1 Hemostatic Mechanisms

Hemostasis maintains blood in the fluid state within the blood vessels and prevents excessive blood loss after vascular injury. It depends on reciprocal and balanced interactions among the tissues, especially the vascular endothelium; blood cells, especially platelets; and blood plasma containing the coagulation proteins. The size and blood flow of the affected blood vessel are also important hemostatic factors.

In response to vascular damage, blood clots to seal the vessel and prevent leakage. Vascular constriction, platelet aggregation, and fibrin formation occur virtually simultaneously. Once the clot has formed and tissue repair has begun, digestion of the clot (fibrinolysis) begins, eventually leading to vascular patency.

The sequence of events leading to clotting is initiated by trauma to the vessel. Reflex vasoconstriction results in reduced blood flow. When the vascular endothelium is damaged, platelets adhere to subendothelial collagen fibers and microfibrils. Tissue factor exposed in the vessel wall initiates clotting. The result of the coagulation mechanism is the generation of thrombin. In addition to aggregating platelets, thrombin converts fibrinogen to fibrin, which is incorporated into the platelet plug. With the cross-linking of fibrin strands by factor XIIIa and contraction of the platelet mass, a stable clot (thrombus) is formed. Thrombi formed in the arterial system are called "white thrombi" and are composed primarily of platelets. Red thrombi, found in the venous circulation, are composed of erythrocytes trapped in fibrin and contain few platelets.

26.2 Physiology and Biochemistry of Hemostasis

26.2.1 Platelets

Platelets are anucleated disc-shaped cytoplasmic fragments, 2-4 μm in diameter, normally present in the peripheral blood. In a Wright-stained blood smear, they are identified by their blue-gray cytoplasm and purplish granules. Platelets are formed in the bone marrow from giant (30-60 μm) polyploid cells called "megakaryocytes." Megakaryocytes mature by a series of nuclear replications within a common cytoplasm (endomitosis), leading to multilobar nuclei, and by differentiation of specific cytoplasmic granules. Following maturation, the megakaryocyte cytoplasm becomes demarcated into platelet subunits, and the platelets are released into the circulation through the marrow sinusoids. i26.1 illustrates platelet and megakaryocyte morphology as seen in a Wright-stained blood smear and marrow aspirate, respectively.

i26.1 Platelet and megakaryocyte morphology

Panel **a** is a peripheral blood smear showing approximately 18 platelets in the field . Panel **b** is a bone marrow aspirate showing 5 megakaryocytes in the field. One of the megakaryocytes is shedding platelets (arrow). *(a,b Wright stain, × 50)*

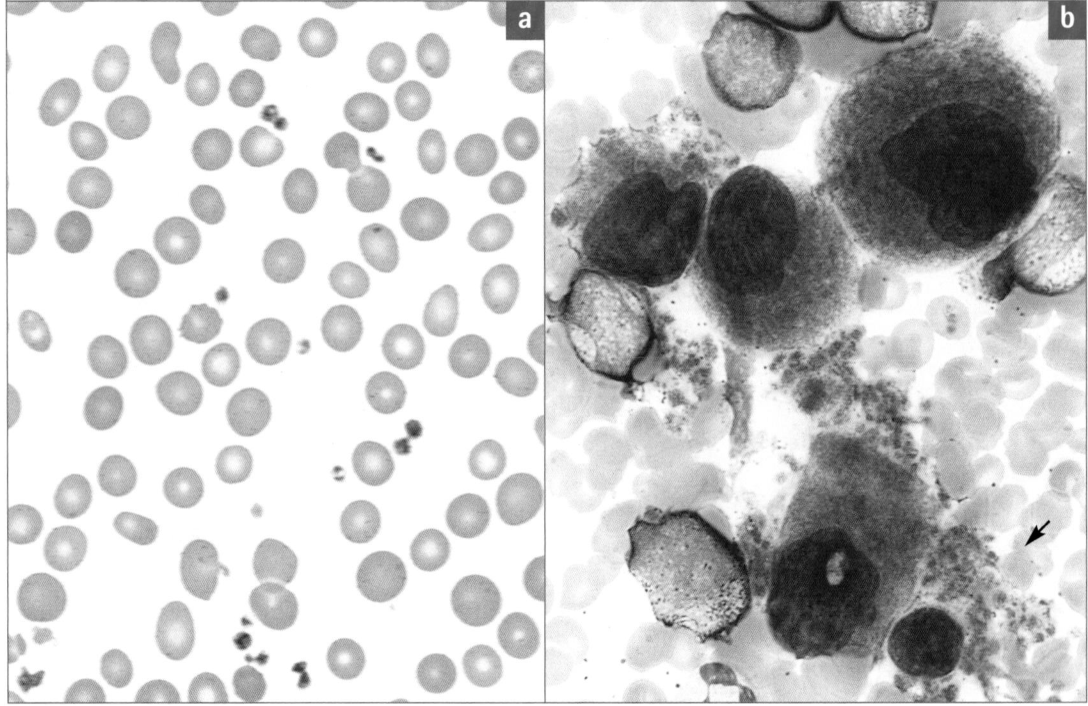

Ordinarily, each megakaryocyte, in its lifetime, produces approximately 1000 platelets. Platelets normally circulate for 9-10 days, and 1/3 of the platelet mass is sequestered in a splenic pool that exchanges freely with the circulatory pool.

Platelets contain 3 types of secretory granules—lysosomes containing acid hydrolases; α-granules containing platelet factor 4 and β-thromboglobulin, platelet-derived growth factor (a mitogen for fibroblasts and smooth muscle cells) and coagulation proteins found in plasma (fibrinogen and von Willebrand factor); and electron-dense bodies (δ-granules) containing adenosine triphosphate, adenosine diphosphate (ADP), calcium, and serotonin.

Adhesion of platelets to the subendothelium initiates the platelet phase of hemostasis (primary hemostasis). Adhesion is mediated when von Willebrand factor binds to subendothelial receptors and to glycoprotein Ib on platelets. Collagen fibers then induce platelets to aggregate by stimulating them to secrete adenosine diphosphate and to synthesize thromboxane A_2. ADP mediates and further amplifies aggregation. Thrombin formed by the soluble coagulation system also activates platelets.

Vasoconstriction is enhanced by the release of serotonin and thromboxane A_2. Platelet activation induces expression of binding sites for coagulation proteins; this activity has been termed "platelet factor 3." In addition to platelet-vessel wall interactions (adhesion), platelet-platelet interactions (aggregation) occur; the latter are mediated by fibrinogen, which links 2 platelets by the fibrinogen receptor, glycoprotein IIb-IIIa. The platelet plug formed is provisional and will not remain hemostatically effective unless a firm fibrin clot forms around it. Platelet actomyosin provides for clot retraction and consolidation.

26.2.2 Blood Coagulation

During blood coagulation, the second phase of hemostasis, soluble plasma fibrinogen is converted to an insoluble fibrin clot as a result of a series of enzymatic interactions leading to the formation of thrombin. These enzymatic interactions involve conversion of a zymogen (enzyme precursor) to a corresponding protease (active enzyme), which is responsible for activation of a subsequent zymogen.

The enzymatic pathways leading to fibrin formation can be initiated by 2 mechanisms f26.1. There is in vivo interdependence between the pathways, and important feedback-activation mechanisms occur. Formation of a normal blood clot requires several plasma coagulation proteins. There are 4 general categories of coagulation factors:

1. Serine endopeptidases (proteases). Factors II (prothrombin), VII, IX, X, XI, XII, and prekallikrein circulate in the zymogen form. Initiation of coagulation results in the activation of each factor. A lower case *a* indicates the active factor (eg, factor Xa). Prothrombin and factors VII, IX, and X, require vitamin K for a posttranslational modification to synthesize fully active coagulation proteins that can bind calcium ions **t26.1**.
2. Cofactors. Cofactors required for activation of some of the procoagulant proteins include high-molecular-weight (HMW) kininogen and factors V and VIII. The 2 latter proteins have minimal activity until activated. Tissue factor also may be considered a cofactor, since factor VIIa is inactive unless complexed with tissue factor.
3. Fibrinogen. Factor I is a soluble protein that becomes the insoluble fibrin clot following cleavage by thrombin.
4. Factor XIII. This is a plasma transglutaminase, which, when activated to factor XIIIa, stabilizes the fibrin clot.

t26.1 The Vitamin K–Dependent Proteins*

Procoagulants	Anticoagulants
Prothrombin (factor II)	Protein C
Factor VII	Protein S
Factor IX	
Factor X	

**Following synthesis of these proteins by the liver, a posttranslational modification (γ-carboxylation of certain glutamic acid residues) occurs, resulting in functional coagulation proteins. This posttranslational modification requires vitamin K. In the absence of vitamin K (vitamin K deficiency) or in the presence of vitamin K antagonists (warfarin sodium [Coumadin]), non-functional coagulation proteins are synthesized.*

Activation of coagulation occurs by 2 mechanisms. Tissue factor initiates the extrinsic pathway of clotting (see f26.1). High concentrations of tissue factor are present in skin, brain, lung, and placenta, as well as in monocytes and the adventitia of large blood vessels. In the basal, unperturbed state, blood is not in contact with tissue factor. Clotting is initiated only by induction of normally latent tissue factor or by exposure of blood to extravascular tissues expressing tissue factor.

Tissue factor initiates clotting by forming a complex with factor VIIa. Tissue factor–factor VIIa complex activates factor X;factor Xa, in the presence of the cofactor (factor Va), activates prothrombin to form thrombin. Excessive activity of the tissue factor-factor VIIa complex is regulated by tissue factor pathway inhibitor. Prothrombin activation

f26.1 The blood coagulation mechanism

In vivo coagulation is initiated by tissue factor expression; the tissue factor–factor VIIa complex activates factors IX and X. When small amounts of factor Xa are generated, tissue factor pathway inhibitor inhibits subsequent tissue factor activity. Thrombin generated by initial tissue factor activates factor XI to initiate intrinsic coagulation and additional thrombin formation. Thrombin generation is amplified by thrombin feedback activation of factors V and VIII. Factor XII initiation of coagulation is important when artificial surfaces are present, but not for in vivo coagulation. The initial fibrin generated by thrombin action on fibrinogen is soluble ($fibrin_s$); hemostatically effective insoluble fibrin ($fibrin_i$) is generated by factor XIIIa.

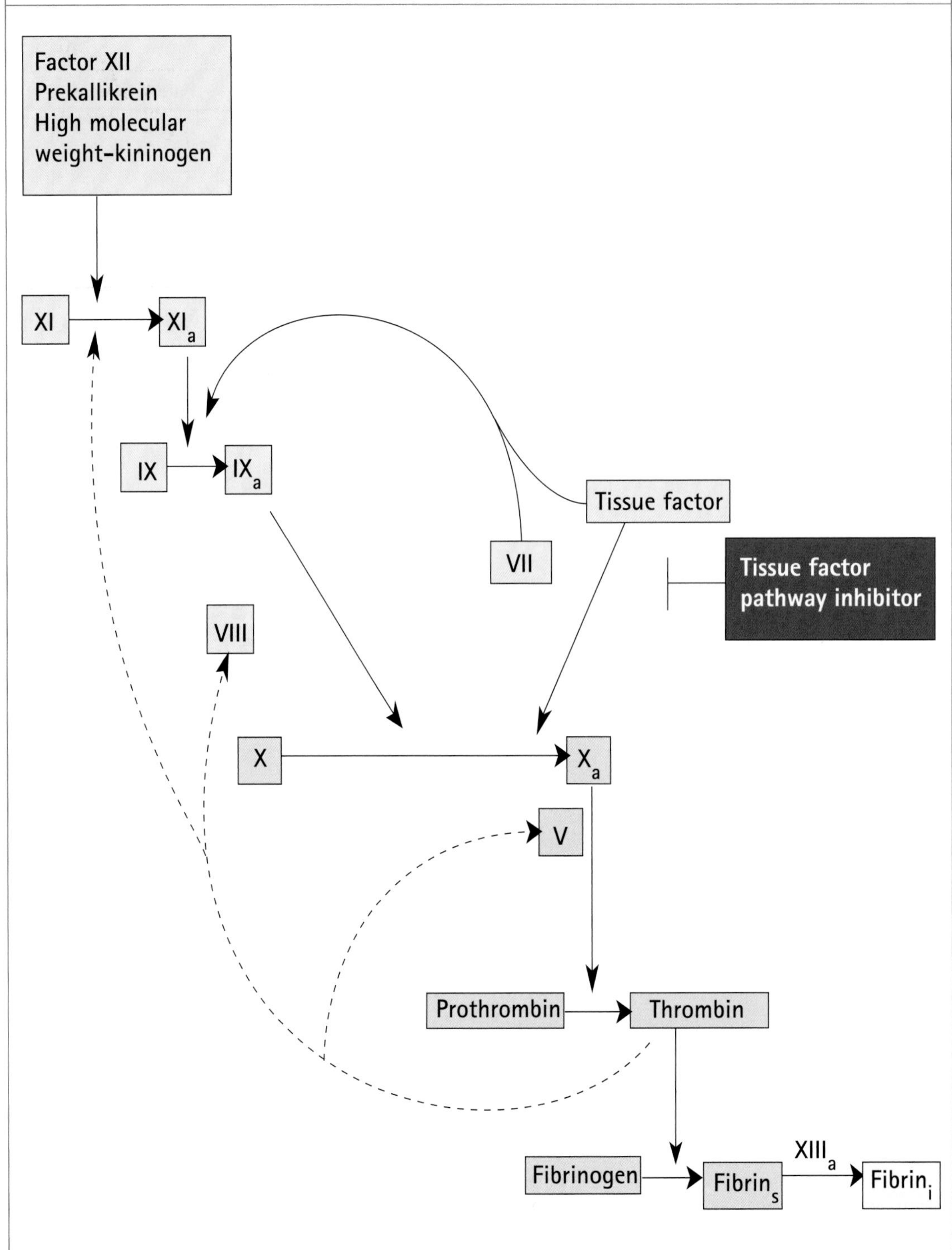

occurs on cellular surfaces of platelets, endothelial cells, smooth muscle cells, and monocytes, and requires calcium and factor Va. Prothrombin activation and thrombin cleavage of fibrinogen constitute the common pathway of coagulation.

Once thrombin is formed, clotting occurs. Thrombin cleavage of fibrinogen results in fibrin monomer formation. Polymerization of fibrin monomers and cross-linking of fibrin by thrombin-activated factor XIIIa lead to generation of the insoluble fibrin clot.

Several feedback-activation mechanisms are important in the amplification of coagulation. For example, thrombin activates factors V and VIII, markedly enhancing thrombin generation. Factor Xa also can activate factor VII to enhance factor X activation by the tissue factor–factor VIIa complex.

The second mechanism for initiating coagulation is the intrinsic pathway (see **f26.1**). Traditionally it has been thought that exposure of subendothelial connective tissue, presumably collagen, activates factor XII. Factor XIIa then converts prekallikrein to kallikrein, which then converts more factor XII to factor XIIa, which in turn activates factor XI. These reactions require a cofactor protein, HMW kininogen. Factor XIa then converts factor IX to factor IXa. Factor XII, prekallikrein, and HMW kininogen are referred to as the contact proteins, because their activation occurs on contact with an abnormal surface (glass or kaolin).

Interdependence between the extrinsic and intrinsic pathways has been demonstrated: the tissue factor–factor VIIa complex can activate factor IX, providing a mechanism for bypassing the initial steps of the intrinsic pathway. Factor IXa activates factor X in a reaction that requires a cofactor (factor VIIIa) and calcium. Like factor V, factor VIII must be activated by thrombin to participate in factor X activation.

It is unclear how the intrinsic pathway of coagulation is initiated in vivo. Patients with a deficiency of factor XII, prekallikrein, or HMW kininogen bleed normally and the necessity of these factors is questionable. However, both pathways are of physiological importance since patients lacking components of either the extrinsic (factor VII) or intrinsic (factors VIII, IX, and XI) pathways have hemorrhagic disease.

Thrombin feedback activation of factor XI may explain how intrinsic coagulation begins in the absence of the contact factors (ie, to explain why patients with contact factor deficiency do not have bleeding disorders). A current model for blood coagulation involves the following steps: First, tissue factor is expressed following vascular injury; complex formation with factor VIIa initiates clotting by activation of factors IX and X. Tissue factor pathway inhibitor then prevents subsequent extrinsic activation of factor X. Thrombin formation is further amplified by feedback activation of factors V, VIII, and XI, leading to persistent activation of intrinsic coagulation. This model has the advantage of explaining both why patients with hemophilia (deficiencies of factors VIII, IX, or XI) bleed and why patients with contact factor deficiency do not.

A summary of the hemostatic events that occur immediately after vascular injury is presented in **f26.2**. In the normal hemostatic response to vascular trauma, the processes of platelet function and blood coagulation are intimately related.

26.2.3 Fibrinolysis

Following hemostatic plug formation and cessation of hemorrhage, vascular repair begins with lysis of the fibrin clot. Local thrombin formation stimulates secretion of vascular endothelial cell tissue plasminogen activator (t-PA). Plasminogen and t-PA diffuse within the thrombus, where t-PA activates plasminogen to plasmin, a protease capable of degrading fibrin in a process called "physiologic fibrinolysis" **f26.3**. Fibrinolysis is restricted to the clot because inhibitors to t-PA and plasmin are present in blood (plasminogen activator inhibitors and α_2-antiplasmin, respectively).

f26.2 Summary of hemostatic events immediately following vascular injury

a Thromboresistant properties of the blood vessel wall (see Chapter 32) maintain blood in a fluid state. Platelets circulate in a non-adhesive state.
b Immediately after vascular injury, exposure of subendothelial components, including collagen fibrils, induces platelet adhesion, mediated by the adhesive plasma protein, von Willebrand factor (vWF), and its platelet receptor, glycoprotein (GP) Ib.
c Platelet activation results from exposure to collagen, leading to thromboxane (Tx) A_2 generation, platelet secretion (release reaction), and formation of thrombin. These events lead to additional platelet recruitment into the platelet plug (aggregation). The platelet-platelet interaction results from fibrinogen binding to its platelet receptor, glycoprotein IIb-IIIa.
d Tissue factor expressed by the subendothelium or by adventitial tissues generates thrombin; thrombin activity results in cross-linked fibrin strands that reinforce the platelet plug. Platelet actomyosin mediates clot retraction.

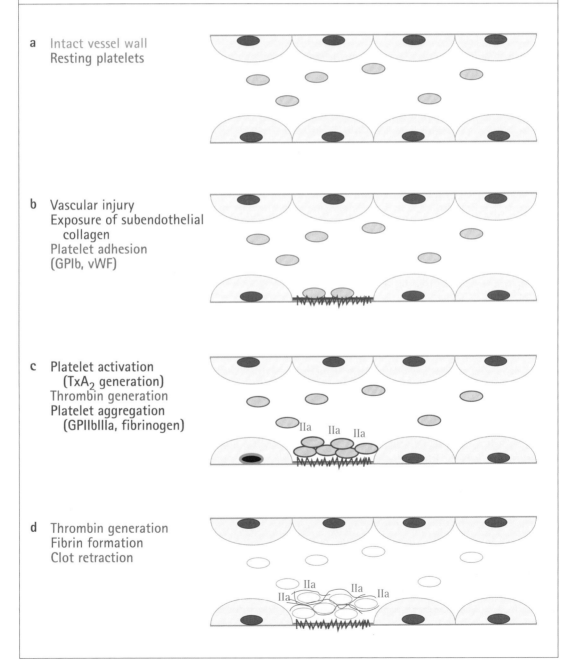

a Intact vessel wall
Resting platelets

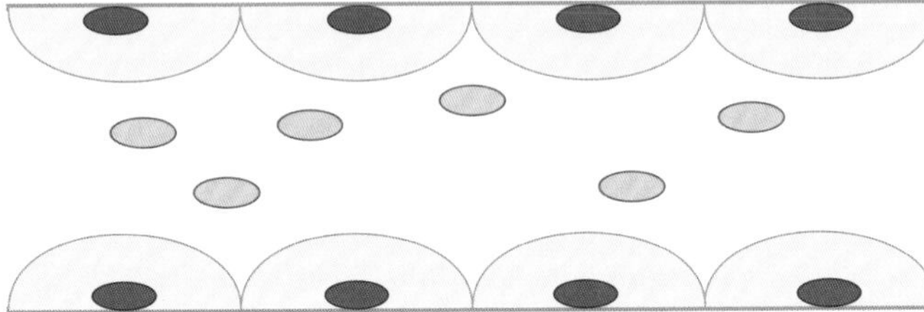

b Vascular injury
Exposure of subendothelial collagen
Platelet adhesion (GPIb, vWF)

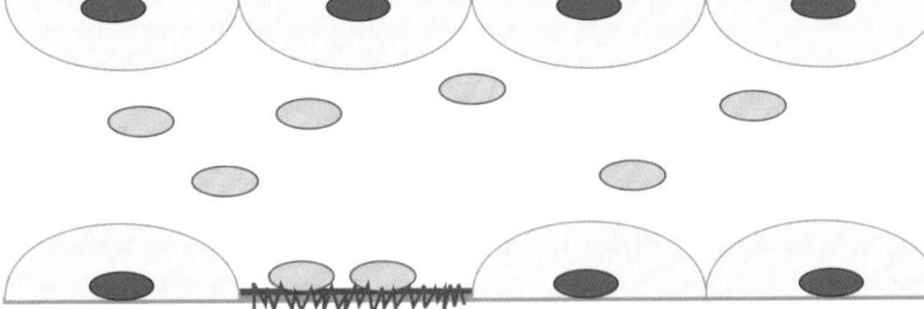

c Platelet activation (TxA_2 generation)
Thrombin generation
Platelet aggregation (GPIIbIIIa, fibrinogen)

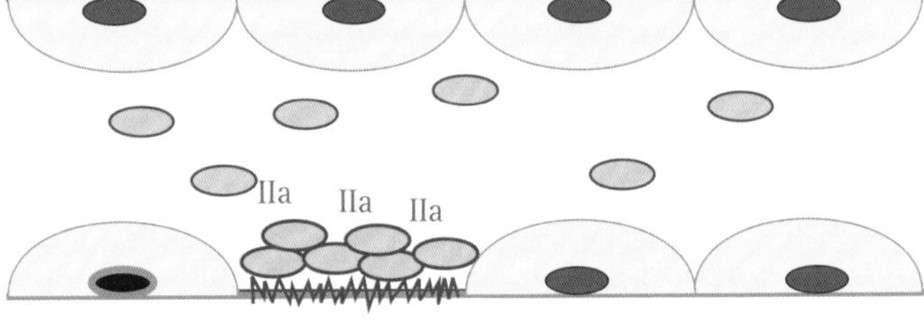

d Thrombin generation
Fibrin formation
Clot retraction

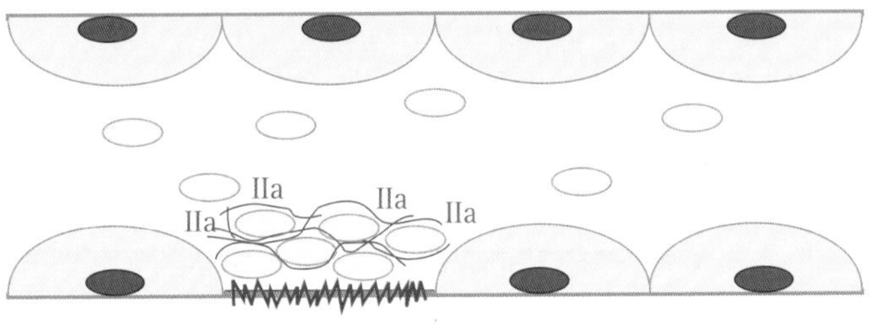

f26.3 Physiologic fibrinolysis

Fibrin formation (shaded area) initiates secretion of vascular endothelial cell tissue plasminogen activator (t-PA). Plasminogen and t-PA assemble on fibrin to generate plasmin, an enzyme that degrades fibrin to fibrin degradation products (FDP). t-PA and plasmin activity are inhibited by plasminogen activator inhibitor and α_2-antiplasmin, respectively, if the active enzymes escape the confines of the clot.

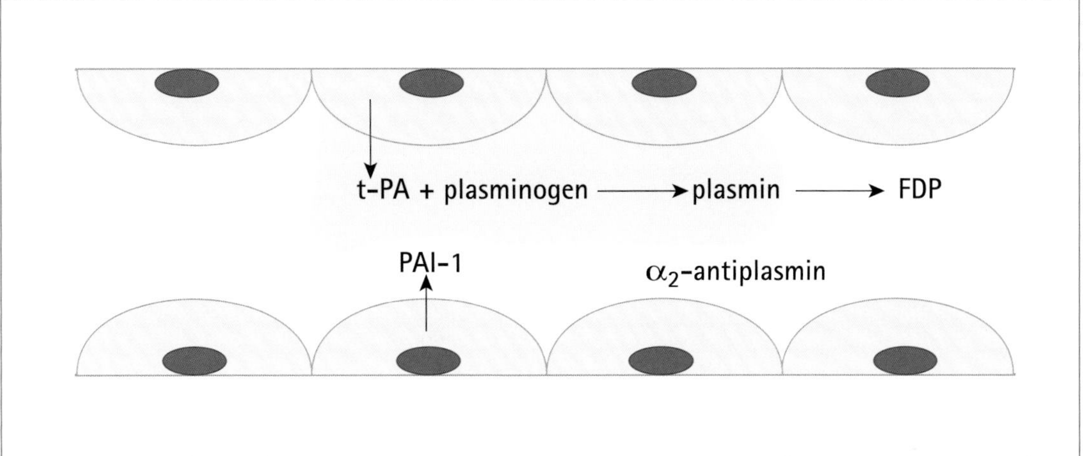

26.3 Approach to the Bleeding Patient

In evaluating a patient with a putative bleeding disorder, answers should be obtained for the following questions as part of the patient history:

1. What is the duration of the bleeding tendency (is it inherited or acquired)?
2. Is there a family history of bleeding? If so, is it transmitted in a dominant or recessive fashion?
3. Is bleeding spontaneous, or is surgery or trauma required to elicit bleeding?
4. What is the location and type of bleeding?

The following questions should be addressed during the physical examination:

1. Is bleeding represented by petechiae or large soft tissue bruises?
2. Are hemarthroses present?
3. Are there telangiectasias?

t26.2 distinguishes the 2 major classes of bleeding disorders—platelet-vascular type and coagulation type—based on information obtained from the patient. Inherited bleeding disorders can be differentiated from acquired disorders by family history, age, and the presence or absence of an underlying disorder. Deficiency of factors VIII and IX (hemophilia A and B, respectively) are both X-linked recessive disorders among men. von Willebrand disease is the most common bleeding disorder and is transmitted in an autosomal dominant fashion. Other inherited bleeding disorders (eg, factor VII deficiency, factor XI deficiency) are usually transmitted in an autosomal recessive manner.

Acquired bleeding disorders usually result from systemic disease, such as leukemia, sepsis, uremia, and liver disease. It is important to remember that abnormalities in blood vessels or their supportive tissues may result in inherited or acquired bleeding (eg, hereditary hemorrhagic telangiectasia, scurvy).

t26.2 Clinical Manifestations in Patients with Bleeding Disorders

Findings	Coagulation Disorders	Platelet or Vessel Disorders
Petechiae	Rare	Characteristic
Deep hematomas	Characteristic	Rare
Hemarthroses	Characteristic	Rare
Delayed bleeding	Common	Rare
Bleeding from superficial cuts	Minimal	Persistent
Patient gender	Most inherited disorders in men	Most inherited disorders in women
Mucosal bleeding	Minimal	Typical

26.4 Laboratory Tests

Coagulation tests are conducted primarily on plasma, which is the anticoagulated, acellular portion of the blood. Trisodium citrate (3.2% or 3.8%), which inhibits clotting by complexing free calcium, is used to anticoagulate the blood for laboratory screening. Consensus guidelines have recommended the use of 3.2% citrate anticoagulant. Most laboratories use silicone-coated glass tubes for collection, although plastic tubes are increasingly used. Unlike many clinical laboratory tests, sample quality is extremely important for coagulation testing. The correct ratio of citrate to plasma and the quality of venipuncture are important factors in the sample collection. Details of the various coagulation tests are given in the following sections, and **t26.3** summarizes test results in common bleeding disorders. **f26.4** illustrates the coagulation mechanism depicted earlier and indicates parts of the mechanism measured by the PT and aPTT.

t26.3 Results of Laboratory Tests for Common Bleeding Disorders

Disorder	PT	aPTT	Platelet Count
von Willebrand disease	Normal	Normal or increased	Normal
Hemophilia A or B	Normal	Usually increased	Normal
Thrombocytopenia	Normal	Normal	Decreased
Vitamin K deficiency	Increased	Normal or increased	Normal

PT = prothrombin time; aPTT = activated partial thromboplastin time

Test 26.4.1 Prothrombin Time Assay

Purpose. The prothrombin time (PT) assay is used to screen for inherited or acquired abnormalities in the extrinsic (factor VII) and common (factors V and X, prothrombin, and fibrinogen) pathways (**t26.4**). It is also used to monitor the effect of oral anticoagulant therapy (see Chapter 33).

Principle. In this assay, clotting is initiated by a commercial tissue factor reagent called "thromboplastin." Plasma, thromboplastin, and calcium are mixed, and the clotting time is determined. The thromboplastin reagent contains phospholipid, so all activities of the extrinsic and common pathways are measured. The PT depends on the concentration of prothrombin; factors V, X, and VII; and fibrinogen. The assay is prolonged when factor levels are low, and normal when factor levels are borderline or normal. Because 3 of the 5 factors measured by the PT are vitamin K-dependent (prothrombin and factors VII and X), this assay is useful in identifying vitamin K deficiency (usually associated with liver disease or oral anticoagulant therapy). The PT assay does not measure the intrinsic factors (factors VIII, IX, and XI; contact factors) or factor XIII activity. Depending on the thromboplastin reagent used, the normal PT reference range is 10-16 seconds.

Specimen. Citrated plasma obtained by clean venipuncture is used.

Procedure. The plasma sample is added to the thromboplastin reagent, which also contains calcium. The test is performed in duplicate and the clotting time average reported.

Interpretation. Numerous commercial thromboplastins are used in the United States and their variable sensitivity in detecting vitamin K deficiency has led to renewed awareness of the pitfalls of comparing results from PT assays using different thromboplastins. A prolongation of the PT usually indicates defective or decreased synthesis of the vitamin K–dependent clotting factors. The PT assay also is sensitive to a decrease in factor V and fibrinogen concentrations, which may occur in end-stage liver disease or in disseminated intravascular coagulation. Another variable affecting the PT reference range is the instrumentation used in the assay. If photo-optical instruments are used

f26.4 The blood coagulation mechanism as screened by the PT and aPTT assays

The PT measures the extrinsic (tissue factor) pathway and common pathway (red loop), while the aPTT measures the intrinsic and common pathways (blue loop). The endpoint of coagulation tests is generation of soluble fibrin, so factor XIII deficiency is not detected by the PT or aPTT tests. PT = prothrombin time; aPTT = activated partial thromboplastin time

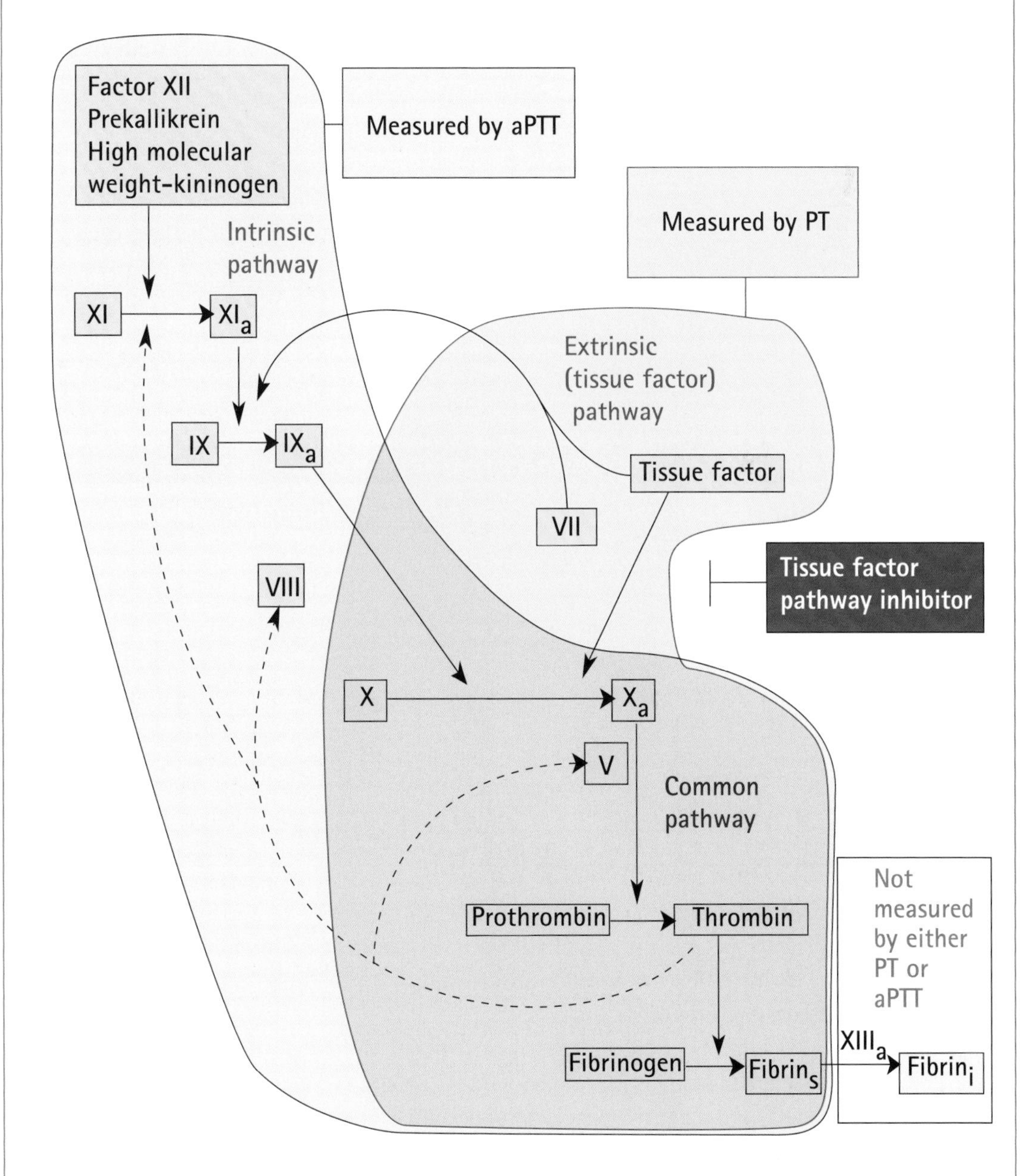

and plasma samples are turbid or icteric, the optical density change induced by clotting may not be detected, and the instruments will record the highest value of which they are capable.

Shortened PT values may be due to poor quality venipuncture, resulting in an activated sample. If this possibility is excluded, shortened values may be caused by chronic disseminated intravascular coagulation (in vivo activation).

An inherited deficiency of one of the factors affecting the PT assay is uncommon. The test may be prolonged due to the presence of antibodies to prothrombin (seen in patients with autoantibodies associated with the lupus anticoagulant) or to factor V, or with specimens from patients with certain abnormal fibrinogens (dysfibrinogenemias).

Notes and Precautions. If a normal plasma sample is left at cold temperatures for several hours, the PT of that sample may be shortened substantially. Contact (factor XII) activation of factor VII may be responsible for this phenomenon. Consensus guidelines recommend that 3.2% citrate be used to anticoagulate blood for coagulation testing (see Chapter 33). Recent data indicate that plastic tubes may be substituted for glass collection tubes with no change in most coagulation reference ranges.

Test 26.4.2 Activated Partial Thromboplastin Time (aPTT)

Purpose. The aPTT assay is used to detect inherited and acquired factor deficiency of the intrinsic pathway, to screen for the lupus anticoagulant, and to monitor heparin therapy.

Principle. The aPTT is an assay of the intrinsic and common pathways. A platelet substitute (crude phospholipid) and a surface-activating agent such as micronized silica (to activate factor XII) are added to plasma. This achieves optimal contact activation. Calcium is then added and the clotting time is recorded. The aPTT assay measures all factors except factors VII and XIII (see **t26.4**). Depending on the reagent used, the aPTT reference clotting time is 25-45 seconds. Because platelet-poor plasma is used, this assay is not influenced by quantitative or qualitative abnormalities in platelets.

t26.4 Coagulation Factors Measured by aPTT and PT Assays

aPTT	PT	Both Tests
XII	VII	X
HMW-K	X	V
Prekallikrein	V	Prothrombin
XI	Prothrombin	Fibrinogen
IX	Fibrinogen	
VIII		
X		
V		
Prothrombin		
Fibrinogen		

aPTT = activated partial thromboplastin time; PT = prothrombin time; HMW-K = high-molecular-weight kininogen

Specimen. Citrated plasma obtained by a clean venipuncture is used.

Procedure. Patient plasma specimen is mixed with an aPTT reagent (containing phospholipid and contact activator), followed by the addition of calcium. The test is performed in duplicate, and the average clotting time is reported.

Interpretation. The aPTT reference range depends on 2 major variables—the aPTT reagent and the instrumentation used. The assay is prolonged when 1 or more of the factors measured is deficient. If the period of contact activation is greater than 2-3 minutes, the aPTT may not detect prekallikrein deficiency.

Many commercial aPTT reagents are insensitive in screening for factor deficiency; mild deficiency (eg, a factor VIII level of 35%) is not detected with most reagents. In addition, reagents vary in detecting the lupus anticoagulant. When evaluating patients for this, it is important to ensure that aPTT plasma samples are prepared so they are platelet-poor. Heparin contamination must be considered in evaluating unexplained prolonged aPTT values, especially when these samples are obtained from patients in intensive care settings.

Specific inhibitors of clotting factors also may prolong the aPTT, the most common being factor VIII antibodies. Isolated prolonged aPTT values of unknown causes should be evaluated with a mixing study. The patient's plasma sample is mixed in equal volume with a normal plasma specimen, and the aPTT assay is run immediately (0 time) and 1-2 hours later. Correction of the prolonged aPTT value to the normal reference range with mixing at both intervals suggests factor deficiency as the cause of the prolonged aPTT value. Failure of the patient's prolonged aPTT value to correct suggests an inhibitor to coagulation, such as heparin, the lupus anticoagulant, or an antibody to a specific coagulation protein. If the patient's sample displays a markedly prolonged thrombin time but not reptilase time, heparin is present in the sample (discussed in the next section). If the mixing study results at 0 and 1-2 hours are similarly prolonged, the lupus anticoagulant is suspected, and corroborative tests for this antiphospholipid antibody can be performed (discussed in Chapter 30). If the mixing study results demonstrate time-dependent prolongation, typically seen with protein-antibody interactions, an antibody to a specific coagulation factor is suggested, and specific factor assays can then be performed.

Shortened aPTT values may be due to poor-quality venipuncture, resulting in an activated sample. Excluding this possibility, two other causes of shortened aPTT values are marked elevation in factor VIII levels or chronic disseminated intravascular coagulation (in vivo activation).

Notes and Precautions. If plasma samples are turbid or icteric, the optical density change induced by clotting may not be detected, and photo-optical instruments will record the highest value of which they are capable. Similarly, if plasma samples have been activated and fibrin formation occurs during the instrument's lag period, the maximal clotting time will be printed. Whenever these maximum clotting time values are obtained on photo-optical instruments, the clotting assay should be repeated using a manual method. Consensus guidelines recommend that 3.2% citrate be used to anticoagulate blood for coagulation testing (see Chapter 34).

Test 26.4.3 Thrombin Time

Purpose. The thrombin time is used to screen for abnormalities in the conversion of fibrinogen to fibrin.

Principle. The addition of thrombin to plasma converts fibrinogen to fibrin, bypassing the intrinsic and extrinsic pathways. The time necessary for fibrinogen to clot is a function of fibrinogen concentration.

Procedure. In this test, thrombin (1-2 U/mL) is added to the patient's plasma sample and the clotting time measured.

Interpretation. The reference range for a normal thrombin time using a final thrombin concentration of ~1 U/mL is 15-20 seconds. A prolongation greater than 3 seconds over the control value is abnormal. Common causes of a prolonged thrombin time include fibrinogen deficiency (quantitative or qualitative), heparin, and elevated fibrin degradation products. Less commonly, certain paraproteins may inhibit fibrin monomer polymerization and prolong the thrombin time. Hyperfibrinogenemia also may prolong the thrombin time, especially if fibrinogen levels are greater than 5 g/L.

Markedly long thrombin time values suggest heparin contamination in the sample and can be confirmed with a normal reptilase time (a reptilase time measures the conversion of fibrinogen to fibrin but is insensitive to heparin). Prolonged thrombin time values not due to heparin can be evaluated using assays for fibrinogen (functional and immunologic) and fibrin degradation products (see Chapter 30).

Notes and Precautions. The concentration of thrombin used in this assay determines the reference range for the test, as well as sensitivity. High concentrations of thrombin result in shorter clotting times and decreased sensitivity.

Test 26.4.4 Automated Coagulation Methods

Purpose. The endpoint of blood coagulation tests can be detected by several methods: mechanical detection of fibrin formation; photometric recording of clot opacity; or the rate of fibrin polymerization.

Procedure. Automated coagulation analyzers can perform large numbers of routine assays, such as PT and aPTT, as well as fibrinogen, antithrombin, and plasminogen. Automated instrument platforms are available to perform a large variety of coagulation methods, allowing cost savings and the capability of laboratories to perform comprehensive testing.

Test 26.4.5 Platelet Count

Purpose. This test is performed routinely on almost all patients using particle counters as part of the routine complete blood count.

Interpretation. The normal platelet count usually ranges from $150 \times 10^3/mm^3$ ($150 \times 10^9/L$) to $440 \times 10^3/mm^3$ ($440 \times 10^9/L$). Bleeding disorders may be associated with either thrombocytopenia or thrombocytosis; a bone marrow examination can frequently help evaluate these disorders.

Test 26.4.6 Bleeding Time

Purpose. The bleeding time has previously been used to screen patients for inherited platelet dysfunction (eg, von Willebrand disease, qualitative platelet abnormalities).

Principle. The bleeding time measures bleeding cessation from a small, superficial wound made under standardized conditions. The bleeding time is mainly affected by primary hemostatic mechanisms (platelet number and function), but is also affected by other conditions (hemotocrit, skin quality, technique).

Procedure. The Ivy bleeding time is the preferred method. A blood pressure cuff is placed around the patient's upper arm and the pressure is raised to 40 mm Hg. Two small punctures are made along the volar surface of the patient's forearm. The drops of blood issuing from the bleeding points are absorbed at intervals of 30 seconds into 2 filter paper disks—one for each puncture wound—until bleeding ceases. The average of the times required for bleeding to stop is taken as the bleeding time.

Several modifications of this technique have attempted to standardize the skin puncture. Perhaps the best and least traumatic of these is a sterile disposable device (Simplate, General Diagnostics, Morris Plains, NJ) that makes 2 uniform incisions 5 × 1 mm using spring-loaded blades contained in a plastic housing. The device is placed firmly on the volar surface of the forearm without pressure and positioned so the incision is parallel to the fold of the elbow, with care taken to avoid superficial veins, scars, and bruises. The blade is then released by depression of the triggering device. The normal bleeding time with this method is less than 8 minutes.

Interpretation. Previous studies using the bleeding time indicated that this test might be an indicator of platelet function and therefore might be helpful in predicting bleeding in individual patients. More recent studies suggest that the bleeding time is determined not only by platelet function but also by hematocrit, certain components of the coagulation mechanism, skin quality, and testing technique. There is no evidence that the bleeding time can predict bleeding, and there is no correlation between a skin template bleeding time and certain visceral bleeding times.

An abnormal bleeding time in patients with a history of lifelong bleeding justifies further hemostatic testing for platelet dysfunction. However, some patients with inherited platelet dysfunction may have normal bleeding times. Given the significant limitations of the bleeding time test, it is preferable to order specific tests to evaluate von Willebrand disease and platelet dysfunction (see Chapter 27).

Antiplatelet drugs usually prolong skin bleeding times (but not necessarily visceral bleeding times). However, patients who are hemostatically normal usually have bleeding times within the normal reference range after aspirin ingestion. In contrast, patients with platelet dysfunction demonstrate marked prolongation of the bleeding time after taking aspirin. **t26.5** lists drug preparations containing aspirin.

t26.5 Aspirin-Containing Drugs*

Alka-Seltzer (extra strength)
Anacin (maximum strength)
Anodynos
APC
Arthritis pain formula
ASA
Ascriptin
(regular or extra strength); A/D
Aspercin (extra)
Aspergum
Aspermin (extra)
Aspirbar
Aspirjen Jr
Aspirtab (maximum strength)
Azdone[†]
Azotal[†]
Bayer Aspirin (genuine; maximum children's) delayed-release Enteric; extended-release 8-hour; plus buffered; plus extra strength buffered; therapy
Buff-A; Buff-A-Comp[†]; Buff-A-Comp 3[†]
Buffaprin (extra)
Buffasal (maximum)
Buffered (therapy)
Bufferin (arthritis strength; extra strength; tri-buffered)
Buffex
Buffinol (extra)
Butalbital compound[†]
Cama arthritis pain reliever
Cope
Damason-P[†]
Darvon compound 65[†]
Doloral[†]
Duradyne
Easprin[†]
Ecotrin (maximum)
Empirin; with codeine (2,[†] 3,[†] 4[†])
Epromate[†]
Equagesic[†]
Equazine[†]
Excedrin (extra strength)
Fiorinal[†]; with codeine[†]
Genprin
Isollyl improved[†]
Lanorinal[†]
Lorprin[†]
Lortab ASA[†]
Magnaprin (arthritis strength)
Maxiprin
Measurin
Meprogesic Q[†]
Midol
Momentum
Norgesic[†]; Forte[†]
Norwich; extra strength
Orphenagesic[†]; Forte[†]
PAC revised formula analgesic
Palagesic
Presalin
Rid-A-Pain with codeine[†]
Robaxisal[†]
Roxiprin[†]
Percodan[†]; Demi[†]
Salecto
Salocol
Sedalgesic inserts[†]
Sine-Off tablets
Soma compound[†]; with codeine[†]
St. Joseph's aspirin (cold tablets for children)
Stanback powder (original formula)
Synalgos-DC[†]
Trigesic
Tri-Pain
Vanquish
Verin
Wesprin buffered
ZORprin[†]

*From Billups NF, ed. American Drug Index 1994. 38th ed. St. Louis, Mo: Facts and Comparisons; 1994.
†Available by prescription only.

Notes and Precautions. The bleeding time test may leave 2 small scars, and the patient should be so informed. The bleeding time test should not be performed on patients with moderate thrombocytopenia (platelet count <50 × 10^3/mm^3 [<50 × 10^9/L]), anemia, or uremia. The College of American Pathologists and the American Society for Clinical Pathology concluded in a position paper that the bleeding time was not effective as a screening test, and that a normal bleeding time does not exclude a bleeding disorder. More recently developed assays such as the Platelet Function Analyzer may be better screening tests for platelet function (see below).

26.5 New Assays of Platelet Function

Limitations of the bleeding time have led to the development of additional tests, including point of care tests. Only one test has been described in multiple reports, the Platelet Function Analyzer (PFA-100). In this technique, citrated blood samples are exposed to high shear rates in a capillary flowing through an aperture with a membrane coated with collagen and either ADP or epinephrine. The endpoint of the test is termed the "closure time," the time for hemostatic plug formation within the aperture. Initial experience with this device suggests that its optimal use will require integrating PFA-100 results with CBC, blood smear, von Willebrand tests, and platelet aggregation findings.

26.6 References

Bennett St, Lehman CM, Rodgers GM, eds. *Laboratory Hemostasis: A Practical Guide for Pathologists.* New York: Springer;2007:1-225.

Broze GJ Jr. The role of tissue factor pathway inhibitor in a revised coagulation cascade. *Semin Hematol.* 1992;29:159-169.

Castellone D. How to deliver quality results in the coagulation laboratory: commonly asked questions. *Lab Med.* 2004;35:208-213.

Hayword CP, Harrison P, Cattaneo M, et al. Platelelet function analyzer (PFA)-100 closure time in the evaluation of platelet function. *J Thromb Haemost.* 2006;4:312-319.

Lehman CM, Blaylock RC, Alexander DP, Rodgers GM. Discontinuation of the bleeding time test without detectable adverse clinical impact. *Clin Chem.* 2001;47:1204-1211.

Peterson P, Hayes TE, Arkin CF, et al. The preoperative bleeding time test lacks clinical benefit. *Arch Surg.* 1998;133:134-139.

Rodgers GM, Lehman CM. The diagnostic approach to the bleeding disorders. In: Greer JP, Foerster J, Rodgers GM, et al, eds. *Wintrobe's Clinical Hematology. 12th ed.* Philadelphia: Lippincott Williams & Wilkins; 2009:1273-1288.

Chapter 27
Thrombocytopenia

George Rodgers, MD, PhD

The typical clinical findings associated with thrombocytopenia include petechial hemorrhage, ecchymoses (bruises), and bleeding from mucous membranes (eg, epistaxis, gum bleeding, menorrhagia).

27.1 Pathophysiology

The causes of thrombocytopenia are summarized in **t27.1** (disorders are classified according to mechanism). Major mechanisms of thrombocytopenia include decreased marrow production, increased platelet destruction, and splenic sequestration. Occasionally, hemodilution results in thrombocytopenia, and artifactual (spurious) thrombocytopenia may occur.

t27.1 Causes of Thrombocytopenia
Failure of marrow production
Reduced megakaryocytes
Marrow infiltration with tumor, infection, or fibrosis
Marrow aplasia (fatty replacement) due to drugs, chemicals, or radiation
Congenital abnormalities (Wiskott-Aldrich syndrome, Fanconi's syndrome)
Ineffective megakaryocytopoiesis
Megaloblastic anemia
Myelodysplasia
Alcohol suppression
Increased platelet destruction
Immune thrombocytopenia
Autoantibody-mediated: systemic lupus erythematosus, lymphomas, drugs, infections, idiopathic (ITP)
Alloantibody-mediated: posttransfusion purpura, fetal-maternal incompatibility
Non-immune thrombocytopenia
Disseminated intravascular coagulation
Thrombotic thrombocytopenic purpura
Mechanical (prosthetic materials)
Splenic sequestration
Hemodilution
Spurious
EDTA-pseudothrombocytopenia

Splenic sequestration usually can be excluded easily by physical examination (palpable splenomegaly is almost always present). The typical evaluation for thrombocytopenia is to distinguish decreased platelet production from increased platelet destruction. If no obvious marrow insult can be identified (chemotherapeutic agents, ionizing radiation, toxic chemicals such as benzene, etc), a bone marrow examination is necessary to categorize the condition. If decreased megakaryocytes are present, the causative disorder should be identifiable, such as leukemia or solid tumor, infection (granuloma), fibrosis, or fatty infiltration, as may be seen in marrow aplasia. In rare cases, an inherited or acquired disorder of ineffective megakaryocytopoiesis may be present.

If normal or increased megakaryocytes are present, peripheral platelet destruction is suggested. This categorization mandates distinguishing possible immune from non-immune mechanisms by considering various disorders, including disseminated intravascular coagulation (DIC), connective tissue diseases, lymphoproliferative disorders, infection, mechanical destruction, drugs, thrombotic thrombocytopenic purpura, and certain alloantibody-mediated thrombocytopenias. If consideration of the disorders associated with increased platelet destruction is non-diagnostic, the patient is diagnosed with idiopathic immune thrombocytopenic purpura (ITP).

Antibody-mediated thrombocytopenia may be associated with autoantibodies or alloantibodies to platelets. Autoantibodies are found in patients with connective tissue or lymphoproliferative diseases. In such cases, antibodies are elicited, which react with target platelet antigens, including platelet membrane receptors such as glycoprotein Ib and the glycoprotein IIb-IIIa complex. Virtually any drug may be associated with immune thrombocytopenia, especially sulfa drugs, quinidine, and heparin. In many cases, the drug acts as a hapten, combining with a serum protein to form an immunogenic complex. Antibody formation is induced against the drug-hapten complex; the antibodies then cross-react with platelets. Certain drugs, such as thiazide diuretics, may cause thrombocytopenia by suppressing platelet production. Antibodies to platelets may develop after viral or bacterial infection, resulting in thrombocytopenia. Regardless of the mechanism, antibody-coated platelets are removed from the circulation by macrophages of the reticuloendothelial system, predominantly in the spleen.

In posttransfusion purpura, patients lacking Pl^{A1} (a high-frequency platelet antigen) receive blood products containing this antigen and develop alloantibody-mediated thrombocytopenia 7-10 days later. For unknown reasons, the alloantibody interacts with the patient's own platelets as well, resulting in severe thrombocytopenia.

Neonatal thrombocytopenia may result from 2 mechanisms. Maternal platelet antibodies may cross the placenta to interact with fetal platelets. In this situation, the mother has underlying immune thrombocytopenia. Alternatively, fetal platelet antigens may immunize the mother to induce maternal platelet antibodies, similar to the situation of Rh hemolytic disease.

27.2 Clinical Aspects

Antecedent viral infections may occur in association with immune thrombocytopenia, especially in children. The acute form of immune thrombocytopenia may present with significant mucocutaneous (or visceral) hemorrhage, whereas chronic immune thrombocytopenia in adults usually is more indolent and limited to bruising. Splenomegaly usually is absent in immune thrombocytopenia. Idiopathic thrombocytopenic purpura is a diagnosis of exclusion; a search for potential underlying causes, including drugs, connective tissue disease, lymphoproliferative disease, and HIV or other infections, is important.

Inherited thrombocytopenic conditions are infrequent and include Fanconi's syndrome and thrombocytopenia with absence of radii, in which megakaryocytic hypoplasia is present. Wiskott-Aldrich syndrome is another inherited (X-linked) disorder characterized by thrombocytopenia, recurrent infections, and eczema. Other inherited thrombocytopenic disorders include Bernard-Soulier syndrome (discussed in Chapter 28), gray platelet syndrome, and May-Hegglin anomaly. A more detailed list of inherited thrombocytopenic disorders is shown in **t27.2**.

t27.2 Inherited Thrombocytopenic Disorders

Autosomal recessive disorders	Clinical features
Bernard-Soulier syndrome	Giant platelets Abnormal GP Ib/V/IX Abnormal RIPA
Congenital amegakaryocytic thrombocytopenia	Severe thrombocytopenia Absent megakaryoytes Evolves to pancytopenia No skeletal abnormalities
Gray platelet syndrome	Large platelets Absent platelet a-granules Agranular platelets by light microscopy Variable aggregation defects
Thrombocytopenia with absent radius (TAR) syndrome	Decreased megakaryocytes Other skeletal abnormalitites present
Autosomal dominant disorders	
May-Hegglin anomaly	Large platelets Leukocyte inclusions (Dõhle bodies)
Quebec platelet disorder	Decreased α-granule proteins Variable aggregation defects Defect-increased u-PA
Epstein's syndrome	Large platelets Nephritis, cataracts, deafness Variable aggregation defects
Fechtner's syndrome	Similar features as Epstein's syndrome with leukocyte inclusions (Döhle bodies)
Sebastian's syndrome	Large platelets Leukocyte inclusions (Döhle bodies)
Montreal platelet syndrome	Large platelets Severe thrombocytopenia Spontaneous platelet aggregation
Hereditary macrothrombocytopenia	Large platelets Deafness Platelets express glycophorin A
X-linked disorders	
Wiskott Aldrich syndrome	Small platelets Immunodeficiency Eczema Deficient platelet calpain
X-linked thrombocytopenia	Similar to WAS, but no eczema or immunodeficency
GATA-1 mutation	Normal or large platelets No immunodeficiency No eczema Dyserythropoiesis

GP = glycoprotein; RIPA = ristocetin-induced platelet aggregation; u-PA = urokinase-type plasminogen activator; WAS = Wiskott Aldrich syndrome

27.3 Approach to Diagnosis

The widespread use of automated blood counters simplifies the diagnosis of thrombocytopenia. However, spurious thrombocytopenia may be observed, especially in blood specimens obtained from patients in whom ethylenediaminetetraacetic acid (EDTA) is used as the anticoagulant. A discrepancy is observed between the platelet count obtained using EDTA-anticoagulated blood and the platelet estimate on the peripheral blood smear, which reveals platelet clumping and/or satellitism (platelets adhere to neutrophils or other leukocytes i27.1). A correct automated platelet count can be obtained in these cases by using citrate or heparin as the anticoagulant.

In addition to confirming the automated platelet count, a survey of the peripheral blood smear may provide clues to underlying disorders (eg, infection, leukemia) that may be associated with thrombocytopenia. f27.1 depicts an algorithm for evaluating patients with thrombocytopenia. If thrombocytopenia is confirmed on evaluation of the peripheral blood smear and there is no obvious reason for its presence, a bone marrow examination is helpful.

The presence or absence of megakaryocytes helps to categorize thrombocytopenia. If megakaryocytes are increased or normal, i27.2, the marrow is otherwise normal, and splenomegaly is not present, specific disorders associated with platelet destruction should be evaluated. DIC should be excluded with a test for fibrinogen and D-dimer. Thrombotic thrombocytopenic purpura is a clinical diagnosis suggested by the presence of microangiopathic hemolysis and thrombocytopenia, the absence of DIC, and other appropriate clinical findings (eg, fever, neurologic abnormalities, renal dysfunction). Some laboratories offer

i27.1 EDTA-dependent pseudothrombocytopenia

Platelet satellitism and platelet clumping in a patient with EDTA-dependent pseudothrombocytopenia. *(courtesy Sherrie Perkins, MD, Wright stain, oil immersion).*

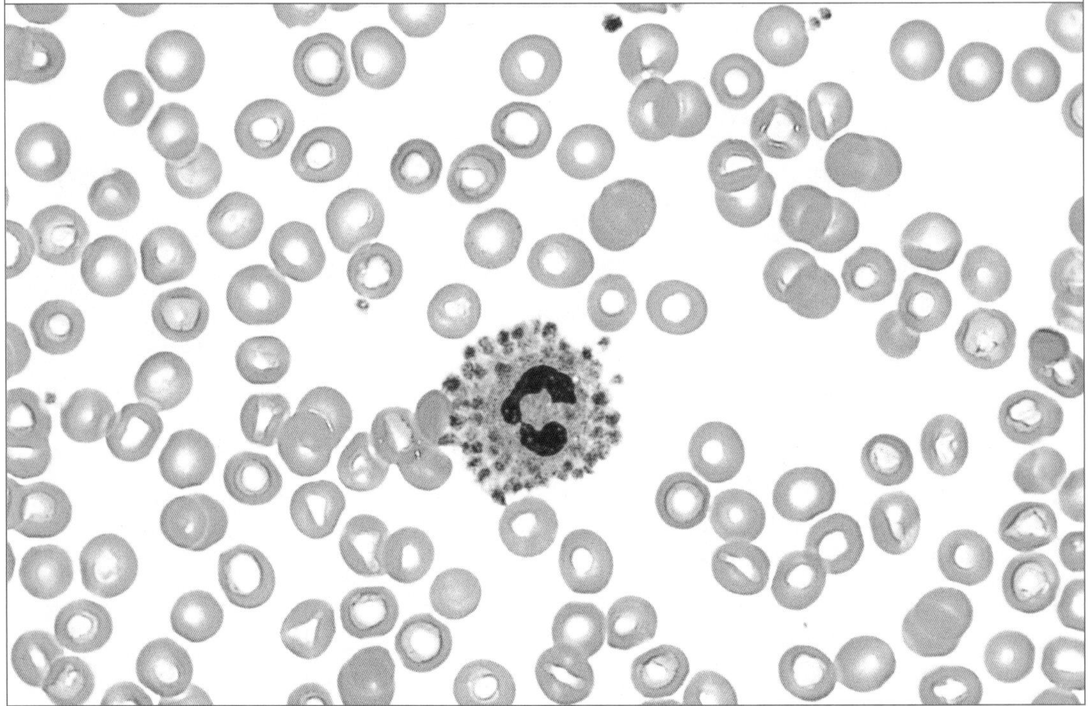

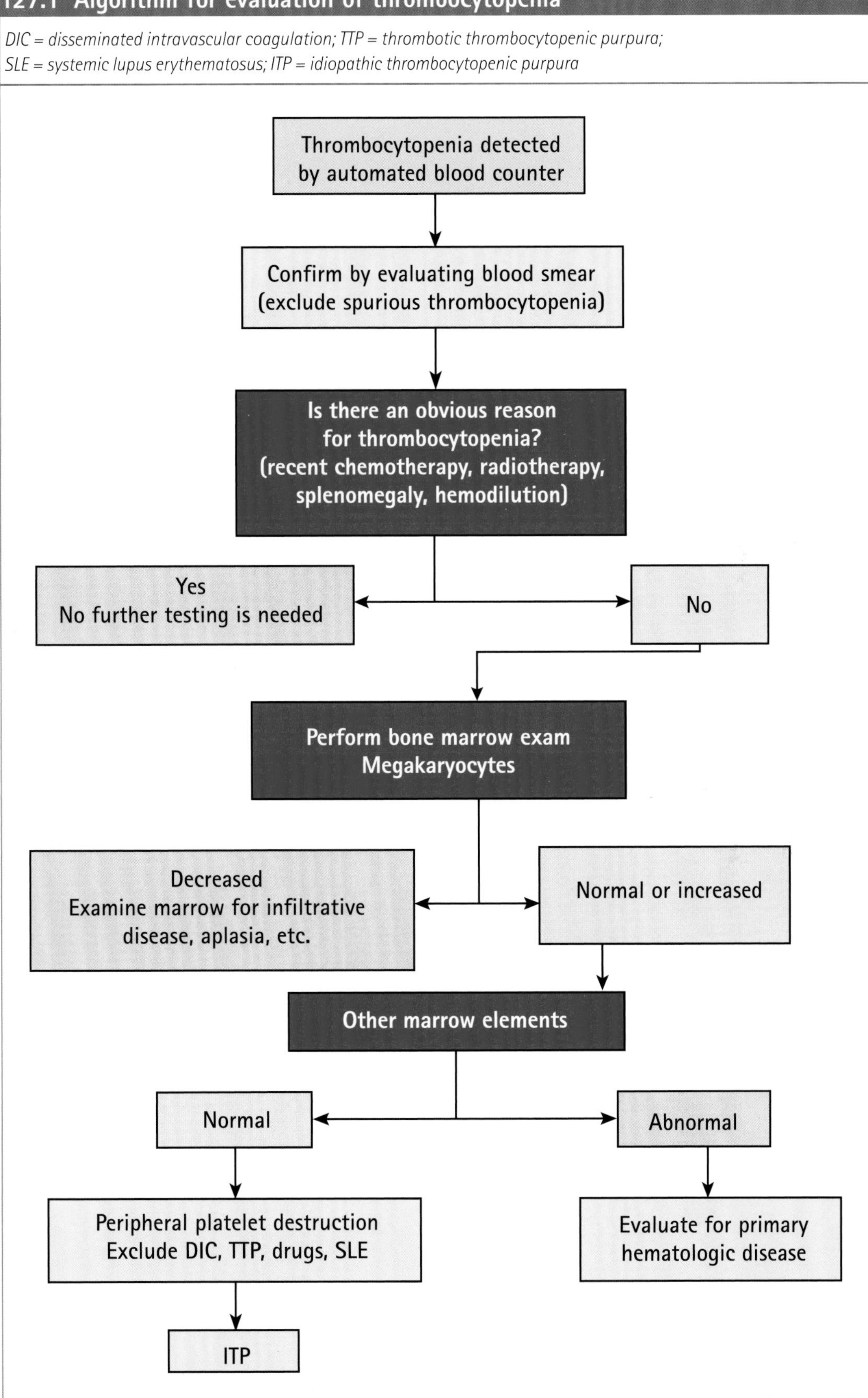
f27.1 Algorithm for evaluation of thrombocytopenia
DIC = disseminated intravascular coagulation; TTP = thrombotic thrombocytopenic purpura;
SLE = systemic lupus erythematosus; ITP = idiopathic thrombocytopenic purpura
Thrombocytopenia detected by automated blood counter
Confirm by evaluating blood smear (exclude spurious thrombocytopenia)
Is there an obvious reason for thrombocytopenia? (recent chemotherapy, radiotherapy, splenomegaly, hemodilution)
Yes
No further testing is needed
No
Perform bone marrow exam
Megakaryocytes
Decreased
Examine marrow for infiltrative disease, aplasia, etc.
Normal or increased
Other marrow elements
Normal
Abnormal
Peripheral platelet destruction
Exclude DIC, TTP, drugs, SLE
Evaluate for primary hematologic disease
ITP

i27.2 Immune thrombocytopenia

Bone marrow biopsy specimen from a patient with immune thrombocytopenia demonstrating increased megakaryocytes. *(H&E)*

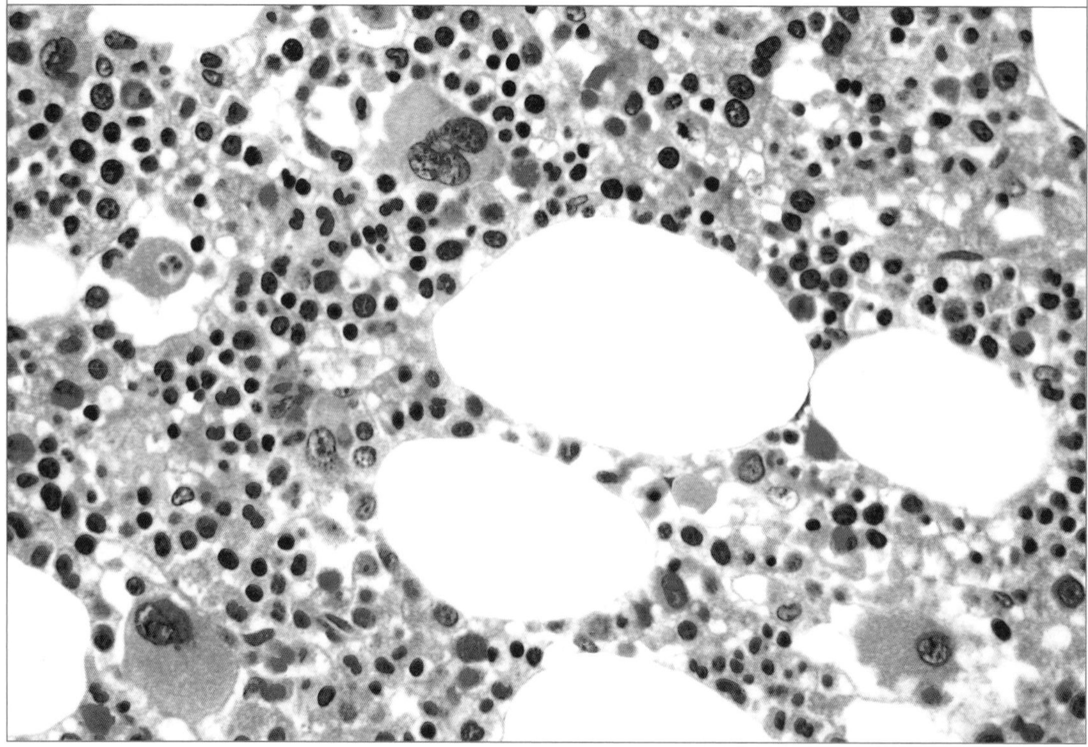

confirmatory tests for TTP (discussed later), but turnaround time for these tests is too long for the clinician to wait before starting treatment. A drug history is helpful, given the large number of medications associated with immune thrombocytopenia. Tests for systemic lupus erythematosus (antinuclear antibodies, anti–double-stranded DNA) may uncover a systemic autoimmune disorder. Because immune thrombocytopenia may be associated with antiphospholipid antibodies, some investigators recommend assays for the lupus anticoagulant and anticardiolipin antibodies. There is no utility in evaluating the bleeding time in thrombocytopenic patients.

Clinically important thrombocytopenia (in the absence of platelet dysfunction) does not occur until the platelet count falls below $100 \times 10^3/mm^3$ ($100 \times 10^9/L$), usually less than $50 \times 10^3/mm^3$ ($50 \times 10^9/L$). Serious hemorrhage should not occur (again, in the absence of platelet dysfunction) unless the platelet count is less than $20 \times 10^3/mm^3$ ($20 \times 10^9/L$).

27.4 Hematologic Findings

27.4.1 Peripheral Blood Smear Morphology

In immune thrombocytopenia, the peripheral blood smear is unremarkable except for absent or decreased platelets that may be larger than normal. If significant hemorrhage has occurred, evidence of iron deficiency also may be present. Atypical lymphocytes suggest a viral origin, such as infectious mononucleosis or HIV infection. Left-shifted myeloid cells (eg, bands, metamyelocytes), together with features of neutrophil toxicity (eg, prominent granules, vacuoles, Döhle bodies), suggest a bacterial infection. Immature cells (ie, myeloblasts, promyelocytes) indicate a leukemic process, whereas in aplastic anemia, neutropenia is present along with thrombocytopenia.

Fragmented RBCs (schistocytes, or helmet cells) i27.3 indicate a microangiopathic hemolytic process such as DIC, thrombotic thrombocytopenic purpura, or hemolytic-uremic syndrome; these disorders are distinguished by results of coagulation tests for DIC, by the clinical picture, and by confirmatory laboratory tests for TTP. Oval macrocytes and hypersegmented neutrophils are seen in megaloblastic anemia (ie, vitamin B_{12} or folic acid deficiency). Thrombocytopenia seen in association with spherocytes, polychromasia, and an elevated reticulocyte count indicates immune hemolysis and thrombocytopenia (Evan's syndrome).

i27.3 Thrombotic thrombocytopenic purpura

Peripheral blood smear of a patient with thrombotic thrombocytopenic purpura (TTP). Numerous RBC fragments (schistocytes) are seen *(Wright stain, oil immersion).*

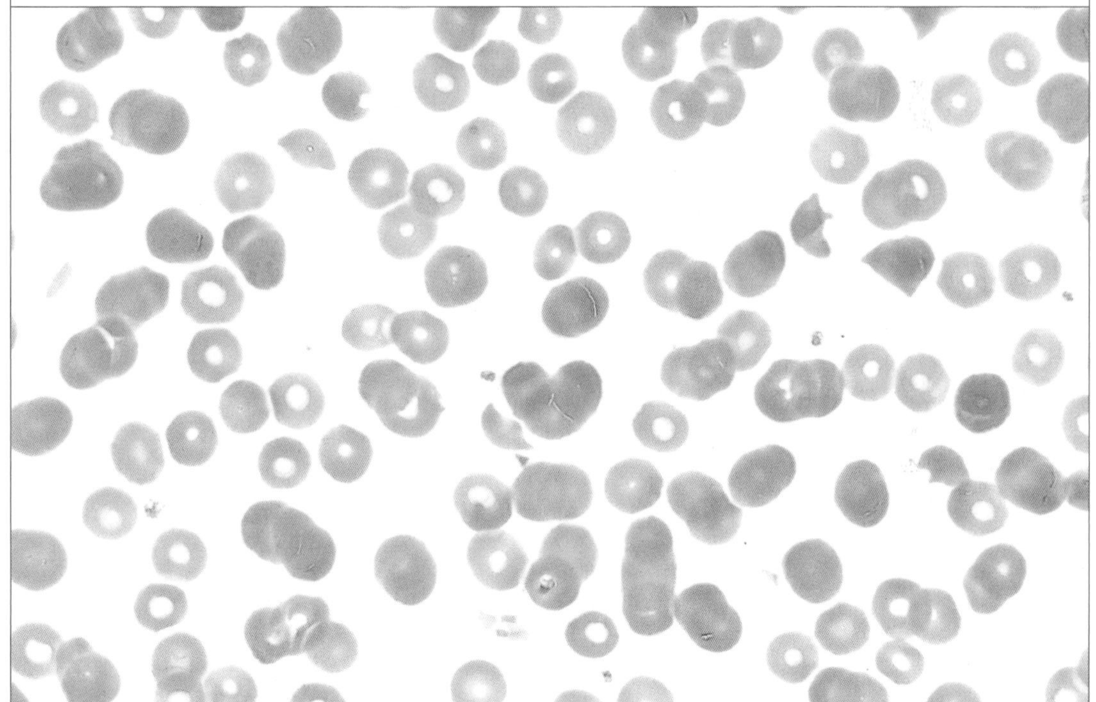

27.4.2 Bone Marrow Examination

This test is helpful in evaluating most cases of thrombocytopenia to exclude a primary hematologic disorder or a systemic disorder affecting the bone marrow. Disorders involving the marrow usually are apparent, whereas the marrow in immune thrombocytopenia is normal except for the possibility of increased and immature megakaryocytes. If the suspicion of marrow disease is low (ie, normal peripheral blood smear except for thrombocytopenia, no obvious systemic disease), a bone marrow aspirate without biopsy may be sufficient. Some physicians believe that a bone marrow examination is not required for the diagnosis of ITP.

27.5 Other Laboratory Tests

Test 27.5.1 Bleeding Time

Interpretation.. The bleeding time should be prolonged in most cases of thrombocytopenia, and no useful clinical information is gained from performing the test.

Test 27.5.2 Prothrombin Time and Activated Partial Thromboplastin Time

Interpretation. These tests yield normal results for immune thrombocytopenia, unless the patient has an additional disorder (liver disease, systemic lupus erythematosus with a lupus anticoagulant, etc). The prothrombin time and activated partial thromboplastin time, fibrinogen, and D-dimer should be evaluated in all patients with unexplained thrombocytopenia to exclude DIC.

Test 27.5.3 Platelet Aggregation Studies

Interpretation. Platelet aggregation studies should not be performed routinely in evaluating thrombocytopenic disorders unless an inherited disorder is suspected. For example, patients with Bernard-Soulier syndrome, an inherited qualitative disorder affecting the von Willebrand factor (vWF) receptor, may have mild thrombocytopenia, and aggregometry identifies these patients. For most patients with acquired thrombocytopenia, little additional clinically useful information is gained with this test.

Test 27.5.4 Test for Heparin-Induced Thrombocytopenia

Purpose. Thrombocytopenia may occur as a serious and diagnostically difficult complication of heparin therapy. About 5% of patients receiving heparin may be affected, and many of these also have an associated arterial or venous thrombosis. Thrombocytopenia typically develops 5-10 days after initiation of heparin therapy, but may occur within 1 day in patients who have received heparin therapy previously.

Principle. Plasma samples from patients with heparin-induced thrombocytopenia initiate ^{14}C-serotonin release from labeled platelets at therapeutic but not high concentrations of heparin.

Specimen. Citrated whole blood is obtained from patients after the development of thrombocytopenia.

Procedure. Platelet-rich plasma is prepared and incubated with ^{14}C-serotonin, then the platelets are washed. The platelet count is adjusted. Test plasma is then mixed with 2 separate heparin concentrations (0.1 U/mL and 100 U/mL final concentration) and with an aliquot of ^{14}C-serotonin–labeled platelets. After incubation and mixing, EDTA is added to terminate the release reaction. The mixture is then centrifuged, and an aliquot of the supernatant is counted in a scintillation counter. The percentage of serotonin release can be calculated from the values for background radioactivity, test sample release, and total radioactivity.

Interpretation. A positive test result occurs when there is more than 20% release at 0.1 U/mL of heparin and less than 20% release at 100 U/mL of heparin.

Notes and Precautions. Although the serotonin release assay is the gold-standard, it is not routinely offered by most laboratories because it involves isotopes and is tedious to perform. If serum samples are used, they must be heat-inactivated to neutralize thrombin. A mechanism for developing heparin-associated thrombocytopenia that involves complex formation between heparin and platelet factor 4 has been described. Antibodies to heparin–platelet factor 4 form immune complexes that react with platelet Fc receptors, leading to thrombocytopenia and platelet activation (see **f27.2**). An enzyme-linked

f27.2 Mechanism for heparin-induced thrombocytopenia and thrombosis

a Injected heparin binds to free platelet factor-4 (PF4). **b** Specific IgG antibodies bind to the heparin-PF4 complex to form immune complexes that subsequently bind to Fc receptors on platelets. **c** Fc-mediated platelet activation triggers release of additional PF4 that binds additional heparin. **d** PF4 may also bind to heparin-like glycosaminoglycans (heparan sulfate) on endothelial cells. **e** These PF4—glycosaminoglycan complexes provide targets for antibody, resulting in immune-mediated endothelial cell injury and thrombosis.

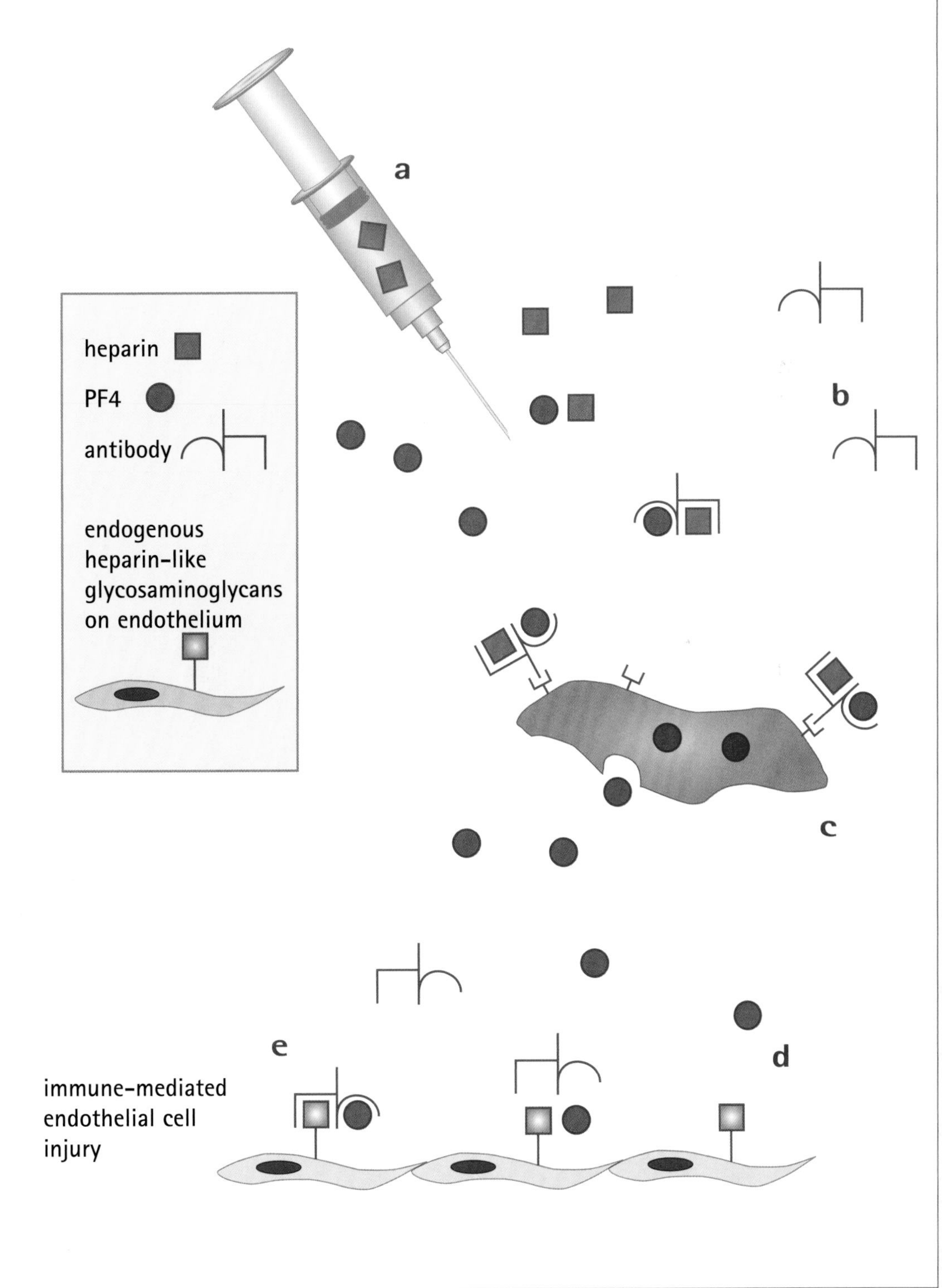

immunosorbent assay (ELISA) is available to identify these patients. The heparin-platelet factor 4 ELISA is recommended for screening; confirmatory testing with an activation assay (such as the serotonin release assay) should be done in patients with a positive ELISA result. False-positive ELISA results are seen; and a positive ELISA result is optimally interpreted only when correlated with clinical risk factors.

Test 27.5.5 Tests for Thrombotic Thrombocytopenic Purpura

Purpose. There are 3 major thrombotic microangiopathies—DIC, TTP, and hemolytic-uremic syndrome (HUS). Distinguishing TTP from HUS may be difficult, but recently, the pathogenesis of TTP was reported. TTP is a disorder of vWF. Vascular endothelium secretes vWF in a form that contains unusually large vWF multimers that are normally processed by a metalloprotease to smaller vWF multimers. Patients with the rare congenital form of TTP have inherited deficiency of the metalloprotease. Patients with acquired TTP have autoantibodies to the metalloprotease. This protease is also referred to in the literature as the vWF cleaving protease, and as ADAMTS-13.

Assays for TTP have in common demonstration of either circulating ultra high-molecular-weight multimers in patient plasma or demonstration of low metalloprotease activity. Patients with HUS generally do not have the metalloprotease defect, therefore, assays for vWF metalloprotease activity provide a means to distinguish TTP from HUS.

Principle. TTP patients have decreased circulating plasma vWF metalloprotease activity resulting in ultra high-molecular-weight multimers of vWF.

Specimen. Citrated plasma is obtained from patients suspected of having TTP prior to plasma exchange.

Procedure. Demonstration of ultra high-molecular weight multimers requires an immunoblot of the plasma sample using agarose gel electrophoresis (see Chapter 28, **Test 28.7.4**). An example of ultra high-molecular weight multimers present in a TTP patient plasma sample is shown in **f27.3**.

Demonstration of decreased plasma activity of the vWF cleaving protease can be accomplished by a number of techniques, including quantitative immunoblotting of vWF substrate degraded by $BaC1_2$–activated vWF cleaving protease, or assays measuring residual collagen binding activity, or residual ristocetin cofactor activity of degraded vWF. Development of a synthetic vWF substrate used in a fluroescence resonance energy transfer assay has led to methods with shorter turn-around times.

Interpretation. There has been controversy in the literature about the level of vWF cleaving protease that is diagnostic for TTP. Most patients with severe TTP will have vWF cleaving protease levels <5-10 U/mL; many will have levels <1 U/mL.

Notes and Precautions. Assays to measure ADAMTS13 activity are available; however, even in the best of laboratories, it may take more than 24 hours for assay results to become available, thus, TTP should still be considered a clinical diagnosis, and treatment should not wait for the laboratory result.

27.6 Course and Treatment

Childhood immune thrombocytopenia is usually a self-limited disorder, and most patients recover with no treatment. Adult immune thrombocytopenia almost always requires treatment. Prednisone (1 mg/kg daily) is usually the initial therapy. If no response occurs or if thrombocytopenia recurs after taper of the prednisone dosage, splenectomy should be considered. Approximately 60%-70% of patients have a normal platelet count after splenectomy.

f27.3 von Willebrand factor (vWF) multimeric analysis in a patient with TTP

Lane 1: normal control plasma

Lane 2: TTP patient plasma

Note the ultra high-molecular-weight multimers present in the TTP plasma sample (arrow).

Plasma samples were electrophoresed in a 1% agarose gel. Gel proteins were transferred to nitrocellulose filter paper. vWF multimers were identified using an immunoperoxidase method.

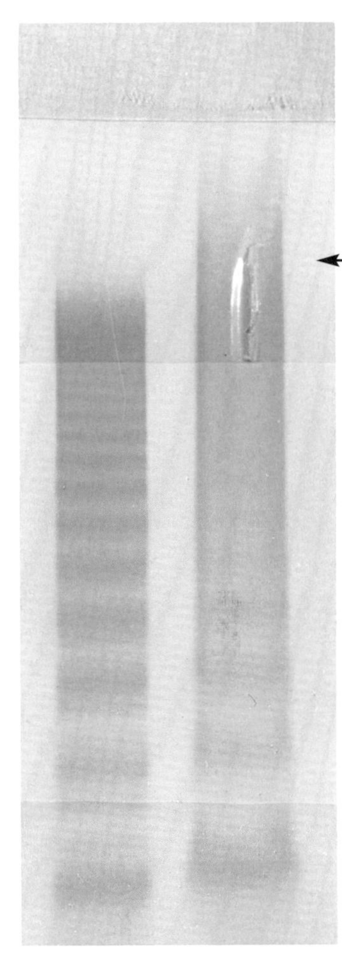

Refractory immune thrombocytopenia can be managed by immunosuppression. Intravenous immunoglobulin is the treatment of choice for emergent bleeding associated with immune thrombocytopenia. Following IgG therapy, patients frequently respond to platelet transfusions.

The primary treatment of thrombocytopenia associated with decreased bone marrow production of platelets or ineffective megakaryocytopoiesis is platelet transfusion. Posttransfusion platelet counts should be obtained within 1 hour after transfusion to document efficacy. Patients with thrombocytopenia due to non-immune platelet destruction (DIC) may not have significant responses to platelet transfusion until the underlying cause of thrombocytopenia has been treated. Platelet transfusion should be avoided in patients with thrombotic thrombocytopenic purpura. Optimal therapy for thrombotic thrombocytopenic purpura includes steriods and plasma exchange. Refractory patients may benefit from plasmapheresis using cryosupernatant, splenectomy, or immunosuppression.

27.7 References

Agarwal N, Rogers GM. Miscellaneous causes of thrombcytopenia. In: Greer JP, Foerster J, Rodgers GM, et al, eds. *Wintrobe's Clinical Hematology. 12th ed.* Philadelphia: Lippincott Williams & Wilkins; 2009: 1326-1334.

George JN, Woolf SH, Raskob GE, et al. Idiopathic thrombocytopenic purpura: a practice guideline developed by explicit methods for the American Society of Hematology. *Blood.* 1996;88:3-40.

Groot E, Hulstein JJ, Rison CN, et al. FRETS-(VWF 7.3): a rapid and predictive tool for thrombotic thrombocytopinic purpura. *J Thromb Haemost.* 2006;4:698-699.

Kokame K, Nobe Y, Kokubo Y, et al. FRETS-VWF 73, a first fluorogenic substrate for ADAMTS13 assay, *Brit J Haematol.* 2005;129:93-100.

Mhawech P, Saleem A. Inherited giant platelet disorders. *Am J Clin Pathol.* 2000;113:176-190.

Rodgers GM. Thrombocytopenia: pathophysiology and classification. In: Greer JP, Foerster J, Rodgers GM, et al, eds. *Wintrobe's Clinical Hematology. 12th ed.* Philadelphia: Lippincott Williams & Wilkins; 2009:1288-1291.

Studt J-D, Böhm M, Budde U, et al. Measurement of von Willdebrand factor-cleaving protease (ADAMTS-13) activity in plasma: a multicenter comparison of different assay methods. *J Thromb Haemost.* 2003; 1:1882-1889.

Tsai H-M. Thrombotic thrombocytopenic purpura, hemolytic-uremic syndrome, and related disorders. In: Greer JP, Foerster J, Rodgers GM, et al, eds. *Wintrobe's Clinical Hematology. 12th ed.* Philadephia: Lippincott Williams & Wilkins; 2009:1314-1325.

Visentin GP, Ford SE, Scott JP, et al. Antibodies from patients with heparin-induced thrombocytopenia/thrombosis are specific for platelet factor 4 complexed with heparin or bound to endothelial cells. *J Clin Invest.* 1994;93:81-88.

Warkentin TE. Platelet count monitoring and laboratory testing for heparin-induced thrombocytopenia. *Arch Pathol Lab Med.* 2002;126:1415-1423.

Warkentin TE, Sheppard Ji, Moore JC, et al. Quantitative interpretation of optical density measurements using PF4-dependent enzyme-immunoassays. *J Thromb Haemost.* 2008;6:1304-1312.

Chapter 28

Qualitative Platelet Disorders and von Willebrand Disease

George Rodgers, MD, PhD

The term "qualitative platelet disorders" refers to bleeding disorders in which platelet dysfunction is associated with a normal platelet count. These disorders and von Willebrand disease (vWD) are characterized clinically by petechiae and purpura, and can be inherited or acquired.

28.1 Pathophysiology of Primary Hemostasis

When platelets are exposed to damaged endothelium, they adhere to the exposed basement membrane collagen and change their shape from smooth disks to spheres with pseudopodia. They then secrete the contents of their granules, a process referred to as the "release reaction." Additional platelets then form aggregates on those platelets that have already adhered to the vessel wall; this constitutes the primary hemostatic plug and arrests bleeding f26.2.

Shape change and release are induced readily in vitro by various stimuli. Thrombin and adenosine diphosphate (ADP) are potent release and aggregation agents; relatively low concentrations of ADP added to platelet-rich plasma induce primary aggregation of platelets, which is reversible. The secretion of ADP from dense bodies in platelets during the release reaction induces the secondary phase, or irreversible aggregation.

Arachidonic acid is formed from platelet phospholipids by the action of phospholipase A_2 whenever platelets are stimulated. Arachidonic acid, in turn, is converted by cyclooxygenase to labile endoperoxide precursors (prostaglandin G_2, prostaglandin H_2), which are converted by thromboxane synthetase to thromboxane A_2. Thromboxane A_2, which has a very short half-life, is a powerful platelet-aggregating agent and vasoconstrictor, and can induce the platelet release reaction. An important controlling mechanism for the release reaction is the concentration of cyclic adenosine monophosphate, which is derived from adenosine triphosphate by adenylate cyclase and is degraded by phosphodiesterase. Cyclic adenosine monophosphate activates a kinase that decreases the sensitivity of platelets to activating stimuli. Theophylline and dipyridamole (Persantine) inhibit phosphodiesterase, and prostacyclin stimulates adenylate cyclase. Both of these actions increase platelet cyclic adenosine monophosphate levels, thereby inhibiting the release reaction.

Prostaglandin synthesis also occurs in endothelial cells with formation of arachidonic acid and labile endoperoxides, but there is no thromboxane synthetase in endothelial cells, so prostacyclin is formed instead of thromboxane A_2. Aspirin irreversibly acetylates and inactivates cyclooxygenase in the platelets, resulting in decreased synthesis of thromboxane A_2 and inhibition of the release reaction. In endothelial cells, however, there is decreased prostacyclin synthesis, resulting in enhancement of the platelet release reaction. Because endothelial cells can synthesize more cyclooxygenase, the aspirin effect on them is relatively short-lived, whereas the effect on platelets is as long as the life span of the affected platelet (9-10 days).

The mechanisms for platelet adhesion and aggregation involve plasma adhesion molecules such as von Willebrand factor (vWF) and fibrinogen, as well as platelet receptors for these adhesion molecules—glycoprotein Ib and the glycoprotein IIb-IIIa complex, respectively. Fibrinogen is required for normal platelet aggregation; vWF is essential for normal platelet adhesion. The fibrinogen receptor (glycoprotein IIb-IIIa) is deficient in the rare inherited qualitative platelet disorder, Glanzmann's thrombasthenia. The receptor for vWF (glycoprotein Ib) is deficient in an inherited platelet disorder known as "Bernard-Soulier syndrome."

The most common bleeding disorder is vWD, which may affect up to 1% of the population. It is characterized by the deficiency or functional abnormality of vWF, the plasma protein essential for normal platelet adhesion. This high-molecular-weight glycoprotein is synthesized by endothelial cells and megakaryocytes, and is present in the alpha granules of platelets and in the subendothelium. It circulates in the blood as a non-covalently linked complex with the procoagulant protein, factor VIII (previously known as factor VIII:C), which is present in only trace amounts. vWF stabilizes factor VIII and plays an important role in the interaction of platelets with the injured vessel wall.

The structure of vWF can be revealed by electrophoretic analysis. Electrophoresis of normal plasma in agarose gels, followed by incubation with labeled antibody to vWF, reveals multiple bands with molecular weights (MWs) ranging from 1×10^6 to 20×10^6, reflecting the presence of large circulating polymers of a single subunit protein (MW 230,000); this technique is known as "multimeric analysis." Incubation of platelets with vWF and the antibiotic ristocetin results in platelet aggregation. It has been shown that the high-molecular-weight multimers of vWF are the most effective in this activity. Ristocetin may mimic the activity of a subendothelial constituent responsible for inducing platelet adhesion.

28.2 Clinical Findings

Most patients with inherited qualitative platelet disorders or vWD usually have a mild to moderate bleeding disorder with excessive bleeding from very small cuts or wounds; mucous membrane bleeding; and easy bruising, which occurs after trivial trauma or (apparently) spontaneously. However, some patients have no symptoms or significant history of bleeding. The ecchymoses are almost invariably superficial, and the deep-tissue hematomas and hemarthroses of severe hemophilia are rare. These disorders are all transmitted in an autosomal manner, but there is an apparent predilection for women, because heavy menses focuses attention on the bleeding disorder. Normally, except in rare severe cases, the easy bruising and excessive bleeding from cuts are not significant enough to cause patients of either sex to seek medical attention. Many cases are so mild that symptoms manifest only when some precipitating factor, such as ingestion of aspirin or mild associated thrombocytopenia following an infection, is present. A careful history of recent medication use is essential, with special attention to aspirin or over-the-counter pain relievers containing aspirin. Patients frequently deny ingestion of aspirin or any medicines containing aspirin, yet on repeated questioning or after an abnormal result is obtained on platelet function testing, they recall taking an over-the-counter aspirin preparation (see **t26.5**).

Many other drugs also may interfere with platelet function; the most important of these are shown in **t28.1**. The thrombocytopenia that can accompany an infectious fever such as infectious mononucleosis may precipitate bleeding in a patient with a previously undiagnosed inherited qualitative platelet disorder or vWD.

t28.1 Drugs That Affect Platelet Function

Anesthetics
- Cocaine (local)
- Procaine (local)
- Volatile general anesthetics

Antibiotics
- Ampicillin
- Carbenicillin
- Gentamicin
- Nitrofurantoin (Furadantin)
- Penicillin G
- Ticarcillin

Anticoagulants
- Dextran
- Heparin

Anti-inflammatory agents and analgesics
- Aspirin
- Colchicine
- Ibuprofen (Motrin)
- Indomethacin (Indocin)
- Naproxen (Naprosyn)
- Phenylbutazone (Butazolidin)
- Sulfinpyrazone (Anturane)

Cardiovascular drugs (ie, vasodilators and antilipemic agents)
- Clofibrate
- Dipyridamole (Persantine)
- Nicotinic acid
- Papaverine (Myobid)
- Theophylline

Genitourinary drugs
- Furosemide (Lasix)

Psychiatric drugs
- Phenothiazines
- Tricyclic antidepressants: imipramine (Tofranil), amitriptyline (Triavil, Elavil)
- Sympathetic blocking agents
- Phenoxybenzamine hydrochloride (Dibenzyline)
- Propranolol (Inderal)

Miscellaneous
- Antihistamines (diphenhydramine hydrochloride)
- Ethanol
- Glyceryl guaiacolate ether (cough suppressant)
- Hashish compounds
- Hydroxychloroquine sulfate

28.3 Approach to Diagnosis

f28.1 shows an algorithm for evaluating patients with suspected platelet-type bleeding disorders. Because patients with Bernard-Soulier syndrome and variant (type 2B) vWD may have mild thrombocytopenia, the presence of mild to moderate thrombocytopenia should not exclude such patients from consideration for platelet function disorders. vWD is suggested when a family history of bleeding compatible with an autosomal dominant disorder is found. Evaluation of vWD is considered initially because it is much more common than inherited platelet disorders. The tests used to diagnose vWD are discussed later in this chapter. Platelet

f28.1 Algorithm for the diagnosis of qualitative platelet disorders or von Willebrand disease (vWD)

Evaluation of vWD is considered first because it is much more common than the inherited qualitative platelet disorders.

DIC = disseminated intravascular coagulation; vWf:Ag = von Willebrand factor antigen; ADP = adenosine diphosphate

Adapted with permission from Rodgers GM. Common clinical bleeding disorders. In: Boldt DH, ed. Update on Hemostasis. *New York: Churchill Livingstone; 1990:75–120.*

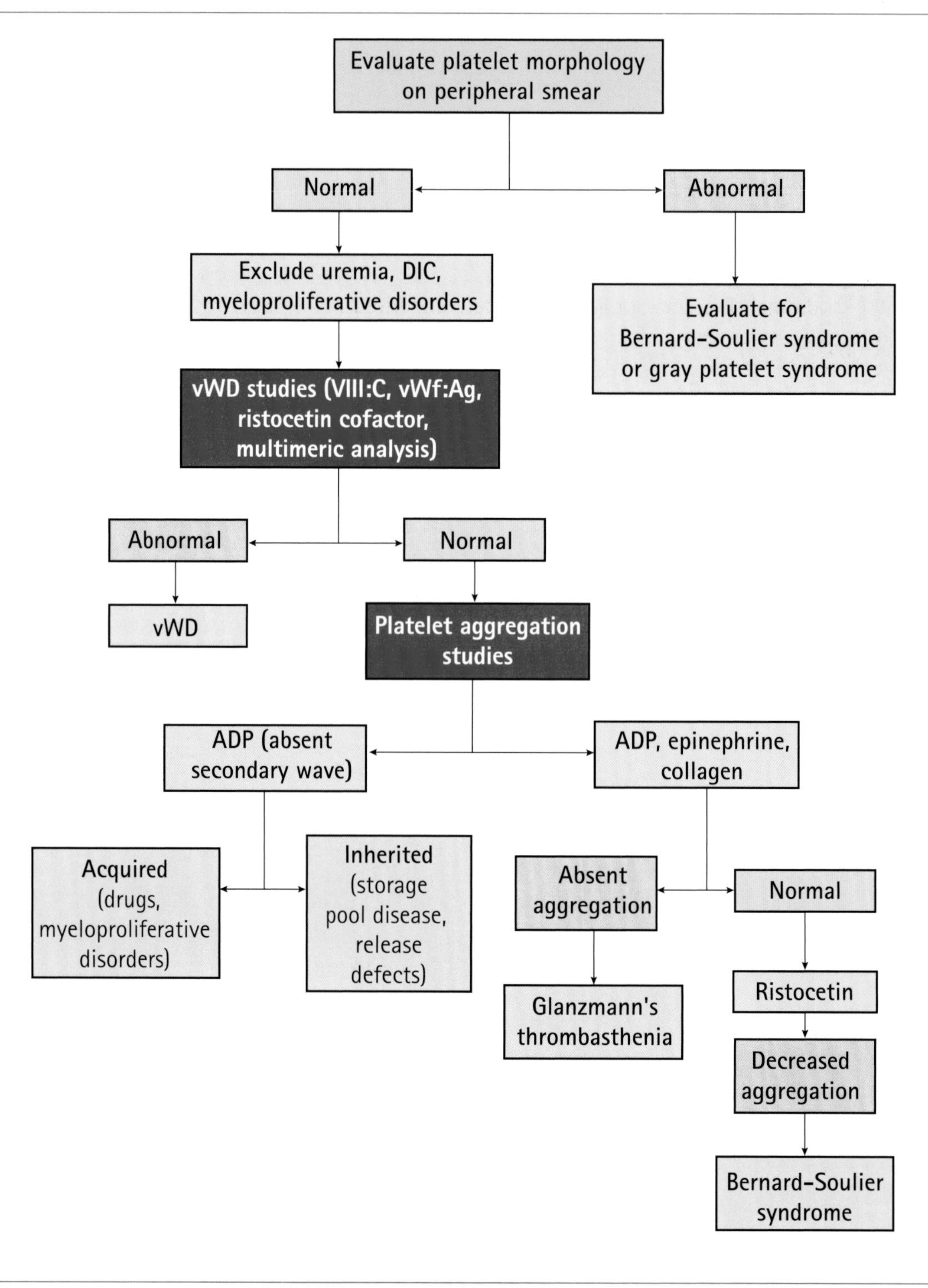

aggregation studies should be reserved for patients in whom vWD has been excluded and who have the potential of an inherited qualitative platelet disorder. Platelet aggregation studies are rarely needed in the diagnosis of acquired disorders of platelet dysfunction (eg, uremia, myeloproliferative disorder).

28.4 Qualitative Platelet Disorders

Inherited platelet disorders may be classified on the basis of findings from platelet aggregation tests (**t28.2, t28.3**; f28.2-f28.6). They fall into 3 main groups: Bernard-Soulier syndrome, Glanzmann thrombasthenia, and the thrombopathies. Bernard-Soulier syndrome is characterized by the failure of platelets to aggregate with ristocetin in the presence of normal plasma; aggregation is normal with ADP, epinephrine, collagen, and thrombin. This aggregation profile is similar to that observed in vWD (see f28.5). Moderate thrombocytopenia may be present in Bernard-Soulier syndrome, and the platelets tend to be very large i28.1. The basic defect is an abnormality of a membrane-specific glycoprotein, GPIb (or of the GP Ib-V-IX complex). Other similar conditions have been called "giant platelet syndromes" (May-Hegglin anomaly, Epstein syndrome). Bernard-Soulier syndrome is inherited in an autosomal recessive manner; it is very rare, and consanguinity is common among the parents of affected individuals. The hemorrhagic manifestations are severe. The diagnosis can also be made using flow cytomery of the peripheral blood; CD42 deficiency is observed in Bernard-Soulier syndrome.

t28.2 Platelet Aggregation Features of vWD and Inherited Qualitative Platelet Disorders

	Aggregation Response				
	ADP or Epinephrine				
Disorders	Primary	Secondary	Collagen	Ristocetin	Special Features
von Willebrand disease	Normal	Normal	Normal	Absent or decreased	Patient's platelets aggregate with ristocetin in the presence of normal plasma. Uncommon variants (2B, platelet-type) exhibit hyperresponsiveness to low-dose ristocetin
Bernard-Soulier syndrome	Normal	Normal	Normal	Absent	Giant platelets seen on smear, clincally severe
Glanzmann thrombasthenia	Absent	Absent	Absent	Normal	Clot retraction poor or absent; clinically severe
Storage pool disease	Normal or decreased	Absent	Normal or decreased	Normal	Decreased or absent dense granules on electron microscopy; platelet ATP:ADP ratio increased
Release defect (aspirin-like disorder)	Normal or decreased	Absent	Normal or decreased	Normal	Normal dense granules on electron microscopy

ADP = adenosine diphosphate; ATP = adenosine triphosphate

t28.3 Inherited Conditions Associated With Abnormal Platelet Aggregation

Glanzmann thrombasthenia
Inherited thrombocytopenia (see Chapter 27)
Storage pool defect (decreased content of ADP)
  Chédiak-Higashi syndrome
  Thrombocytopenia with absent radii (TAR syndrome)
  Wiskott-Aldrich syndrome
  Hermansky-Pudlak syndrome
Aspirin-like defect
  Cyclooxygenase deficiency
  Thromboxane synthetase deficiency
Inborn errors of metabolism
  Homocystinuria
  Wilson disease
  Glycogen storage disease, type I
Connective tissue abnormalities
  Ehlers-Danlos syndrome (collagen*)
  Pseudoxanthoma elasticum (collagen*)
  Osteogenesis imperfecta (collagen*)
  Marfan syndrome
  Constitutional abnormality of collagen (patient's collagen only*)
Afibrinogenemia
Bernard-Soulier syndrome (ristocetin*)
von Willebrand disease (ristocetin*)
Gray platelet syndrome

**The abnormal aggregation patterns are obtained only when this aggregation reagent is used.*
ADP = adenosine diphosphate; TAR = thrombocytopenia-absent radius.

Glanzmann thrombasthenia is another rare condition in which there is no aggregation with any concentration of ADP, epinephrine, or collagen (see **f28.4**); however, aggregation with ristocetin is normal. The basic defect is an abnormality or absence of the platelet surface glycoprotein IIb-IIIa. The platelets, while failing to aggregate, undergo most of the normal changes, including the release reaction when stimulated by collagen or thrombin. The platelets on the peripheral blood film are round and isolated but are otherwise unremarkable. Like Bernard-Soulier syndrome, Glanzmann thrombasthenia is associated with severe bleeding manifestations and is inherited in an autosomal recessive manner. Periheral blood flow cytometry in Glanzmann thrombasthenia demonstrates deficiency of CD41/CD61.

Thrombopathies, characterized by abnormalities in the release reaction, are common, in contrast to Bernard-Soulier syndrome and Glanzmann thrombasthenia. They can be divided into 2 subgroups: storage pool disease, in which there is a deficiency of the specialized pool of ADP, and defects in the mechanism responsible for the release of the storage pool contents. Both of these subgroups are characterized by the absence of a secondary wave of aggregation with epinephrine or ADP; aggregation with ristocetin is normal (see **f28.6**). Differentiation of the 2 subgroups requires special tests or procedures not usually available in most coagulation laboratories. In storage pool disease, electron microscopy shows a decrease in dense granules. In the second subgroup, the dense granules appear normal, but fail to release their constituents when the platelets are exposed to ADP, epinephrine, or collagen. This is by far the most frequently encountered type of inherited qualitative platelet abnormality, and the platelet defects closely resemble those seen after ingestion of aspirin. Many patients with this condition have bleeding primarily after aspirin ingestion; this type of case has been referred to as an intermediate syndrome of platelet dysfunction. For convenience, however, this condition may be considered a very mild type of release defect. Its importance lies in the fact that

f28.2 Platelet aggregation tracing: correlation with platelet function events

Following addition of ADP, several distinct phases of aggregation are seen. First, **a** there is a small increase in light transmittance following addition of the agonist due to dilution. Next, **b** the agonist induces platelet shape change, followed by **c** the initial (primary) wave of platelet aggregation. Once a threshold value is achieved, **d** platelet secretion occurs (release reaction), leading to **e** the secondary wave of platelet aggregation.

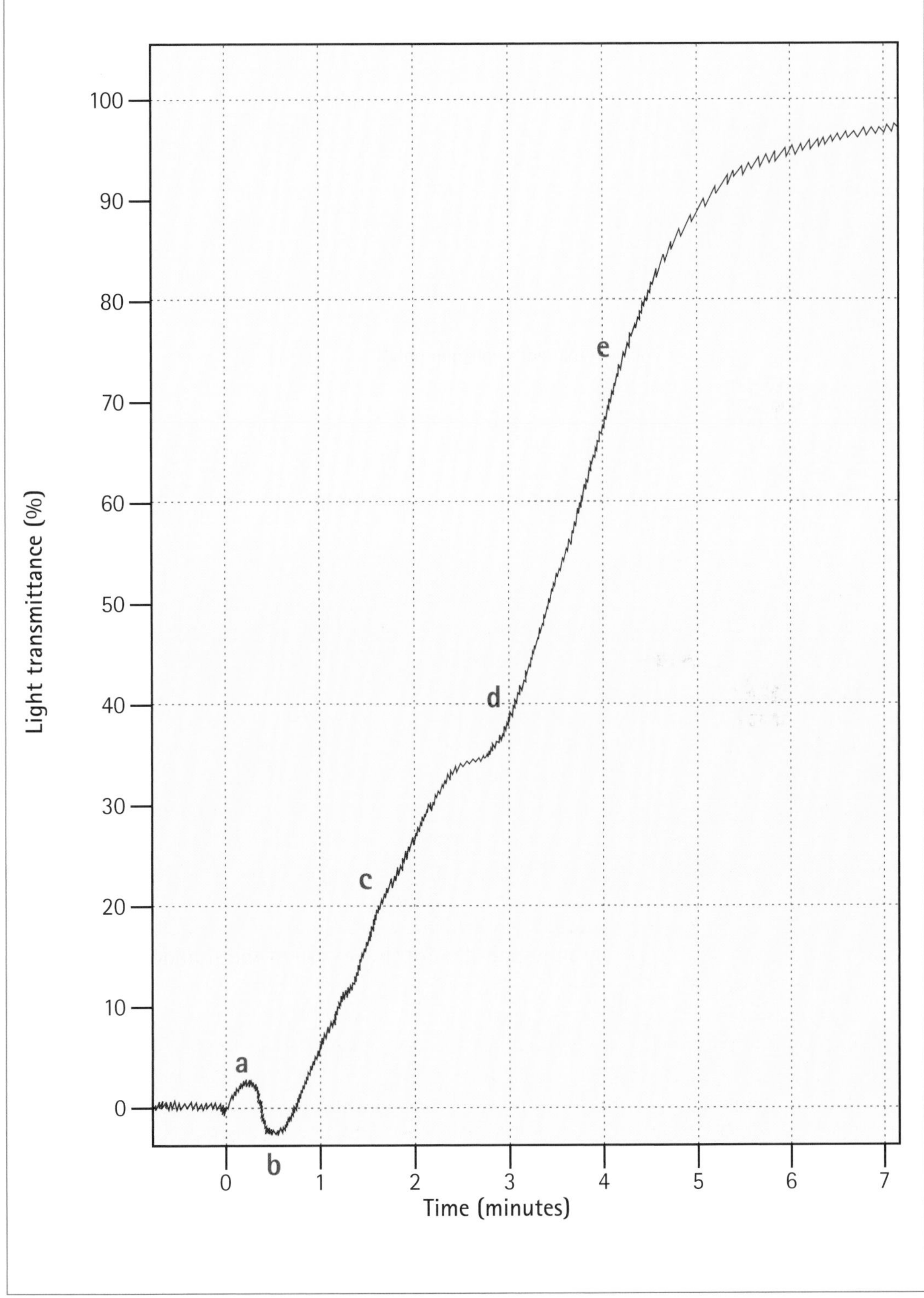

f28.3 Platelet aggregation studies: normal tracings

Adenosine diphosphate (ADP), epinephrine, collagen, and ristocetin are used as agonists.

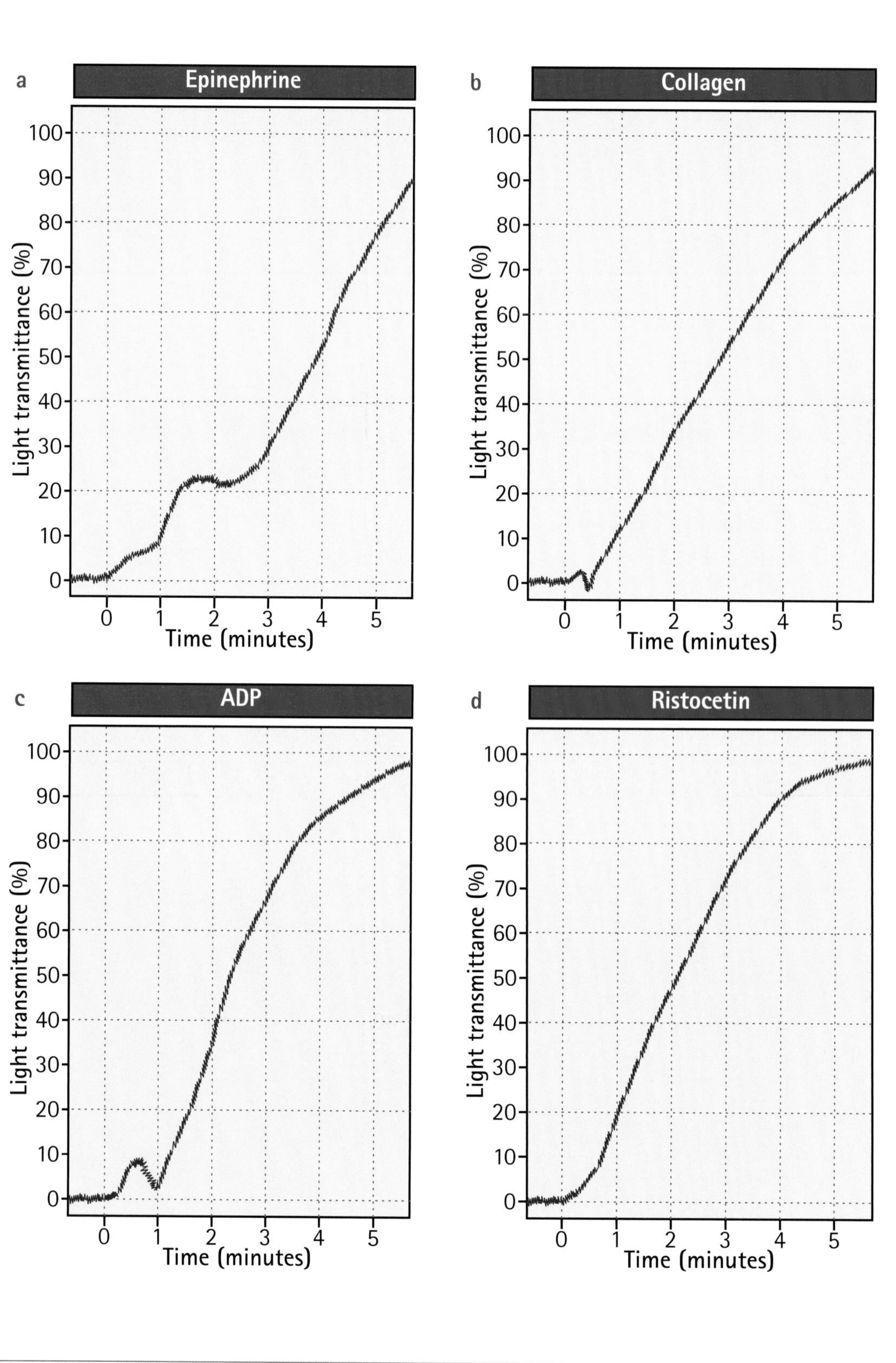

f28.4 Platelet aggregation studies: Glanzmann thrombasthenia

Note the absence of aggregation with epinephrine, collagen, and adenosine diphosphate (ADP), but normal aggregation with ristocetin.

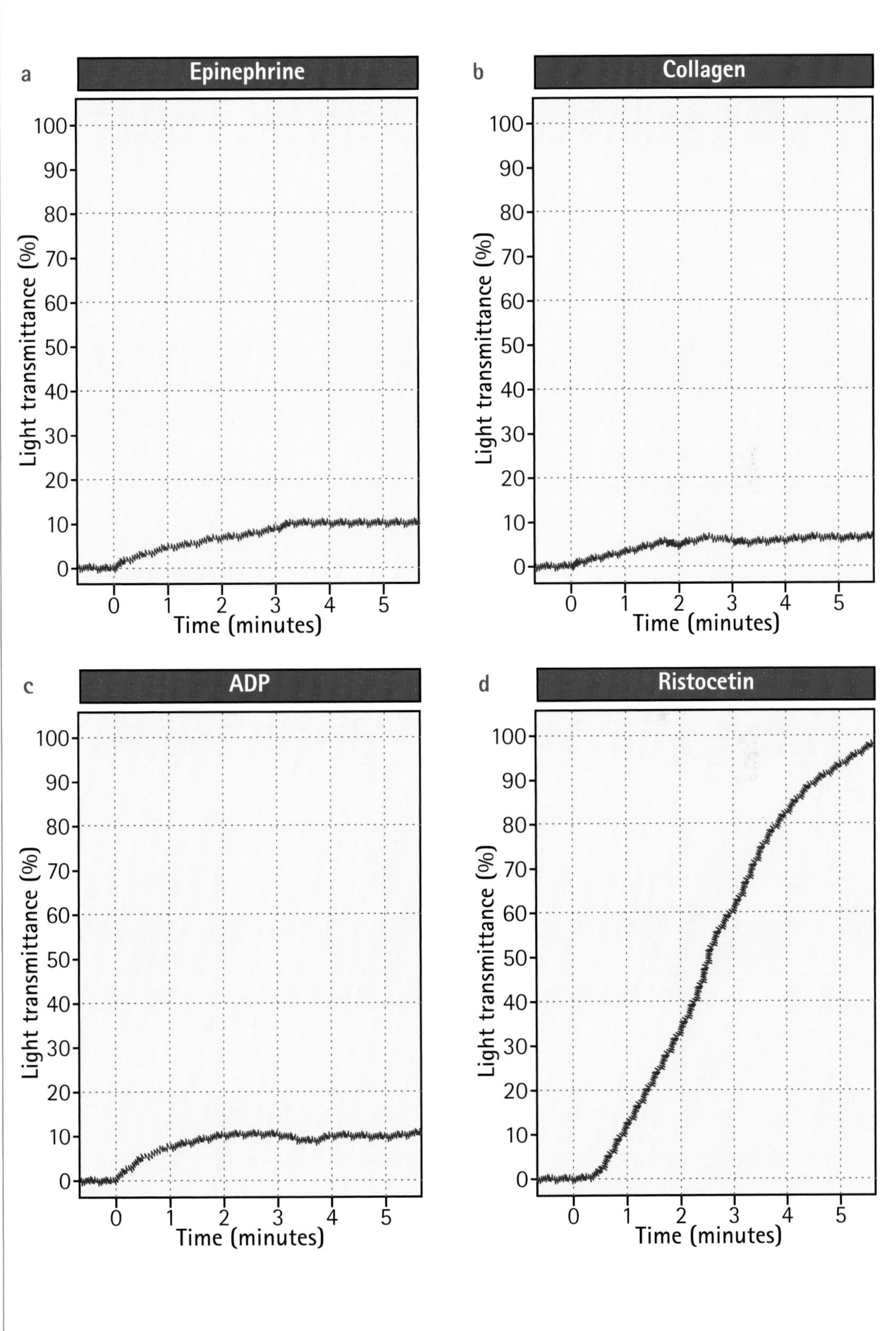

f28.5 Platelet aggregation studies: von Willebrand disease (vWD)

Note the absence of aggregation with ristocetin, but normal aggregation with epinephrine, collagen, and adenosine diphosphate (ADP). In milder cases, ristocetin aggregation is diminished but not absent. A similar pattern is seen in the inherited qualitative platelet disorder, Bernard-Soulier syndrome. Decreased ristocetin cofactor activity in vWD distinguishes it from Bernard-Soulier syndrome.

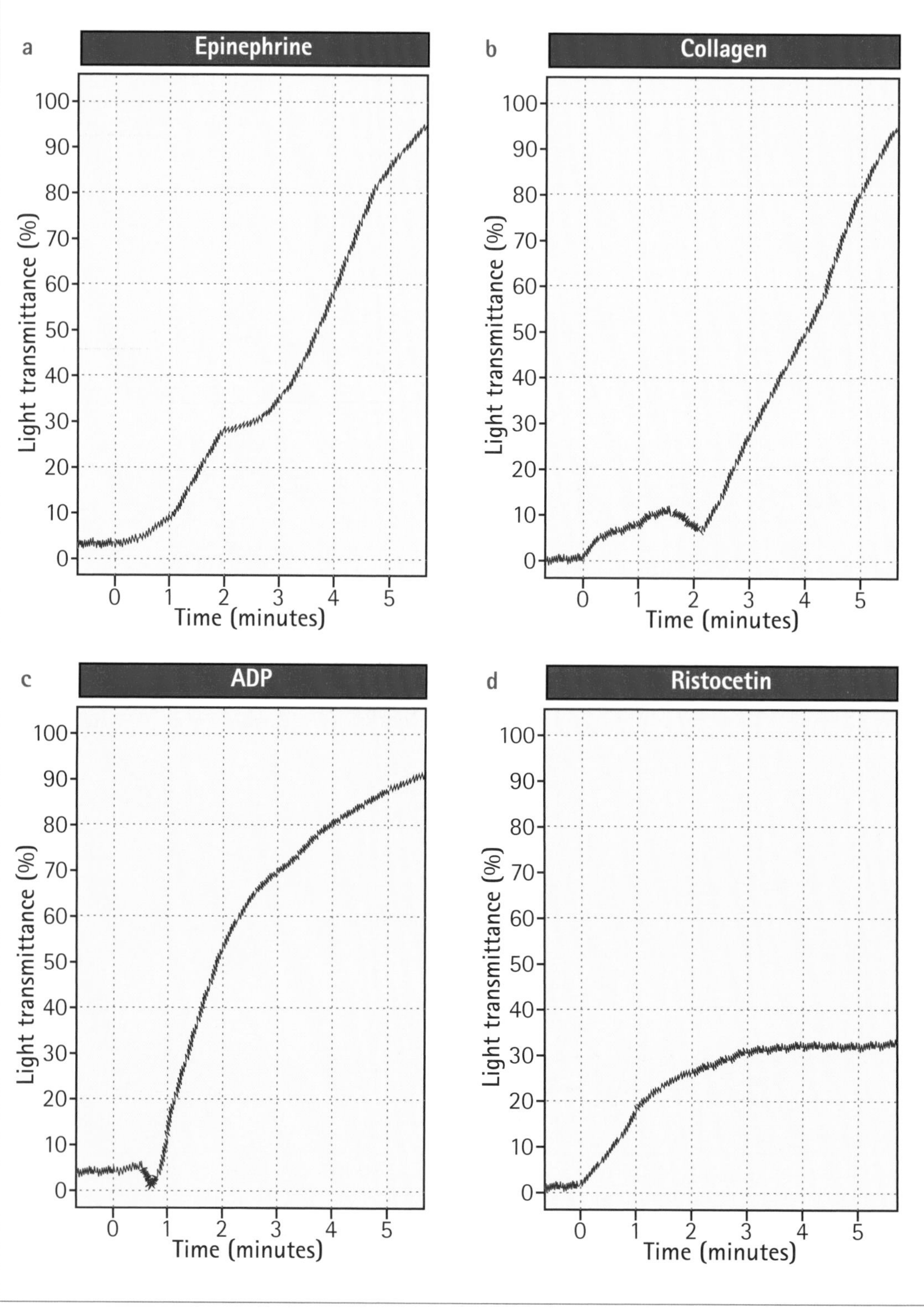

f28.6 Platelet aggregation studies: storage pool disease

Primary aggregation waves are seen with epinephrine, collagen, and adenosine diphosphate (ADP), whereas secondary waves are absent. The response to ristocetin is normal. Similar tracings may be seen with aspirin ingestion or defects in the platelet release reaction (secretion).

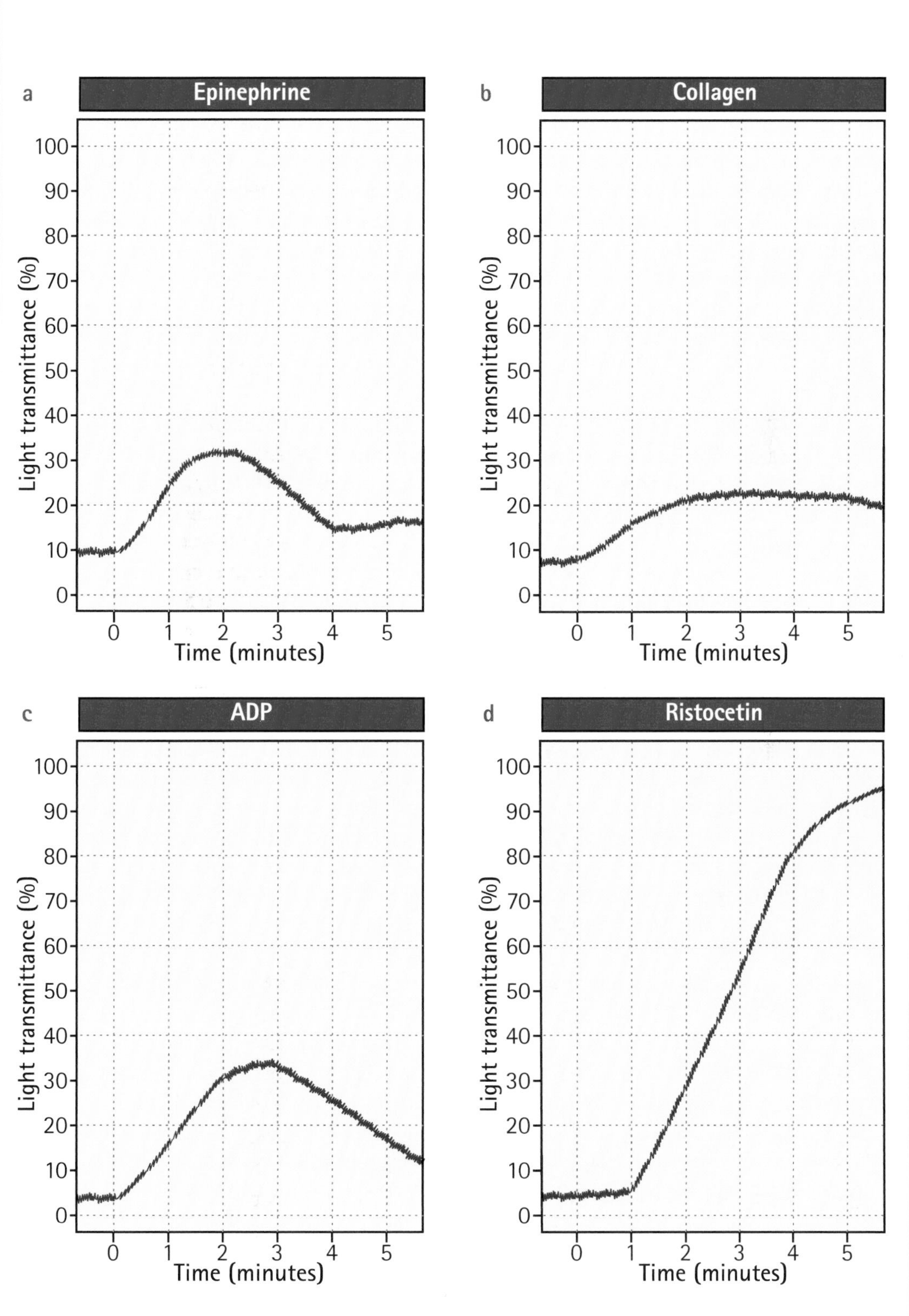

postoperative bleeding can be avoided in affected patients by abstinence from drugs known to interfere with platelet function. The condition may not be recognized with routine screening tests for hemostasis.

Qualitative platelet abnormalities have been reported in patients with type I glycogen storage disease and Wilson disease, as well as in some patients with inherited connective tissue disorders, including Ehlers-Danlos and Marfan syndromes (see **t28.3**).

28.5 von Willebrand Disease

There are several variants of vWD. Most patients exhibit a quantitative deficiency of vWF. The activity of this protein as determined by ristocetin cofactor activity is reduced in proportion to the protein (vWF antigen) as measured with immunologic methods, usually by Laurell immunoelectrophoresis or ELISA. In addition, factor VIII coagulant activity in affected patients is reduced to a similar extent.

This most frequently encountered type of vWD is referred to as "type 1." Multimeric analysis reveals all polymeric forms for vWF, but the intensity of the bands is decreased **f28.6**. Asymptomatic or mild forms of this type of vWD are frequently found, in which the level of vWF falls between 40% and 60%.

Another vWD type is referred to as "type 2A." In this form, there is a qualitative defect of vWF, although the amount of protein synthesized may be normal. The defect is manifested by loss of intermediate and high-molecular-weight multimers, which is revealed on multimeric analysis (see **f28.7**) or on crossed-immunoelectrophoresis. In type 2A, the factor VIII level is decreased or normal.

The recognition of type 2B vWD is considered important because these patients may not respond to desmopressin (1-desamino-8-D-arginine vasopressin [DDAVP]). In this form of vWD, the vWF antigen is usually reduced, whereas the level of ristocetin cofactor activity is somewhat lower than that of the antigen. The diagnostic feature is a concentration of ristocetin that is too low to induce aggregation in normal platelet-rich plasma but does so in the patient's platelet-rich plasma. In this form of the disease, the highest molecular weight multimers appear to be absent (see **f28.7**), and it resembles another rare form (pseudo-vWD, or platelet-type vWD) in which there are abnormal platelet receptors for vWF. The laboratory findings for type 2B and platelet-type vWD are similar, showing enhanced responsiveness of platelet-rich plasma to lower-than-normal concentrations of ristocetin. Direct binding of vWF to the patient's platelets with aggregation in the absence of another agonist, however, has been demonstrated in platelet-type vWD. Genetic assays or a monoclonal antibody assay have been developed to distinguish between platelet-type vs 2B vWD.

Two other vWD variants, types 2M and 2N, have been described. In type 2M vWD, there is decreased interaction of vWF with platelets not due to deficiency of high-molecular-weight multimers. The laboratory profile of type 2M vWD is similar to that of type 2A vWD, but multimeric analysis of type 2M vWF is normal. In type 2N vWD, there is decreased binding of factor VIII to vWF. The laboratory profile of type 2N vWD is normal except for low factor VIII levels, and multimeric analysis is normal. Specialized genetic or biochemical tests are necessary to diagnose types 2M and 2N vWD.

Patients with type 3 vWD have a severe bleeding disorder resembling hemophilia A. These patients have very low levels of factor VIII, vWF antigen, and ristocetin cofactor activity. The laboratory features of vWD are summarized in **t28.4**.

Acquired forms of vWD may result from development of an autoantibody to vWF, appearing in a previously healthy individual without any apparent cause or in an individual with systemic lupus erythematosus or other autoimmune disease. Acquired vWD also may occur with lymphoma or multiple myeloma due to the presence of an abnormal protein that in some way inhibits a phys-

f28.7 Multimeric analysis of von Willebrand factor

Plasma was obtained from a normal subject (N), and from patients with various types of von Willebrand disease (1, 2A, 2B, and 3). Plasma was electrophoresed in an agarose gel, then von Willebrand factor was identified using an immunoperoxidase method. The dark bands at the top of the gel (N) represent the high-molecular-weight multimers most important in platelet adhesion. Note the generalized decrease in band intensity characteristic of type 1 disease, the loss of intermediate and high-molecular-weight multimers in type 2A, the loss of only high-molecular-weight multimers in type 2B, and the virtual absence of all multimers in type 3.

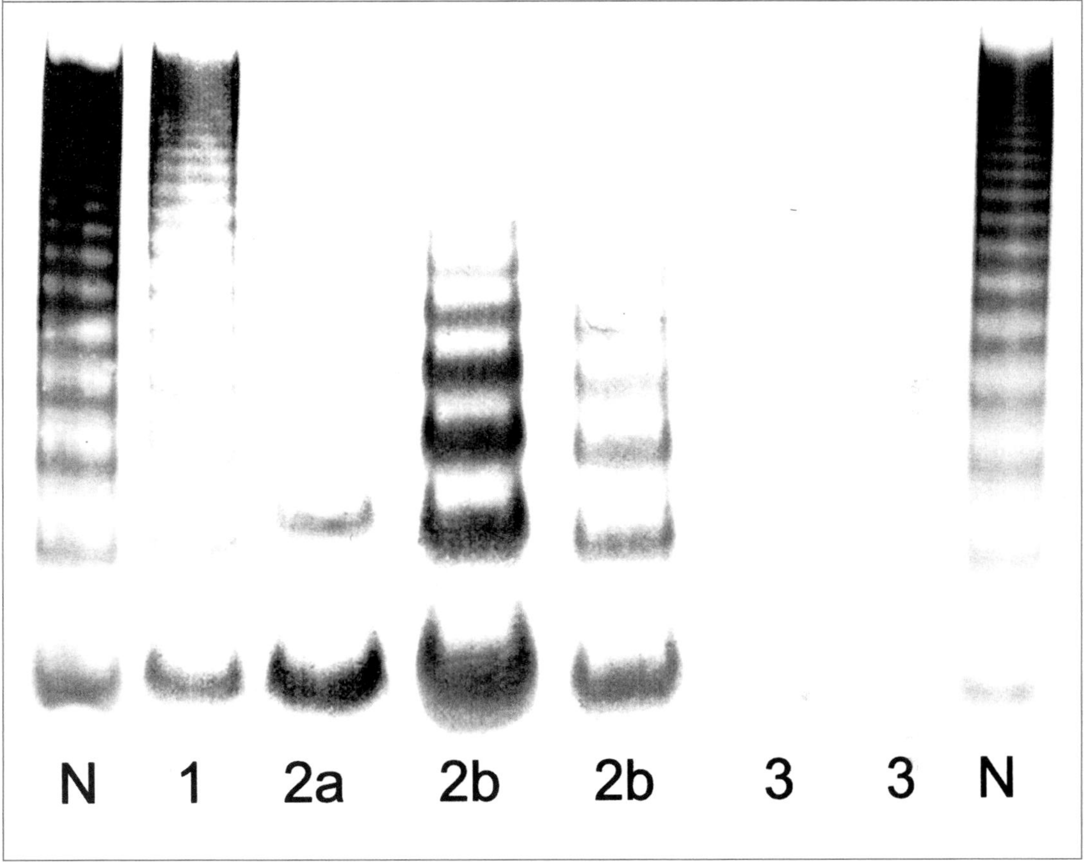

t28.4 Laboratory Features of von Willebrand Disease*

	Type 1	Type 2A	Type 2B	Type 2M	Type 2N	Type 3	Platelet-Type
Factor VIII activity	D	D or N	D or N	D	D	D	D or N
von Willebrand factor antigen	D	N or D	N or D	D	N	D	D or N
Ristocetin cofactor activity	D	D	D or N	D	N	D	D
Ristocetin-induced platelet aggregation	D or N	D	I†	D	N	D	I†
Multimeric analysis	N	A	A	N	N	A	A

**The bleeding time may be normal or abnormal in vWD. Because patients with mild vWD may have borderline normal test results, repeated testing may be necessary to establish the diagnosis.*

†Increased aggregation is seen in response to low concentration of ristocetin.

I = increased; D = decreased; N = normal; A = abnormal

iologic counterpart of ristocetin, with valvular heart disease that results in shearing of vWF, or disorders associated with marked thrombocytosis, where there is increased platelet binding of vWF.

Qualitative abnormalities of platelets are encountered in patients with myeloproliferative disorders (especially essential thrombocytosis) and, to a lesser extent, in those with polycythemia vera and myelofibrosis with myeloid metaplasia. Mild abnormalities are found in patients with uremia and cirrhosis. Certain acquired platelet function disorders are caused by in vivo platelet activation and result in an acquired storage pool defect (certain disorders associated with antiplatelet antibodies or immune complexes, disseminated intravascular coagulation, cardiopulmonary bypass, hairy cell leukemia).

Evaluation of these disorders proceeds as follows:

1. Hematologic evaluation is conducted with particular attention paid to platelet number and morphology.
2. Screening tests for hemostasis, including the activated partial thromboplastin time (aPTT), prothrombin time (PT), and platelet count, are performed. In general, a coagulation-type bleeding abnormality may be excluded if the aPTT and PT are normal. If results of 1 or both of these tests are prolonged, specific factor assays are performed (see Chapter 29).
3. von Willebrand disease is evaluated by testing the 3 components of the von Willebrand panel—factor VIII activity, vWF antigen, and ristocetin cofactor activity. Classification of vWD subtypes is performed using multimeric analysis.
4. Platelet aggregation tests, which are non-quantitative, are primarily used for the diagnosis of qualitative platelet disorders. Less commonly, some patients with vWD have a normal von Willebrand panel but exhibit abnormal ristocetin-induced platelet aggregation. An abnormal ristocetin-induced platelet aggregation test indicates that the patient has

i28.1 Bernard-Soulier syndrome

Giant platelet is present. *(Wright stain)*

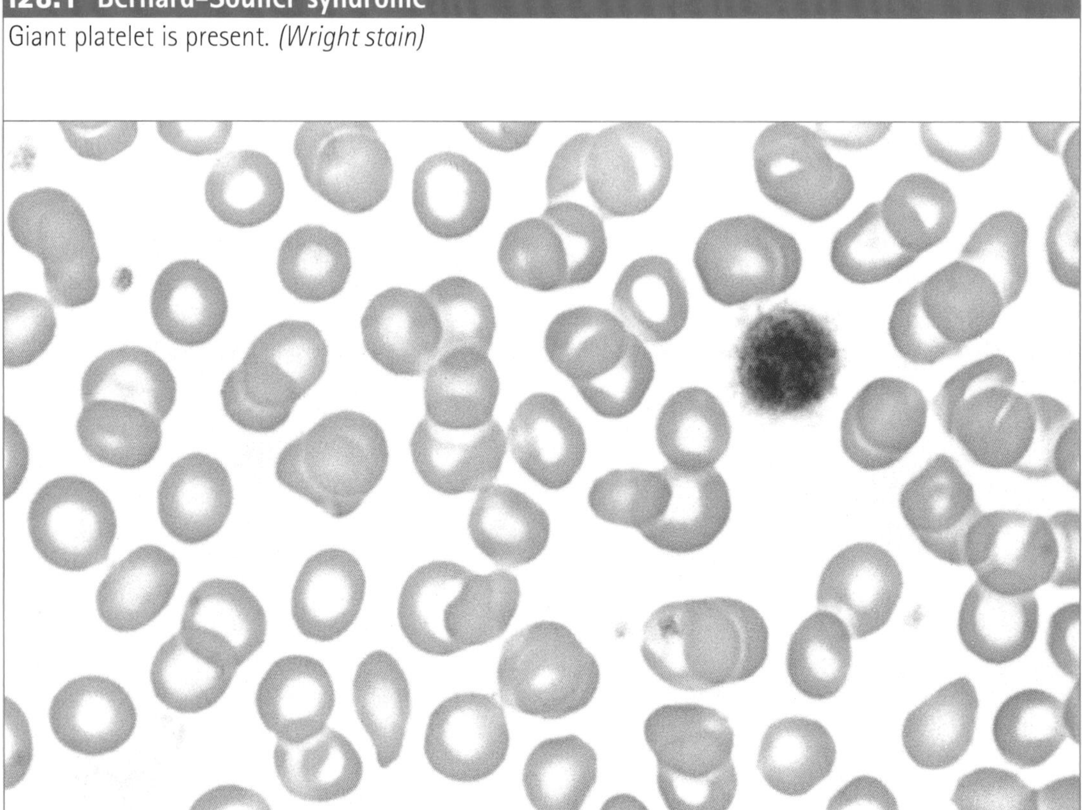

vWD or, rarely, Bernard-Soulier syndrome. A ristocetin cofactor activity test is then performed, using the patient's plasma specimen and freshly washed or formalin-fixed normal platelets. This test measures the vWF activity in the plasma specimen. It is normal in Bernard-Soulier syndrome, because normal platelets are used in the test; the defect in Bernard-Soulier syndrome resides in the platelets, whereas the plasma is normal. This is the reverse of vWD, in which the plasma ristocetin cofactor activity is reduced.

28.6 Hematologic Findings

General features are usually unremarkable and, apart from Bernard-Soulier syndrome in which giant platelets are seen i28.1, abnormal platelets are rarely seen on the smear. Occasionally, hematologic features may be consistent with iron-deficiency anemia.

28.6.1 Peripheral Blood Smear Morphology

The number of platelets in the peripheral blood should be estimated and the presence of any large platelets noted. Unless there has been significant bleeding, the red and white blood cells will be normal. A direct platelet count should be performed.

28.6.2 Bone Marrow Examination

Characteristic changes in bone marrow are seen with acquired platelet defects secondary to myeloproliferative or myelodysplastic disorders, or in association with lymphoproliferative disorders.

28.7 Other Laboratory Tests

Many of the laboratory tests described in this section are not routinely performed by most laboratories, and will be available only in reference coagulation laboratories. As discussed in Chapter 26, the bleeding time is not a useful test. Patients with features of a platelet-type bleeding disorder should have direct testing for vWD, and if necessary, platelet dysfunction using platelet aggregation.

Test 28.7.1 Platelet Aggregation Test

Purpose. Platelet aggregation tests are used to detect abnormalities in platelet function (see f28.2-f28.6). Such defects, which may be inherited or may result from the ingestion of certain drugs, can cause bleeding in certain patients.

Principle. When an aggregating agent is added to an initially turbid platelet-rich plasma specimen in the cuvette of an aggregometer, the specimen clears as platelets clump, permitting more light to pass through the plasma. The aggregometer is basically a photo-optical instrument; the amount of light transmitted through the cuvette is recorded. f28.2 depicts a typical aggregation tracing and indicates the sequence of events following the addition of an agonist to platelet-rich plasma.

Specimen. A platelet-rich plasma specimen is prepared from whole blood anticoagulated with sodium citrate. The responsiveness of the platelets to aggregating agents is influenced by the time elapsing from collection, and the tests should be completed within 1-3 hours of collection. The temperature at which the specimen is prepared, as well as the temperature at which the actual aggregation tests are carried out, have a significant influence on the rate and extent of aggregation. Platelets prepared at room temperature are more sensitive to ADP than are platelets stored at 37°C. Due to the large number of medications that can affect platelet function, it is recommended that all medications (including over-the-counter drugs and supplements) be discontinued at least 1 week prior to testing.

Procedure. Platelet-rich plasma is obtained by the slow centrifugation of whole blood anticoagulated with sodium citrate. This procedure is carried out in plastic tubes at room temperature, and at no time should the plasma be cooled. The supernatant (platelet-rich plasma) is pipetted off and retained. The remaining portion of anticoagulated blood is recentrifuged at high speed to obtain a platelet-poor plasma specimen. The platelet-rich plasma specimen is then mixed with the platelet-poor plasma specimen to obtain a final platelet count of $250 \times 10^3/mm^3$ ($250 \times 10^9/L$). The aggregation agents used are ADP, collagen suspensions, epinephrine, and ristocetin (see f28.3-f28.6); some laboratories also use arachidonic acid or calcium ionophore. A blank value is obtained by using a platelet-poor plasma sample from the patient. The adjusted platelet-containing plasma sample is placed in the cuvette and warmed to 37°C, the aggregating agent is added, and the contents of the cuvette are stirred constantly by means of a small Teflon-coated stirring rod.

Interpretation. The results with each aggregation agent may be recorded as the slope of the curve, the absolute magnitude of the transmittance change, or the percentage change of the transmittance, or of the optical density. In most laboratories, however, the results are not reported in a quantitative manner, but merely in descriptive terms (normal vs abnormal aggregation), with a comment as to the type of abnormality.

The results depend on the concentration of the aggregating agents, which should be stated in the report. With relatively low doses of ADP (1-2 µg/mL), 2 waves of aggregation are seen. The first, or primary, wave is induced by the ADP added to the patient's plasma, whereas the secondary wave is attributed to the release of relatively large amounts of intrinsic ADP from the storage pool within the platelets (release reaction) (see f28.2). With even lower concentrations of ADP (0.5 µg/mL), the release reaction does not occur, the platelets disaggregate, and only a primary wave is seen; with relatively large doses of ADP (10-20 µg/mL), a single broad wave is seen. A biphasic response occurs with epinephrine in up to 80% of healthy persons. However, 20%-30% of healthy people exhibit abnormal epinephrine aggregation. Because collagen acts by inducing a release of ADP, a primary wave is not seen. In thrombasthenia, aggregation occurs with ristocetin, but not with any concentration of ADP, epinephrine, or collagen (see f28.4). In storage pool disease and release defects (aspirin-like disorders), the secondary waves with ADP and epinephrine are absent (see f28.6), and aggregation with collagen is reduced or absent; ristocetin aggregation is normal.

More subtle changes may be clinically significant when ristocetin is used as the aggregating agent, and the slope should be compared with that of the control. A normal tracing with ristocetin does not exclude a moderate vWF deficiency. Thus, when vWD is suspected, a quantitative ristocetin cofactor activity must be performed. In addition to the usual concentration of ristocetin, a lower concentration (0.5 mg/mL or less final concentration) also should be used in the platelet aggregation test to detect the rare type 2B or platelet-type vWD. In these conditions, aggregation occurs with the patient's platelet-rich plasma specimen and the lower concentration of ristocetin, whereas aggregation with the normal control platelet-rich plasma specimen and the low ristocetin concentration is not seen.

Notes and Precautions. Specimens left at room temperature for more than 4 hours may lose their ability to aggregate. Platelets stored at 0°C sometimes undergo spontaneous aggregation. Plasma should not be lipemic or icteric. Whenever an unexpectedly abnormal result is obtained, the test should be repeated on another specimen collected several days later. Numerous medications, including antibiotics, antidepressants, and antihistamines, can markedly influence in vitro platelet function. Abnormal aggregation results in patients taking medications should be assumed to be due to antiplatelet drug effects.

Whole blood aggregation methods that are less laborious than the method described here have been reported. Aggregometer instruments (lumi-aggregometers) that report aggregation results combined with release reaction (secretion) data are also available.

Test 28.7.2 von Willebrand Factor–Ristocetin Cofactor Activity Test

Purpose. This test is used to measure the biologic activity of vWF.

Principle. The ability of the patient's plasma specimen to aggregate normal platelets in the presence of ristocetin is compared with that of a normal pooled plasma specimen.

Specimen. Plasma specimens used for the aPTT or PT tests are satisfactory; the specimens may be stored for several weeks at -70°C without losing activity.

Procedure. A standard curve is prepared by making serial dilutions of plasma in saline. An aliquot of each is then added to a fixed amount of a saline suspension of washed platelets in the cuvette of an aggregometer. Ristocetin is then added and the slope of the wave determined (maximum change in light transmittance). By plotting slope against the dilution of the plasma on log-log paper, a straight line is obtained. A dilution of the patient's plasma specimen is then tested, and the equivalent dilution of the normal plasma specimen that would give the same slope is read from the straight-line curve. For example, if a 1:10 dilution of the patient's plasma specimen gives the same slope as a 1:20 dilution of normal plasma specimen, the vWF activity in the patient's plasma specimen is 50% of normal.

Interpretation. A decrease in vWF parameters in a patient with a lifelong history of bleeding is diagnostic of vWD. Acquired deficiencies caused by antibodies to vWF and certain paraproteins also may result in a decrease in vWF levels.

Notes and Precautions. The ristocetin cofactor assay already described is very time-consuming. Simpler methods based on enzyme-linked immunosorbent assay (ELISA), in which a monoclonal antibody recognizes a functional epitope of vWF, are also available.

Test 28.7.3 Laurell Immunoelectrophoresis Assay for vWF Antigen

Purpose. Historically, the immunoelectrophoresis assay has been used for the diagnosis of vWD. In this disease, vWF antigen is usually decreased.

Principle. A precipitating rabbit antibody is used to quantitate vWF. The immunoassay is usually performed using the Laurell technique, which is an electroimmunodiffusion method for the quantitation of proteins in which rocket-shaped anodic immunoprecipitates are formed. The height of the rocket is proportional to the concentration of vWF.

Specimen. The patient's plasma or serum sample may be used, but the former is preferable. A plasma sample collected for the aPTT or PT test is satisfactory.

Procedure. The antibody is mixed with liquid agarose, which is then poured onto a plate and allowed to solidify by cooling. Holes are punched on one side of the plate, which is then placed in an electrophoresis chamber. Serial dilutions of normal pooled plasma in saline (1:2, 1:4, 1:8, etc) are made to prepare the standard curve. The 1:2 and 1:4 dilutions of the plasma being tested are prepared and placed in the wells. Electrophoresis of the sample is then performed, and when the run is completed, the plate is examined. The rocket-shaped immunoprecipitates are sometimes difficult to see, but visibility can be increased by immersing the plates in tannic acid for a few minutes.

Interpretation. A value below 40% is consistent with vWD, and values between 40% and 60% are borderline. Both vWF antigen and ristocetin cofactor activity are increased by exercise, hepatitis, hormone replacement estrogen therapy, and pregnancy. Patients with vWD in one or more of these situations may have normal levels of vWF. Repeated testing may be necessary to diagnose vWD.

Notes and Precautions. The determination of vWF antigen, previously referred to as "factor VIII-related antigen," should be distinguished from the determination of the factor VIII antigen. The latter is the antigen corresponding to the factor VIII coagulant protein, which is decreased in at least 90% of patients with hemophilia A. The test to determine factor VIII antigen is currently available in some reference laboratories.

vWF antigen also can be measured using ELISA-based methods.

Test 28.7.4 von Willebrand Factor Multimeric Analysis

Purpose. This test measures the qualitative (structural) aspects of vWF.

Principle. The patient's vWF is separated by gel electrophoresis and identified with immunologic methods. The patient's multimeric pattern is compared with those of normal patients.

Specimen. Plasma specimens used for the aPTT and PT assays are satisfactory. Plasma frozen at −70°C for several weeks also may be used.

Procedure. An agarose gel (0.7%-1%) is prepared, and patient and normal plasma samples are electrophoresed. The electrophoresed plasma proteins are then transferred to nitrocellulose paper and incubated with an antibody to vWF. Immunodetection of multimers can be performed with a ^{125}I label on the antibody, followed by autoradiography, or with the avidin-biotin-peroxidase technique, or with chemiluminescence.

Interpretation. Samples from patients with type 1 vWD have the full range of multimers, but in reduced quantities. Those from type 2A patients have no intermediate or high-molecular-weight bands, while those from type 2B patients do not exhibit the highest-molecular-weight bands. Platelet-type vWD cannot be distinguished from type 2B by multimeric analysis; therefore, patient samples that demonstrate loss of high-molecular-weight multimers should be interpreted as being consistent with either type 2B or platelet-type vWD. Type 3 patient samples show a virtual absence of all bands (see **f28.7**). Patients with TTP may exhibit ultra-high-molecular-weight multimers on multimeric analysis (Chapter 27).

Notes and Precautions. This is a laborious technique and is usually performed by coagulation reference laboratories. Cold storage of citrated blood may result in significant loss of factor VIII and vWF activities, potentially leading to misdiagnosis.

28.8 References

Bennett JS. Platelet aggregation. In: Williams WJ, Beutler E, Erslev AJ, Lichtman MA, eds. *Hematology. 4th ed.* New York, NY: McGraw-Hill; 1990:1778-1781.

Bennett JS. Hereditary disorders of platelet function. Hoffman R, Benz EJ, Shattil SJ, et al, eds, *Hematology: Basic Principles and Practice. 3rd ed.* New York, NY: Churchill Livingstone; 2000:2154-2172.

Böhm M, Täschner S, Kretzschmar E, et al. Cold storage of citrated whole blood induces drastic time-dependent losses in factor VIII and von Willebrand factor: potential for misdiagnosis of haemophilia and von Willebrand disease. *Blood Coagul Fibrinolysis.* 2006;17:39-45.

Goodall AH, Jarvis J, Chand S, et al. An immunoradiometric assay for human factor VIII/von Willebrand factor (VIII:vWf) using a monoclonal antibody that defines a functional epitope. *Br J Haematol.* 1985;59:565-577.

Ingerman-Wojenski CM, Silver MJ. A quick method for screening platelet dysfunctions using the whole blood lumi-aggregometer. *Thromb Haemost.* 1984;51:154-156.

Friedman KD, Rodgers GM. Inherited coagulation disorders. In Greer JP, Foerster J, Rodgers GM, et al, eds. *Wintrobe's Clinical Hematology. 12th ed.* Philadelphia: Lippincott Williams & Wilkins; 2009;1379-1424.

Rodgers GM. Testing for inherited bleeding disorders. In Bennett ST, Lehman CM, Rodgers GM. *Laboratory Hemostasis: A Practical Guide for Pathologists.* New York: Springer;2007;103-120.

Scott JP, Montgomery RR. The rapid differentiation of type IIb von Willebrand's disease from platelet-type (pseudo-) von Willebrand's disease by the "neutral" monoclonal antibody binding assay. *Am J Clin Pathol.* 1991;96:723-728.

Zhou L, Schmaier AH. Platelet aggregation testing in platelet-rich plasma. *Am J Clin Pathol.* 2005;123:172-183.

Chapter 29

Inherited Coagulation Disorders

George Rodgers, MD, PhD

Inherited coagulation disorders result from quantitative deficiency or qualitative abnormality of a clotting factor. Deficiency of factors VIII or IX (hemophilia A or B, respectively) constitute the vast majority of patients with inherited coagulation disorders. Von Willerand disease is discussed in Chapter 28.

29.1 Pathophysiology

When a small vessel is punctured or cut, a hemostatic plug formed from aggregated platelets seals the leak, and the plug is subsequently reinforced by fibrin. When the formation of fibrin is abnormal, the hemostatic plug may be relatively weak and unstable, resulting in delayed bleeding, sometimes for several days following the injury. Based on the severity of symptoms for the same level of reduced activity, factors VIII and IX appear to be the 2 most important procoagulant factors required for normal hemostasis. Factor XI deficiency results in mild or asymptomatic conditions; patients with deficiencies of fibrinogen, prothrombin, factors V, VII, or X experience symptoms of intermediate severity. Deficiencies of the contact factors, other than factor XI, are not associated with any clinically important hemostatic abnormalities, which may be explained by bypass mechanisms (see Chapter 26).

29.2 Clinical Findings

The characteristic clinical features of a bleeding disorder caused by an abnormality of a blood clotting factor (features that distinguish them from platelet disorders) are outlined in **t26.2**.

The great majority of inherited coagulation-type disorders are relatively benign, and bleeding occurs only when the hemostatic mechanism is severely challenged. A history of easy bruising and excessive bleeding after minor surgery such as tonsillectomy or tooth extraction usually exists. Such bleeding is troublesome but rarely life-threatening. Hemarthroses are usually seen only in severe cases but may occur in mild cases following joint injury. The clinical differentiation of a coagulation-type disorder from a platelet-type disorder may be difficult, but a history of bleeding from a wound or injury starting after an interval of several hours or days suggests the former. The lifelong nature of the bleeding disorder is usually sufficient to permit its categorization as inherited rather than acquired. **t29.1** summarizes the inherited coagulation disorders associated with bleeding. Acquired disorders of coagulation are discussed in Chapter 30.

t29.1 Inherited Coagulation Disorders Associated with Bleeding

Deficiency of Procoagulants	Increased Fibrinolytic Activity
Factor VIII deficiency (hemophilia A)	α_2-antiplasmin deficiency
Factor IX deficiency (hemophilia B)	Plasminogen activator inhibitor deficiency
Factor XI deficiency	(increased levels of tissue plasminogen activator)
Factor X deficiency	
Factor VII deficiency	
Factor V deficiency	
Prothrombin deficiency	
Fibrinogen deficiency (afibrinogenemia)	
(dysfibrinogenemia)	
Factor XIII deficiency	

Platelet-type bleeding disorders are discussed in Chapter 28. Deficiencies of factor XII, prekallikrein, and high-molecular-weight kininogen are not associated with bleeding. Rare combined inherited disorders such as deficiency of factors V and VIII and combined deficiency of the vitamin K-dependent factors are not included in this table

29.3 Diagnostic Approach

Hemarthroses in a man may be considered the hallmark of a severe coagulation disorder. If this is sex-linked, the patient has either hemophilia A or hemophilia B; exceptions to this rule are rare (type 3 vWD). All that is then needed to establish the diagnosis is a specific assay of factor VIII and, if the results are normal, an assay for factor IX. Petechiae or purpura are rare in a coagulation disorder and suggest von Willebrand disease (vWD), thrombocytopenia, or a qualitative platelet disorder. Heparin use should be excluded.

Evaluation of inherited coagulation disorders proceeds as follows:

1. Hematologic evaluation is conducted to exclude thrombocytopenia and anemia.
2. Coagulation tests, including activated partial thromboplastin time (aPTT) and prothrombin time (PT), are performed. The necessity for and nature of subsequent studies depend on the results of these tests **t29.2, t29.3**. If the diagnosis of an inherited coagulation disorder is uncertain, bleeding disorders such as vWD or qualitative platelet dysfunction should be considered (see Chapter 28).
3. An isolated prolonged PT suggests factor VII deficiency, which can be confirmed with a specific assay for factor VII.
4. An isolated prolonged aPTT in a patient with lifelong bleeding suggests deficiency of factor VIII, IX, or XI. Von Willebrand disease also should be considered, especially if an autosomal dominant pattern of bleeding exists in the family history. Because deficiencies of factor XII, high-molecular-weight kininogen (HMW-K), and prekallikrein are not associated with excessive bleeding, their routine assay is not necessary to evaluate prolonged aPTT values in patients with bleeding disorders. Heparin use should be excluded.

t29.2 Results of aPTT and PT Assays in inherited Deficiencies of Clotting Factors

Factor	aPTT	PT
HMW-K, prekallikrein, XII, XI, IX, VIII	Increased	Normal
V, X, prothrombin, hypofibrinogenemia	Increased	Increased
VII	Normal	Increased
Dysfibrinogenemia	Increased or normal	Increased or normal
XIII deficiency	Normal	Normal
α_2-antiplasmin	Increased or normal	Increased or normal

HMW-K = high-molecular-weight kininogen; PT = prothrombin time; aPTT = activated partial thromboplastin time

t29.3 Use of aPTT and PT Tests for Screening for Inherited Bleeding Disorders

aPTT	PT	Further Tests to Be Performed
Normal	Normal	Platelet aggregation studies, vWD studies, factor XIII screen, α_2-antiplasmin, exclude heterozygous deficiency of factors VIII, IX, XI, X, VII, V, and prothrombin
Increased	Normal	Factor VIII assay; if normal, assays for factor IX, then factor XI; if factor VIII is low, assays for vWF:Ag and ristocetin cofactor activity; exclude inhibitor/heparin
Increased	Increased	Thrombin time; if normal, assays for factors V and X and prothrombin; if thrombin time is prolonged, assay for fibrinogen by functional and antigenic methods; exclude heparin
Normal	Increased	Factor VII assay

aPTT = activated partial thromboplastin time; PT = prothrombin time; vWD = von Willebrand disease; vWF = von Willebrand factor; Ag = antigen

5. If both the aPTT and PT assays are prolonged, deficiency of prothrombin, fibrinogen, or factor V or X is possible. A prolonged thrombin time in such cases suggests hypofibrinogenemia or dysfibrinogenemia, and specific fibrinogen assays (functional and antigenic) can identify these patients. A normal thrombin time in such cases necessitates specific assays for factors V and X and prothrombin to identify the deficient factor. A mixing study should be performed to exclude an inhibitor to coagulation. Heparin use should be excluded.
6. If the aPTT, PT, and thrombin time are normal, a test for clot solubility in 5 mol/L of urea should be performed to exclude factor XIII deficiency.
7. When the aPTT is prolonged and the PT is normal, the aPTT should be repeated using a mixture of equal parts of the patient's plasma and normal plasma. This test is called an "inhibitor screen," or "mixing study," and is useful to screen for antibodies or other inhibitors (eg, heparin). It is, however, relatively insensitive and non-specific, and a specific test for the presence of an antibody to factor VIII should be performed for all patients with a known factor VIII deficiency. In patients with other types of inherited deficiencies, the development of an antibody specifically directed against the deficient factor is rare. Accordingly, unless there are unusual circumstances, such as a failure to respond to treatment with the appropriate concentrate or a positive aPTT inhibitor screen, a specific search for antibody is not part of a routine evaluation for hereditary deficiencies of clotting factors other than factor VIII.
8. In some patients with vWD, the clinical and laboratory findings may mimic those seen in mild hemophilia **t29.4**. It is therefore necessary to consider testing for vWD in all patients with decreased levels of factor VIII in whom there is no clear-cut sex-linked family history.

t29.4 Distinguishing von Willebrand Disease From Hemophilia A

Characteristic	von Willebrand Disease	Hemophilia A
Inheritance	Autosomal dominant	Sex-linked recessive
Hemarthroses or joint damage	Rare	Present in most severe cases
Clinical severity	Usually mild and rarely dangerous or crippling	Mild to severe
Factor VIII activity	Usually 6%-50%	0-35%
vWF antigen	<50%	>50%
Ristocetin cofactor activity	Abnormal	Normal

vWF = von Willebrand factor

9. Patients with mild bleeding disorders may have normal results on screening studies. If vascular disorders such as hereditary hemorrhagic telangiectasia are excluded, the following hemostatic disorders should be considered: vWD, carriers for factor VIII or IX deficiency, factor XI deficiency, dysfibrinogenemia, factor XIII deficiency, platelet dysfunction, and α_2-antiplasmin deficiency. Remember that normal coagulation screening results do not exclude a significant hemostatic defect. If the above tests are normal, assays to evaluate platelet procoagulant activity should be done.
10. Molecular biology techniques are not useful to identify genetic defects resulting in inherited coagulation disorders. These bleeding disorders are due to genotypically heterogeneous mutations, which require tedious mutation analysis. Consequently, the coagulation tests described are preferred for initial diagnosis. On the other hand, if the molecular defect in a given patient is known, molecular techniques to identify carriers in the family and to determine whether a fetus would be affected are useful and are superior to coagulation tests. This is especially true for evaluation of hemophilia carriers.

f29.1 summarizes one approach to evaluating isolated, prolonged aPTT values in patients with bleeding disorders. f29.2 depicts an algorithm for evaluating patients with a likely inherited bleeding disorder who have normal hemostasis screening studies.

29.4 Hematologic Findings

Apart from the exclusion of anemia and thrombocytopenia, the morphology of the formed elements in the blood is usually unremarkable. Blood counts and red blood cell morphology may be consistent with chronic blood loss.

29.5 Other Laboratory Tests

Test 29.5.1 Assay for Factor VIII

Purpose. The determination of factor VIII level is necessary for the diagnosis of hemophilia A and vWD. The level usually correlates well with clinical severity. Assays also are used for monitoring response to therapy. Factor VIII is usually decreased in vWD in proportion to the level of von Willebrand factor (vWF). Although hemophilia A carriers have decreased levels of factor VIII, their vWF antigen level is normal. Stress or pregnancy in hemophilia A carriers may cause factor VIII to rise to normal, but the ratio of vWF antigen to factor VIII activity remains increased. Factor VIII deficiency also must be considered in every patient who has an acquired coagulopathy with a prolonged aPTT and a normal PT associated with bleeding.

Principle. The ability of dilutions of a sample of patient plasma deficient in factor VIII to correct the prolonged aPTT of commercially deficient plasma is compared with that of normal pooled plasma. For example, if a 1:20 dilution of normal plasma shortens the clotting time of deficient plasma to the same extent as a 1:5 dilution of the patient's plasma, the latter sample has 25% of normal activity.

Specimen. The plasma sample collected for the PT or aPTT assay is used. Factor VIII activity is fairly stable, and the test may be performed on a plasma sample frozen within 30 minutes of collection and stored at -30°C.

Procedure. The deficient plasma sample used is obtained from a patient known to have less than 1% factor VIII. It may be kept for several years if stored at –70°C. Dilutions of normal pooled plasma (1:10, 1:20, 1:40, 1:80, and 1:160) and the patient's plasma sample (1:10 and 1:20) in saline are prepared. One part of each dilution is added to one part of the deficient plasma, and an aPTT is performed in duplicate. A typical standard curve is shown in f29.3.

f29.1 Evaluation of a patient with bleeding and prolonged activated partial thromboplastin times

This algorithm refers only to patients with clinical bleeding who are candidates for an inherited disorder and who have isolated prolonged aPTT values.

PT = prothrombin time; aPTT = activated partial thromboplastin time; vWF = von Willebrand factor

**Patients with clinical bleeding but normal diagnostic studies should be evaluated further for lupus anticoagulants associated with either platelet dysfunction or thrombocytopenia.*

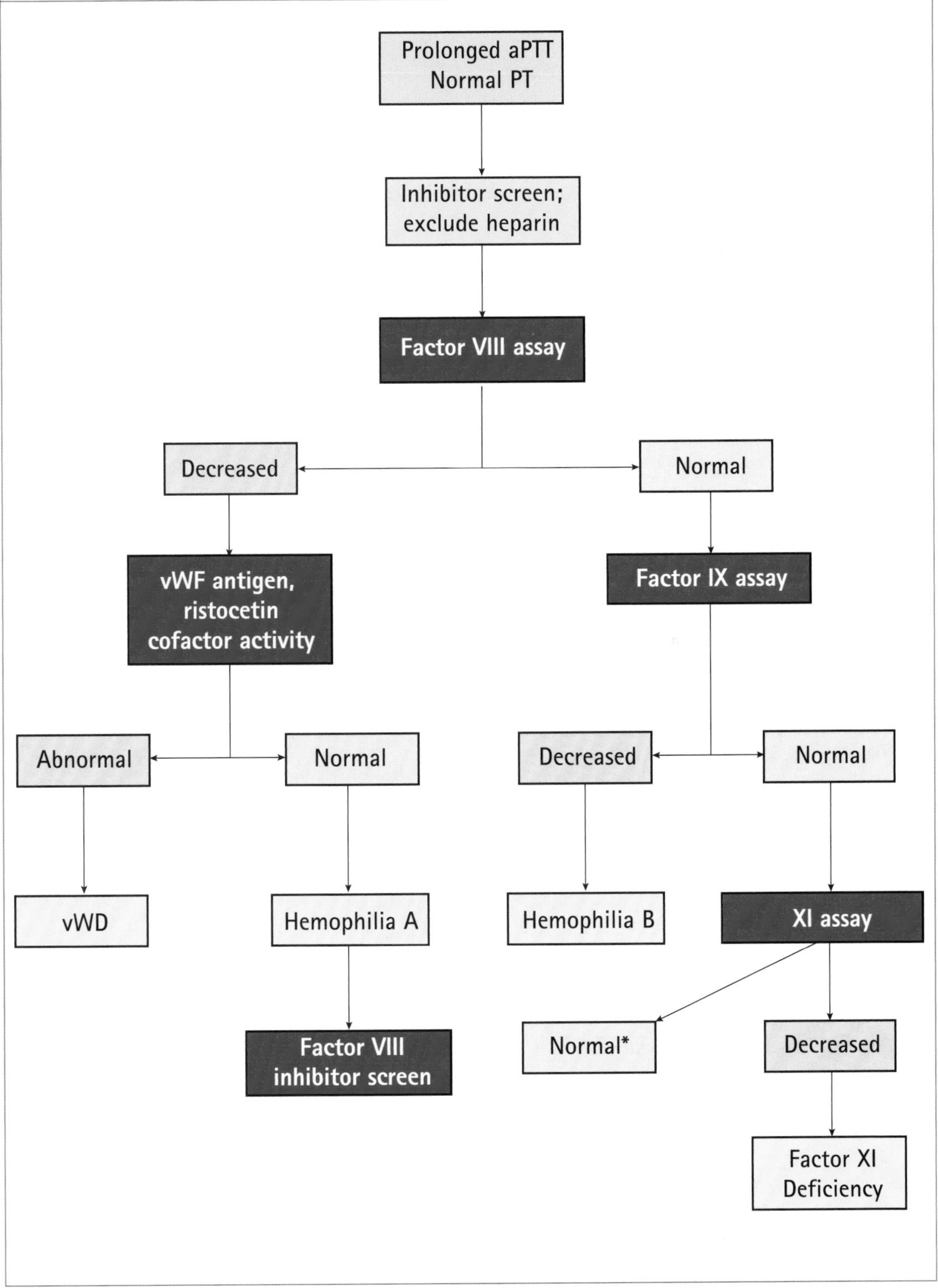

f29.2 Algorithm to evaluate patients with a likely inherited bleeding disorder and normal screening studies

The type of bleeding (ie, soft tissue, mucosal, vascular) is used to determine the initial laboratory strategy.

PT = prothrombin time; PTT = partial thromboplastin time; vWD = von Willebrand disease

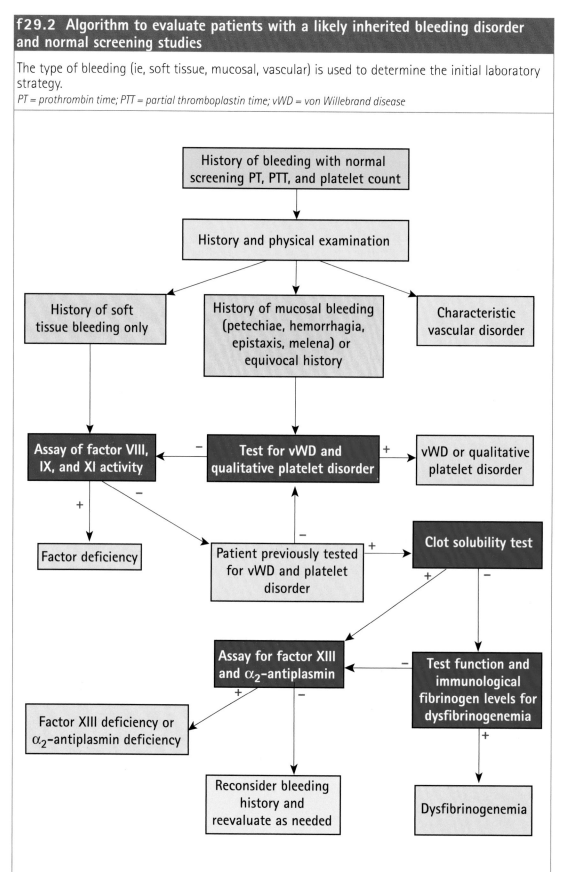

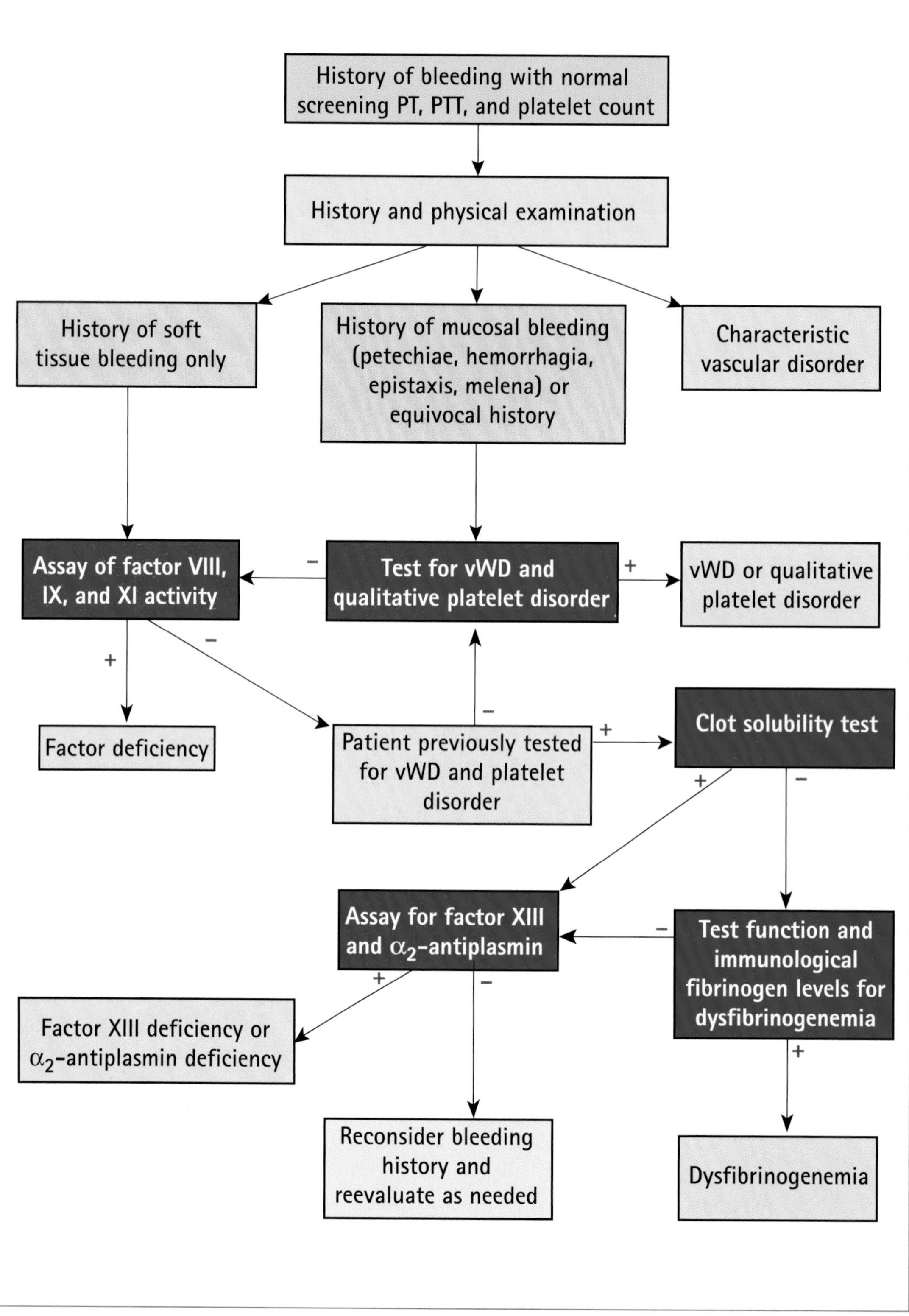

f29.3 A typical factor assay standard curve

Dilutions of normal pooled plasma are made (1:10-1:320) and clotting times measured. Results of clotting times vs factor concentration are plotted on log-log paper, and the best-fit line is drawn. Patient plasma is diluted 1:10 and 1:20, and clotting times measured. As shown in the figure, the 1:10 dilution of patient plasma had a clotting time of 71 sec (red "x"). Interpolation from the standard curve yields a factor value of 37%. These curves can be prepared manually using fibrometer methods, or fully automated instruments can be used to prepare dilutions, add reagents, measure clotting times, plot standard curves, and calculate patient results.

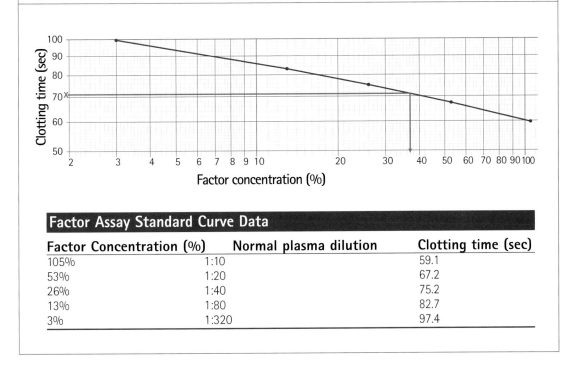

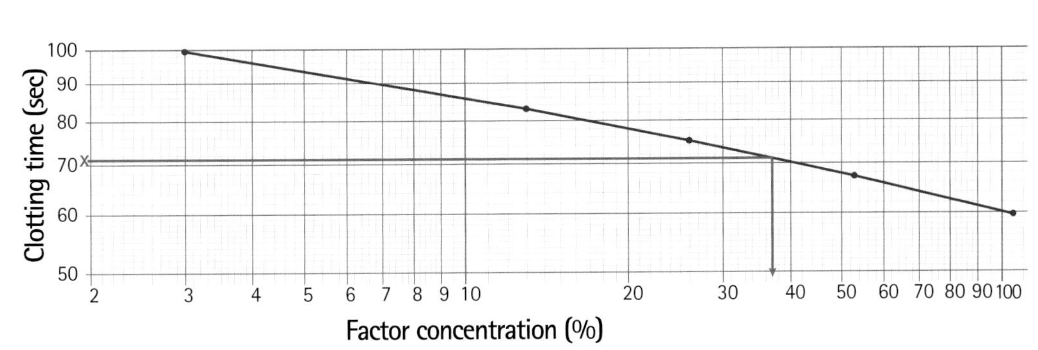

Factor Assay Standard Curve Data

Factor Concentration (%)	Normal plasma dilution	Clotting time (sec)
105%	1:10	59.1
53%	1:20	67.2
26%	1:40	75.2
13%	1:80	82.7
3%	1:320	97.4

Interpretation. The 1:10 dilution of the normal pooled plasma sample is arbitrarily taken as 100% activity, the 1:20 as 50%, the 1:40 as 25%, and so forth. A line of best fit is obtained on log-log paper when clotting times are plotted against percentage concentration of normal plasma. The normal plasma concentrations that would give the same clotting times as the 1:10 and 1:20 dilutions of the patient's plasma sample are determined from the graph. The percentage concentration obtained with the 1:10 dilution is the actual concentration of factor VIII in the patient's plasma sample; the value obtained with the 1:20 dilution must be multiplied by two. The mean of the 2 values is reported. If the value with the 1:20 dilution is significantly higher than that of the 1:10 dilution, an inhibitor should be suspected, but the assay should be repeated to exclude a technical error. The normal range for factors VIII and IX is approximately 60%-150%.

Notes and Precautions. The activity of factor VIII may be increased significantly by trace amounts of thrombin that can form if the blood is collected too slowly or if mixing with the anticoagulant is incomplete. Factor VIII activity also is sometimes increased in low-grade disseminated intravascular coagulation (DIC), presumably owing to thrombin activation. Exercise may double or even triple the level, which may remain high for several hours. Patients with chronic elevations of factor VIII >150% of normal may have a thrombotic risk (see Chapter 33).

Test 29.5.2 Assays for Other Factors Involved in Intrinsic Coagulation Only

Purpose. Assays for other factors (ie, factors, IX, XI, XII, prekallikrein, and HMW-K) involved in the intrinsic pathway may reveal the cause of a prolonged aPTT not attributable to factor VIII deficiency.

Specimen. The plasma sample collected for the PT or aPTT assay is used.

Principle. The principle is the same as that underlying the one-stage procedure for the factor VIII assay described previously. The relative ability of plasma to shorten prolonged aPTTs of commercially deficient plasma is compared with that of pooled normal plasma.

Procedure. The procedure is the same as that described for the factor VIII assay, using the appropriate factor-deficient plasma in place of factor VIII–deficient plasma. For the prekallikrein assay, the preincubation period in the aPTT test after addition of contact activator should not exceed 3 minutes; longer incubation periods cause the aPTT of prekallikrein-deficient plasma to approach the normal value. Accordingly, certain automated instruments in which the preincubation period exceeds 3 minutes cannot be used.

In the HMW-K assay, the 1:20 dilution of normal plasma may be as effective in shortening the aPTT of the HMW-K–deficient plasma as the 1:5 dilution. Therefore, in performing this assay, it is advisable to start at a 1:20 dilution and to continue up to a 1:640 dilution. The unknown is tested at 1:5 dilution up to a 1:20 dilution.

Interpretation. The normal range for factors IX, XI, XII, prekallikrein and HMW-K is approximately 60%-150%.

Notes and Precautions. The deficient plasma may be commercially obtained. Prekallikrein- and HMW-K–deficient plasmas are rare, so few coagulation laboratories perform these assays, although they are technically quite simple. In most instances, however, a provisional diagnosis of these 2 deficiencies may be made by a process of exclusion. Thus, if the patient has a prolonged aPTT, normal PT, normal levels of the relevant intrinsic factors (factors VIII, IX, and XI), and a negative bleeding history, a deficiency of factor XII, prekallikrein, or HMW-K should be considered. Prekallikrein-deficient plasma shortens progressively on incubation with kaolin (Celite) in an aPTT assay and may be normal after 8 minutes of preincubation, thereby distinguishing it from HMW-K deficiency or factor XII deficiency.

Certain intrinsic clotting factors exhibit age-dependent normal ranges, so interpretation of a pediatric result as normal or abnormal requires comparison of the result to specific age normal ranges.

Test 29.5.3 Assays for Prothrombin and Factors V, VII, and X

Purpose. Assays for prothrombin and factors V, VII, and X are performed to determine the specific cause(s) of a prolonged PT.

Principle. The principle is the same as that for the assays described previously, but the PT is used instead of aPTT.

Specimen. Blood is collected in the same manner as for the factor VIII assay. The assay for factor V should be performed within 4 hours of collection because it is relatively labile. Assays for factor VII are best performed as soon as possible after collection because factor VII may increase in activity when the plasma is stored in the refrigerator (cold activation).

Procedure. The actual technique using plasma samples from patients deficient in prothrombin and factors V, VII, and X is simple; however, these deficient states are rare, and deficient plasma samples usually are prepared artificially and are commercially available. For example, factor V–deficient plasma is prepared by aging plasma at 37°C. The assays are performed in the same manner as the assays for the intrinsic factors (eg, factor VIII) using the PT instead of aPTT. The ability of the patient's plasma to shorten the prolonged PT of commercially deficient plasma is compared with that of normal plasma.

Interpretation. The normal range for prothrombin and factors V, VII, and X is approximately 60%-150%. Pediatric normal ranges may differ from adult normal ranges. Elevated levels of prothrombin may be associated with a thrombotic risk (see Chapter 33).

Test 29.5.4 Inhibitor Screening Test

Purpose. The inhibitor screening test detects clotting inhibitors, usually immunoglobulins or heparin-like substances.

Principle. The addition of plasma containing an inhibitor of a factor involved in intrinsic clotting prolongs the aPTT of normal plasma.

Specimen. The same plasma specimen for the aPTT test is used.

Procedure. One part of the plasma being tested is incubated with an equal part of normal plasma. The aPTTs of the mixture are determined immediately and after incubation at 37°C for 1-2 hours.

Interpretation. When 1 part of plasma that is congenitally deficient in a clotting factor such as factor VIII is mixed with an equal part of normal plasma, the aPTT of the mixture should be normal. Failure of the aPTT to correct to within the normal reference range suggests the presence of heparin or an antibody. The 2 most common types of inhibitors (excluding heparin) encountered by the coagulation laboratory are the lupus anticoagulant (antiphospholipid antibody) and antibodies to factor VIII. In many cases, these 2 possibilities can be distinguished using the inhibitor screening test at 2 incubation times. The lupus anticoagulant frequently exhibits immediate prolongation of the aPTT (0 time) with similar values observed at the 2-hour incubation time. In contrast, antibodies to factor VIII exhibit time dependence, with increasing aPTT values seen in the 2-hour sample.

The presence of an inhibitor (especially the lupus anticoagulant) may result in spuriously low values of the intrinsic factors. Consequently, inhibitor screening should be considered a routine procedure in evaluating an isolated prolonged aPTT value.

Notes and Precautions. The time-dependence criteria mentioned above are not absolute in distinguishing lupus anticoagulants from antibodies to coagulation factors. Thus, for patients with bleeding symptoms and an isolated prolonged PTT that does not correct with mixing, specific tests for factor VIII antibodies should be done, regardless of the mixing study profile.

Test 29.5.5 Factor VIII Antibody Screening Test

Purpose. Antibodies to factor VIII develop in up to 30% of patients with hemophilia A. The titer of antibody increases after infusions of factor VIII concentrates, and detection is important because the patient may become refractory to treatment. Factor VIII antibodies are an important cause of severe bleeding in previously healthy individuals; in patients with a background of immunologic disorders such as systemic lupus erythematosus, rheumatoid arthritis, and penicillin sensitivity; and in women following parturition. An antibody to factor VIII should be considered in every patient found during a preoperative workup to have an inhibitor. Although the vast majority of inhibitors are lupus-like (see Chapter 30) and do not give rise to excessive bleeding, surgery in a patient with a factor VIII inhibitor is dangerous and may be fatal.

Principle. If a plasma specimen suspected of containing a factor VIII inhibitor is incubated with an equal volume of normal plasma specimen, the factor VIII concentration of the mixture will be significantly decreased below normal after a period of incubation.

Specimen. The plasma specimen collected for the aPTT is used; the antibodies are remarkably stable and are present in both plasma and serum.

Procedure. One part of patient plasma is mixed with an equal volume of normal pooled plasma (used as the 100% standard). After incubation for 2 hours at 37°C, the mixture is diluted with saline in a 1:5 ratio and assayed for factor VIII.

Interpretation. If the factor VIII concentration of the mixture is 35% or more, the patient does not have an inhibitor or the inhibitor is too weak to be significant.

Notes and Precautions. To detect a low-titer inhibitor, it is advisable to obtain plasma specimens several days after, as well as before, replacement therapy.

Test 29.5.6 Factor VIII Antibody Titer

Purpose. Quantitation of the level of a factor VIII antibody is important in clinical treatment of hemophiliac patients.

Principle. Serial dilutions of a plasma specimen containing the inhibitor are incubated with a normal plasma specimen for a specified period, and the residual factor VIII activity is determined. Factor VIII inhibitor titers are commonly expressed in Bethesda units, which are defined as the reciprocal of the plasma dilution that, when incubated with normal plasma for 2 hours, neutralizes half of the factor VIII activity.

Specimen. Blood is collected as for the aPTT test or factor VIII assay.

Procedure. Serial dilutions of the patient plasma sample in saline (1:2, 1:4, etc) are incubated with an equal volume of normal plasma for 2 hours at 37°C. The residual factor VIII in each of the incubation mixtures is determined. The inhibitor titer in Bethesda units is the reciprocal of the dilution of the test plasma sample that gives 50% inhibition; this may be determined by drawing a curve relating the activity of residual factor VIII to the reciprocal of the dilution or by a rough approximation made from inspection of the data.

Interpretation. A factor VIII antibody titer up to 5 Bethesda units is considered a low-titer inhibitor, whereas a value greater than 5 Bethesda units is considered a high-titer inhibitor. The clinical importance of quantitating the titer of a factor VIII antibody is that it may determine therapy. Low-titer inhibitors usually can be overcome by infusion of factor VIII, but this therapy is less effective in patients with high-titer inhibitors.

There is considerable heterogeneity between the factor VIII antibodies of different patients. The antibodies seen in non-hemophiliacs may differ strikingly from those seen in hemophiliac patients. For example, some of the antibodies seen in non-hemophiliacs may neutralize only 80% of the available factor VIII in normal plasma over a period of 12 hours, reaching a plateau. Yet when the factor VIII concentration of the mixture is increased to 100% by addition of factor VIII concentrate, the level again falls to only 20%, indicating that the antibody was only partially neutralized. Moreover, if a factor VIII concentrate is given to a patient with a factor VIII antibody, the factor VIII level determined in the laboratory may not be a true reflection of the level at the time the plasma was drawn, because neutralization of factor VIII activity occurs in vitro between the time of collection and actual performance of the assay.

Other test systems with different unit definitions are used to assay factor VIII antibodies. The results obtained using different test systems are generally poorly correlated; however, each method gives useful information with respect to the relative potency of the antibody in any single patient over time. The standard Bethesda assay does not control pH, allowing variable low-level inactivation of factor VIII by non-immunologic mechanisms. A modified assay, the Nijmegen modification, has been described for controlling pH and improving classification of positive and negative samples. A Bethesda assay of patient plasma can also be performed against porcine factor VIII; if anti-porcine antibody levels are low, porcine factor VIII can be a treatment option.s

Test 29.5.7 Alpha$_2$-Antiplasmin Determination

Purpose. An α_2-antiplasmin determination is performed for patients with an acquired or inherited bleeding diathesis who have normal platelet function and normal levels of the known coagulation factors.

Principle. A known amount of plasmin is added to the patient's plasma specimen and, after a short interval, the amount of residual plasmin activity is measured. The method for determining the plasmin level is essentially the same as that used in the plasminogen assay, in which a fluorescent or chromogenic substrate is used (see Chapter 33). The percentage of plasmin inhibited provides a measure of the α_2-antiplasmin level, which also may be measured with immunologic methods.

Specimen. Citrated plasma is used for this test.

Procedure. Aliquots of a standardized and stable preparation of human plasmin are added to patient and control plasma samples and to a saline control sample. After exactly 1 minute, the mixture containing the plasmin is then added to a fluorescent or chromogenic synthetic substrate as described for the plasminogen assay (see Chapter 33). The residual plasmin is the difference between the values obtained for the plasma test sample and the control containing saline instead of plasma. A normal range has to be established for each laboratory and is usually 80%-120%.

Interpretation. Heterozygotes with inherited α_2-antiplasmin deficiency at levels between 25% and 60% of normal may bleed excessively following surgery. In acquired deficiencies—which are seen with liver disease and thrombotic states, especially DIC—plasminogen activity is depressed concomitantly.

Notes and Precautions. Alpha$_2$-antiplasmin levels cannot be determined in patients who are receiving fibrinolytic inhibitor therapy (eg, ε-aminocaproic acid [Amicar]).

Test 29.5.8 Factor XIII Screening Test

Purpose. Factor XIII deficiency is an uncommon bleeding disorder associated with normal screening tests of hemostasis.

Principle. Clots cross-linked by factor XIII resist denaturation by high concentrations of urea or acid. Factor XIII deficiency is associated with premature clot lysis.

Specimen. Citrated plasma is used in this test.

Procedure. Patient and control plasmas are recalcified separately to induce a clot. The clots are suspended in 5 mol/L urea (or trichloroacetic acid) for 24 hours. Clot stability is examined visually after 24 hours of incubation.

Interpretation. Clot lysis suggests factor XIII deficiency.

Notes and Precautions. This assay is a screening test. Abnormal results should be confirmed with a repeat assay, as well as a quantitative factor XIII assay. A mixing study using this assay should be done to exclude inhibitors to factor XIII in patients with a positive screening test. Deficiency of α_2-antiplasm may also cause an abnormal clot lysis result.

29.6 Course and Treatment

The specific treatment for bleeding associated with inherited coagulation disorders is to increase deficient or defective protein above the minimum concentration believed adequate for normal hemostasis (ie, approximately 30%-50% of the mean normal level for most factors). To achieve this level with plasma alone in a patient with a very low baseline value is virtually impossible; therefore, concentrated forms of clotting factors are necessary. Monoclonal-purified factor VIII and IX preparations are available; these products, in addition to being highly purified, appear to be sterile regarding transmission of viral infections. Recombinant preparations of factors VIII and IX are also available. Concentrates to treat deficiencies of factors V, XI, or XIII are not yet widely available, so fresh-frozen plasma is used for affected patients. A solvent-treated plasma product currently is available and appears to offer safety from viral infection.

The dosage schedules depend on the half-life of the factor being replaced, which is roughly 12 hours for factor VIII and 24 hours for factor IX. Replacement therapy is indicated for life-threatening hemorrhages (eg, central nervous system or intraperitoneal bleeds), surgery, and the early treatment of hemarthroses and deep-tissue hematomas.

Almost all patients with mild hemophilia A and many patients with vWD (with the exception of those with variant vWD) respond well to intravenous or subcutaneous administration of desmopressin, a synthetic analog of vasopressin given as 0.3 µg/kg over a period of 15-30 minutes. This drug often increases factor VIII and vWF as much as twofold or threefold above the basal level, often without any side effects. Thus, plasma or plasma concentrates are rarely required by affected patients when they have minor bleeding. Desmopressin is also available as a nasal spray.

Epsilon-aminocaproic acid or tranexamic acid are sometimes useful for minor bleeding episodes associated with coagulation disorders and are very effective in the treatment of α_2-antiplasmin deficiency. Patients with vWD and significant bleeding or who require major surgery should receive sterile products that contain both factor VIII and vWF activity, such as Humate-P.

29.7 References

Giddings JC, Peake IR. The investigation of factor VIII deficiency. In: Thomson JM, ed. *Blood Coagulation and Haemostasis: A Practical Guide.* New York, NY: Churchill-Livingstone; 1985:135-207.

Freidman KD, Rodgers GM. Inherited coagulation disorders. In: Greer JP, Foerster J, Rodgers GM, et al, eds. *Wintrobe's Clinical Hematology. 12th ed.* Philadelphia: Lippincott Williams & Wilkins; 2009:1379-1424.

Santoro SA, Eby CS. Laboratory evaluation of hemostatic disorders. In: Hoffman R, Benz EJ, Shattil SJ, et al, eds. *Hematology: Basic Principles and Practice. 3rd ed.* New York, NY: Churchill-Livingstone; 2000:1841-1850.

Verbruggen B, Novakova I, Wessels H, et al. The Nijmegen modification of the Bethesda assay for factor VIII:C inhibitors: improved specificity and reliability. *Thromb Haemost.* 1995;73:247-251.

Chapter 30

Acquired Coagulation Disorders

George Rodgers, MD, PhD

The most common causes of acquired clotting factor deficiencies associated with hemorrhagic manifestations are decreased or abnormal synthesis of clotting factors caused by liver disease or disseminated intravascular coagulation (DIC). The latter is seen in many severe illnesses, including metastatic carcinoma and infectious diseases. Vitamin K deficiency is an important and common cause of hemorrhagic diathesis. Lupus anticoagulants are encountered frequently and are linked with abnormal coagulation tests and are associated with thrombosis and recurrent miscarriage; their laboratory identification is important despite no association with excessive bleeding. Antibodies to prothrombin and factors V, VIII, and XIII, although rare, may arise de novo in individuals with no previous hemorrhagic disorder and cause severe bleeding.

30.1 Pathophysiology

30.1.1 Liver Disease and Vitamin K Deficiency

The liver is the major site of clotting factor synthesis, and a hemorrhagic diathesis can occur in severe hepatitis or cirrhosis. In these conditions, the vitamin K–dependent procoagulant clotting factors (ie, prothrombin and factors VII, IX, and X; see Chapter 26), and anticoagulant proteins (ie, protein C and protein S; see Chapter 33) are usually the first to be reduced, followed by factor V. Factor VIII is not synthesized by hepatic parenchymal cells, and levels of this protein are actually increased in liver disease as an acute-phase response. Similarly, von Willebrand factor, synthesized in vascular endothelial cells, is elevated in liver disease. In addition to altered coagulation protein levels, other hemostatic defects exist with liver disease, including decreased clearance of activated clotting factors and increased levels of degradation products of fibrinogen and fibrin. Fibrin degradation products inhibit hemostasis by interfering with both platelet function and fibrin formation. Fibrinolysis also may be enhanced in liver disease.

Significant liver disease, with associated portal hypertension and splenomegaly, can result in mild to moderate thrombocytopenia. Splenomegaly results in splenic sequestration of platelets. Hepatoma and cirrhosis may also be associated with synthesis of qualitatively abnormal fibrinogen (dysfibrinogen).

The coagulopathy of liver disease is complex and affects global hemostasis, including platelet number and function, coagulation, and fibrinolysis. These defects usually result in a bleeding tendency.

When vitamin K is absent, vitamin K–dependent clotting factors do not bind calcium and, although synthesized in normal amounts, are inactive. Naturally occurring vitamin K is fat soluble, and bile is essential for its absorption from the gastrointestinal tract. In any condition in which the influx of bile into the gut is impeded, a hemorrhagic diathesis may ensue. The absorption of vitamin K occurs in the small intestine and may be deficient in diseases of the intestinal wall as regional ileitis and non-tropical sprue. Sterilization of the bowel resulting from the administration of antibiotics also may result in vitamin K deficiency, because bacterial flora are important in vitamin K synthesis.

30.1.2 Disseminated Intravascular Coagulation

The delicate hemostatic balance between the procoagulant factors and the natural inhibitors necessary for the maintenance of blood fluidity may be disturbed in many diseases **t30.1**. This may result in an uncontrolled generation of thrombin in the blood, leading to formation of thrombi in the microcirculation, a process referred to as DIC. This term is usually used to include a paradoxical hypocoagulable state, which is the natural sequela of DIC and is attributable to the consumption of platelets, fibrinogen, and other procoagulant factors in the formation of the thrombi. Thrombi removal, essential for survival, is accomplished by fibrinolysis, and this mechanism, although an appropriate secondary response and primarily protective, may aggravate bleeding. The formation of thrombin is believed to be essential to DIC. Its presence is presumed by the recognition of products of thrombin action on fibrinogen. These products include fibrinopeptides A and B, fibrin monomer, and D-dimer. Whereas some of the fibrin monomers polymerize and form fibrin, others form soluble complexes with native fibrinogen and with the degradation products that result from the lysis of formed fibrin. The fibrinopeptides have half-lives of only a few minutes, which limits their usefulness as an index of DIC. However, the soluble fibrin monomer complexes remain in the circulation for several hours. Fibrinolysis occurs as a consequence of thrombin generation and results in the formation of several fibrin degradation products, of which products D and E are the most stable and readily measured **f30.1**.

t30.1 Causes of Disseminated Intravascular Coagulation

Excessive tissue factor activity
Metastatic carcinoma (adenocarcinomas)
Tissue injury (eg, brain tissue destruction)
Extensive burn injury
Heat stroke
Promyelocytic leukemia

Infections
Gram-negative endotoxemia
Severe gram-positive septicemia
Rocky Mountain spotted fever
Viral infections

Obstetric disorders
Amniotic fluid embolism
Retained dead fetus
Hypertonic saline abortion
Placental abruption
Hemolytic transfusion reactions

Endothelial cell injury (vasculitis)
Giant hemangioma
Venomous snakebites

f30.1 Generation of cross-linked fibrin by thrombin and factor XIIIa following activation of coagulation, and consequences of plasmin degradation of cross-linked fibrin

a Following activation of coagulation, thrombin activates the transglutaminase, factor XIII to factor XIIIa, and cleaves fibrinopeptides A and B from fibrinogen to generate fibrin monomers.
b Fibrin monomers align longitudinally and with adjacent monomers to form fibrin polymers.
c Factor XIIIa cross-links the D-domains of fibrin monomers to form rigid fibrin polymers.
d Plasminogen activators (TPA or UK) convert plasminogen to plasmin; plasmin degrades cross-linked fibrin to fibrin degradation products, including fragment D, fragment E, and D-dimer, in addition to other products.

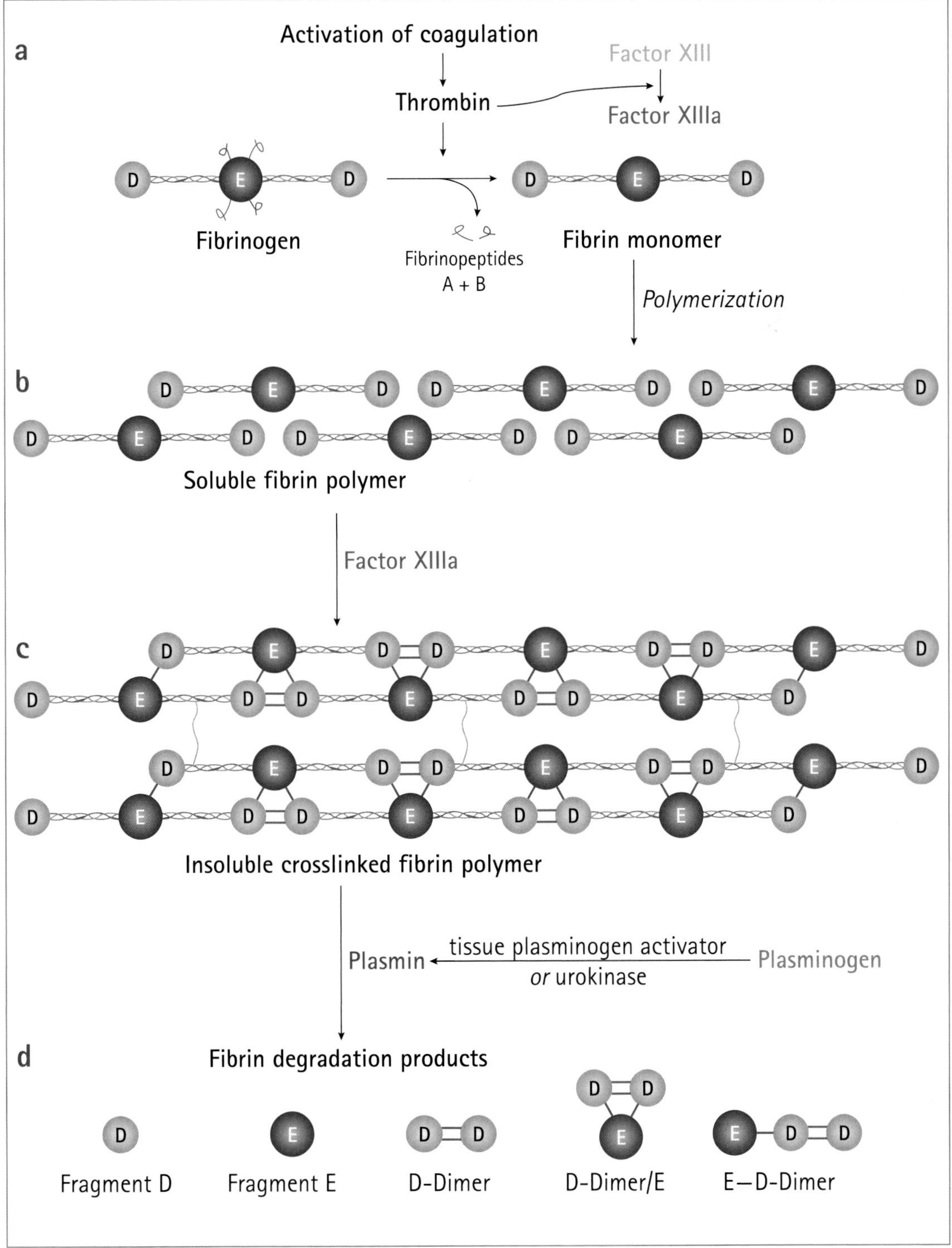

Fibrin is cross-linked by the action of factor XIIIa (transglutaminase). One of the major soluble degradation products is referred to as "D-dimer" (f30.1). Specific monoclonal antibodies to the cross-linked domains of this degradation product are used to detect D-dimer; such antibodies do not react with fibrinogen or fibrinogen degradation products because they lack specific covalent bonds. Fibrinogen degradation products also are generated when urokinase or streptokinase is infused intravenously (fibrinolytic therapy) to convert plasminogen into plasmin and dissolve thrombi. The plasmin may not be neutralized completely by α_2-antiplasmin and can degrade fibrinogen, factor V, and other plasma proteins. If therapy is efficacious, the thrombus lyses and D-dimer is found, as are fibrinogen degradation products derived from the action of the plasmin on fibrinogen.

One of the consequences of intravascular fibrin deposition is the fragmentation of RBCs by strands of fibrin in the microcirculation, resulting in schistocytes or helmet cells. When associated with significant hemolytic anemia, this is referred to as microangiopathic hemolytic anemia. This process is prominent in a group of conditions called "thrombotic microangiopathies," which are characterized by hyaline microthrombi composed of fibrin and aggregated platelets in terminal arterioles and capillaries. The thrombotic microangiopathies include DIC, thrombotic thrombocytopenic purpura, and the hemolytic-uremic syndrome.

A common cause for many cases of DIC is tissue factor expression, either by tumor tissue (eg, promyelocytic leukemia, adenocarcinoma), damaged normal tissue (eg, obstetric emergencies, extensive burns), or activated monocytes and vascular endothelium (eg, gram-negative sepsis). Initiation of contact activation is not usually an important mechanism for DIC.

30.1.3 Abnormal Fibrinolysis

Abnormal fibrinolysis, also called primary fibrinolysis, is an uncommon bleeding disorder in which excessive plasmin is generated in the absence of initiation of coagulation and thrombin formation. Patients with DIC can have secondary fibrinolysis, which is an appropriate response to thrombin generation; this contrasts with primary fibrinolysis in which there is no laboratory evidence for thrombin formation (D-dimer test is negative). t30.2 summarizes disorders or conditions associated with excessive fibrinolysis, in which tests for DIC are usually negative. The diagnosis of primary fibrinolysis is suggested by a low fibrinogen level, elevated FDP levels, a negative D-dimer, and an underlying cause consistent with excessive fibrinolysis. The PT and aPTT may be prolonged if hypofibrinogenemia is substantial or if FDP levels are markedly elevated. The platelet count is usually normal in primary fibrinolysis.

t30.2 Causes of Excessive Fibrinolysis

Condition	Comments
DIC	Fibrinolysis is secondary to thrombin generation. D-dimer test is positive.
α_2-antiplasmin deficiency	An inherited disorder. D-dimer test is negative.
Certain malignancies	Tumors of the genito-urinary tract and gynecologic tumors secrete excess amounts of urokinase (u-PA). D-dimer test is negative. Acute promyelocytic leukemia may have elements of DIC and/or fibrinolysis. Elevated FDP levels with a normal D-dimer level suggests excessive fibrinolysis without DIC.
Liver disease	Excessive fibrinolysis results from decreased liver clearance of plasminogen activators. Usually associated with other hemostatic defects (thrombocytopenia, vitamin K deficiency). D-dimer test is negative unless the patient also has infection or cancer.
Fibrinolytic drugs	All of these drugs induce the "lytic state" (hypofibrinogenemia, elevated FDP levels).
Cardiac bypass	Uncertain mechanisms(s).

DIC=disseminated intravascular coagulation; u-PA = urokinase type plasminogen activator; FDP = fibrin(ogen) degradation products

30.2 Clinical Findings

The bleeding found in thrombocytopenia and functional disorders of the platelets is purpuric, whereas the bleeding manifestations of acquired deficiencies of coagulation factors are of the coagulation type (see **t26.2**). In DIC, however, features of both types of bleeding may be present.

Hemorrhagic disease of the newborn caused by vitamin K deficiency has been virtually eliminated as a result of prophylactic vitamin K therapy. The bleeding typically occurs during the second to sixth day after delivery. Hemorrhagic disease of the newborn is an exaggeration of physiologic hypoprothrombinemia, a temporary state that reaches its maximum point of bleeding on the second or third day after birth and usually returns to normal within 1 week. The onset of bleeding is usually abrupt, and the most common symptoms include melena with hematemesis, umbilical bleeding, epistaxis, submucosal hemorrhage affecting the buccal cavity, intraventricular hemorrhage, and urethral and vaginal bleeding. The disease also may present as excessive bleeding at circumcision or persistent bleeding following a heel prick. Multiple ecchymoses may be found. Petechial hemorrhages are unusual and suggest thrombocytopenia. Premature infants are particularly prone to excessive bleeding, because immaturity of the liver results in decreased synthesis of vitamin K-dependent factors, which is enhanced by vitamin K deficiency.

30.3 Diagnostic Approach

30.3.1 Disseminated Intravascular Coagulation

If a patient with a severe illness, such as metastatic carcinoma or fulminant septicemia or viremia, develops purpuric manifestations, the likely cause is DIC (see **t30.1**). Fibrinogen is an acute-phase reactant protein, and the fibrinogen level may be very high in many conditions that can cause DIC. Therefore, a significant decrease in the concentration may not be apparent from a single fibrinogen determination, as it may be normal or high, depending on the baseline level. Serial fibrinogen determinations to follow the course of the process should therefore be performed. Factor VIII also is an acute-phase reactant protein and its level may remain above normal in DIC despite a significant fall. Thrombin is believed to activate factor VIII and also may cause a high factor VIII level. Factor V activity usually is decreased but rarely sufficiently to raise the prothrombin time (PT) by more than 1 or 2 seconds. Milder depressions of the other factor levels, such as that of factor XIII, also occur, but these changes are of little or no diagnostic value.

A falling platelet count is of considerable diagnostic and prognostic importance and is consistent with DIC. Probably the parameter used most often, however, is the presence of fibrin degradation products, of which the D-dimer appears to be the most specific. D-dimer is more helpful in diagnosing DIC than measurement of other fibrin (fibrinogen) degradation products, because the latter are elevated in both liver disease and DIC, but D-dimer is a specific marker for the presence of thrombin in blood. The presence of microangiopathic hemolytic anemia confirms a diagnosis of DIC, but many patients with DIC may not have morphologic evidence of RBC fragmentation.

30.3.2 Vitamin K Deficiency and Liver Disease

The PT response to the parenteral administration of vitamin K in patients who lack vitamin K-dependent factors is useful in differentiating hepatocellular diseases from other forms of vitamin K deficiency (malnutrition, biliary disease, etc). The PT remains prolonged in hepatocellular disease, but returns to normal in the other conditions unless some associated liver parenchymal damage is also present. In a previously healthy individual who has developed a bleeding diathesis, a prolonged PT with otherwise normal liver function test results often can be attributed to ingestion of warfarin sodium (Coumadin) or rodenticides (superwarfarins).

30.3.3 Antibodies to Coagulation Factors

The development of a coagulation-type bleeding disorder in an individual with previously normal hemostasis is often manifested by deep-tissue hematoma and suggests an antibody specifically directed against factor VIII, factor V, or, more rarely, one of the other clotting factors. Antibodies to specific factors are encountered far less frequently than the lupus anticoagulant **t30.3**.

t30.3 Acquired Coagulation Inhibitors

Type	Clinical Associations	Nature of Antibody	Clinical Findings and Course	Laboratory Findings
Specific antibodies to factor VIII	Previously healthy elderly persons; patients with autoimmune disorders; postpartum patients	IgG, monoclonal	May be persistent, especially in elderly patients; life-threatening bleeding can occur	Increased aPTT; normal PT; decreased factor VIII, positive mixing study
Specific antibodies to factor V	Usually preceded by streptomycin administration; may develop after massive blood transfusion or exposure to bovine thrombin	IgG or IgM, polyclonal	Bleeding tendency usually disappears in weeks or months	Increased aPTT; increased PT decreased factor V; positive mixing study
Specific antibodies to prothrombin	Usually associated with lupus anticoagulant	IgG	Bleeding tendency usually disappears in weeks	Increased aPTT; increased PT; positive mixing study; decreased prothrombin
Specific antibodies to factor XIII or XIIIa	Therapy with isoniazid	IgG	Bleeding tendency usually disappears in weeks or months	Normal aPTT; normal PT; clot soluble in 5 mol/L of urea; positive clot solubility mixing study
Specific antibody to vWF	Myeloma; lymphoproliferative disorders; connective tissue disorders	IgG	Mild bleeding tendency	Decreased ristocetin cofactor activity; normal or decreased factor VIII
Lupus anticoagulant	Procainamide, chlorpromazine, quinidine, lupus erythematosus, pregnancy, HIV infection, no apparent disease	Usually IgG, sometimes IgM, or both	Bleeding tendency absent; patients may have thromboembolic events or recurrent abortions	Increased aPTT; usually normal PT; positive mixing study, positive DRVVT or KCT with phospholipid correction

aPTT = activated partial thromboplastin time; PT = prothrombin time; vWF = von Willebrand factor; DRVVT = dilute Russell's viper venom time; KCT = kaolin clotting time

The lupus anticoagulant results in a prolongation of the activated partial thromboplastin time (aPTT) and occasionally the PT. Patients with this non-specific antibody rarely bleed excessively, even while undergoing major surgery. Because such an antibody was first found in a patient with systemic lupus erythematosus, it is referred to as the "lupus anticoagulant," even though lupus erythematosus is now known to be an uncommon cause. The lupus anticoagulant may be seen in individuals who are taking certain drugs, such as quinidine, procainamide, and chlorpromazine (often an IgM antibody), and in viral infections, such as HIV.

The lupus anticoagulant also is commonly found in individuals in whom no causative factor can be determined (often an IgG antibody). The Venereal Disease Research Laboratory (VDRL) test may give a false-positive result in these patients. The lupus anticoagulant probably comprises a heterogeneous group of antibodies with different actions—IgG or IgM—that may be targeted against negatively charged phospholipid-protein complexes. When the lupus anticoagulant results in a marked prolongation of the aPTT, the aPTT of an equal part of both patient and control plasma usually exceeds that of the normal reference range. The coagulant activities of factors VIII, IX, XI, and XII appear reduced when assayed at a 1:5 dilution, but when assayed at higher dilutions, they usually increase significantly. This phenomenon is attributed to "diluting out the inhibitor." Factor VIII usually appears to be reduced the least and factors XI and XII the most. Weak lupus anticoagulants that result in only a slight prolongation of the aPTT are difficult to diagnose. In these cases, mixing studies may demonstrate correction of the prolonged aPTT, and additional specific tests for the lupus anticoagulant such as the dilute Russell's viper venom time (DRVVT) or the kaolin clotting time (KCT) may be necessary for diagnosis.

In rare cases, a lupus anticoagulant may be associated with a prothrombin deficiency and normal levels of factors V, VII, and X. This is attributable to another autoantibody that binds to but does not neutralize prothrombin, with rapid in vivo clearance of the antibody-prothrombin complex. Patients with this condition may develop a bleeding tendency. A lupus anticoagulant can develop in a patient with a preexisting congenital or acquired coagulation abnormality and give rise to diagnostic problems. Optimal detection of the lupus anticoagulant probably requires at least 2 phospholipid-dependent assays and demonstration of phospholipid correction. **t30.4** summarizes consensus recommendations for laboratory diagnosis of the lupus anticoagulant.

t30.4 ISTH Criteria for the Laboratory Diagnosis of the Lupus Anticoagulant

Prolongation of at least 1 phospholipid-dependent coagulation test with the use of platelet-poor plasma (eg, aPTT, DRVVT, KCT).
Failure to correct the prolonged coagulation time by mixing patient and normal plasma.
Confirmation of the lupus anticoagulant by demonstrating correction of the prolonged coagulation time by addition of excess phospholipid or freeze-thawed platelets.
Exclusion of alternative coagulopathies (eg, factor VIII antibodies).

Diagnostic criteria from: Levine JS, et al. N Engl J Med. *2002;346:752-763; and Brandt JT, et al.* Thromb Haemost. *1995; 74:1185-1190.*
ISTH=International Society on Thrombosis and Haemostasis; aPTT= activated partial thromboplastin time; DRVVT=dilute Russell viper venom time; KCT= kaolin clotting time

A rare cause of an acquired hemorrhagic diathesis that can result in severe bleeding is the acquired deficiency of factor X seen in primary amyloidosis.

Evaluation of the acquired coagulation disorders proceeds as follows:

1. Hematologic evaluation is conducted, with particular attention paid to platelet number, RBC morphology indicative of DIC, and WBC count and differential.
2. Samples are screened for bleeding disorders using platelet count, aPTT, and PT. These tests help differentiate thrombocytopenic purpuras and the acquired diathesis caused by inhibitors, liver disease, vitamin K deficiency, or DIC **t30.5**.

t30.5 Use of Screening Tests in Acquired Bleeding Disorders

Disorder	Platelet Count	aPTT	PT
Thrombocytopenic purpura*	Decreased	Normal	Normal
Liver disease	Normal or decreased	Normal or increased	Increased
Vitamin K deficiency	Normal	Normal or increased	Increased
Factor VIII antibody	Normal	Increased	Normal
Lupus anticoagulant	Normal (usually)	Increased	Normal or increased
DIC†	Decreased	Normal or increased	Increased

aPTT = activated partial thromboplastin time; PT = prothrombin time; DIC = disseminated intravascular coagulation
**See Chapter 27*
†Patients with low-grade chronic DIC may have normal screening test results.

3. In all instances in which the aPTT is significantly prolonged, perform inhibitor screening on a mixture of equal parts of normal plasma and patient plasma (sometimes referred to as a 50:50 mix). Failure of the addition of normal plasma to correct the prolonged aPTT is evidence of a circulating anticoagulant. This is in contrast to the finding in deficient states, in which the aPTT value of the 50:50 mix with normal plasma rarely exceeds the aPTT reference range. Correction, however, does not necessarily exclude the presence of an inhibitor. This is particularly applicable when the aPTT of the patient plasma alone is only a few seconds outside the upper limit of the normal range. If a plasma sample containing a potent lupus anticoagulant is diluted with a normal plasma sample to shorten the aPTT to approximately 40 seconds, it often is difficult to demonstrate the presence of a lupus anticoagulant in the resulting plasma mixture based solely on a failure to correct. In this instance, a specific test for the lupus anticoagulant, such as DRVVT or other phospholipid-dependent assays, may be helpful. In the case of some very slow-acting factor VIII inhibitors, correction may be observed, particularly if the aPTT test is performed within a few minutes of preparing the 50:50 mix with normal plasma. However, the 1-hour incubation sample should indicate the presence of an antibody.
4. If an inhibitor is present or cannot be excluded on the basis of the aPTT of the 50:50 mix and the PT is normal, the presence of a factor VIII inhibitor must be excluded if the patient is bleeding. One practice is to perform assays for factors VIII, IX, and XI routinely in all such cases when the patient has clinical bleeding. If the factor VIII level is normal, a factor VIII inhibitor can be excluded. However, if the factor VIII level is significantly

decreased and does not appear to increase when tested at a higher dilution (eg, 1:20), a specific test for a factor VIII inhibitor is performed (see Chapter 29). When both the aPTT and PT are prolonged and neither is corrected in the 50:50 mix, a specific factor V inhibitor should be considered. If the factor V level is normal, assays for factor X and prothrombin should be performed. If they are all normal, the cause of the PT prolongation may be an unusual type of lupus anticoagulant, or a dysfibrogenemia. If prothrombin is the only factor whose level is decreased, a prothrombin inhibitor should be considered. The diagnosis of a lupus anticoagulant should be made using DRVVT, the kaolin clotting time test, or other phospholipid-dependent assays, and confirmed using a phospholipid correction assay.

5. Assay of D-dimer or fibrin monomer (using the protamine sulfate paracoagulation test), as well as serial fibrinogen determinations, are useful if DIC is suspected.
6. Serial PT assays after vitamin K therapy can confirm vitamin K deficiency due to warfarin sodium ingestion or malnutrition if the PT corrects.

30.4 Hematologic Findings

A platelet count is performed and the morphology of RBCs (schistocytes, etc) is evaluated by peripheral blood smear. If platelets are absent or markedly reduced, the patient is evaluated for thrombocytopenic purpura (see Chapter 27). A moderate to severe reduction, however, can be found in liver disease or DIC and may be associated with schistocytes i30.1 and spherocytes in the peripheral blood smear for DIC.

i30.1 Peripheral blood smear of a patient with disseminated intravascular coagulation

Numerous RBC fragments (schistocytes) are present. (*Oil immersion, Wright stain*)

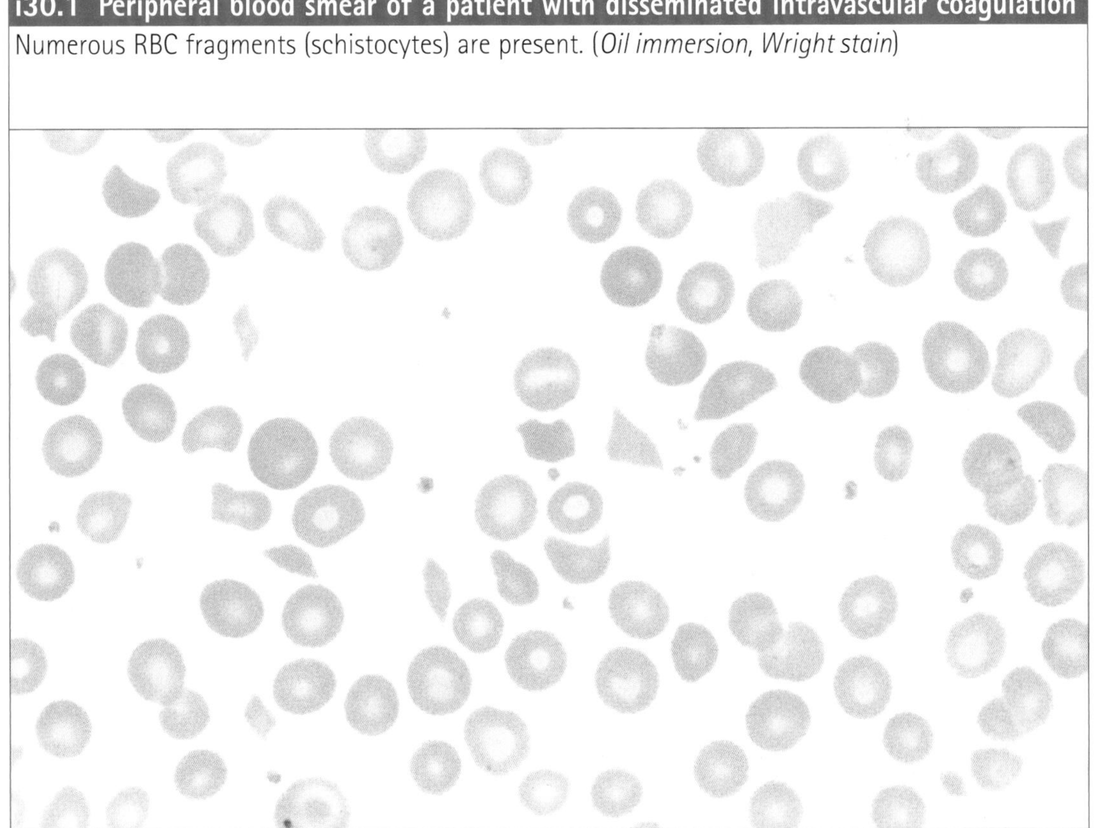

30.5 Other Laboratory Tests

Test 30.5.1 Protamine Sulfate Paracoagulation Test

Purpose. This test detects fibrin monomer in plasma and is used for the diagnosis of DIC.

Principle. Soluble complexes of fibrin monomer with fibrin (fibrinogen) degradation products or fibrin dissociate with the addition of protamine sulfate. The fibrin monomers then polymerize, forming a fibrin web.

Specimen. Platelet-poor plasma, as collected for the aPTT test, is used.

Procedure. Ten drops of plasma are placed in a small glass test tube warmed to 37°C. One drop of 1% protamine sulfate is added and, after gentle shaking, incubated for 20 minutes.

Interpretation. Fibrin webs or strands indicate a positive result. A finely granular, non-cohesive precipitate is usually interpreted as a weak-positive result.

Notes and Precautions. False-positive results may be obtained if there is difficulty with venipuncture or a delay in mixing the blood with anticoagulant because of the formation of small amounts of thrombin in vitro. A test should not be performed on oxalated or heparinized blood, but therapeutic administration of heparin does not interfere with the test. Many hospital laboratories have replaced the protamine sulfate test with the D-dimer test.

Test 30.5.2 Latex Particle Agglutination Test for Fibrin or Fibrinogen Degradation Products

Purpose. This test detects the presence of fibrin or fibrinogen degradation products (FDPs) and is used in the diagnosis of DIC.

Principle. Antibodies to fibrin (fibrinogen) degradation products are bound to latex particles, which clump in the presence of the antigen. If an antiserum to highly purified fibrinogen fragments D and E is employed in the FDP test, a positive result is obtained with fibrinogen and fibrinogen degradation products as well as with fibrin degradation products.

Specimen. In some FDP tests, only serum samples may be used. The blood specimen must be obtained by careful and clean venipuncture and placed in a special sample collection tube that contains soybean trypsin inhibitor plus thrombin or reptilase. After formation of a clot, the tube is incubated at 37°C for approximately 30 minutes before separating the serum by centrifugation.

Procedure. The FDP test uses 1:5 and 1:20 dilutions of serum in buffer. The normal serum level of degradation products derived from fibrinogen or fibrin is less than 10 μg/mL, and the reagents are adjusted so a serum sample with less than this concentration will give no agglutination with either 1:5 or 1:20 dilutions of normal serum.

Interpretation. In DIC, the level of FDPs exceeds 10 μg/mL and in most cases may exceed 40 μg/mL.

Notes and Precautions. Degradation products of fibrinogen or fibrin may be incorporated into the clots formed in vitro during the preparation of the serum sample, thereby giving a normal (negative) result or a spuriously low value. False-positive results may be seen with the FDP test in patients with dysfibrinogenemia when residual fibrinogen remains in the serum. The FDP test may give positive results following surgical procedures or in patients with deep-vein thrombosis and pulmonary embolism.

Because FDPs are cleared by the liver, patients with liver disease have elevated FDP levels. False-positive results can be seen in patients with rheumatoid factors (IgM molecules). Because of these limitations of the FDP test in diagnosing DIC, the D-dimer test is preferred.

Test 30.5.3 Tests for D-Dimer

Purpose. This test is used to diagnose disseminated intravascular coagulation (DIC). Modifications of this assay are used to diagnose or exclude venous thromboembolism.

Principle. Antibodies to the D-dimer epitope of plasmin-digested, cross-linked fibrin are bound to latex particles, which clump in the presence of the antigen. Semi-quantitative assays for D-dimer use visual agglutination as the end-point of the test, while sensitive, quantitative D-dimer assays use photometric detection of bead agglutination as the endpoint.

Specimen. Citrated plasma, as collected for the PT and aPTT assays is used. Special tubes as used for the FDP assay are not necessary.

Procedure. In the semi-quantitative D-dimer assay, the undiluted plasma sample, a 1:2 dilution in buffer, and a 1:4 dilution in buffer are added to the suspension of antibody-coated beads on a glass slide. The suspensions are rotated on the slides for a precise number of minutes, then inspected for macroscopic agglutination. Known positive or negative control samples are also tested.

In the quantitative D-dimer assay, patient plasma is used undiluted. An automated instrument measures agglutination of latex particles by photometry. The increase in absorbance (turbidity) is correlated with the D-dimer level in the sample. If the patient results fall outside of the assay's working range, the instrument dilutes the sample for retesting.

Interpretation. The normal plasma concentration is less than 200 ng/mL. In the semi-quantative assay, assaying serial dilutions of the test plasma is done to determine the highest dilution titer that remains positive. Typically, values greater than or equal to 4 µg/mL by the semi-quantatative method are seen in DIC. Values less than 4 µg/mL, but greater than the upper limit of normal are seen in patients who are acutely ill, postoperative state, and in patients with venous thromboembolism.

For the quantitative D-dimer assay, each method may have different assay characteristics. For example, the STA-Liatest D-Di (Diagnostica Stago) has as its upper limit of normal reference range, 0.5 µg/mL. Values >10 µg/mL are typically seen in DIC, while values between 0.5-10 µg/mL can be seen in hospitalized medical or surgical patients, with or without thrombosis.

The quantitative D-dimer assay has been adapted for use in the exclusion diagnosis of venous thromboembolism. When combined with clinical criteria in the outpatient setting, a normal quantitative D-dimer value is helpful in excluding thromboembolism.

Test 30.5.4 Functional Fibrinogen Determination

Purpose. This test quantitates functional plasma fibrinogen levels and is most commonly used in the diagnosis of DIC. Less commonly, it is used to diagnose inherited fibrinogen disorders (eg, dysfibrinogenemia, afibrinogenemia).

Principle. A thrombin time-based clotting assay is used. Thrombin directly cleaves fibrinogen to fibrin monomer; fibrin monomers then polymerize. The clotting time is inversely proportional to the amount of fibrinogen in the sample when read off a standard curve.

Specimen. Citrated plasma sample, as collected for the PT or aPTT assay, is used.

Procedure. A calibration curve is constructed using serial dilutions of a fibrinogen reference preparation. Serial dilutions of patient plasma are prepared. Thrombin is added, and clotting times are measured in duplicate. Patient fibrinogen levels are determined from the standard curve.

Interpretation. The reference range for normal fibrinogen levels is 150-350 mg/dL (1.5-3.5 g/L). Fibrinogen is an acute-phase reactant with elevated levels occurring in liver disease and inflammatory diseases. Low levels are seen in end-stage liver disease, DIC, dysfibrinogenemias, and the inherited disorders, afibrinogenemia/hypofibrinogenemia, as well as conditions associated with excessive fibrinolysis.

Notes and Precautions. Large concentrations of heparin in the plasma sample or high levels of FDP may prolong the clotting time and falsely indicate low fibrinogen levels. When evaluating patients for dysfibrinogenemia, functional and antigenic fibrinogen levels should be tested on the same sample.

Test 30.5.5 Dilute Russell Viper Venom Time (DRVVT)

Purpose. The DRVVT test can identify the presence of the lupus anticoagulant in patients with positive findings on inhibitor screening or in patients with negative findings on inhibitor screening in whom the lupus anticoagulant is strongly suspected.

Principle. A modified PT assay is used in which clotting is initiated by a snake venom (Russell viper venom) and dilute phospholipid. Russell viper venom directly converts factor X to factor Xa. Factor Xa, factor V, and phospholipid convert prothrombin to thrombin. By diluting the venom and the phospholipid, the assay is more sensitive in detecting antiphospholipid antibodies that inhibit coagulation (lupus anticoagulant).

Specimen. Platelet-poor plasma, as collected for the aPTT assay, is used. Because platelets can neutralize antiphospholipid antibodies in these plasma samples, it is critical that measures be taken to ensure that the sample has a very low platelet count ($<10 \times 10^3$/mm3 [$<10 \times 10^9$/L]). This can be achieved using centrifugation or filtration methods.

Procedure. Normal or patient plasma samples are mixed with a phospholipid source (eg, aPTT reagent) and the dilute Russell viper venom reagent. Clotting times are then measured. If the patient's clotting time is prolonged, the clotting time test is repeated after mixing patient plasma sample with a normal pooled plasma sample. The DRVVT reference range in the author's laboratory is 36-42 seconds.

Interpretation. A prolonged DRVVT result in a plasma sample with a normal PT is suspicious for the lupus anticoagulant. A mixing study with a normal plasma sample that also results in a prolonged DRVVT is diagnostic of the lupus anticoagulant.

Notes and Precautions. Obtaining platelet-poor plasma samples is important in maintaining the sensitivity of this test. Samples with prolonged PT values (eg, from patients on oral anticoagulant therapy) exhibit prolonged DRVVT values even in the absence of the lupus anticoagulant. For patients who have prolonged PT values and in whom the lupus anticoagulant is suspected, anticardiolipin antibodies may be a helpful surrogate test since many patients with the lupus anticoagulant will have positive results for anticardiolipin antibodies. Alternatively, the kaolin clotting time or a dilute PT assay may be a useful test.

A consensus group recommends additional testing to demonstrate phospholipid neutralization of prolonged coagulation tests, definitively diagnosing the lupus anticoagulant. Current practice is to use multiple phospholipid-dependent assays to increase the likelihood of diagnosing the lupus anticoagulant. The choice of a "gold standard" coagulation assay to detect lupus anticoagulants is controversial. Many laboratories use the DRVVT assay or a combination of phospholipid-dependent assays.

Test 30.5.6 Confirmatory Tests for the Lupus Anticoagulant

Purpose. These tests can confirm whether a screening test result for the lupus anticoagulant (eg, the DRVVT) is indeed due to this antiphopholipid antibody.

Principle. Several phospholipid-dependent coagulation assays can be utilized to confirm the lupus anticoagulant, including the aPTT, DRVVT, or the hexagonal phase assay. All assays have in common the principle that a prolonged coagulation assay due to the lupus anticoagulant will shorten or correct when phospholipid is added to the test reagents.

Specimen. Platelet-poor citrated plasma, as collected for the aPTT assay is used (see Test 30.5.5 above).

Procedure. If the aPTT is used as the assay, platelet lysate (a source of phospholipid) is added to the aPTT assay reagent. If the DRVVT is used as the assay, a DRVVT reagent containing excess phospholipid is used. This DRVVT assay is available commercially as LA Sure®. For both the aPTT and DRVVT assays, shortening of the clotting times is confirmation of the lupus anticoagulant.

For the hexagonal phase assay, test plasma is incubated with and without hexagonal phase phosphatidyl-ethanolamine (HPE). Next, an aPTT is performed on both tubes. If a lupus anticoagulant is present in the plasma sample, it would be neutralized by the HPE, resulting in shortening of the aPTT clotting time. This assay is available commercially as Sta Clot®.

Interpretation. Each laboratory should validate these tests to establish clotting time values to correctly classify patients.

Notes and Precautions. As mentioned earlier, the use of platelet-poor plasma samples is key for sensitive lupus anticoagulant assays. Some commercial assays (LA Sure®, Sta-Clot®) contain a heparin-neutralizing agent so that heparin interference is minimized.

30.6 Course and Treatment

Treatment for DIC is directed at the primary cause. For patients with significant thrombocytopenia and hypofibrinogenemia, platelet transfusion and cryoprecipitate may be helpful. Patients who have DIC and primarily thrombotic symptoms may benefit from heparin therapy. New therapies are being developed to inhibit thrombin and other coagulation proteases important in DIC.

Patients with the coagulopathy of liver disease and clinical bleeding rarely respond to vitamin K therapy owing to significant hepatocellular damage; these patients may benefit transiently from fresh-frozen plasma. Other disorders associated with vitamin K deficiency (eg, malnutrition, biliary obstruction, antibiotics, warfarin sodium ingestion) should reverse with vitamin K therapy.

Usually no treatment is required for the lupus anticoagulant, unless it is associated with significant thrombocytopenia, thrombosis, or recurrent miscarriage. In these cases, anticoagulant therapy or immunosuppression (steroids) may be helpful. Antibodies to specific coagulation factors (especially acquired factor VIII antibodies) are best treated with immunosuppression (steroids plus rituximab or cyclophosphamide), because major bleeding is common in affected patients. Low-titer factor VIII antibodies may be overcome with factor VIII concentrate therapy, in amounts 2-3 times the usual 100% dosage. High-titer factor VIII antibodies can be treated with prothrombin complex concentrates, porcine factor VIII, or recombinant factor VIIa.

30.7 References

Brandt JT, Triplett DA, Alving B, et al. Criteria for the diagnosis of lupus anticoagulants: an update. *Thromb Haemost.* 1995;74:1185–1190.

Carey MJ, Rodgers GM. Disseminated intravascular coagulation: clinical and laboratory aspects. *Am J Hematol.* 1998;59:65–73.

Exner T, Burridge J, Power P, et al. An evaluation of currently available methods for plasma fibrinogen. *Am J Clin Pathol.* 1979;71:521–527.

Greenberg CS, Devine DV, McCrae KM. Measurement of plasma fibrin D-dimer levels with the use of a monoclonal antibody coupled to latex beads. Am J Clin Pathol. 1987;87:94–100.

Hougie C. Latex particle agglutination tests for fibrin or fibrinogen degradation products. In: Williams WJ, Beutler E, Erslev AJ, et al, eds. *Hematology.* 4th ed. New York, NY: McGraw-Hill; 1990:1770–1773.

Lehman CM, Wilson LW, Rodgers, GM. Analytical validation and clinical evaluation of the utility of the STA LIATEST D-dimer assay for the diagnosis of disseminated intravascular coagulation. *Am J Clin Pathol.* 2004;122:178-184.

Martin BA, Branch DW, Rodgers GM. Sensitivity of the activated partial thromboplastin time, the dilute Russell's viper venom time, and the kaolin clotting time for the detection of the lupus anticoagulant: a direct comparison using plasma dilutions. *Blood Coag Fibrinolysis.* 1996;7:31–38.

Rodgers GM. Acquired coagulation disorders. In: Greer JP, Foerster J, Rodgers GM, et al, eds. *Wintrobe's Clinical Hematology. 12th ed.* Philadelphia: Lippincott Williams & Wilkins; 2009:1425-1463.

Thiagarajan P, Pengo V, Shapiro SS. The use of the dilute Russell viper venom time for the diagnosis of lupus anticoagulants. *Blood.* 1986;68:869–874.

Turkstra F, van Beek EJR, Cate JW, Buller HR. Reliable rapid blood test for the exclusion of venous thromboembolism in symptomatic outpatients. *Thromb Haemost.* 1996;76:9–11.

Chapter 31

Laboratory Evaluation of the Patient With Bleeding

George Rodgers, MD, *PhD*

Chapters 26 through 30 discussed specific diseases and their associated laboratory tests. Evaluation of a patient with a hemostatic bleeding disorder is summarized in this chapter. Screening test results with possible differential diagnoses are summarized in t31.1. Structural bleeding (eg, esophageal varices or surgical bleeding due to a lacerated blood vessel) should always be considered before embarking on a potentially expensive hemostasis evaluation.

The appropriate confirmatory tests are suggested by the differential diagnosis. For example, an isolated prolonged prothrombin time (PT) is most commonly evaluated by liver function studies or by obtaining a history of warfarin use or malnutrition. An isolated prolonged activated partial thromboplastin time (aPTT) should be evaluated by an inhibitor screen and assays for factors VIII, IX, and XI, after excluding heparin contamination. For patients with prolonged PT and aPTT values in whom disseminated intravascular coagulation is suspected, fibrinogen and D-dimer values should be obtained.

Patients with bleeding and normal laboratory screening test results are challenging, because normal test results do not exclude mild factor deficiency (eg, carriers of factors VIII or IX deficiency), or mild factor XI deficiency. In addition, many patients with mild von Willebrand disease have normal screening test results. For these patients, extensive investigation to evaluate uncommon bleeding disorders, including abnormal fibrinolysis, vascular disorders, factor XIII deficiency, dysfibrinogenemia, autoerythrocyte sensitization, and disorders of platelet procoagulant activity may be required before a diagnosis is confirmed.

31.1 References

Rodgers GM. The diagnostic approach to the bleeding disorders. In: Greer JP, Foerster J, Rodgers GM, et al, eds. *Wintrobe's Clinical Hematology. 12th ed.* Philadelphia: Lippincott Williams & Wilkins; 2009:1273-1288.

t31.1 Hemostasis Screening Test Results in Patients With Bleeding Disorders

PT	aPTT	Platelet Count	Frequency	Differential Diagnosis
I	N	N	Common	Factor VII deficiency (early liver disease, early vitamin K deficiency, early warfarin therapy)
			Rare	Factor VII inhibitor, dysfibrinogenemia, inherited factor VII deficiency, some cases of DIC, certain factor X variants, superwarfarin ingestion
N	I	N	Common	Deficiency or inhibitor of factors VIII, IX, or XI; vWD; heparin
			Rare	Lupus inhibitor with qualitative platelet defect, certain factor X variants
I	I	N	Common	Vitamin K deficiency, liver disease, warfarin, heparin, superwarfarin ingestion
			Rare	Deficiency or inhibitor of factors X or V, prothrombin, or fibrinogen; lupus inhibitor with hypoprothrombinemia; DIC; primary fibrinolysis; dysfibrinogenemia
I	I	D		DIC, liver disease, heparin therapy with associated thrombocytopenia
N	N	D	Common	Increased platelet destruction, decreased platelet production, splenomegaly, hemodilution
			Rare	Certain inherited platelet disorders (Wiskott-Aldrich syndrome, Bernard-Soulier syndrome)
N	N	I		Myeloproliferative disorders
N	N	N	Common	Mild vWD, acquired qualitative platelet disorders (eg, uremia, antiplatelet medications)
			Rare	Inherited qualitative platelet disorders; vascular disorders; fibrinolytic disorders; factor XIII deficiency; autoerythrocyte sensitization; dysfibrinogenemia; mild deficiency of factors VIII, IX, and XI; disorders of platelet procoagulant activity

PT = prothrombin time; aPTT = activated partial thromboplastin time; I = increased; D = decreased; N = normal; vWD = von Willebrand disease; DIC = disseminated intravascular coagulation

This table addresses the differential diagnosis of hemostasis screening test results in patients with a history of bleeding. Diagnoses of patients with abnormal coagulation test results and no bleeding history are omitted.

Modified from Rodgers GM. Common clinical bleeding disorders. In: Boldt DH, ed. Update on Hemostasis. *New York: Churchill-Livingstone; 1990:75–120.*

Chapter 32
Preoperative Hemostasis Screening

George Rodgers, MD, PhD

The use of screening coagulation tests in preoperative patients is controversial. Large amounts of money are routinely spent to obtain few positive results. However, the outcome of major surgery in a patient with an unknown hemostatic defect may be catastrophic. One sensible approach is to balance the costs of preoperative testing with the extent of surgery to be done and with the amount of bleeding that can be tolerated safely. This approach places critical importance on obtaining a thorough hemostasis history. Patients scheduled for minor procedures (eg, oral surgery, skin biopsy) do not need routine screening tests if they have a negative history. Patients undergoing neurosurgery or procedures that may induce a hemostatic defect (eg, cardiothoracic surgery with a bypass pump) and those with a positive bleeding history need a hemostasis evaluation by the laboratory.

t32.1 summarizes Rapaport's suggested guidelines for evaluating preoperative patients. Based on the patient's bleeding history and the type of surgery, 4 levels are identified. Based on these levels of concern, recommendations are made as to the intensity of suggested hemostasis evaluation. Assays for factors VIII, IX, and XI are suggested in the level IV evaluation, because most aPTT reagents are insensitive in detecting a mild factor deficiency; factor levels of 20%-30% may not be detected, and these patients would bleed with surgery. The thrombin time screens for dysfibrinogens, and the α_2-antiplasmin assay screens for deficiency of this fibrinolysis inhibitor. The bleeding time is not recommended as a preoperative screening test because it is not reliable in distinguishing patients with bleeding disorders from the normal population. Other platelet function tests such as the Platelet Function Analyzer-100 may be useful in screening preoperative patients, but evidence supporting widespread use is lacking.

t32.1 Guidelines for Preoperative Hemostasis Evaluation

Level	Bleeding History	Surgical Procedure	Recommended Hemostasis Evaluation
I	Negative	Minor	None
II	Negative	Major	Platelet count, aPTT
III	Equivocal	Major, involving hemostatic impairment	PT, aPTT, platelet count, factor XIII assay, ECLT
IV	Positive	Major or minor	Level III tests; if negative, then factors VIII, IX, and XI assays, thrombin time, α_2-antiplasmin assay; consider vWD and platelet aggregation testing, as well as uncommon disorders listed in **t31.1**

aPTT = activated partial thromboplastin time; PT = prothrombin time;
ECLT = euglobulin clot lysis time (a screen for abnormal fibrinolysis); vWD = von Willebrand disease

32.1 Reference

Rapaport SI. Preoperative hemostatic evaluation: which tests, if any? *Blood.* 1983;61:229–232.

Part VII

Thrombotic Disorders

Chapter 33

Inherited Thrombotic Disorders

George Rodgers, MD, PhD

Thrombosis is the formation of a blood clot in the circulatory system during life. Arterial thrombi, especially those in the smallest vessels, are composed primarily of platelets, whereas fibrin is the predominant component of venous thrombi. "Hypercoagulability" refers to changes associated with an abnormal tendency toward thrombosis. It should never refer to conditions in which the clotting time is shortened or procoagulant factor levels are increased, unless these changes are associated with an abnormal tendency toward thrombosis.

33.1 Pathophysiology

Hemostasis is a complex process in which the vascular endothelial cell surface plays a pivotal role in maintaining blood fluidity. The coagulation cascade is modulated by many regulatory mechanisms. f33.1 summarizes the anticoagulant properties of the endothelium. One of the regulatory mechanisms shown is the protein C pathway, which consists of 2 vitamin K–dependent plasma proteins—protein C and protein S **t33.1**. Protein C is converted to an active form (APC); this activation is mediated by a receptor, thrombomodulin, which is present on endothelial cell surfaces. Thrombomodulin forms a stoichiometric complex with thrombin on the endothelial cell surface, and this complex activates protein C generating APC, which in turn inactivates factors Va and VIIIa. Protein S binds to the endothelial cell surface, providing a receptor for APC. Protein S circulates in a free form that exhibits anticoagulant activity and a form bound to C4b-binding protein, which has no anticoagulant activity. A factor V mutation (factor V Leiden) that results in thrombosis due to the inability of APC to degrade the abnormal factor Va molecule (APC resistance) has been described.

Antithrombin is another naturally occurring plasma protein with anticoagulant activity. It irreversibly binds to and inactivates certain activated clotting factors such as factor Xa and thrombin. This inactivation is catalyzed (enhanced) by heparin-like glycosaminoglycans on the endothelial cell surface (see f33.1) or by commercial heparin used in therapy.

Fibrin formation is essential in wound healing as well as in hemostasis, but its removal is equally important. This removal is accomplished by the fibrinolytic mechanism, which, like the coagulation system, is composed of activators and inhibitors in a delicate balance. Moreover, this system, which is part of the overall hemostatic mechanism, functions cooperatively with the coagulation system. Both may be triggered in the same way, and the formation of fibrin greatly enhances fibrinolysis activation.

Well-characterized components of the fibrinolytic system **t33.2** include the active serine protease plasmin, which is derived from the inactive zymogen, plasminogen; α_2-antiplasmin, an inhibitor that neutralizes free plasmin almost instantaneously; tissue-plasminogen activator (t-PA); and the major plasminogen activator inhibitor (PAI-1).

f33.1 Antithrombotic properties of the blood vessel wall

The major antithrombotic properties are depicted. Heparin-like glycosaminoglycans (GAG) present on the luminal surface catalyze inactivation of coagulation proteases, including thrombin, by antithrombin III (AT III). Complex formation of the endothelial cell membrane protein (thrombomodulin) with thrombin generates activated protein C (APC). Binding of APC to endothelial cell-bound protein S promotes proteolysis of factors Va and VIIIa, resulting in inhibition of coagulation. Tissue plasminogen activator (t-PA) is secreted by endothelial cells to initiate fibrinolysis. Vascular endothelium also secretes 2 antiplatelet substances—prostacyclin (PGI_2) and nitric oxide (not shown). Endothelial cells also express CD39, an ADPase with antiplatelet properties (not shown). Modified with permission from Rodgers GM. Hemostatic properties of normal and perturbed vascular cells. *FASEB*. 1988;2:116-123.

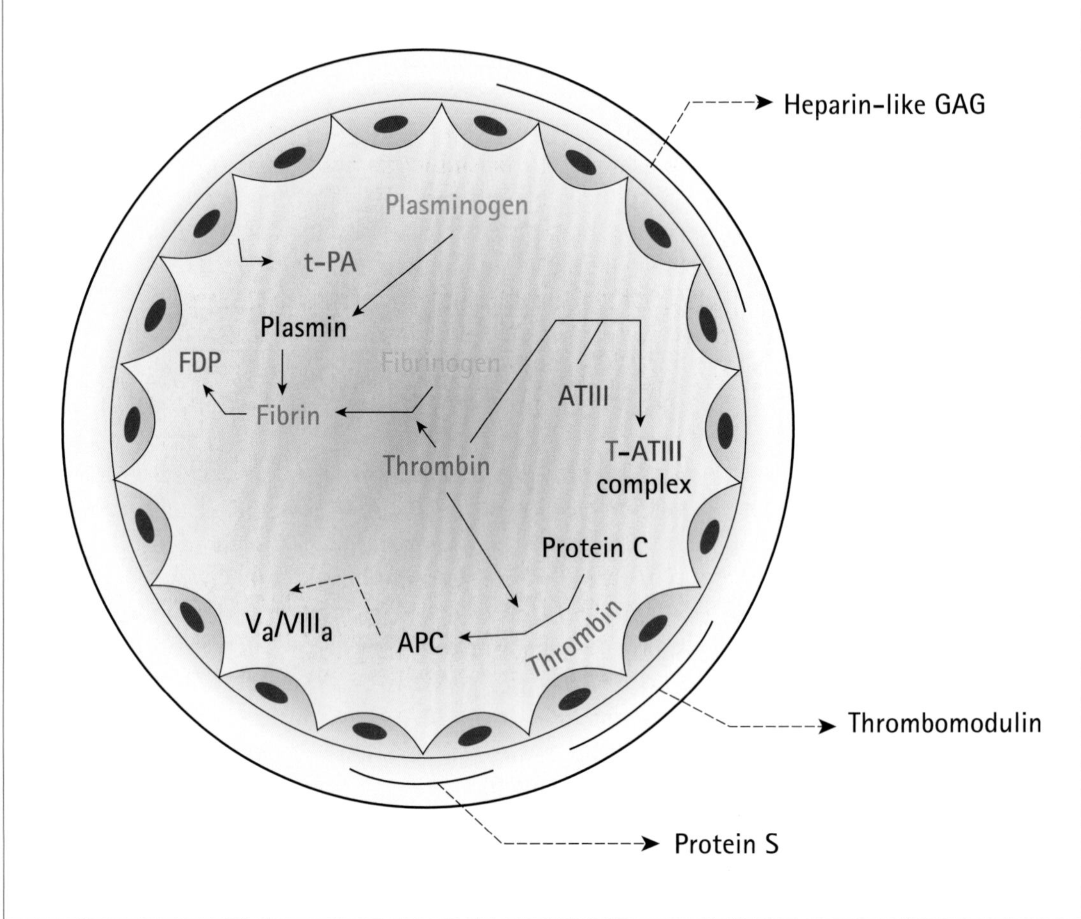

t33.1 Features of Vitamin K-Dependent Anticoagulant Proteins

	Protein C	Protein S
Activation	Zymogen activated by thrombin-thrombomodulin complex	None required
Function	Inactivation of factors Va and VIIIa	Cofactor of APC; binds to C4b-binding protein
Inactivation	APC inhibitor	Thrombin cleavage

APC = activated protein C

t33.2 Components of the Fibrinolytic Mechanism

Protein	Site of Synthesis	Comments
Plasminogen	Liver	Precursor of plasmin
t-PA	Endothelial cells	Most inactivated by PAI-1; high concentrations released from endothelial cells by occlusion, exercise, epinephrine, etc
PAI-1	Endothelial cells, platelets	t-PA inhibitor
Alpha$_2$-antiplasmin	Liver	Potent plasmin inhibitor

t-PA = tissue plasminogen activator; PAI-1 = plasminogen activator inhibitor-1

The fibrinolytic system may be initiated by the coagulation cascade or by tissue injury. As soon as fibrin is formed, it binds plasminogen, plasminogen activators, and α_2-antiplasmin. Plasminogen activation occurs in the fibrin clot, but any plasmin formed may be neutralized by α_2-antiplasmin, which is present in the clot at the equivalent molar concentration as the fibrin-bound plasminogen. The state of equilibrium is such that when clots are formed in vitro, they do not lyse under normal conditions. In the circulation, however, plasminogen activators are released from the endothelial cell surface in contact with the clot and are absorbed into the thrombus so the equilibrium then favors fibrinolysis (see f33.1). In congenital or acquired states in which the activity of the fibrinolytic inhibitor α_2-antiplasmin is decreased, excessive clot lysis occurs at a site of injury, and the hemostatic plugs break down prematurely, resulting in bleeding.

Fibrin plays an integral role in the interplay between t-PA, plasminogen, and α_2-antiplasmin. Tissue plasminogen activator has little effect on plasminogen in the absence of fibrin. The affinity of plasminogen for fibrin is attributable to lysine-rich binding sites and is inhibited by lysine, ε-aminocaproic acid (Amicar), and tranexamic acid. Even a hundredfold increase of free t-PA activity, such as occurs in good responders after strenuous exercise, does not result in the presence of free plasmin in the blood.

Of the classic triad of Virchow (ie, the risk factors predisposing to thrombosis—endothelial cell damage, stasis, and hypercoagulability), endothelial cell damage is by far the most important factor in arterial thrombosis. Because platelets adhere to damaged endothelium, thrombosis may be considered the natural sequela of arterial disease; the most common cause of this is atherosclerosis. Thrombotic episodes, usually arterial and involving the smaller vessels, are frequent in myeloproliferative disorders, especially in polycythemia vera and essential thrombocytosis when the platelet count is very high. The vessel wall regulates platelet activation and aggregation by secreting 2 mediators, prostacyclin (PGI_2) and nitric oxide, as well as expressing an endothelial cell protein, CD39, an ADPase that can inhibit platelet activation. However, the clinical importance of these mediators in preventing arterial thrombosis in vivo is uncertain.

In contrast to arterial thrombosis, in which underlying vascular disease is of major importance, stasis and hypercoagulability are critical factors in venous thrombosis. Thus, even in normal individuals, venous thrombosis in the lower extremity occurs with surprising frequency whenever the leg is immobilized for a number of hours (eg, during a long plane journey), but the fibrinolytic system almost always lyses the thrombi. Abnormalities or decreases in the activity of natural anticoagulants, protein C, protein S, or antithrombin, or the presence of the factor V Leiden mutation, may be associated with an increased incidence of primarily venous thrombosis. The therapeutic infusion of antifibrinolytic agents or activated clotting factors may also result in massive venous thrombosis.

33.2 Clinical Findings

Symptoms of arterial thrombosis or embolism depend on the size of the vessel, the state of the vessel wall, the degree and length of time of occlusion, the adequacy of a collateral circulation, and the organ involved. For example, if the thrombus or embolus occludes the retinal artery, permanent loss of sight may result; however, occlusion of a small branch of a renal artery may be asymptomatic. The consequences of venous thrombosis usually are less severe, thus, thrombi in the lower calf veins are often asymptomatic. Because deep venous thrombosis is so frequently asymptomatic, a high index of suspicion is usually required for its recognition, and the differential diagnosis is often difficult. The diagnosis is best established by objective testing, such as ultrasonography or venography. Quantitative D-dimer testing is useful in the exclusion of venous thromboembolism.

33.3 Summary of the Inherited Thrombotic Disorders

t33.3 classifies the inherited thrombotic disorders and briefly describes their prevalence, inheritance patterns, and clinical features. Abnormalities of the protein C pathway (protein C, protein S, APC resistance (factor V Leiden), thrombomodulin) constitute almost half of all cases of inherited thrombosis. In general, inherited disorders are transmitted in an autosomal dominant manner, and venous thromboembolism is the common clinical feature. The clinical importance of inherited t-PA deficiency or excess PAI-1 activity is uncertain.

Another common inherited thrombotic disorder is the prothrombin mutation–this disorder may account for up to 10% of patients with recurrent thrombosis. Some patients with this mutation have elevated plasma prothrombin levels.

Homocysteinemia (homocystinuria) is a metabolic disorder associated with thrombosis. The prevalence of homocysteinemia in patients with inherited thrombosis is uncertain because this diagnosis has not been considered routinely, but estimates indicate that 10-20% of patients with recurrent thrombosis have homocysteinemia. Although pediatric patients present clinically with the homozygous defect, adult patients heterozygous for homocysteinemia have primarily premature arterial disease. Heterozygous homocysteinemia may account for a significant number of patients with premature vascular disease in the absence of traditional risk factors (eg, tobacco use, hypertension, hyperlipidemia). It has been estimated that 1%-2% of the general population has heterozygous homocysteinemia.

Another recently described inherited risk factor for thrombosis is elevated factor VIII activity levels. Although factor VIII is an acute-phase reactant, studies indicate that 10%-20% of patients with recurrent thrombosis have elevated factor VIII levels as their only risk factor. However, the genetic basis for this risk factor is not understood.

Increased levels of other coagulation factors, including fibrinogen, factor IX, and factor XI have been associated with thrombosis. However, routine laboratory testing of these analytes is not recommended by the CAP Consensus Conference on Thrombophilia (see **t33.4**).

33.4 Diagnostic Approach

Obesity, diabetes, smoking, hyperlipidemia, and hypertension are associated with an increased risk of atherosclerosis and of arterial thrombosis. Venous thrombosis is particularly common after surgical procedures associated with tissue injury, after fractures of the neck of the femur, and in the postpartum period; immobilization of the lower limbs in these situations also is an important causative factor. When one or more of these conditions is present, a special

t33.3 A Summary of the Inherited Thrombotic Disorders

Classification and Disorders	Inheritance	Estimated Prevalence*	Clinical Features
Deficiency or qualitative abnormalities of inhibitors to activated coagulation factors			
AT deficiency	AD	1%–2%	Venous thromboembolism (usual and unusual sites), heparin resistance
TM deficiency	AD	1%–5%	Venous thrombosis
Protein C deficiency	AD	1%–5%	Venous thromboembolism
Protein S deficiency	AD	1%–5%	Venous and arterial thromboembolism
APC resistance (factor V Leiden)	AD	20%–50%	Venous thromboembolism
Abnormality of coagulation zymogen or cofactor			
Prothrombin mutation	AD	5%–10%	Venous thromboembolism
Elevated factor VIII	Unknown	20%–25%	Venous thromboembolism
Elevated factor IX	Unknown	~10%	Venous thromboembolism
Elevated factor XI	Unknown	~10%	Venous thromboembolism
Impaired clot lysis			
Dysfibrinogenemia	AD	1%–2%	Venous thrombosis > arterial thrombosis
Plasminogen deficiency	AD, AR	1%–2%	Venous thromboembolism
t-PA deficiency	AD	?	Venous thromboembolism
Excess PAI-1 activity	AD	?	Venous thromboembolism and arterial thrombosis
Metabolic defect			
Homocysteinemia	AR	1 in 300,000 live births; 10-25% of patients with recurrent thrombosis	Arterial and venous thrombosis (homozygous patients); premature development of coronary and cerebral arterial thrombotic disease (heterozygous patients)

AT = antithrombin; APC = activated protein C; t-PA = tissue plasminogen activator; PAI-1 = plasminogen activator inhibitor-1; TM = thrombomodulin; AD = autosomal dominant; AR = autosomal recessive; ? = uncertain prevalence of abnormal fibrinolysis

**Prevalence data are estimated by pooling information from studies in which large groups of patients with thrombosis were screened for these disorders. Results are expressed in terms of a percentage that each disorder might constitute of the total patient population with inherited thrombosis. (Assays for thrombomodulin mutations are not widely available.)*

hemostasis workup is rarely indicated. However, when there is no predisposing cause, the venous thrombosis occurs at a very early age or an unusual site (eg, axillary vein), there have been several episodes, or there is a family history of venous thrombosis, the possibility of an inherited or primary hypercoagulable state should be considered. Six key points to address in the laboratory evaluation of these patients include the following:

1. The laboratory evaluation should be deferred until 2-3 months after the acute thrombotic event when the patient is clinically well and preferably has not been receiving anticoagulant therapy for 2 weeks. Thrombosis induces an acute-phase response that may make interpretation of certain test results difficult. Optimal data are obtained in the absence of anticoagulants, because these drugs alter levels of important factors to be

assayed. If anticoagulants cannot be discontinued, symptomatic family members who are not receiving anticoagulants can be tested. However, DNA-based tests (for the factor V Leiden or the prothrombin gene mutations) are unaffected by acute phase changes of thrombosis. Similarly, homocysteine testing will not be affected by anticoagulant therapy. Factor VIII activity testing should be deferred until 6 months after the thrombotic event.

2. The likelihood of obtaining positive results is increased if the patient population being evaluated is restricted to young patients with recurrent thrombosis or patients under 50 years of age with a single event and a positive family history.
3. Functional coagulation assays are preferable to immunologic assays. Functional assays detect patients with either a deficient or abnormal protein. However, functional assays are affected more than immunologic assays by anticoagulant therapy.
4. Assays for components of the protein C pathway should be performed initially, because abnormalities of these components (protein C, protein S, APC resistance [factor V Leiden]) are found in up to half of the patients with inherited thrombosis.
5. If fibrinolytic assays are to be performed, optimal assay techniques are critical. The CAP Thrombophilia Consensus panel does not recommend testing patients for fibrinolytic defects.
6. Heterozygous homocysteinemia should be considered as a cause for thrombosis in middle-aged patients with premature vascular disease. Immunoassays for this metabolite are now available.

Establishing a specific diagnosis of inherited thrombosis may be important, because it allows a single test to be performed on the patient's siblings and children who also may be at risk for thrombosis, since most disorders are transmitted in a dominant fashion. A positive test result in a woman may affect certain clinical decisions such as the method of contraception and pregnancy counseling in her and her female children.

33.4.1 Perspective on Laboratory Testing for Inherited Thrombotic Disorders

Widespread testing of thrombosis patients for inherited disorders has resulted from the identification of new genetic predispositions and the availability of thrombosis test panels by many laboratories. Testing the likely patient population with optimal assays should identify an inherited predisposition to thrombosis in over 50% of patients. However, such results may not have a significant impact on patient management. There are no data that intensity or duration of anticoagulation are affected by the presence or absence of inherited disorders. On the other hand, positive test results may have clinical implications for family members of affected patients, especially females.

33.5 Strategy of Laboratory Evaluation of Inherited Thrombosis

Patients with arterial thrombosis should be evaluated initially by assays for PAI-1 or homocysteinemia, depending on their age f33.2. In contrast, patients with venous thromboembolism are initially evaluated by assays of the protein C pathway (protein C, protein S, APC resistance); if these are normal, other causes of inherited thrombosis (eg, prothrombin mutation, homocysteinemia, antithrombin deficiency, dysfibrinogenemia, abnormal fibrinolysis) can be considered. f33.3 summarizes one approach to the laboratory evaluation of these patients. The exact sequence of test ordering may vary, depending on test availability in a given laboratory, and whether the patient is on anticoagulant therapy. Factor VIII tests should be deferred for at least 6 months to minimize any acute-phase effects.

f33.2 Suggested algorithm for evaluation of inherited arterial thrombosis

Excluding common acquired etiologies for arterial disease (hyperlipidemia, diabetes, myeloproliferative disease, lupus anticoagulants, etc), possible etiologies for inherited arterial thrombosis include abnormal fibrinolysis, homocysteinemia, and protein S deficiency. Up to 30% of patients have no identifiable cause of thrombosis, whereas others may have 2 or more abnormalities.

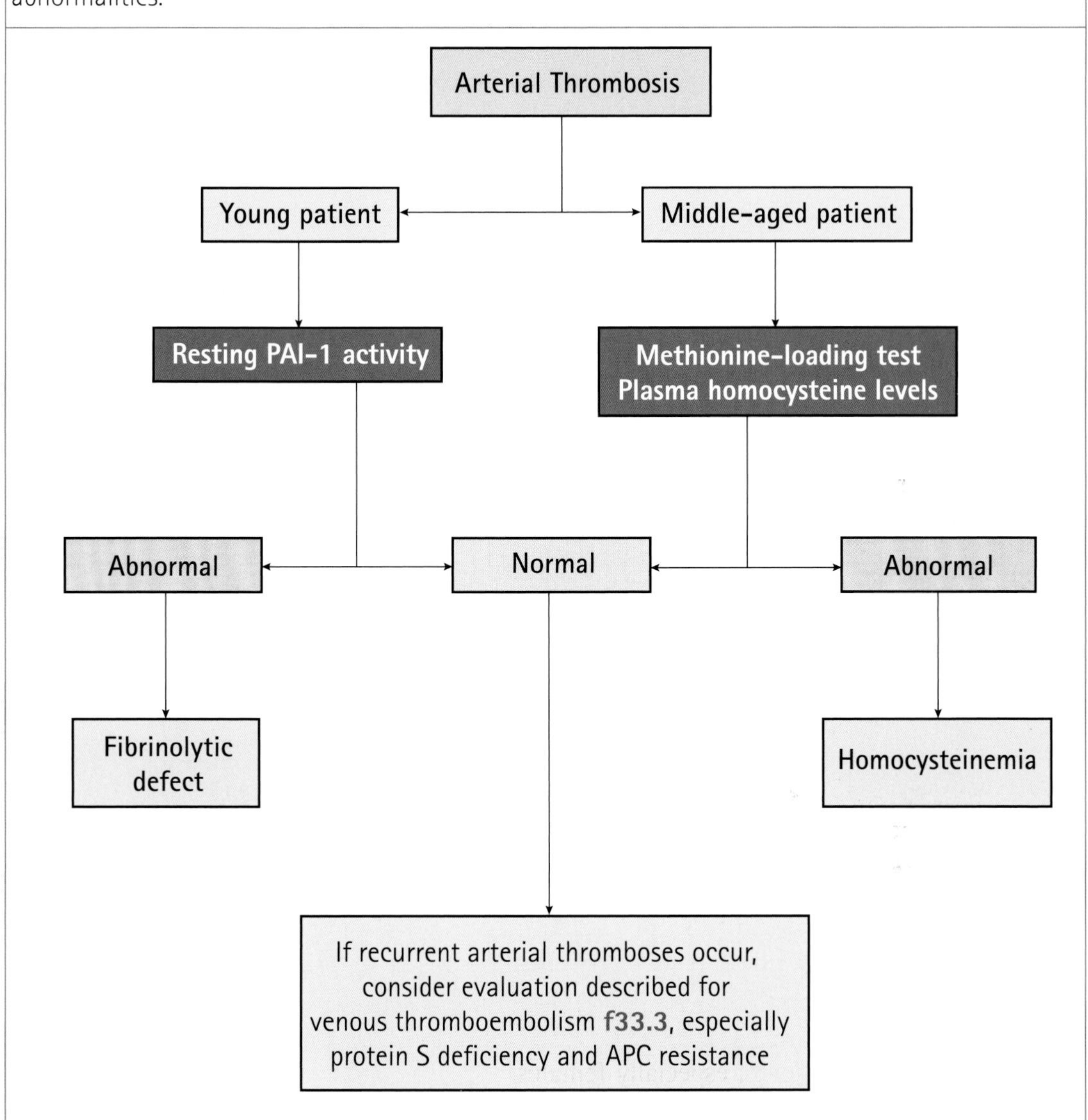

33.6 The CAP Recommendations on Laboratory Testing for Inherited Thrombosis

The recommendations of the CAP Consensus Conference XXXVI on Thrombophilia were published in 2002 and are summarized in **t33.4**. Specfic details for testing methods are given in the references cited in the consensus document or in the laboratory section below. Commercial kits are available for most of these assays.

f33.3 Suggested algorithm for evaluation of patients with inherited venous thrombosis

In this approach, patients with an appropriate personal and family history are tested several weeks after the acute thrombotic event, preferably at a time when they are not taking anticoagulants. Because APC resistance is common in patients with inherited thrombosis, consideration should be given to assaying for this disorder in the initial evaluation. DNA-based assays can be done for the factor V Leiden mutation in lieu of clotting assays for APC resistance. Assays for elevated factor VIII activity can be performed 6 months after the thrombotic event when anticoagulant therapy has been discontinued. Modified with permission from Rodgers GM, Chandler WL. Laboratory and clinical aspects of inherited thrombotic disorders. *Am J Hematol.* 1992;41:113-122.

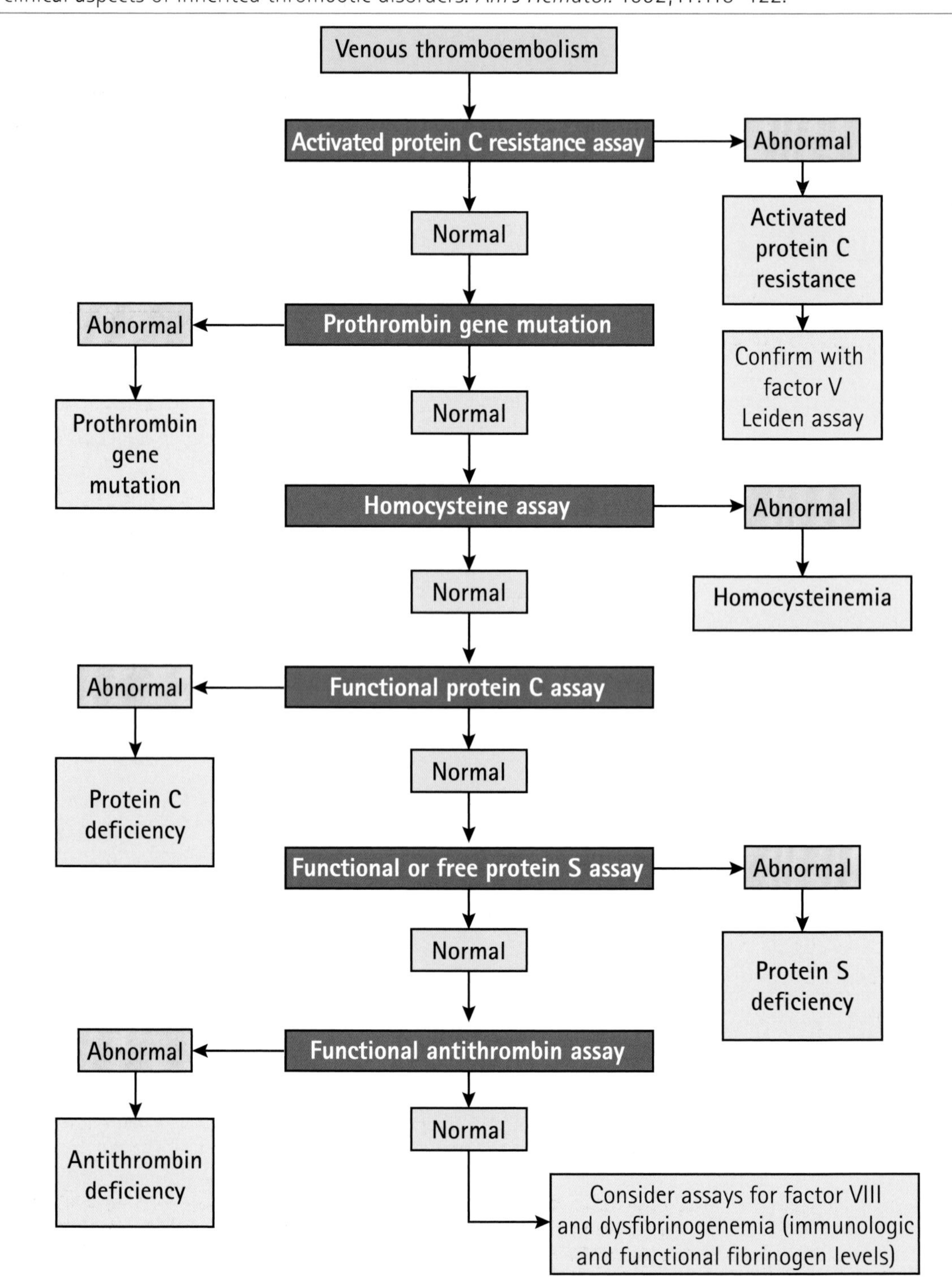

t33.4 Summary of the College of American Pathologists' Recommendations on Laboratory Testing for Inherited Thrombosis

Thrombotic Disorder	Who Should Be Tested?	Test Method(s)	Comments
FVL	1st VTE at age <50 years; recurrent VTE; 1st unprovoked VTE; 1st VTE, unusual site; 1st VTE, positive family history; 1st VTE related to pregnancy or hormonal therapy; unexplained 2nd or 3rd trimester miscarriage	APC resistance assay using factor-V deficient plasma or DNA-based assay	Patients with relatives who are known to have FVL should be tested directly with DNA-based assays. Patients with positive APC resistance assays should have confirmatory DNA tests.
Prothrombin gene mutation	As above	DNA-based assay	Prothrombin activity assays should not be used
Homocysteinemia	Arterial vascular disease controversial for VTE	HPLC or immunoassays	Genotyping for MTHFR mutations is not recommended. Fasting or methionine loading may not be necessary. Sample processing is crucial.
Protein C deficiency	Infants with neonatal purpura fulminans; VTE patient from a family with known PC deficiency	Chromogenic substrate assays are preferred	Avoid testing during acute thrombosis or anticoagulant therapy. Exclude causes of acquired PC deficiency. Consider age-dependent reference ranges.
	Asymptomatic female from a known PC-deficient family prior to hormonal therapy	Functional assays are useful; immunologic assays are discouraged	
Protein S deficiency	Patient with VTE from a family with known PS deficiency	Functional assay or immunoassay for free PS; total PS antigen assays not recommended	Abnormal functional assay results should be confirmed with an immunoassay for free PS. Exclude acquired causes of PS deficiency. Avoid testing during acute thrombosis, anticoagulant therapy, and pregnancy. Consider age- and gender-dependent reference ranges.
Antithrombin deficiency	Patient with VTE from a family with known AT deficiency Asymptomatic female from a known AT- deficient family prior to hormonal therapy	Chromogenic substrate assays are preferred; AT antigen assays not recommended	Exclude acquired causes of AT deficiency. Avoid testing during acute thrombosis or anticoagulant therapy.
Elevated factor VIII levels	Controversial	Factor VIII activity assay	Test 6 months after thrombosis. Avoid anticoagulant therapy.
Dysfibrinogenemia	Not recommended		
Heparin cofactor II	Not recommended		
Factor XIII polymorphisms	Not recommended		
Plasminogen activator inhibitor-1	Not recommended		
Plasminogen deficiency	Test in non-deep vein thrombosis (DVT) patients with ligneous conjunctivitis		

Information in this table is taken from the College of American Pathologists' Consensus Conference on Thrombophilia. Arch Pathol Lab Med. *2002; 126:1277-1433.*

FVL = factor V Leiden; VTE = venous thromboembolism; APC = activated protein C; HPLC = high performance liquid chromatography; MTHFR =methylenetetrahydrofolate reductase; PC = protein C; PS = protein S; AT = antithrombin

33.7 Laboratory Tests

Test 33.7.1 Antithrombin Determination

Purpose. Antithrombin determinations detect hypercoagulable states associated with venous thrombotic episodes. This assay also may be useful for evaluating patients who appear to be resistant to heparin therapy, or who have thrombosis in an unusual location (intra-abdominal thrombosis).

Principle. A known amount of thrombin is added to a patient plasma sample, and the residual thrombin activity is determined. Antithrombin antigen levels also may be measured by the Laurell immunoelectrophoresis or radial diffusion methods using specific antibodies, but the functional assay is preferred.

Specimen. Citrated plasma is used in synthetic substrate methods. In clotting assay methods, either citrated plasma or serum may be used, but plasma should be defibrinated.

Procedure. A known amount of thrombin is added to the plasma sample in the presence of heparin; after a timed interval, an aliquot is removed and added to a specific synthetic chromogenic or fluorescent thrombin substrate. In the chromogenic method, colored p-nitroaniline is liberated from the colorless substrate by the thrombin and measured spectrophotometrically. In the fluorescence method, a fluorescent compound is released and measured in a fluorometer. This assay is automated.

Interpretation. The normal range appears to be relatively narrow (85%-122% based on a normal pool). The level is slightly decreased by oral contraceptives; it is also decreased in the last trimester of pregnancy, but the levels rarely fall below 75% of normal. Such minor decreases may have no clinical relevance. Prolonged use of heparin can result in marked decreases in antithrombin levels; such decreases also may occur following a thrombotic event or in association with disseminated intravascular coagulation (DIC). Low values are also seen with liver disease. In inherited deficiency states, the levels are usually in the 40%-65% range. The antigen level may be normal in approximately 10% of patients with antithrombin deficiency, so a functional measurement should be performed, at least initially, to exclude these variants.

Notes and Precautions. Serum samples give values approximately 30% lower than plasma samples. Long-term warfarin therapy may increase plasma antithrombin levels in certain patients. One disadvantage of functional antithrombin assays is that the presence of heparin cofactor II in the plasma may result in overestimation of antithrombin activity. Assays using bovine thrombin and lower heparin concentrations (3 U/mL) may minimize thrombin inhibition by heparin cofactor II. Assays based on inhibition of factor Xa rather than thrombin yield more accurate results. Acquired causes of antithrombin (AT) deficiency should be considered **t33.5**.

Test 33.7.2 Protein C Determination

Purpose. This test detects hypercoagulable states associated with protein C deficiency. The functional assay can detect both quantitative and qualitative abnormalities in protein C.

Principle. Protein C in plasma is most commonly activated by a specific snake venom (Protac). The APC is then assayed by its ability to prolong the aPTT of normal plasma (clotting assay) or to cleave a specific synthetic substrate. Specific antibodies are commercially available, and antigenic determinations can be performed using Laurell immunoelectrophoresis or the enzyme-linked immunosorbent assay (ELISA).

Specimen. Citrated plasma is used for this test.

Procedure. The protein C in the plasma sample is activated directly with Protac. The APC is then assayed using either a clotting method or an amidolytic method with a chromogenic substrate. The chromogenic assay is recommended.

Interpretation. The normal range in adults is 78%-232%; however, the normal range is age-dependent for younger patients. Numerous acquired conditions can result in protein C deficiency **t33.5**.

t33.5 Acquired Causes of Deficiency of Protein C, Protein S, and Antithrombin

Analyte	Causes of Deficiency
Protein C	DIC Acute thrombosis Vitamin K deficiency, including oral anticoagulant therapy Newborn infants, children Liver disease Post-operative state
Protein S	DIC Acute thrombosis Inflammatory illness of any cause Vitamin K deficiency, including oral anticoagulant therapy Newborn infants, children Liver disease Pregnancy Nephrotic syndrome
Antithrombin	DIC Acute thrombosis Liver disease Oral contraceptives Nephrotic syndrome Pregnancy Heparin (therapeutic levels)

Conditions, drugs, or diseases listed in this table may result in acquired deficiency of protein C or S, or antithrombin. These causes should be considered before evaluating patients for inherited deficiency.
DIC=disseminated intravascular coagulation

The level is reduced in patients with hepatocellular disease, and even a moderate disturbance of liver function may reduce the level to 30%. Heterozygotes have levels of 30%-65%. Homozygotes are born with DIC (neonatal purpura fulminans) and have protein C levels less than 5% of normal; their parents are heterozygotes. A normal antigenic level does not exclude heterozygosity, because in rare variants there is synthesis of an abnormal protein. Because protein C is a vitamin K–dependent protein with a very short half-life, it is depressed early during oral anticoagulant therapy, leading to a transient hypercoagulable state. The ratio of protein C activity to protein C antigen is reduced by warfarin therapy, even in the absence of an inherited abnormality of protein C. The protein C level is reduced in DIC and is lower in serum than in plasma. Newborn infants have physiologically low levels of protein C that rise slowly after birth; the levels are even lower in premature infants. Acute thrombosis also may result in low protein C levels.

Protein C can be assayed in patients receiving stable oral anticoagulation; however, identification of protein C deficiency in patients receiving warfarin therapy requires comparison of these patients' laboratory values with those of patients who receive warfarin and do not have protein C deficiency. Most commonly, ratios of protein C activity to prothrombin activity are compared.

Notes and Precautions. Disadvantages of the Protac functional protein C assay include the inability of chromogenic substrate assays to measure all functional aspects of protein C activity in patients receiving oral anticoagulants. Clot-based functional protein C assays have the advantage of measuring complete biologic functions of APC. However, clotting assays are hampered by acute elevations in plasma factor VIII activity, which result in false-low protein C values, and by heparin treatment. Some clotting assays for protein C determination contain heparin neutralizers and are not affected by heparin. Therapeutic heparin levels do not affect the functional chromogenic substrate assay. Age-dependent reference ranges should be used to correctly classify patients.

Test 33.7.3 Protein S Determination

Purpose. This test detects hypercoagulable states associated with protein S deficiency. The functional assay can detect both quantitative and qualitative abnormalities in protein S.

Principle. Protein S acts as a cofactor for APC. Protein S deficiency should be considered in patients evaluated for an inherited disorder of thrombosis.

Specimen. Citrated plasma is used for this determination.

Procedure. Immunologic methods are currently used, including ELISA and Laurell immunoelectrophoresis. A functional assay is based on aPTT with activated factor V as a substrate for APC. Protein S–deficient plasma is mixed with a reference or test plasma sample. Factor Va and APC are added prior to recalcification. Immunoassays for free protein S are also available.

Interpretation. Heterozygotes with protein S levels between 30% and 60% of the normal range may have recurrent venous thrombotic episodes. The functional protein S assay detects quantitative deficiency and qualitative abnormality of protein S. Abnormal functional assay results should be confirmed with an immunoassay for free protein S.

Notes and Precautions. Spuriously low protein S values may be obtained in patients with APC resistance who are tested using the functional assay. Numerous acquired conditions result in protein S deficiency **t33.5**. Low protein S levels are seen in acute thrombosis, because C4b-binding protein is an acute-phase reactant, whose elevated levels suppress protein S activity. Because protein S is a vitamin K–dependent protein, liver disease and warfarin therapy also reduce protein S levels. Age- and gender-dependent reference ranges should be considered to correctly classify patients.

Test 33.7.4 APC Resistance Assay

Purpose. APC resistance due to the factor V Leiden mutation appears to be the major cause of inherited venous thrombosis. This disorder can be diagnosed using clotting assays or molecular diagnostics. This section discusses clotting assays.

Principle. APC is an anticoagulant. When added to normal plasma, clotting times are prolonged; when added to plasma from a patient with the factor V Leiden mutation, clotting times are less prolonged.

Specimen. Citrated plasma is used.

Procedure. Both aPTT- and PT-based assays are available. They are performed with and without APC. Reference range values are determined with a normal population. If the patient's baseline aPTT value is normal (no lupus anticoagulant or anticoagulant therapy), a normalized ratio (aPTT + APC/aPTT) is sufficient. For patients with lupus anticoagulants or those on anticoagulant therapy, PT- or aPTT-based assays in which the patient sample is diluted in factor V–deficient plasma are preferred.

Interpretation. In affected patients, the APC-dependent clotting time is prolonged less than the mean minus 2 standard deviations of the normal population.

Notes and Precautions. Because patients with APC resistance may have spuriously low functional protein S levels, APC resistance should be considered in protein S–deficient patients who were diagnosed with a functional assay. Because APC resistance appears to be the most common cause of inherited thrombosis, this disorder should be evaluated initially. A polymerase chain reaction–based assay that detects most patients with APC resistance (discussed later in this chapter) has been described. If the laboratory has large numbers of samples from patients taking heparin or warfarin therapy, this DNA-based test may be a more appropriate assay. The CAP consensus panel recommends that patients with positive test results for activated protein C resistance have confirmatory testing for the factor V Leiden mutation.

Test 33.7.5 Plasminogen Determination

Purpose. In addition to identifying inherited plasminogen deficiency, this test is also used to distinguish inherited from acquired deficiencies of α_2-antiplasmin. In inherited deficiencies, plasminogen is normal, but in acquired states (eg, liver disease, DIC), plasminogen and α_2-antiplasmin are reduced proportionately.

Principle. Plasminogen is converted to its active form, plasmin, by the addition of an activator. The plasmin is then assayed by the release of a chromophore or fluorescent molecule from a small synthetic peptide substrate. Specific antibodies are commercially available, and immunologic assays may be used.

Specimen. Citrated plasma is used.

Procedure. Streptokinase is usually added to the plasma sample, converting inactive plasminogen to plasmin. The plasmin is then assayed by removing an aliquot and adding a small synthetic peptide substrate bound either to a fluorescent molecule or to a p-nitroanilide compound. The release of fluorescence is measured by a fluorometer; the release of the colored p-nitroanilide compound from the colorless substrate is followed by measurement of optical density at 405 nm in a spectrophotometer.

Interpretation. The normal plasminogen level is 70%-113%. Striking decreases are found in primary and secondary fibrinolysis (DIC). Plasminogen levels are decreased in liver disease and may be very low or absent following treatment with t-PA, urokinase, or streptokinase.

Notes and Precautions. The test cannot be performed on patients who have received fibrinolytic inhibitors (eg, ε-aminocaproic acid) or on plasma samples containing these types of inhibitors. Antigenic assays give higher values than functional methods, probably because of the action of natural inhibitors in the latter. Several different substrates such as fibrin or casein may be used, but these have been almost completely replaced in routine coagulation laboratories by methods using synthetic chromogenic or fluorescent substrates. Methods to measure α_2-antiplasmin levels are described in Chapter 29. Testing thrombosis patients for plasminogen deficiency is not recommended by the CAP consensus panel.

Test 33.7.6 Tissue Plasminogen Activator Determination

Purpose. This test identifies a fibrinolytic disorder associated with inherited thrombosis.

Principle. Functional assays for t-PA use a plasminogen-chromogenic substrate assay. Total t-PA antigen (free t-PA and t-PA complexed with PAI-1) is measured using an ELISA. Assays for t-PA need to consider the collection, time, and processing issues necessary for optimal results.

Specimen. Activity of t-PA is unstable in normal plasma. For optimal measurements, citrated blood must be acidified immediately and the RBCs rapidly removed. Acidification prevents neutralization of t-PA by PAI-1 and prevents PAI-1 from interfering in the assay. Citrated plasma can be used to measure t-PA antigen levels. Because of diurnal variation in fibrinolysis, samples should be obtained between 8:00 AM and 9:00 AM. Some investigators recommend obtaining postvenous occlusion samples for optimal identification of normal individuals from patients with abnormal fibrinolysis.

Procedure. Citrated blood must be acidified with 0.5 M acetate buffer, pH 4.2 (0.5 mL blood:0.25 mL acetate buffer), mixed, and centrifuged. The acidified plasma is collected immediately. For the assay, acidified plasma is incubated with plasminogen, cyanogen-bromide cleaved fibrinogen fragments, and a chromogenic substrate for plasmin. The change in absorbance at 405 nm is proportional to the t-PA activity in the sample; a standard curve is prepared using purified single-chain t-PA.

Interpretation. Low t-PA levels indicate diminished fibrinolysis and may represent a risk factor for thrombosis. Elevated t-PA levels have been associated with excessive fibrinolysis and a bleeding tendency.

Notes and Precautions. As previously mentioned, optimal results require attention to sample collection and timing. Otherwise, it may be difficult to correctly classify patients who may have abnormal findings on fibrinolysis assays. A literature survey by Prins and Hirsh evaluated the evidence for an association between venous thromboembolism and abnormal fibrinolysis. The authors concluded that the published evidence does not prove such an association except in the postoperative setting. Therefore, the association remains unestablished, and the utility of routinely testing patients with inherited thrombosis for fibrinolytic defects remains uncertain. The CAP consensus panel does not recommend testing thrombosis patients for t-PA deficiency.

Test 33.7.7 Plasminogen Activator Inhibitor–1 Determination

Purpose. Elevated levels of PAI-1 have been linked to recurrent thrombosis, and abnormal fibrinolysis has been suggested as a common cause for thrombosis.

Principle. PAI-1 activity is measured using a back-titration method with t-PA. PAI-1 antigen levels can be measured using ELISA.

Specimen. Citrated plasma can be used to measure PAI-1 activity and antigen levels. Acidification of plasma is not necessary. Some investigators suggest obtaining postvenous occlusion samples to optimally distinguish normal individuals from patients with abnormal fibrinolysis.

Procedure. PAI-1 activity is measured by using multiple dilutions of citrated plasma to which a standard amount of purified-single-chain t-PA is added. After incubation, the plasma samples are acidified (to inhibit α_2-plasmin inhibitor), and residual t-PA activity is measured as described previously, using the chromogenic substrate assay.

Interpretation. Elevated PAI-1 levels may be associated with thrombosis.

Notes and Precautions. Sample collection and timing are important variables in fibrinolysis assays. Because an association between inherited thrombosis and abnormal fibrinolysis has not been demonstrated conclusively, the routine use of these assays in evaluating patients for inherited thrombosis is not recommended.

Test 33.7.8 Homocysteine Measurement

Purpose. The metabolic disorder heterozygous homocysteinemia is a common risk factor for arterial and venous thrombosis.

Principle. Various methods have been described to measure homocysteine levels, including high performance liquid chromatography (HPLC) and fluorescence polarization immunoassay.

Specimen. Most methods use a fasting plasma or serum sample. The most sensitive method to identify heterozygous homocysteinemic patients uses serum measurements before and after oral methionine loading. Collected blood samples should be placed on ice, and plasma or serum must be separated promptly from the RBCs.

Procedure. This assay is typically performed in a clinical chemistry reference laboratory. A common method treats the plasma sample with a reducing agent to reduce homocystine to homocysteine. Perchloric acid is added to remove disulfide-bound homocysteine from protein. Next, a fluorographic reagent is added, chromatography is performed, and total homocysteine is quantitated by a fluorescence detector. Details of the biochemical measurement of homocysteine are provided in the review articles cited in the references.

Interpretation. Reference ranges in the author's laboratory are 4-12 µmol for men and 4-10 µmol for women. The risk for vascular disease (arterial or venous) increases progressively with homocysteine concentration.

Notes and Precautions. A routine fasting homocysteine level may not identify 40% of patients with heterozygous homocysteinemia; these patients are best identified by homocysteine measurements before and after oral methionine loading. Less expensive and easier assays to measure plasma homocysteine levels are available, including fluorescent polarization enzyme immunoassay and a microtiter enzyme immunoassay. These methods will likely replace the HPLC methods.

In evaluating patients for venous thrombosis, the author typically reserves the evaluation of homocysteinemia for patients who test negative for APC resistance (factor V Leiden), protein C, protein S, antithrombin deficiency, and the prothrombin mutation. The CAP consensus panel recommends homocysteine testing for patients with arterial thrombosis, but not venous thrombosis. The genotyping assay for methylenetetrahydrofolate reductase mutations is not recommended.

Test 33.7.9 Molecular Diagnostic Testing for Inherited Thrombosis

Molecular diagnostic methods have not been clinically relevant for the general evaluation of hemostatic and thrombotic disorders because most of these disorders (von Willebrand disease, the hemophilias, protein C and S deficiencies, etc) are genetically heterogeneous. However, with the discovery of APC resistance and the prothrombin mutation, each of which is due to highly conserved point mutations in the factor V or prothrombin gene, respectively, these methods have become more useful. This is especially true for the laboratory evaluation of thrombosis in patients receiving anticoagulant therapy, because standard clotting assays are less reliable in diagnosing these patients.

Test 33.7.10 Factor V Leiden Mutation Detection

Purpose. The factor V Leiden mutation is the most common cause of APC resistance and the most common etiology for inherited thrombosis. Patients on anticoagulant therapy can be evaluated reliably by this DNA-based method.

Principle. Several polymerase chain reaction–based assays have been used to diagnose the factor V Leiden mutation (Arg^{506}♦Gln). In the original method described by Bertina et al, the restriction enzyme *MnI* was used to digest a 267-bp amplified fragment of patient DNA. Normal DNA digestion results in 3 fragments, whereas the factor V Leiden mutation results in 2 fragments. Various modifications for detecting this mutation have been reported (see reference list).

Specimen. A blood specimen anticoagulated by ethylenediaminetetraacetic acid (EDTA) is used. The sample should be refrigerated if DNA isolation cannot be done promptly.

Procedure. Details of DNA isolation and PCR methodologies can be found in the references and in Chapter 34.

Interpretation. If DNA isolation and amplification as well as restriction enzyme digestion are successful, 3 results are possible:

1. Negative. The patient does not have the factor V Leiden mutation (the major cause of APC resistance).
2. Heterozygous. The patient has 1 allele positive for the factor V Leiden mutation.
3. Homozygous. The patient has 2 alleles positive for the factor V Leiden mutation.

A negative test result for the factor V Leiden mutation does not exclude APC resistance due to other genetic defects (~5% of patients with APC resistance).

Notes and Precautions. This DNA-based test costs more than the clotting assay for the disorder. Before genetic testing is done, consideration should be given to counseling the patient and obtaining informed consent, particularly because genetic tests have implications for patients and their families. The CAP consensus panel recommends that patients with positive assays for activated protein C resistance have confirmatory testing for the factor V Leiden mutation.

33.8 References

Bertina RM, Koeleman BPC, Koster T, et al. Mutation in blood coagulation factor V associated with resistance to activated protein C. *Nature.* 1994;369:64-67.

Chandler WL, Trimble SL, Loo SC, et al. Effect of PAI-1 levels on the molar concentrations of active tissue plasminogen activator (t-PA) and the t-PA/PAI-1 complex in plasma. *Blood.* 1990;76:930-937.

Chandler WL, Rodgers GM, Sprouse JR, Thompson AR. Elevated hemostatic factor levels as potential risk factors for thrombosis. *Arch Pathol Lab Med.* 2002;126:1405-1414.

Deitcher SR, Rodgers GM. Thrombosis and antithrombotic therapy. In: Greer JP, Foerster J, Rodgers GM, eds. *Wintrobe's Clinical Hematology. 12th ed.* Philadelphia; Lippincott Williams & Wilkins; 2009:1464-1508.

de Ronde H, Bertina RM. Laboratory diagnosis of APC-resistance: a critical evaluation of the test and the development of diagnostic criteria. *Thromb Haemost.* 1994;72:880-886.

Florell SR, Rodgers GM. Inherited thrombotic disorders: an update. *Am J Hematol.* 1997;54:53-60.

Goodwin AJ, Rosendaal FR, Kottke-Marchant K, Bovill EG. A review of the technical, diagnostic, and epidemiologic considerations for protein S assays. *Arch Pathol Lab Med* 2002; 126:1349-1366.

Hirsh J. Congenital antithrombin III deficiency: incidence and clinical features. *Am J Med.* 1989;87(suppl 3B):34-38.

Koster T, Blann AD, Briët E, et al. Role of clotting factor VIII in effect of von Willebrand factor on occurrence of deep-vein thrombosis. *Lancet.* 1995;345:152-155.

Kottke-Marchant K, Comp PC. Laboratory issues in diagnosing abnormalities of protein C, thrombomodulin, and endothelial cell protein C receptor. *Arch Pathol Lab Med.* 2002;126:1337-1348.

Nagy PL, Schrijver I, Zehnder JL. Molecular diagnosis of hypercoagulable states. *Lab Med.* 2004; 35: 214-221.

Poort SR, Rosendaal FR, Reitsma PH, et al. A common genetic variation in the 3'-untranslated region of the prothrombin gene is associated with elevated plasma prothrombin levels and an increase in venous thrombosis. *Blood.* 1996;88:3698-3703.

Prins MH, Hirsh J. A critical review of the evidence supporting a relationship between impaired fibrinolytic activity and venous thromboembolism. *Arch Intern Med.* 1991;151:1721-1731.

Robetorye RS, Rodgers GM. Update on selected inherited venous thrombotic disorders. *Am J Hematol.* 2001;68:256-268.

Rodgers GM. Testing for inherited and acquired thrombotic disorders. In: Bennett ST, Lehman CM, Rodgers GM, eds. *Laboratory Hemostasis: A Practical Guide for Pathologists.* New York: Springer; 2007;143-166.

Rosendaal FR. Venous thrombosis: a multicausal disease. *Lancet.* 1999;353:1167-1173.

Segal JB, Brotman DJ, Necochea AJ, et al. Predictive value of factor V Leiden and prothrombin G20210A in adults with venous thromboembolism and in family members of those with a mutation: a systematic review. *JAMA.* 2009; 301:2472-2485.

Ueland PM, Refsum H, Stabler SP, et al. Total homocysteine in plasma or serum: methods and clinical applications. *Clin Chem.* 1993;39:1764-1779.

Part VIII

Anticoagulant Therapy

Chapter 34

Laboratory Monitoring of Anticoagulant and Fibrinolytic Therapy

George Rodgers, MD, PhD

Anticoagulant therapy is designed to inhibit the formation of thrombi and to prevent the extension and propagation of existing thrombi. The goal of fibrinolytic therapy is to dissolve or lyse a recent thrombus. Antiplatelet therapy is aimed at reducing the platelets' ability to adhere to one another (aggregate) or to adhere to the damaged endothelium and thereby inhibit thrombosis.

34.1 Pathophysiology

Rudolph Virchow, a German pathologist, postulated in the mid-nineteenth century that thrombosis resulted from 3 factors (Virchow's triad): stasis of blood flow, vascular injury, and "intrinsic alterations in the nature of the blood itself" (hypercoagulability).

Endothelial cell damage is the most important factor in arterial thrombosis. Because this damage is almost always induced by atherosclerosis, measures designed to reverse or halt this process may be considered antithrombotic. Platelets adhere to the damaged endothelial cell lining, forming the foundation for a thrombus; platelets also can form aggregates in the circulation that may be large enough to block a small artery. In contrast to arterial thrombosis, endothelial cell damage is not essential to venous thrombosis. Stasis is relatively more important because it hinders the flowing blood from removing activated coagulation proteases from the site of the thrombus. Thus, immobilization of the lower limbs, particularly in bedridden patients or following surgery or childbirth, may precipitate venous thrombosis.

The oral anticoagulants comprise derivatives of coumarin and include warfarin (Coumadin) and a closely related compound used in Europe, phenindione. These drugs inhibit the synthesis of vitamin K–dependent proteins by the liver. The vitamin K–dependent proteins involved in coagulation are the procoagulants: factors II (prothrombin), VII, IX, and X; and the anticoagulant proteins C and S. Vitamin K is essential for a posttranslational event in which glutamic acid residues are carboxylated, allowing the protein to bind calcium and to phospholipid of cell surfaces. Because the half-lives of the various vitamin K–dependent factors differ, their levels decrease at different rates after warfarin is started f34.1. Factor VII and protein C have half-lives of less than 6 hours and are the first to decrease with therapy and to reappear after cessation, while prothrombin has the longest half-life (3 days) and is the last to decrease and reappear.

The other type of widely used anticoagulant is heparin, a heterogeneous substance consisting of glycosaminoglycans of widely varying, but high average molecular weight. Several low-molecular-weight heparins also are available. Heparin, which is negatively charged, binds to antithrombin and sterically modifies this molecule so that its ability to bind to and inactivate thrombin and factors IXa and Xa is greatly enhanced. Heparin is rapidly neutralized by protamine

f34.1 Half-lives of the vitamin K-dependent procoagulant proteins after initiation of warfarin therapy

Warfarin inhibits synthesis of functional vitamin K-dependent proteins. The coagulant activity of these proteins in plasma declines as a function of their half-life. The half-lives of factors VII, IX, X and prothrombin are 6, 24, 40, and 60 hours, respectively. As shown, even though a single warfarin dose will prolong the PT assay (due to the rapid fall in factor VII activity), therapeutic anticoagulation requires ~5 days to achieve. Vitamin K-dependent protein activity levels of 10%-20% of normal are roughly equivalent to the desired warfarin therapeutic range (INR 2.0–3.0).

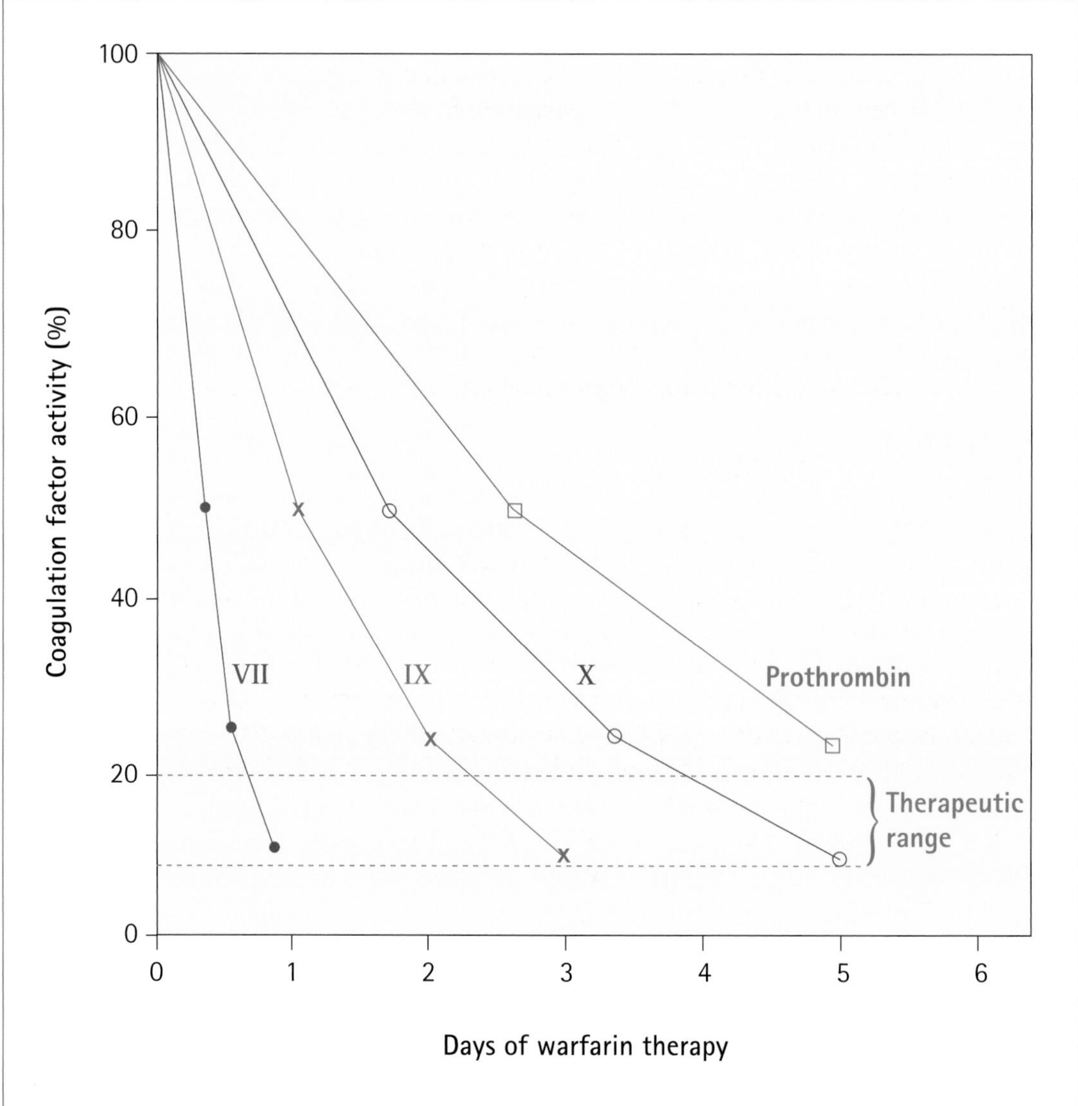

sulfate, which is positively charged. Administration is usually intravenous and may be subcutaneous, but is never intramuscular.

Fibrinolytic agents (also called "thrombolytic agents") include urinary plasminogen activator (u-PA) or urokinase, streptokinase, and tissue plasminogen activator (t-PA). Various recombinant analogs of these agents have also been developed. Treatment with fibrinolytic agents may result in bleeding from previous venipuncture sites, indicating dissolution of the hemostatic plugs and the effectiveness of these agents.

When oral anticoagulation medications exceed a toxic level, bleeding is almost inevitable, and purpura is a frequent complication. Similarly, a patient receiving heparin is likely to bleed from an open wound. Despite the hemorrhagic complications associated with these drugs, their efficacy in preventing or treating thrombotic disease is well established, and they are among the most commonly used drugs in treating hospitalized patients. The advent of low-molecular-weight heparin (LMWH) also allows anticoagulation of patients in the outpatient setting.

34.2 Clinical Indications

Heparin is used for the prophylaxis and treatment of venous thromboembolism, unstable angina, acute myocardial infarction, and chronic disseminated intravascular coagulation (DIC). It is also used in hemodialysis and cardiac bypass surgery and to maintain catheter patency. Warfarin is used in the treatment and prophylaxis of venous thromboembolism and in the prevention of systemic embolism in the settings of tissue heart valves, mechanical heart valves, acute myocardial infarction, and atrial fibrillation.

Common indications for fibrinolytic therapy include acute myocardial infarction, massive venous thrombosis or pulmonary embolism, peripheral arterial thromboembolism, and restoration of catheter patency.

Indications for aspirin and other antiplatelet drugs include primary and secondary prophylaxis of arterial vascular disease (stroke, myocardial infarction, and peripheral vascular disease).

34.3 Administration Methods

Anticoagulant therapy in patients with acute venous thrombosis initially consists of unfractionated heparin or LMWH administration. Unfractionated heparin is best given intravenously, starting with a bolus of 5000 or 10,000 units followed by a constant infusion of at least 1300 units/hour. LMWH is given subcutaneously on a body weight basis. After therapeutic anticoagulation has been achieved (preferably within the first 24 hours), oral warfarin is started, usually at dosages of 5-10 mg/day. There should be at least a 5-day overlap of heparin and warfarin so the patient remains anticoagulated until attaining therapeutic vitamin K deficiency with warfarin f34.1. When unfractionated heparin is used prophylactically, the usual regimen is 5000 units, given subcutaneously, every 8-12 hours.

Fibrinolytic agents are administered intravenously. Streptokinase and urokinase are given in bolus form, followed by continuous infusion over 12-72 hours; t-PA is given in a shorter intravenous infusion.

34.4 Laboratory Monitoring

With the increasing use of anticoagulant drugs in treating thrombotic disease, accurate laboratory methods to monitor anticoagulant intensity is important. Recognition of laboratory variables that may result in inaccurate monitoring has led to attempts to standardize these assays. Consensus guidelines for monitoring heparin therapy and warfarin therapy have been published and are summarized in this chapter. In general, for all coagulation assays described, 3.2% citrate is the recommended anticoagulant for specimen collection.

34.4.1 Monitoring Unfractionated Heparin Therapy

The effect of heparin can be monitored by various assays, but the standard method is the activated partial thromboplastin time (aPTT) test. Heparin should be given in doses sufficient to prolong the aPTT from 1.5-2.5 times the mean laboratory control aPTT (mean of the normal range). This recommendation assumes that the aPTT reagent is responsive to heparin so that plasma heparin levels of 0.2-0.4 U/mL (measured by protamine titration) or 0.35-0.7 U/mL (measured by anti-factor Xa activity) result in the aPTT being prolonged in the suggested range. However, because aPTT reagents may vary widely in terms of heparin responsiveness, each laboratory should establish its own therapeutic range so it corresponds to the plasma heparin levels given here. The most appropriate method for determining the therapeutic range is direct comparison of the aPTT with heparin concentrations in plasma samples from patients receiving heparin. Details of the College of American Pathologists consensus guidelines on the standardization of aPTT assays have been summarized by Olson et al and are shown in **t34.1**.

The timing and type of sample collected for monitoring heparin therapy is important. The aPTT should be checked 6 hours after heparin bolus or after a change in infusion rate so steady-state levels are measured. Samples drawn from indwelling lines may give nonrepresentative results. If prophylactic subcutaneous heparin or LMWH is used, laboratory monitoring is usually not necessary.

t34.1 Consensus Recommendations on Laboratory Monitoring of Unfractionated Heparin Therapy

Using the aPTT assay

Therapeutic UFH requires monitoring using a method with a defined therapeutic range.

Specimens used for monitoring UFH therapy should be collected from a different extremity than that used for drug infusion.

Clinicians should be informed of the method used to monitor UFH therapy, as well as the recommended therapeutic range.

The coagulation laboratory should be notified when the hospital pharmacy changes the UFH lot. The new UFH lot should be evaluated to define the new therapeutic range.

The coagulation laboratory should define the new therapeutic range when the aPTT reagent lot is changed.

The therapeutic range of UFH therapy for the laboratory aPTT reagent-instrument combination should be determined by:

- comparison of ex-vivo specimens with an appropriately validated heparin assay (anti-factor X_a or protamine sulfate neutralization).
- comparison of ex-vivo specimens to a previously calibrated aPTT, using a method of control for reagent drift.

Using heparin levels

Heparin levels can be used to monitor UFH therapy.

The UFH used to calibrate the assay should be linked to an approved international standard UFH, preferably the WHO standard.

Heparin levels are most useful when:

- large doses of UFH are required (>2000 U/h), as may occur in heparin resistance.
- the baseline aPTT is prolonged (eg, lupus anticoagulant).

Data in this table are taken from Olson JD, et al. Laboratory monitoring of unfractionated heparin therapy. Arch Pathol Lab Med. *1998;122:782-798.*
UFH = unfractionated heparin; WHO = World Health Organization

Heparin (or low-molecular-weight heparin) monitoring also can be done using heparin levels (anti-factor Xa activity). This assay is usually reserved for patients receiving heparin in whom the aPTT assay is not reliable (eg, lupus anticoagulant) or for patients receiving low-molecular-weight heparin who accumulate the drug abnormally (eg, renal failure). Platelet counts should be monitored during heparin administration, because heparin-induced thrombocytopenia is a potentially serious complication. Heparin-induced thrombocytopenia is much less likely with low-molecular-weight heparin therapy. Consensus guidelines on low-molecular-weight heparin monitoring are summarized in **t34.2**.

t34.2 Consensus Recommendations on Laboratory Monitoring of Low-Molecular-Weight Heparin Therapy

Uncomplicated patients receiving LMWH in prophylactic or therapeutic doses do not require laboratory monitoring.

Laboratory monitoring of LMWH therapy may be useful for pediatric patients, patients with renal disease, and patients receiving long-term therapy.

Samples for LMWH monitoring should be obtained 4 hours (peak level) after a subcutaneous dose.

The target therapeutic range for peak LMWH therapy in patients receiving twice-daily dosing for venous thromboembolism is 0.5-1.1 U/mL when measured by an anti-factor Xa method.

LMWH therapy should be monitored with a chromogenic anti-factor Xa assay.

The standard curve used to measure LMWH levels should be constructed using the LMWH in clinical use.

This table is used with permission from Laposata M, et al. The clinical use and laboratory monitoring of low-molecular-weight heparin, danaparoid, hirudin and related compounds, and argatroban. Arch Pathol Lab Med. *1998; 122:799-807.*
LMWH = low-molecular-weight heparin

Newer anticoagulants such as the direct thrombin inhibitors (hirudin and its analogs, argatroban) can be monitored using the aPTT. For example, lepuridin and argatroban therapy should prolong the patient's aPTT 1.5-2.5 times the mean of the aPTT reference range.

34.4.2 Monitoring Warfarin Therapy

Patients receiving warfarin (or other oral anticoagulants) should be monitored using the prothrombin time (PT) assay with calculation of the international normalized ratio (INR). The INR is used because different tissue extracts, or "tissue thromboplastins," can give different PT values with different pathologic plasma samples, although the normal control times may be the same. Even extracts prepared by the same method from the same tissue do not always give identical results with a pathologic plasma, although the differences are minimized. In general, human brain extracts, now rarely used, give longer clotting times than rabbit brain extracts. When the PT test was first devised by Quick, it was believed to measure prothrombin specifically, provided the concentration of fibrinogen was above a certain critical level, and the results were often recorded in percentage of prothrombin activity. With the subsequent discovery of factors V, VII, and X, which are also measured by the test along with prothrombin, this method of reporting became invalid. In addition, laboratories traditionally used several reporting methods to quantify oral anticoagulation intensity. These differences in assays and reporting methods resulted in inadequate anticoagulation or excessive anticoagulation with adverse consequences.

An important advance was the adoption of a World Health Organization (WHO) international reference thromboplastin preparation. Each new batch of thromboplastin can be calibrated against the primary WHO reference material by using each batch to determine the PTs of plasma samples from different patients whose conditions have been stabilized with long-term oral anticoagulant therapy. The unknown preparation of thromboplastin is found to give PT values that are the same as, longer (higher ratios), or shorter (lower ratios) than those obtained with the standard thromboplastin, but a consistent and reproducible pattern is obtained. These results are used to calculate the relative sensitivity of the unknown preparation compared with the standard (International Sensitivity Index [ISI]). f34.2 illustrates how ISI values are derived. From this value, an INR, defined as the PT ratio that would have been obtained if the WHO international reference thromboplastin had been used, can be determined for any ratio obtained with the unknown thromboplastin (INR = [PT ratio]^{ISI}) f34.3. f34.4 illustrates the relationship between the PT ratio and the INR.

The manufacturer should calibrate each new lot of thromboplastin, and a table enabling conversion to the equivalent INR should be included in the product insert. This table is valid only for the particular instrument-reagent combination used by the manufacturer. The laboratory report should always state the PT value in seconds, as well as the INR. Only then can a result be interpreted by a physician at another institution without having to first consult the pathologist performing the test. In the past, many physicians endeavored to maintain the PT ratio at 2, but with some reagents, this represented an excessive degree of anticoagulation and resulted in a relatively high incidence of hemorrhagic manifestations; with other reagents, this ratio provided relatively little pro-

f34.2 Derivation of an International Sensitivity Index (ISI) value for a thromboplastin preparation

Log prothrombin time (PT) values are determined using a reference thromboplastin reagent and the commercial laboratory thromboplastin reagent. Patients receiving stable oral anticoagulants are tested, as are a group of normal volunteers. The best-fit line is determined, and the slope of this line multiplied by the ISI of the reference thromboplastin reagent is the ISI value for the commercial thromboplastin reagent.

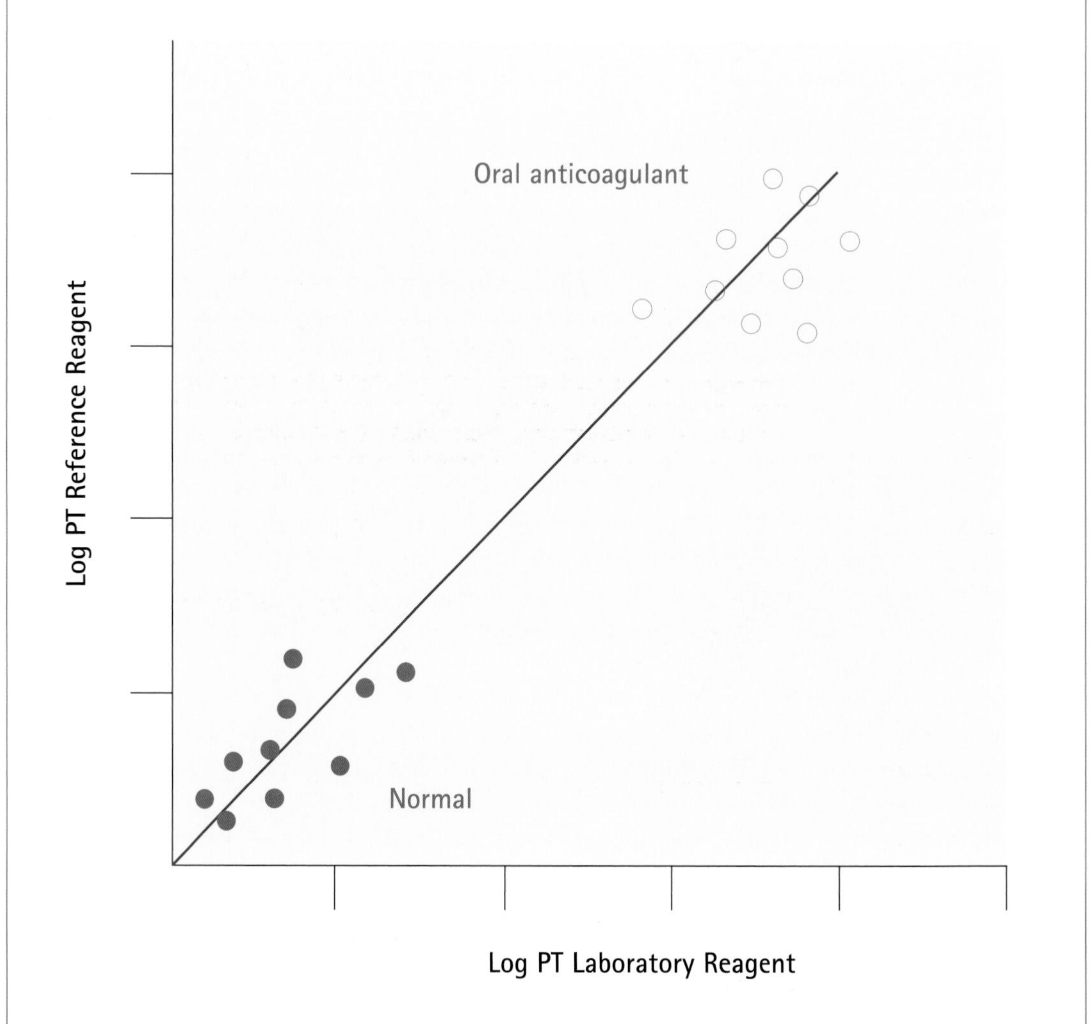

f34.3 Relationship between the prothrombin time (PT) ratio and the International Normalized Ratio (INR) for thromboplastin reagents over a range of International Sensitivity Index (ISI) values

The example shown is for a PT ratio of 1.3-1.5 for a thromboplastin preparation with an ISI value of 2.3. From the formula, INR = [PT ratio]^{ISI}, the INR is calculated as $1.3^{2.3}$ to $1.5^{2.3}$, or 1.83-2.54. Adapted with permission from Hirsh J. Oral anticoagulant drugs. *N Engl J Med.* 991;324:1865–1875. (Copyright © 1991 Massachusetts Medical Society. All rights reserved.)

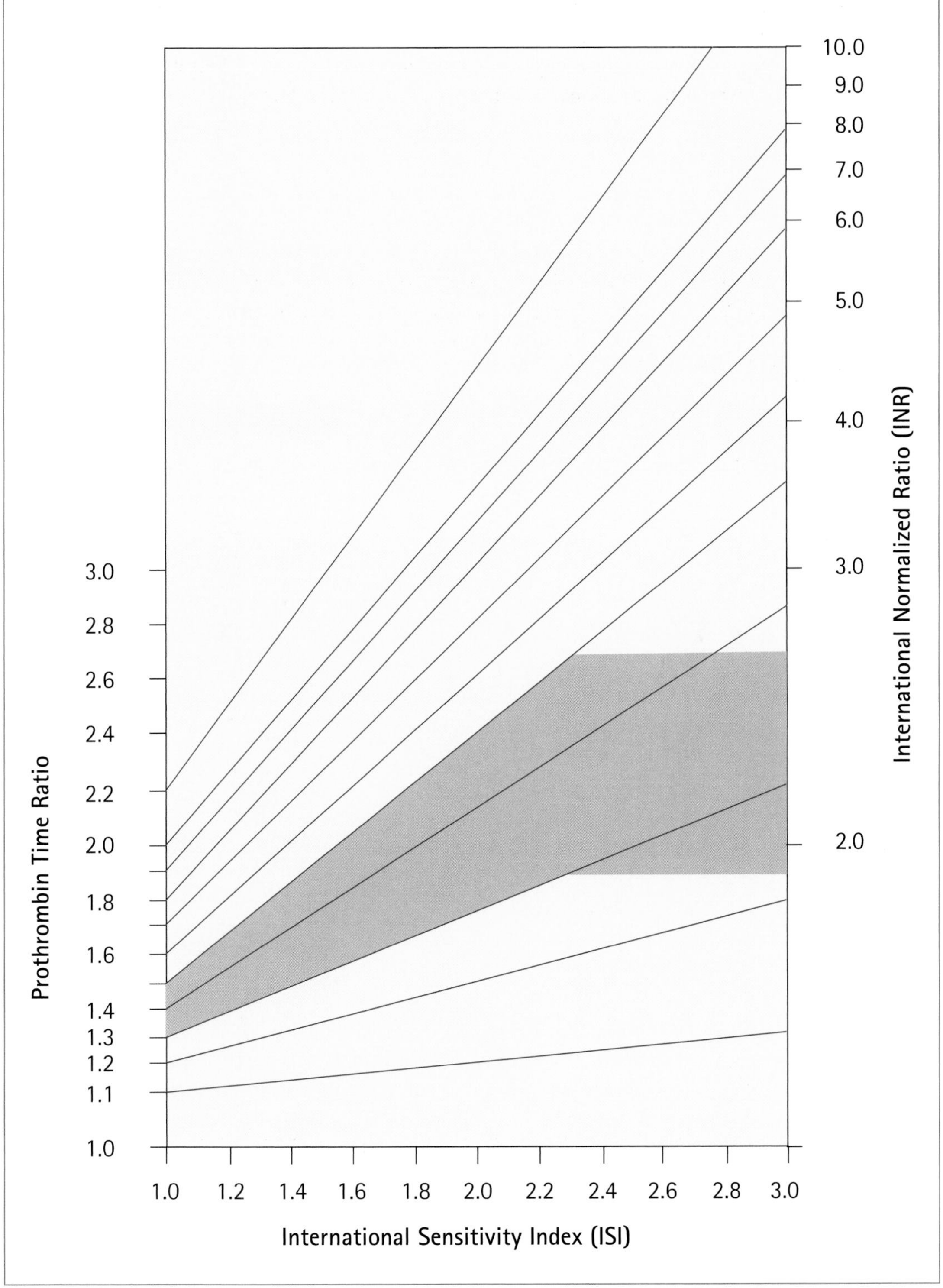

f34.4 Relationship between the prothrombin time (PT) ratio of a patient on warfarin therapy and the corresponding INR value

The slope of the line represents the International Sensitivity Index (ISI) value of the particular thromboplastin preparation used in the laboratory's PT assay. In this example, for low-intensity warfarin therapy (INR=2.0-3.0), a PT ratio between 1.5-1.75 would be required. Thromboplastins with higher ISI values would have slopes greater than that shown and would be less sensitive PT reagents, whereas thromboplastins with lower ISI values would have slopes less than that shown and would be more sensitive reagents.

From Greenberg PL, Negrin R, Rodgers GM. Hematologic disorders. In Melmon KL, Morrelli HF, Hoffman BB, Nierenberg DW, eds. *Clinical Pharmacology: Basic Principles in Therapeutics. 3rd ed.* New York: McGraw Hill;1992:524-599.

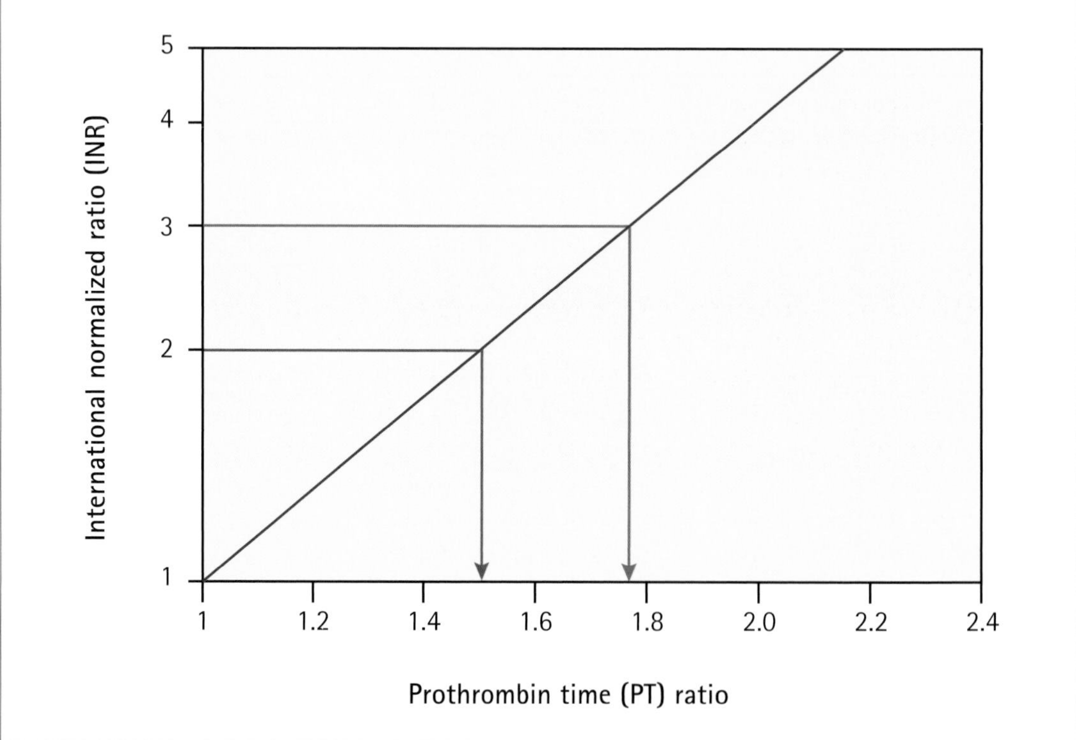

tection against thrombosis. **t34.3** summarizes the guidelines issued by a consensus conference (American College of Chest Physicians–National Heart Lung and Blood Institute, 2008); the therapeutic ranges in terms of INR are shown. Prothrombin time ratios are less useful because the ISI values of thromboplastins used in the United States still differ dramatically. With the exception of treating patients with high-risk prosthetic (metal) heart valves or patients with recurrent embolism, standard warfarin therapy is targeted at an INR of 2.0-3.0.

With more widespread use, limitations in using the INR format have been reported. Manufacturers of thromboplastin reagents do not provide ISI values derived for all instrument-reagent combinations. Consequently, the thromboplastin ISI package insert is not accurate for all laboratories. Less sensitive thromboplastins (higher ISI values) yield INR results with greater variability than do more sensitive thromboplastins (lower ISI values), because determination of PT results using less sensitive thromboplastins is associated with higher coefficients of variation. More optimal INR values are obtained if the coagulation laboratory uses a sensitive thromboplastin (ISI 1.0-1.5) and ensures that the ISI value is correct, either by calibrating the reagent or by using a thromboplastin whose ISI is appropriate for the laboratory's instrumentation. Many manufacturers now provide sensitive thromboplastins, and recombinant thromboplastins with ISI values of 1.0 also are available.

t34.3 Recommended Therapeutic Range for Warfarin Therapy

Indication	International Normalized Ratio
Treatment of venous thrombosis Treatment of pulmonary embolism Prevention of systemic embolism Tissue heart valves Acute myocardial infarction Atrial fibrillation	2.0 - 3.0 (low intensity)
Recurrent embolism Mechanical heart valves (high-risk)	2.5 - 3.5 (high intensity)

From a consensus conference report published in Chest. *2001;119(suppl):8S–21S. These recommendations were confirmed in a 2008 report in* Chest *2008; 133 (suppl).*

Unfractionated heparin therapy may variably affect the PT/INR values. This latter effect results from some, but not all, thromboplastin manufacturers including heparin-neutralizing substances (such as polybrene) in their reagents.

Some laboratories do not correctly establish the mean normal prothrombin time (the denominator in the PT ratio of the INR equation). Ideally, the laboratory should derive the mean normal PT from a minimum of 20 healthy donors of both sexes and over a range of ages. Plasma samples from these donors should be assayed with the same instrument-reagent combination as patient samples, and a geometric mean PT should be determined. Using a laboratory normal control mean value is not acceptable, and can introduce significant error into the INR calculation.

How can these problems be overcome to enable the coagulation laboratory to provide reliable INR results? One approach is the use of local calibration using certified plasmas that have assigned PT/INR values; these plasmas can be used to generate a local laboratory ISI or to construct a standard curve to determine INR values. A plasma calibrant should: be derived from patients on stable oral anticoagulant therapy; be frozen and not lyophilized; have at least 12 calibrant samples; have a consistent plasma citrate concentration of the calibrants; be performed over several days; and calibrant samples must have assigned PT/INR values. Details of using calibrants to generate a local ISI or a standard curve to determine INR values are presented in the review by Adcock and Duff.

Many other drugs or medical conditions, particularly liver disease, alter the effect of oral anticoagulants **t34.4**. Recent ingestion of such a drug or the presence of one of these illnesses should be suspected whenever the PT changes unexpectedly in a patient whose condition was previously stabilized. For individuals with marginal dietary vitamin K intake, sterilization of the gut by an antibiotic can result in increased sensitivity to oral anticoagulants; this is perhaps the most common adverse interaction that occurs with warfarin.

Alternative methods to monitor oral anticoagulant therapy, including fingerstick-monitor devices, have been investigated. Although early studies found some of the fingerstick devices to be problematic for monitoring warfarin therapy, more recent reports have indicated that these devices are safe and effective. If these devices are to be used, the laboratory must validate them against a reference PT method to ensure their reliability. Consensus guidelines have been published on laboratory monitoring of oral anticoagulation using PT methods and fingerstick-monitor devices. These recommendations include (1) using 3.2% citrate as the anticoagulant for coagulation testing, (2) processing and testing PT specimens within 24 hours for room temperature storage, (3) using a thromboplastin with a low ISI value (~1.0), (4) using thromboplastin reagents with known reagent-instrument ISI relationships, and (5) being aware that lupus anticoagulants and heparin may affect the PT/INR. **t34.5** provides a detailed listing of the College of American Pathologists recommendations on oral anticoagulation monitoring.

t34.4 Drugs and Medical Conditions Affecting the Potency of Warfarin

Drugs	Conditions
Increased Potency	
Antibiotics	Age
Aspirin	Liver disease
Cimetidine	Malabsorption
Allopurinol	Congestive heart failure
	Malnutrition
Decreased Potency	
Barbiturates	Excess dietary vitamin K
Vitamin K	Nephrotic syndrome

34.4.3 Monitoring Fibrinolytic Therapy

The systemic intravenous infusion of streptokinase has been used since 1959 to dissolve arterial or venous clots. Streptokinase, however, is a bacterial product derived from streptococci and, because many individuals have significant titers of antistreptokinase antibodies as a result of a previous streptococcal infection, this complicates therapy and may result in severe side effects. Until recently, urokinase and t-PA were derived only from human sources, making them scarce and expensive; however, these drugs are now available as recombinant products.

Fibrinolytic drugs can be administered systemically to treat venous thromboembolism or myocardial infarction, or infused locally to lyse catheter clots. Local infusions do not require routine laboratory monitoring. However, when these agents are used systemically, it is useful to ensure that a "lytic effect" is achieved. This is especially true for streptokinase therapy, because of possible neutralizing antibodies. The lytic state is most easily monitored using the thrombin time assay; prolongation of the thrombin time to values between 2 and 5 times over baseline indicates the presence of the lytic state. Since there is no correlation between efficacy of therapy and changes in coagulation or fibrinolytic assays, no additional testing is necessary if an appropriate increase in the thrombin time occurs. For patients with myocardial infarction who receive short-term t-PA infusion, laboratory monitoring is not usually necessary. If the patient receives concomitant heparin therapy, the thrombin time will not be useful, and the reptilase test or fibrinogen assays should be used to monitor the lytic state.

t34.5 Consensus Recommendations on Laboratory Monitoring of Oral Anticoagulant (Warfarin) Therapy

PT specimens may be stored at room temperature, centrifuged, or not centrifuged, but should be processed and tested within 24 hours.

PT reagents (thromboplastins) with an ISI between 0.9-1.7 are recommended, and it is desirable to use reagents with an INR close to 1.0.

Laboratories should use PT reagent-instrument combinations for which the ISI is known.

INR variation can be reduced by using lyophilized calibrator plasmas or INR-certified plasmas.

UFH can variably increase the PT/INR. Laboratories should use a thromboplastin that is insensitive to therapeutic UFH.

Lupus anticoagulants can variably affect the PT/INR. Alternative assays (prothrombin or factor X measured by clotting or chromogenic methods) may be needed for some patients with the lupus anticoagulant.

Whole blood INR monitors can be used to monitor oral anticoagulation. These devices should be appropriately validated against reference methods. Patients and providers who use these devices should be properly educated in quality control procedures.

Data for this table are taken from Fairweather RB, et al. Laboratory monitoring of oral anticoagulant therapy. Arch Pathol Lab Med. *1998; 122:768-781.*

PT = prothrombin time; ISI = International Sensitivity Index; INR = international normalized ratio; UFH = unfractionated heparin

34.4.4 Aspirin and Other Antiplatelet Therapy

Aspirin is used extensively to treat arterial thromboembolic disease and to prevent occlusion of arterial grafts and formation of thrombi on prosthetic heart valves. It reduces thromboxane production for the life of the platelet, thereby decreasing platelet aggregation. However, it also diminishes the production of prostacyclin by the endothelium, albeit for a relatively shorter time, thereby enhancing aggregation. Extensive studies have been performed to evaluate the possibility of using low-dose aspirin therapy selectively to inhibit platelet thromboxane synthesis without affecting vascular prostacyclin formation. In recent clinical trials, the daily dose has varied from 80 mg ("baby aspirin") to 650 mg. Antiplatelet therapy is not routinely monitored by laboratory testing. However, patients with recurrent arterial thrombosis can be evaluated for "aspirin resistance" using standard platelet aggregation tests, which currently are the gold-standard assays for platelet function. Typically, inhibition of arachidonic acid aggregation to <20% of normal indicates aspirin efficacy. Point of care tests are being developed to assay for aspirin resistance.

Causes of aspirin resistance include non-compliance with therapy, abnormal bioavailability (altered metabolism or absorption), and mutations in cyclooxygenase-1. Clinical trials are ongoing in patients with cardiovascular disease to determine the utility of aspirin resistance testing in affecting clinical outcomes. As of mid-2009, insufficient data is available to recommend routine testing for aspirin resistance. Other antiplatelet therapies currently used include an antibody to the platelet fibrinogen receptor (abciximab, Reo-Pro), as well as several peptide inhibitors to this receptor. Inhibitors to the platelet ADP receptor such as ticlopidine and clopidogrel are also widely used. Insufficient data exists to justify testing for resistance to these drugs.

34.5 Laboratory Reporting

Results of anticoagulation tests should be reported in a standard format, as shown in **t34.6**. The therapeutic range for the coagulation laboratory should always be listed, as well as appropriate interpretive comments (eg, for oral anticoagulation intensity).

t34.6 Laboratory Reporting of Anticoagulation Tests

Drug	Laboratory Test	Therapeutic Range/Comments
Oral anticoagulants	PT/INR	INR=2.0-3.0 (standard therapy) for prophylaxis of venous thromboembolism, prevention of systemic embolism (atrial fibrillation, valvular heart disease, bioprosthetic heart valves, acute myocardial infarction) INR=2.5-3.5 (high intensity); for prophylaxis of mechanical prosthetic heart valves, recurrent systemic embolism
UFH	aPTT	59-94 sec
	Heparin level, UFH (anti-Xa)	0.35-0.70 U/mL
LMWH	Heparin level, LMWH (anti-Xa)	0.5-1.1 U/mL This range is based on peak levels obtained 4 hr after subcutaneous injection
Direct thrombin inhibitors		
Lepirudin	aPTT	56-75 sec*
Argatroban	aPTT	56-94 sec*

**reference range for ARUP Laboratories*
PT = prothrombin time; INR = international normalized ratio; UFH = unfractionated heparin; aPTT = activated partial thromboplastin time; LMWH = low-molecular-weight heparin

34.6 Laboratory Tests

Test 34.6.1 Heparin Level

Purpose. Occasionally it is necessary to determine plasma heparin levels to monitor heparin anticoagulation in patients for whom the aPTT is not a reliable assay (those with lupus anticoagulant), or in those patients requiring very large heparin doses to achieve a therapeutic aPTT.

Principle. The ability of dilutions of patient plasma to inhibit factor Xa is compared with that of standard concentrations of heparin in normal pooled plasma.

Specimen. Citrated plasma collected during stable heparin infusion is used. Blood specimens should not be drawn from indwelling catheters.

Procedure. The manual (fibrometer) method for assaying heparin levels is tedious. Dilutions of heparin are made in saline and normal pooled plasma. Calcium, the aPTT reagent, and factor Xa are added and clotting times measured. Control and patient plasma standard curves are constructed, and a best-fit line is drawn. Plasma heparin levels are determined from these curves.

Interpretation. The therapeutic heparin level from this assay is 0.35-0.7 U/mL. The heparin used to construct laboratory standard curves should be the same brand and lot number as that for which the sample is being tested.

Notes and Precautions. Automated methods to measure heparin levels are available. In these methods, a chromogenic substrate assay is used to quantitate inhibition of bovine factor Xa by heparin–antithrombin. With the increasing use of LMWH, some patients with renal failure who receive these drugs require monitoring using this assay. A calibrated LMWH should be used to establish the standard curve for the assay to measure LMWH. The target concentration for the peak LMWH level in patients treated with twice-daily dosing (ie, enoxaparin) for acute deep-vein thrombosis should be 0.5-1.1 U/mL **t34.2**.

34.7 References

Adcock DM, Duff S. Enhanced standardization of the international normalized ratio through the use of plasma calibrants: A concise review. *Blood Coag Fibrinol.* 2000;11:583-590.

Cattaneo M. Laboratory detection of "aspirin resistance": what test should we use (if any)? *Eur Heart J.* 2007;28:1673-1675

Deitcher SR, Rodgers GM. Thrombosis and antithrombotic therapy. In: Greer JP, Foerster J, Lukens JN, et al, eds. *Wintrobe's Clinical Hematology. 12th ed.* Philadelphia: Lippincott Williams & Wilkins; 2009:1464-1508.

Fairweather RB, Ansell J, van den Besselaar AMHP, et al. College of American Pathologists Conference XXXI on Laboratory Monitoring of Anticoagulant Therapy: laboratory monitoring of oral anticoagulant therapy. *Arch Pathol Lab Med.* 1998;122:768-781.

Hirsh J. Oral anticoagulant drugs. *N Engl J Med.* 1991;324:1865-1875.

Hirsh J. Heparin. *N Engl J Med.* 1991;324:1565-1574.

Hirsh J, Dalen JE, Anderson DR, et al. Oral anticoagulants: mechanism of action, clinical effectiveness, and optimal therapeutic range. *Chest.* 2001;119(suppl):8S-21S.

Hirsh J, Poller L. The international normalized ratio: a guide to understanding and correcting its problems. *Arch Intern Med.* 1994;154:282-288.

Laposata M, Green D, Van Cott EM, et al. College of American Pathologists Conference XXXI on Laboratory Monitoring of Anticoagulant Therapy: The clinical use and laboratory monitoring of low-molecular-weight heparin, danaparoid, hirudin and related compounds, and argatroban. *Arch Pathol Lab Med.* 1998;122:799-807.

Ng VL, Valdes-Camin R, Gottfried EL, et al. Highly sensitive thromboplastins do not improve INR precision. *Am J Clin Pathol.* 1998:109:335-345.

Olson JD, Arkin CF, Brandt JT, et al. College of American Pathologists Conference XXXI on Laboratory Monitoring of Anticoagulant Therapy: Laboratory monitoring of unfractionated heparin therapy. *Arch Pathol Lab Med.* 1998;122:782-798.

Shojania AM, Tetreault J, Turnbull G. The variations between heparin sensitivity of different lots of activated partial thromboplastin time reagent produced by the same manufacturer. *Am J Clin Pathol.* 1988;89:19-23.

Yang DT, Robetorye RD, Rodgers GM. Home prothrombin time monitoring: a literature analysis. *Am J Hematol.* 2004;77:177-186.

Appendix

Hematology Reference Values

Table 1 Hematology Reference Values in Adults for Common Tests*

Test	Men: Conventional Units	Men: SI Units	Women: Conventional Units	Women: SI Units
Hemoglobin	13-18 g/dL	130-180 g/L	12-16 g/dL	120-160 g/L
Hematocrit	40%-52%	0.40-0.52	35%-47%	0.35-0.47
Red blood cell count	4.4-5.9 × 10^6/mm^3	4.4-5.9 × 10^{12}/L	3.8-5.2 × 10^6/mm^3	3.8-5.9 × 10^{12}/L
White blood cell count	3.8-10.6 × 10^3/mm^3	3.8-10.6 × 10^9/L	3.6-11.0 × 10^3/mm^3	3.6-10.6 × 10^9/L
MCV	80-100 μm^3	80-100 fL	80-100 μm^3	80-100 fL
MCH	26-34 pg	26-34 pg	26-34 pg	26-34 pg
MCHC	32-36 g/dL	320-360 g/L	32-36 g/dL	320-360 g/L
Platelet count	150-440 × 10^3/mm^3	150-440 × 10^9/L	150-440 × 10^3/mm^3	150-440 × 10^9/L
Reticulocyte count	0.8%-2.5%	0.008-0.025	0.8%-4.0%	0.008-0.04
Reticulocyte count	18,000-158,000/mm^3	18-158 × 10^9/L	18,000-158,000/mm^3	18-158 × 10^9/L
Sedimentation rate†	0-10 mm/h	0-10 mm/h	0-20 mm/h	0-20 mm/h
Zeta sedimentation rate	40-52	40-52	40-52	40-52

Modified from: Wintrobe MM. Clinical Hematology. 8th ed. *Philadelphia: Lea & Febiger; 1984.*
Henry JB. Clinical Diagnosis and Management by Laboratory Methods. 17th ed. *Philadelphia: WB Saunders Co; 1984.*
Miale JB. Laboratory Medicine: Hematology. 6th ed. *St Louis, Mo: CV Mosby; 1982.*
Williams WJ, Beutler E, Erslev AJ, Lichtman MA. Hematology. 3rd ed. *New York, NY: McGraw-Hill Book Co; 1983.*
†*May be age dependent, according to method.*
MCV = mean corpuscular volume; MCH = mean corpuscular hemoglobin;
MCHC = mean corpuscular hemoglobin concentration

Table 2 Automated Hematology Reference Values in Normal Men at 4500 ft*

Test	Coulter S+ STKR (80 Men): Mean	Coulter S+ STKR (80 Men): Central 95% Range	Technicon HI (64 Men): Mean	Technicon HI (64 Men): Central 95% Range
White blood cells (× 10^3/mm^3)	6.6	3.5-9.8	6.7	4.4-8.2
Platelets (× 10^3/mm^3)	280	147-412	285	147-422
Red blood cells (× 10^6/mm^3)	5.4	4.76-6.04	5.54	4.87-6.20
Hemoglobin (g/dL)	16.4	14.7-18.1	16.2	14.6-17.8
Hematocrit (%)	48.7	43.7-53.6	48.7	43.6-53.8
MCV (μm^3)	90.3	83.3-97.2	88.0	80.9-95.2
MCH (pg)	30.5	28.1-32.9	29.3	27.0-31.7
MCHC (g/dL)	33.8	33.0-34.6	33.3	32.1-34.6
RDW	12.4	11.5-13.4	12.8	12.0-13.6
Mean platelet volume	8.4	6.8-10.0	8.9	7.6-10.2

Data are based on measurements from healthy male medical students, age range 23-31 years, at an altitude of 4500 ft.
From Wintrobe MM. Wintrobe's Clinical Hematology. 9th ed. *Philadelphia: Lea & Febiger; 1993.*
MCV = mean corpuscular volume; MCH = mean corpuscular hemoglobin;
MCHC = mean corpuscular hemoglobin concentration; RDW = red cell distribution width

Table 3 Effect of Altitude on VPRC in Normal Men*

Altitude			
Feet	Meters	No. of Subjects	VPRC (L/L)
0	0	721	0.47
4400	1340	744	0.495
7457	2280	100	0.51
12,240	3740	40	0.54
14,900	4540	32	0.61
17,800	5430	10	0.69

**Mean values in males.*

From Wintrobe MM. Wintrobe's Clinical Hematology. 9th ed. *Philadelphia: Lea & Febiger; 1993.*

VPRC = volume packed red cells

Table 4 Manual White Blood Cell Differential Count, Reference Values in Adults

	Conventional Units		SI Units	
Cell Type	Relative	Absolute Counts	Relative	Absolute Counts
Segmented neutrophils	50%-70%	2400-7560/mm^3	0.5-0.7	2.40-7.56 × 10^6/L
Bands	2%-6%	96-648/mm^3	0.02-0.06	0.10-0.65 × 10^6/L
Lymphocytes	20%-44%	960-4752/mm^3	0.2-0.44	0.96-4.75 × 10^6/L
Monocytes	2%-9%	96-972/mm^3	0.02-0.09	0.10-0.97 × 10^6/L
Eosinophils	0-4%	0-432/mm^3	0.0-0.04	0.00-0.43 × 10^6/L
Basophils	0-2%	0-216/mm^3	0.0-0.02	0.00-0.22 × 10^6/L

Table 5 Automated Leukocyte Differential Counts, Reference Values in Normal Male Adults*

	Coulter S+ STKR (80 Men)		Technicon HI (64 Men)	
Differential (%)	Mean	Central 95% Range	Mean	Central 95% Range
Lymphocytes	36.1	22.3-49.9	31.3	18.3-44.2
Monocytes	4.1	0.7-7.5	5.5	2.6-8.5
Granulocytes	59.7	45.5-74.0	–	–
Neutrophils	–	–	58.8	45.5-73.1
Eosinophils	–	–	1.9	0.0-4.4
Basophils	–	–	0.7	0.2-1.2
Large unstained cells (LUC)	–	–	1.8	0.0-4.9
Absolute Numbers				
Lymphocytes (× 10^3/mm^3)	2.4	1.2-3.5	2.06	0.9-3.22
Monocytes (× 10^3/mm^3)	0.3	0.0-0.5	0.37	0.12-0.62
Granulocytes (× 10^3/mm^3)	4.0	1.4-6.6	–	–
Neutrophils (× 10^3/mm^3)	–	–	4.01	1.31-6.71
Eosinophils (× 10^3/mm^3)	–	–	0.13	0.00-0.30
Basophils (× 10^3/mm^3)	–	–	0.05	0.01-0.09
LUC (× 10^3/mm^3)	–	–	0.12	0.00-0.31

**Data are based on measurements from healthy male medical students, age range 23-31 years, at an altitude of 4500 ft.*

From Wintrobe MM. Wintrobe's Clinical Hematology. 9th ed. *Philadelphia: Lea & Febiger; 1993.*

Table 6 Hematologic Reference Ranges in Racial and Ethnic Subgroups (2.5th to 97.5th Percentiles) in Men*

	Range		Range	
Test	White (n = 181)	Black (n = 172)	Latino (n = 141)	Asian (n = 72)
WBCs (× $10^3/mm^3$)	3.7-10.4	3.5-9.6	4.1-11.5	3.4-11.5
RBCs (× $10^6/mm^3$)	4.3-5.8	4.0-5.8	4.4-5.6	4.0-6.2
Hemoglobin (g/dL)	13.0-17.3	11.9-16.7	13.7-17.0	12.5-17.0
MCHC (g/dL)	32.4-35.4	32.1-35.2	32.5-35.6	32.1-35.3
Platelets (× $10^3/mm^3$)	176-372	167-408	176-397	223-422
MPV (μm^3)	7.7-1.2	7.5-12.4	7.4-11.3	7.4-10.9
Hematocrit (%)	38-49	36-48	40-50	36-50
MCV (μm^3)	81.6-96.6	71.8-99.8	82.0-96.5	67.3-96.3
MCH (pg)	27.2-33.4	23.3-33.9	26.7-33.2	21.6-33.4
RDW (%)	11.9-14.3	12.1-16.2	12.1-14.7	11.8-14.6
Three-part differential cell count	**(n = 106)**	**(n = 114)**	**(n = 101)**	**(n = 46)**
Lymphocytes (× $10^3/mm^3$)	1.26-3.05	1.20-3.17	1.12-3.36	1.03-3.38
Monocytes (× $10^3/mm^3$)	0.13-0.66	0.14-0.77	0.14-0.68	0.08-0.77
Granulocytes (× $10^3/mm^3$)	1.78-7.72	1.49-6.56	2.41-8.33	1.51-7.26
Manual differential cell count	**(n = 80)**	**(n = 72)**	**(n = 48)**	**(n = 43)**
Segmented neutrophils (× $10^3/mm^3$)	1.51-7.00	1.11-6.70	2.40-7.59	2.02-5.50
Band cells (× $10^3/mm^3$)	0.00-0.07	0.00-0.07	0.00-0.21	0.00-0.06
Lymphocytes (× $10^3/mm^3$)	0.65-2.80	0.97-3.30	0.94-4.22	0.90-3.50
Monocytes (× $10^3/mm^3$)	0.00-0.51	0.02-0.83	0.00-0.68	0.00-0.53
Eosinophils (× $10^3/mm^3$)	0.00-0.42	0.00-0.47	0.00-0.80	0.00-0.32
Basophils (× $10^3/mm^3$)	0.00-0.16	0.00-0.16	0.00-0.17	0-0.14

**From Saxena S, Wong ET. Heterogeneity of common hematologic parameters among racial, ethnic, and gender subgroups.* Arch Pathol Lab Med. *1990;114:715-719.*

MCHC = mean corpuscular hemoglobin concentration; MPV = mean platelet volume; MCV = mean cell volume; MCH = mean corpuscular hemoglobin; RDW = red cell distribution width

Table 7 Hematologic Reference Ranges in Racial and Ethnic Subgroups (2.5th to 97th Percentiles) in Women*

	Range		Range	
Test	**White (n = 482)**	**Black (n = 525)**	**Latina (n = 394)**	**Asian (n = 175)**
WBCs (× 10^3/mm^3)	3.8-10.6	3.4-11.2	4.1-11.8	3.5-9.7
RBCs (× 10^6/mm^3)	3.8-5.0	3.6-5.3	3.7-5.1	3.7-5.4
Hemoglobin (g/dL)	11.4-15.5	10.6-14.9	10.3-15.1	11.3-15.0
MCHC (g/dL)	32.7-35.3	31.9-35.0	32.0-35.3	32.2-35.5
Platelets (× 10^3/mm^3)	188-438	193-485	198-460	193-417
MPV (μm^3)	7.7-11.5	7.7-11.6	7.8-11.5	7.6-11.1
Hematocrit (%)	34-45	31-44	31-44	33-44
MCV (μm^3)	78.0-98.0	72.9-97.5	69.6-95.8	72.4-97.0
MCH (pg)	25.9-33.8	23.7-33.1	22.3-33.0	22.1-33.8
RDW (%)	11.7-15.2	12.0-17.3	11.9-16.4	11.6-16.6
Three-part differential cell count	**(n = 284)**	**(n = 375)**	**(n = 295)**	**(n = 130)**
Lymphocytes (× 10^3/mm^3)	1.14-3.19	1.28-3.29	1.07-3.44	0.94-2.75
Monocytes (× 10^3/mm^3)	0.10-0.74	0.10-0.67	0.11-0.67	0.09-0.51
Granulocytes (× 10^3/mm^3)	2.03-7.46	1.43-7.68	2.19-8.24	1.93-6.13
Manual differential cell count	**(n = 216)**	**(n = 175)**	**(n = 114)**	**(n = 50)**
Segmented neutrophils (× 10^3/mm^3)	2.023-7.33	1.50-8.14	1.85-7.57	1.60-7.33
Band cells (× 10^3/mm^3)	0.00-0.13	0.00-0.09	0.00-0.13	0.00-0.11
Lymphocytes (× 10^3/mm^3)	1.01-3.38	1.05-3.48	0.89-3.73	1.24-2.59
Monocytes (× 10^3/mm^3)	0.00-0.82	0.02-0.72	0.06-0.66	0.00-0.65
Eosinophils (× 10^3/mm^3)	0.00-0.52	0.00-0.46	0.00-0.50	0.00-0.49
Basophils (× 10^3/mm^3)	0.00-0.16	0.00-0.20	0.00-0.15	0.00-0.16

**From Saxena S, Wong ET. Heterogeneity of common hematologic parameters among racial, ethnic, and gender subgroups.* Arch Pathol Lab Med. *1990;114:715-719.*

MCHC = mean corpuscular hemoglobin concentration; MPV = mean platelet volume; MCV = mean cell volume; MCH = mean corpuscular hemoglobin; RDW = red cell distribution width

Table 8 Red Blood Cell Values at Various Ages: Mean and Lower Limit of Normal (-2 SD)*†

Age	Hemoglobin (g/dL)		Hematocrit (%)		RBCs ($\times 10^6$/mm^3)		MCV (μm^3)		MCH (pg)		MCHC g/dL)	
	Mean	-2 SD	Mean	-2 SD	Mean	-2 SD	Mean	-2 SD	Mean	-2 SD	Mean	-2 SD
Birth (cord blood)	16.5	13.5	51	42	4.7	3.9	108	98	34	31	33	30
1-3 d (capillary)	18.5	14.5	56	45	5.3	4.0	108	95	34	31	33	29
1 wk	17.5	13.5	54	42	5.1	3.9	107	88	34	28	33	28
2 wk	16.5	12.5	51	39	4.9	3.6	105	86	34	28	33	28
1 mo	14.0	10.0	43	31	4.2	3.0	104	85	34	28	33	29
2 mo	11.5	9.0	35	28	3.8	2.7	96	77	30	26	33	29
3-6 mo	11.5	9.5	35	29	3.8	3.1	91	74	30	25	33	30
0.5-2 y	12.0	10.5	36	33	4.5	3.7	78	70	27	23	33	30
2-6 y	12.5	11.5	37	34	4.6	3.9	81	75	27	24	34	31
6-12 y	13.5	11.5	40	35	4.6	4.0	86	77	29	25	34	31
12-18 y												
Female	14.0	12.0	41	36	4.6	4.1	90	78	30	25	34	31
Male	14.5	13.0	43	37	4.9	4.5	88	78	30	25	34	31
18-49 y												
Female	14.0	12.0	41	36	4.6	4.0	90	80	30	26	34	31
Male	15.5	13.5	47	41	5.2	4.5	90	80	30	26	34	31

**From Wintrobe MM.* Wintrobe's Clinical Hematology. 9th ed. *Philadelphia: Lea & Febiger; 1993.*

†These data were compiled from several sources. Emphasis is on recent studies employing electronic counters and on the selection of populations that are likely to exclude individuals with iron deficiency. The mean ±2 SD can be expected to include 95% of the observations in a normal population. (From Dallman PR. In: Rudolph A, ed. Pediatrics. 16th ed. *East Norwalk, Conn: Appleton-Century-Crofts; 1977. Lubin BH. Reference values in infancy and childhood. In: Nathan DG, Oski FA, eds.* Hematology of Infancy and Childhood. 3rd ed. *Philadelphia: Saunders Co; 1987.)*

Table 9 Hematology Reference Values During the First Month of Life in the Term Infant*

Value	Cord Blood	Day 1	Day 3	Day 7	Day 14	Day 28
Hemoglobin (g/dL)	16.8	18.4	17.8	17.0	16.8	15.6
Hematocrit (%)	53	58	55	54	52	45
RBCs ($\times 10^6$/mm^3)	5.25	5.8	5.6	5.2	5.1	4.7
MCV (μm^3)	107	108	99	98	96	91
MCH (pg)	34	35	33	32.5	31.5	31
MCHC (g/dL)	31.7	32.5	33	33	33	32
Reticulocytes (%)	3-7	3-7	1-3	0-1	0-1	0-1
Nucleated RBCs ($\times 10^3$/mm^3)	500	200	0-5	0	0	0
Platelets ($\times 10^3$/mm^3)	290	192	213	248	252	240

**From Oski F, Naiman JL.* Hematologic Problems in the Newborn. 2nd ed. *Philadelphia: Saunders Co; 1972.*

MCV = mean corpuscular volume; MCH = mean corpuscular hemoglobin; MCHC = mean corpuscular hemoglobin concentration

Table 10 Leukocyte Counts and Differential Counts: Reference Values in Children*†

Age	Total Leukocytes Mean	Total Leukocytes (Range)	Neutrophils Mean	Neutrophils (Range)	Neutrophils %	Lymphocytes Mean	Lymphocytes (Range)	Lymphocytes %	Monocytes Mean	Monocytes %	Eosinophils Mean	Eosinophils %
Birth	18.1	(9.0-30.0)	11.0	(6.0-26.0)	61%	5.5	(2.0-11.0)	31%	1.1	6%	0.4	2%
12 Hours	22.8	(13.0-38.0)	15.5	(6.0-28.0)	68%	5.5	(2.0-11.0)	24%	1.2	5%	0.5	2%
24 Hours	18.9	(9.4-34.0)	11.5	(5.0-21.0)	61%	5.8	(2.0-11.5)	31%	1.1	6%	0.5	2%
1 Week	12.2	(5.0-21.0)	5.5	(1.5-10.0)	45%	5.0	(2.0-17.0)	41%	1.1	9%	0.5	4%
2 Weeks	11.4	(5.0-20.0)	4.5	(1.0-9.5)	40%	5.5	(2.0-17.0)	48%	1.0	9%	0.4	3%
1 Month	10.8	(5.0-19.5)	3.8	(1.0-9.0)	35%	6.0	(2.5-16.5)	56%	0.7	7%	0.3	6%
Months	11.9	(6.0-17.5)	3.8	(1.0-8.5)	32%	7.3	(4.0-13.5)	61%	0.6	5%	0.3	3%
1 Year	11.4	(6.0-17.5)	3.5	(1.5-8.5)	31%	7.0	(4.0-10.5)	61%	0.6	5%	0.3	3%
2 Years	10.6	(6.0-17.0)	3.5	(1.5-8.5)	33%	6.3	(3.0-9.5)	59%	0.5	5%	0.3	3%
4 Years	9.1	(5.5-15.5)	3.8	(1.5-8.5)	42%	4.5	(2.0-8.0)	50%	0.5	5%	0.3	3%
6 Years	8.5	(5.0-14.5)	4.3	(1.5-8.0)	51%	3.5	(1.5-7.0)	42%	0.4	5%	0.2	3%
8 Years	8.3	(4.5-13.5)	4.4	(1.5-8.0)	53%	3.3	(1.5-6.8)	39%	0.4	4%	0.2	2%
10 Years	8.1	(4.5-13.5)	4.4	(1.8-8.0)	54%	3.1	(1.5-6.5)	38%	0.4	4%	0.2	2%
16 Years	7.8	(4.5-13.0)	4.4	(1.8-8.0)	57%	2.8	(1.2-5.2)	35%	0.4	5%	0.2	3%
21 Years	7.4	(4.5-11.0)	4.4	(1.8-7.7)	59%	2.5	(1.0-4.8)	34%	0.3	4%	0.2	3%

From Wintrobe MM. Wintrobe's Clinical Hematology. 9th ed. *Philadelphia, Lea & Febiger; 1993.*

†*These data were compiled from several sources. Emphasis is on recent studies employing electronic counters and on the selection of populations that are likely to exclude individuals with iron deficiency. The mean ±2 SD can be expected to include 95% of the observations in a normal population. (From Dallman PR. In: Rudolph A, ed.* Pediatrics. 16th ed. *East Norwalk, Conn: Appleton-Century-Crofts; 1977. Lubin BH. Reference values in infancy and childhood. In: Nathan DG, Oski FA, eds.* Hematology of Infancy and Childhood. 3rd ed. *Philadelphia: Saunders Co; 1987.)*

Table 11 Hematology Reference Values in Adults for Ancillary Tests*

Test	Men: Conventional Units	Men: SI Units	Women: Conventional Units	Women: SI Units
Serum iron	70-201 μg/dL	12.7-35.9 μmol/L	62-173 μg/dL	11-30 μmol/L
Total iron-binding capacity	250-450 μg/dL	45.2-77.7 μmol/L	253-435 μg/dL	45.2-77.7 μmol/L
Ferritin	20-250 ng/mL	20-250 μg/L	10-200 ng/mL	10-200 μg/L
Serum B_{12}	200-1000 pg/mL	150-750 pmol/L	200-1000 pg/mL	150-750 pmol/L
Serum folate	2-10 ng/mL	4-22 nmol/L	2-10 ng/mL	4-22 nmol/L
Red cell folate	140-960 ng/mL	550-2200 nmol/L	140-960 ng/mL	550-2200 nmol/L
Methylmalonic acid	0.00-0.40 μmol/L	0.00-0.40 μmol/L	0.00-0.40 μmol/L	0.00-0.40 μmol/L
Homocysteine	4.0-12.0 μmol/L	4.0-12.0 μmol/L	4.0-12.0 μmol/L	4.0-12.0 μmol/L
Hemoglobin A2	<3.5%	<0.035	<3.5%	<0.035
Hemoglobin F	<2%	<0.02	<2%	<0.02

Modified from: Wintrobe MM. Clinical Hematology. 11th ed. *Lippincott Williams & Wilkins; 2004. Henry JB.* Clinical Diagnosis and Management by Laboratory Methods. 17th ed. *Philadelphia: Saunders Co; 1984. Burtis CA, Ashwood ER, Bruns DE.* Tietz Textbook of Clinical Textbook of Clinical Chemistry and Molecular Diagnostics. 4th ed. *2006.*

Table 12 Age Related Coagulation Reference Interval Values

Coagulation Test	Age			
	5 d	90 d	1-5 y	7-9 y
PT (sec)	–	–	–	13.0-15.4
PTT (sec)	–	–	–	27-38
Fibrinogen (g/L)	1.62-4.62	1.50-3.79	1.70-40.5	1.98-4.13
Prothrombin (U/mL)	0.33-0.93	0.45-1.05	0.71-1.16	0.78-1.25
Factor V (U/mL)	0.45-1.45	0.48-1.32	0.79-1.27	0.69-1.32
Factor VII (U/mL)	0.35-1.43	0.39-1.43	0.55-1.16	0.67-1.45
Factor VIII (U/mL)	0.50-1.54	0.50-1.25	0.59-1.42	0.76-1.99
Factor IX (U/mL)	0.15-0.91	0.21-1.13	0.47-1.04	0.70-1.33
Factor X (U/mL)	0.19-0.79	0.35-1.07	0.58-1.16	0.74-1.30
Factor XI (U/mL)	0.23-0.87	0.41-0.97	0.56-1.50	0.70-1.38
vWF antigen* (U/mL)	0.50-2.54	0.50-2.06	0.60-1.2	0.62-1.80
Ristocetin cofactor (U/mL)	–	–	–	0.52-1.76
Antithrombin (U/mL)	0.41-0.93	0.73-1.21	0.82-1.39	0.90-1.35
Protein C (U/mL)	0.20-0.64	0.28-0.80	0.40-0.92	0.70-1.42
Protein S male (U/mL)	–	–	–	0.66-1.40
Protein S female (U/mL)	–	–	–	0.62-1.51
Plasminogen (U/mL)	–	–	0.78-1.18	0.76-1.16
α2-antiplasmin (U/mL)	–	–	0.93-1.17	0.88-1.47

**vWF antigen assay results are based on an antigenic method. All other results are based on functional coagulation assays.*
Data in this table are from two sources. There are no data for children 6 y of age.
Values from children aged 5 d through 1-5 y are from:
Andrew M, et al. Maturation of the hemostatic system during childhood. Blood. *1992; 80:1998; and*
Andrew M, et al. Development of the hemostatic system in the neonate and young infant. Am J Pediatr Hematol Oncol. *1990; 12:95.*

Age				
10–11 y	**12–13 y**	**14–15 y**	**16–17 y**	**Adult**
13.0-15.6	13.0-15.2	12.8-15.4	12.6-15.7	12.3-14.4
27-38	27-39	26-36	26-35	26-38
1.97-4.10	2.15-3.78	2.04-3.92	2.08-4.38	2.11-4.41
0.78-1.20	0.72-1.23	0.75-1.35	0.77-1.30	0.86-1.50
0.66-1.36	0.66-1.35	0.61-1.29	0.65-1.31	0.62-1.40
0.71-1.63	0.78-1.60	0.74-1.80	0.63-1.63	0.80-1.81
0.80-2.09	0.72-1.98	0.69-2.37	0.63-2.21	0.56-1.91
0.72-1.49	0.73-1.56	0.80-1.61	0.86-1.76	0.78-1.84
0.70-1.34	0.69-1.33	0.63-1.46	0.74-1.46	0.81-1.57
0.66-1.37	0.68-1.38	0.57-1.29	0.65-1.59	0.56-1.53
0.63-1.89	0.60-1.89	0.57-1.99	0.50-2.05	0.52-2.14
0.60-1.95	0.50-1.84	0.50-2.03	0.49-2.04	0.51-2.15
0.90-1.34	0.90-1.32	0.90-1.31	0.87-1.31	0.76-1.28
0.68-1.43	0.66-1.62	0.69-1.70	0.70-1.71	0.83-1.68
0.69-1.39	0.72-1.39	0.68-1.45	0.77-1.67	0.66-1.43
0.65-1.42	0.70-1.40	0.55-1.45	0.51-1.47	0.57-1.31
0.74-1.17	0.66-1.14	0.71-1.24	0.75-1.32	0.71-1.44
0.90-1.44	0.87-1.42	0.83-1.36	0.77-1.34	0.82-1.33

Values from children aged 7-17 and adults are from:
Flanders M, et al. Pediatric reference intervals for seven common coagulation assays. Clin Chem. *2005; 51:1738-1742;*
Flanders M, et al. Pediatric reference intervals for ten coagulation assays. Blood. *2003; 104:816a-17a; and*
Flanders M, et al. Pediatric reference intervals for five coagulation assays. J Thromb Haemost. *2005; Suppl, poster 1272.*
PT, prothrombin time; PTT, partial thromboplastin time; vWF, von Willebrand factor

Index Volume 1

Numbers in *italics* refer to pages on which tables or figures appear.

Numbers in **boldface** refer to pages on which lab tests or images appear.

A

D

G

H

I

J

K

L

M

N

O

P

Q

R

S

U

V

W

Z